BSAVA Manual of Rodents and Ferrets

Editors:

Emma Keeble

BVSc DZooMed (Mammalian) MRCVS
RCVS Recognised Specialist in Zoo and Wildlife Medicine
Exotic Animal and Wildlife Service, Royal (Dick) School of
Veterinary Studies, Hospital for Small Animals, Easter Bush
Veterinary Centre, Roslin, Midlothian, EH25 9RG

and

Anna Meredith

MA VetMB CertLAS DZooMed MRCVS
RCVS Recognised Specialist in Zoo and Wildlife Medicine
Exotic Animal and Wildlife Service, Royal (Dick) School of
Veterinary Studies, Hospital for Small Animals, Easter Bush
Veterinary Centre, Roslin, Midlothian, EH25 9RG

Published by:

British Small Animal Veterinary Association
Woodrow House, 1 Telford Way, Waterwells
Business Park, Quedgeley, Gloucester GL2 2AB

A Company Limited by Guarantee in England.
Registered Company No. 2837793.
Registered as a Charity.

Illustrations 16.6 17.6 and 19.5 were drawn by S.J. Elmhurst BA Hons
(www.livingart.org.uk) and are printed with her permission.

Stock photography: Dreamstime.com; © Lockstockbob, © Jiri Castka

A catalogue record for this book is available from the British Library.

ISBN 978 1 905319 08 4

The publishers, editors and contributors cannot take responsibility for information
provided on dosages and methods of application of drugs mentioned or referred to
in this publication. Details of this kind must be verified in each case by individual
users from up to date literature published by the manufacturers or suppliers of those
drugs. Veterinary surgeons are reminded that in each case they must follow all
appropriate national legislation and regulations (for example, in the United Kingdom,
the prescribing cascade) from time to time in force.

Printed in the UK by Severn, Gloucester GL2 5EU – a carbon neutral printer
Printed on ECF paper made from sustainable forests

18933PUBS23

Titles in the BSAVA Manuals series:

Manual of Avian Practice: A Foundation Manual
Manual of Backyard Poultry Medicine and Surgery
Manual of Canine & Feline Abdominal Imaging
Manual of Canine & Feline Abdominal Surgery
Manual of Canine & Feline Advanced Veterinary Nursing
Manual of Canine & Feline Anaesthesia and Analgesia
Manual of Canine & Feline Behavioural Medicine
Manual of Canine & Feline Cardiorespiratory Medicine
Manual of Canine & Feline Clinical Pathology
Manual of Canine & Feline Dentistry and Oral Surgery
Manual of Canine & Feline Dermatology
Manual of Canine & Feline Emergency and Critical Care
Manual of Canine & Feline Endocrinology
Manual of Canine & Feline Endoscopy and Endosurgery
Manual of Canine & Feline Fracture Repair and Management
Manual of Canine & Feline Gastroenterology
Manual of Canine & Feline Haematology and Transfusion Medicine
Manual of Canine & Feline Head, Neck and Thoracic Surgery
Manual of Canine & Feline Musculoskeletal Disorders
Manual of Canine & Feline Musculoskeletal Imaging
Manual of Canine & Feline Nephrology and Urology
Manual of Canine & Feline Neurology
Manual of Canine & Feline Oncology
Manual of Canine & Feline Ophthalmology
Manual of Canine & Feline Radiography and Radiology: A Foundation Manual
Manual of Canine & Feline Rehabilitation, Supportive and Palliative Care: Case Studies in Patient Management
Manual of Canine & Feline Reproduction and Neonatology
Manual of Canine & Feline Shelter Medicine: Principles of Health and Welfare in a Multi-animal Environment
Manual of Canine & Feline Surgical Principles: A Foundation Manual
Manual of Canine & Feline Thoracic Imaging
Manual of Canine & Feline Ultrasonography
Manual of Canine & Feline Wound Management and Reconstruction
Manual of Canine Practice: A Foundation Manual
Manual of Exotic Pet and Wildlife Nursing
Manual of Exotic Pets: A Foundation Manual
Manual of Feline Practice: A Foundation Manual
Manual of Practical Animal Care
Manual of Practical Veterinary Nursing
Manual of Practical Veterinary Welfare
Manual of Psittacine Birds
Manual of Rabbit Medicine
Manual of Rabbit Surgery, Dentistry and Imaging
Manual of Raptors, Pigeons and Passerine Birds
Manual of Reptiles
Manual of Rodents and Ferrets
Manual of Small Animal Practice Management and Development
Manual of Wildlife Casualties

For further information on these and all BSAVA publications, please visit our website: **www.bsava.com**

Contents

Contributors

R. Avery Bennett DVM MS DipACVS
Department of Veterinary Clinical Medicine, College of Veterinary Medicine, University of Illinois,
1008 West Hazelwood Drive, Urbana, IL 61802, USA

Vittorio Capello DVM
Clinica Veterinaria San Siro, Clinica Veterinaria Gran Sasso, Milano, Italy

John Chitty BVetMed CertZooMed MRCVS
Strathmore Veterinary Clinic, Andover, Hants SP10 2PH

Ricardo de Matos LMV DipABVP (Avian)
Section of Wildlife and Exotic Animal Medicine, Department of Clinical Sciences,
College of Veterinary Medicine, Cornell University, Ithaca, NY 14853, USA

Peter G. Fisher DVM
Pet Care Veterinary Hospital, Virginia Beach, VA 23462, USA

Paul Flecknell MA VetMB PhD DLAS DipECVA DECLAM (Hon) DACLAM (Hon) FRCVS
Comparative Biology Centre, Medical School, Framlington Place, Newcastle NE2 4HH

Simon J. Girling BVMS DZooMed CBiol MIBiol MRCVS
RCVS Recognised Specialist in Zoo and Wildlife Medicine
Cotgreen Road, Tweedbank, Galashiels

Gidona Goodman DVM MSc (Wild Animal Health) MRCVS
Exotic Animal and Wildlife Service, Royal (Dick) School of Veterinary Studies,
Hospital for Small Animals, Easter Bush Veterinary Centre, Roslin, Midlothian EH25 9RG

Michelle G. Hawkins VMD Dip ABVP (Avian Practice)
Assistant Professor, Companion Avian and Exotic Animal Medicine and Surgery,
Department of Medicine and Epidemiology, School of Veterinary Medicine, University of California,
Davis, CA 95616, USA

Heidi Hoefer DVM DipABVP
Head of Exotic Pet Services, Island Exotic Veterinary Care, Huntington, NY 11746, USA

Simon Hollamby BA BVSc (Hon II) MS MRCVS
Royal (Dick) School of Veterinary Studies, Hospital for Small Animals,
Easter Bush Veterinary Centre, Roslin, Midlothian, EH25 9RG

Vladimír Jekl MVDr PhD
Avian and Exotic Animal Clinic, Faculty of Veterinary Sciences, University of Veterinary and
Pharmaceutical Sciences Brno, Palackeho 1-3, 61242 Brno, Czech Republic

Cathy A. Johnson-Delaney BS DVM DipABVP
Eastside Avian & Exotic Animal Medical Center, 13603 100th Avenue NE, Kirkland, WA 98034, USA

Emma Keeble BVSc DZooMed (Mammalian) MRCVS
RCVS Recognised Specialist in Zoo and Wildlife Medicine
Exotic Animal and Wildlife Service, Royal (Dick) School of Veterinary Studies,
Hospital for Small Animals, Easter Bush Veterinary Centre, Roslin, Midlothian, EH25 9RG

La'Toya Latney DVM
Matthew J. Ryan Veterinary Hospital, University of Pennsylvania, School of Veterinary Medicine,
3900 Delancey Street, Philadelphia, PA 19104, USA

Angela Lennox DVM DipABVP(Avian)
Avian and Exotic Animal Clinic of Indianapolis, 9330 Waldemar Road, Indianapolis, IN 46268, USA

William Lewis BVSc CertZooMed MRCVS
The Wylie Veterinary Centre, 196 Hall Lane, Upminster, Essex RM14 1TD

Marla Lichtenberger DVM DipACVECC
Milwaukee Emergency Center for Animals and Referral Services, 3670 South 108th Street,
Milwaukee, WI 53092, USA

Lesa Longley MA BVM&S DZooMed (Mammalian) MRCVS
Royal (Dick) School of Veterinary Studies, University of Edinburgh, Easter Bush Veterinary Centre,
Roslin, Midlothian, EH25 9RG

Rebecca Malakoff DVM DipACVIM (Cardiology)
Angell Animal Medical Center, 350 South Huntington Avenue, Boston, MA 02130, USA

Anna Meredith MA VetMB CertLAS DZooMed MRCVS
RCVS Recognised Specialist in Zoo and Wildlife Medicine
Head of Exotic Animal and Wildlife Service, Royal (Dick) School of Veterinary Studies,
Hospital for Small Animals, Easter Bush Veterinary Centre, Roslin, Midlothian EH25 9RG

Fabiano Montiani-Ferreira MV MCV PhD Dipl.
Brazilian CVO Professor Adjunto de Clínica Médica de Pequenos Animais e Oftalmologia,
Veterinária Departamento de Medicina Veterinária, Universidade Federal do Paraná,
Rua dos Funcionários, 1540 80035-050, Curitiba-PR, Brazil

James Morrisey DVM DipABVP (Avian)
Section of Wildlife and Exotic Animal Medicine, Department of Clinical Sciences,
College of Veterinary Medicine, Cornell University, Ithaca, NY 14853, USA

Connie Orcutt DVM DipABVP (Avian)
Avian and Exotic Animal Medicine Service, Angell Animal Medical Center, Boston, MA 02130, USA

Hannah Orr BVM&S CertLAS MRCVS
Rowett Research Institute, Greenburn Road, Bucksburn, Aberdeen AB21 9SB

Claire Richardson BSc BVM&S CertLAS MRCVS
Comparative Biology Centre, Medical School, Framlington Place, Newcastle NE2 4HH

Nico J. Schoemaker DipECAMS Dip ABVP(Avian)
Division of Zoological Medicine, Department of Clinical Sciences of Companion Animals,
Utrecht University, Yalelaan 108, 3584 CM Utrecht, The Netherlands

Sam Silverman DVM PhD DipACVR
2330 Marinship #180, Sausalito, CA 94965, USA

Michelle L. Ward BSc BVSc(Hons I) DZooMed (Mammalian) MRCVS
RCVS Recognised Specialist in Zoo and Wildlife Medicine
Royal (Dick) School of Veterinary Studies, Hospital for Small Animals,
Easter Bush Veterinary Centre, Roslin, Midlothian, EH25 9RG

Petra Wesche DVM MSc (Wild Animal Health) MRCVS
Finn Pathologists, One Eyed Lane, Weybread, Diss, Norfolk IP21 5TT

Allison Zwingenberger DVM DipACVR DipECVDI
University of California–Davis, 1 Shields Avenue, Davis, CA 95616, USA

Foreword

The *BSAVA Manual of Rodents and Ferrets* is another in a series of well planned, well designed, practical books for those who wish to see some of the more charming animals in practice.

For more than twenty years, veterinarians have been raising the level of medicine and surgery we can offer to owners of ferrets and rodents. This newest addition to the cause continues the tradition of informative presentations that allow both the novice to these special species and those who have been working with them for years to better understand the complexities of these animals.

This Manual is separated into logical sections. The biology, husbandry and clinical techniques of rodents and then ferrets are dealt with separately from the diseases of each group. The beauty of this design is that you can read the book, cover to cover, to learn about these animals in depth. Or you can use this book as a reference, to have in your library, to pull out and jump right to the appropriate section when a rodent comes in with such maladies as skin or neurologic disorders.

The usefulness of this Manual is not only the depth the authors go into to describe each procedure or disease, but also that we have a truly international selection of authors who bring expertise from all corners of the world. It is a testament to the achievements of the editors that they are able to bring together this amazing collection of internationally recognized veterinary talent that in the end allows us to give our patients the same level of excellence of care that their patients are lucky enough to receive.

Karen Rosenthal DVM MS DipABVP (Avian)
University of Pennsylvania, Philadelphia, PA, USA

Preface

In recent years the number of rodents and ferrets kept as pets has grown considerably, with a consequent growth in demand for appropriate veterinary care. Many owners of pet rodents and ferrets develop a strong emotional attachment to their pets and expect high-quality medical care from the veterinary surgeon. For veterinarians, the small size, susceptibility to stress-related problems and short natural life expectancy of these species present challenges compared with traditional companion animals.

Much of the veterinary information available for rodents and ferrets is based on laboratory animal medicine and consequently there is a lack of up-to-date reference texts on medicine and surgery of pet rodents and ferrets. The practitioner needs to have an accessible book that provides information about the biology, husbandry, clinical approach and main disease conditions likely to be encountered in these species. This new BSAVA Manual provides just this, covering the medicine and surgery of rodents and ferrets in much greater depth and breadth than any existing BSAVA publication, in a manner that is easy to read, assimilate and apply to the clinical situation.

The Manual covers the most commonly encountered rodent species – mice, rats, hamsters, gerbils, guinea pigs, chinchillas and degus – in detail, as well as containing a separate chapter on the less commonly owned rodent species. In recognition of the very fundamental differences between the rodent group of species and ferrets, the book is presented in two distinct sections.

The first section is devoted to rodents and is divided into two parts. The first part covers biology, husbandry and clinical techniques in rodents (including anaesthesia and surgery, as well as the more unusual rodent species). The second part contains chapters based on common diseases of pet rodents by clinical system. These describe aetiology, clinical signs, diagnosis, treatment and prevention/management where relevant. The second section focuses on ferrets and is again divided into two parts following the same format as those for the rodent section, including a separate chapter on systemic viral diseases of ferrets. The final part of the book contains a useful appendix on differential diagnoses based on clinical signs in rodents, and in ferrets.

It is well illustrated with many high-quality colour images and contains numerous quick-reference tables, as well as detailed well referenced text. The Manual is aimed at veterinarians, veterinary students and veterinary nurses in practice worldwide as a general reference, but is also useful for those individuals wanting to study this field in greater depth.

An international field of contributing authors with extensive practical experience in their subject has resulted in a comprehensive and easy-to-use manual. The editors are very grateful for the expertise, hard work and punctual manuscript delivery of all the authors. We would also like to thank Marion Jowett and her team at BSAVA for all their encouragement, patience and technical assistance. In particular we would both like to thank our partners and families for all their support and encouragement over the past year.

Emma Keeble and Anna Meredith
October 2008

Rodents: biology and husbandry

Emma Keeble

Introduction

Rodents comprise the largest order of mammals with 33 families and to date 2,277 different species (Wilson and Reeder, 2005). New species are still being discovered around the world as well as new data and interpretations, making this a dynamic continually changing group of animals. Classification of rodents has always been controversial, with dispute between authors over the Hystricomorpha suborder. There are four other suborders (Figure 1.1) and it is the suborders Hystricomorpha and Myomorpha that include the species in this chapter: the former covers chinchillas, guinea pigs and degus; while mice, rats, hamsters and gerbils are myomorphs (or mouse-like rodents).

The word rodent is derived from the Latin verb *rodere*, meaning 'to gnaw'. This refers to rodents' characteristic dentition with elongated chisel-shaped incisors (see later and Chapter 8). Traditionally rodents have been associated with disease transfer and they act as reservoir hosts for many infectious diseases.

More recently they have been widely used as models for laboratory research, from which the majority of veterinary information has arisen. There is an increasing trend for keeping rodents as pets and correspondingly high client expectation that their pet will receive quality veterinary care. As such it is important for the veterinary surgeon in practice to have up-to-date knowledge when dealing with this mammal group. The aim of this chapter is to outline some of the basic biological, anatomical and physiological features of rodents and give information on their basic housing, nutrition, reproduction and preventive health care.

Biology

Rodents are highly successful mammals with a worldwide distribution, being absent only in the Antarctic, New Zealand and some small oceanic islands. They inhabit a diverse range of environments from deserts to Arctic tundra and tropical rainforests. They are

Suborder	Group type	Examples of families in this suborder	Common name	Examples of pet species
Sciuromorpha	Squirrel-like	Sciuridae	Squirrels	Siberian chipmunk (*Eutamias sibiricus*) Black-tailed prairie dog (*Cynomys ludovicianus*)
Castorimorpha	Beaver	Castoridae	Beavers	
Anomaluromorpha	Scaly-tailed squirrel	Pededitae	Springhares	
Myomorpha	Mouse-like	Muridae	True mice	Domestic mouse (*Mus musculus*) Domestic rat (*Rattus norvegicus*)
		Cricetidae	Burrowing rodents	Syrian or golden hamster (*Mesocricetus auratus*) Russian Dwarf Campbell hamster (*Phodopus campbelli*) Russian Dwarf Winter White hamster (*P. sungorus*) Roborovski hamster (*P. roborovskii*) Chinese hamster (*Cricetulus griseus*) Mongolian gerbil (*Meriones unguiculatus*) Duprasi or fat-tailed gerbil (*Pachyuromys duprasis*) Jirds
Hystricomorpha	Porcupine-like	Hystricidae	Porcupines	
		Chinchillidae	Chinchillas	Chinchilla (*Chinchilla* spp.)
		Caviidae	Cavies, capybaras	Guinea pig (*Cavia aperea f. porcellus*)
		Dasyproctidae	Agoutis	
		Octodontidae	Octodonts	Degu (*Octodon degus*)

1.1 Classification of rodents (order Rodentia) and examples of families from each suborder.

extremely adaptable and have developed variable abilities such as gliding, swimming, tree-climbing, digging and jumping. They may be active during the day, night, dawn or dusk, depending on the species. Most are sociable, living in pairs or groups, though there are exceptions. Their diet varies according to species and includes seeds and fruits, tubers, grasses and leaves, insects, worms, fish and carcasses. Some species undergo periods of hibernation (e.g. Syrian hamsters (*Mesocricetus auratus*) hibernate at temperatures below 5°C). Most species are small, weighing on average between 20 g and 1 kg (Figure 1.2). The largest of all rodents is the capybara (*Hydrochoerus hydrochaeris*), weighing 30–50 kg.

Anatomy and physiology

Despite occupying such diverse geographical locations, rodents have retained a fairly uniform body structure with generally a small body size, short legs and various tail adaptations depending on their mode of existence. For example, the tails of beavers (*Castor* spp.) are flattened and oar-like as an adaptation to their semi-aquatic lifestyle. Dormice (family Gliridae) have prehensile tails to enable them to climb tall grasses. The anatomy of the foot varies according to the mode of locomotion, with most rodents being plantigrade. Beavers have webbing between the toes to aid swimming, while jumping mice, such as jerboa, have fused metatarsal bones and reduced numbers of digits to aid jumping. Rodents do not have sweat glands and are therefore prone to heat exhaustion.

The one major anatomical feature that characterizes all rodents is their dentition (see Chapter 8), primarily their large and continuously growing paired upper and lower incisors. These are chisel shaped with curved roots, which occupy most of the mandibular and maxillary skeleton. The tooth composition varies, with the labial surface consisting of hard-wearing enamel and the inner buccal surface of softer dentine. This results in greater wear on the buccal surface forming a chisel-shaped cutting edge to aid gnawing. The incisors have open apical pulp cavities and are constantly growing and erupting. This is termed aradicular (open-rooted) elodont (elongating teeth) dentition. All rodents lack canine teeth and have a diastema caudal to the incisors. The cheek teeth are variable in shape and classification (heterodont). Some rodents, such as the Chinchillidae and Caviidae, have continuously growing cheek teeth whereas others, such as the Sciuridae and Muridae, have rooted teeth.

Dental formulae vary between rodent families (see Chapter 8).

Rodents have a simple digestive tract comprising a simple stomach, large sacculated caecum (involved in the bacterial digestion of cellulose) and elongated colon. The hamster is different in that it has two distinct parts to the stomach: a non-glandular forestomach (cardiac stomach), similar in function to a rumen, and a glandular region (pyloric stomach) separated by muscular folds. Coprophagy is common practice for rodent species. Vomiting and regurgitation do not occur, due to a muscular ridge at the junction of the distal oesophagus and the stomach. (See also Chapter 11.)

Female rodents have separate vaginal and urethral orifices, with the vaginal opening usually being non-patent until oestrus.

The following sections highlight some anatomical and physiological differences between the species.

Rats

Rats do not have gall bladders. Albino varieties have poor vision and rely on their vibrissae for navigation. Yellowing of the fur is common and normal in aged animals.

Scientific name	Common name	Body weight (g)	Average life expectancy (years)	Body temperature (°C)	Respiratory rate (per minute)	Heart rate (beats per minute)
Mus musculus	Mouse	20–40	1–2.5	37.5	84–230	500–725
Rattus norvegicus	Rat	400–800	3	38	66–114	280–500
Mesocricetus auratus	Syrian hamster	100–200	1.5–2	38 Hibernates	100–250	276–425
Cricetulus griseus/ Phodopus sungorus	Chinese/Russian hamster	20–40	1.5–2	38	–	–
Meriones unguiculatus	Gerbil	70–130	1.5–2.5	38	70–120	260–600
Cavia aperea f. porcellus	Guinea pig	750–1000	4–7	38–39	69–150	226–300
Chinchilla laniger	Chinchilla	400–500	10–15	38–39	40–100	100
Octodon degus	Degu	200–300	5–7	37.9	–	–
Tamias sibiricus	Chipmunk	80–150	3–5	38 Hibernates	–	–

1.2 Biological data for selected species.

Hamsters

Hamsters have large paired cheek pouches extending caudally as far as the scapulae. These are muscular and are lined with oral mucosa. Their primary function is for food storage and transport of material. Hamsters dislike swimming but if forced to will inflate their cheek pouches with air to help them float.

Syrian hamsters have bilateral pigmented sebaceous glands (flank glands; Figure 1.3), which are more prominent in male animals, particularly when sexually aroused. Dwarf hamsters possess a ventral scent gland (Figure 1.4). The scent glands are involved in territorial marking and mating behaviour.

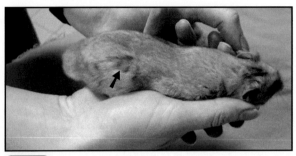

1.3 Flank glands on a Syrian hamster.

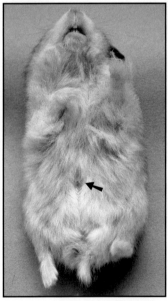

1.4

Normal ventral scent gland in a Djungarian or Russian dwarf hamster. (Courtesy of Hannah Orr.)

Gerbils

Gerbils possess a large ventral scent gland mid-abdomen (Figure 1.5) which is under gonadal hormone control and is thought to be involved in territorial marking. Secretions from this gland are used to mark objects within the territory and will identify an individual animal to others, depending on the composition of the secretion.

Concentration of urine, an adaptation to an arid environment, occurs in desert species such as the Mongolian gerbil (*Meriones unguiculatus*). This species also drinks very little, obtaining most of its water from its food and metabolism (see also Chapter 13).

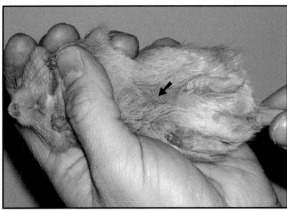

1.5 Ventral abdominal scent gland in a gerbil. Note also the obvious testicles in this male.

The habitat of the Mongolian gerbil undergoes wide temperature variations and gerbils have adapted to tolerate these temperature extremes. The Harderian gland has an important role in thermoregulation. Secretions from the gland are mixed with saliva and groomed on to the coat from the nares. If the animal is too cold the lipid and protoporphyrin pigments from the Harderian gland act as an insulation layer when groomed on to the coat. If the animal is too hot the Harderian gland secretion is reduced and saliva is groomed on to the coat, removing the lipid and providing evaporative cooling.

Gerbil blood normally contains high levels of serum cholesterol, even when the animal is fed a moderately low fat diet. Gerbils have been used to study cholesterol metabolism and atherosclerosis. High cholesterol levels are thought to be a consequence of reduced faecal excretion of steroids and differences in liver enzymes involved in cholesterol metabolism. The gerbil's red blood cells have extremely short life spans (10 days) and consequently show pronounced basophilic stippling on blood smears. See also Chapter 4.

Guinea pigs

Guinea pigs possess sebaceous glands along the dorsum, rump and perianal area which are involved in territorial marking. Despite having no tail, guinea pigs do have four to six coccygeal vertebrae. The tympanic bullae are large. The front feet each have four digits and the hind feet have three. The gastrointestinal system occupies most of the abdominal cavity, with the small intestine on the right side and the large caecum on the left. The latter is sacculated, due to three longitudinal bands of muscle (taeniae coli) that extend along the whole of the large intestine. Guinea pigs possess a gall bladder. The thymus extends from the mediastinum to subcutaneously in the neck. Male guinea pigs have extremely large seminiferous vesicles (Figure 1.6) that extend from the pubis into the abdomen and could potentially be confused with uterine horns on laparotomy. They have one pair of mammary glands.

Gastric emptying time is 2 hours in the guinea pig, with total gut transit time typically between 12 and 15 hours in all rodent species. Caecal fermentation yields volatile fatty acids.

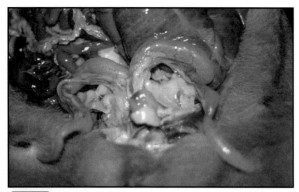

1.6 Large seminiferous vesicles in a guinea pig on post-mortem examination.

Chinchillas

Chinchillas are renowned for their dense fur and are still intensively farmed for the fur trade in some countries. Each hair follicle may grow up to 90 hairs. Each of the front and hind feet possesses four digits and the base of each foot is hairless. Tympanic bullae are large. Chinchillas have a large coiled caecum and a sacculated colon.

Degus

The front and hind feet each have five digits. Degus have long tails with brush-like hair at the tip. Degloving of the tail is common in this species with incorrect handling. Degus are diurnal and have excellent vision. Their retinas contain two different types of cone and behavioural studies have shown that they can discriminate ultraviolet light from the wavelengths visible to humans. This may be involved in social behaviour, since both the fur on their ventrum and their urine are highly UV-reflective.

Degus are prone to spontaneous diabetes, since their insulin and glucagon structure is different from that of other mammals (Nishi and Steiner, 1990). They are also often found to have islet amyloidosis. For this reason they have been used for laboratory research in this field. See also Chapter 16.

Being a diurnal species, degus have been used to research circadian rhythms, in particular for jet lag studies.

Characteristics and varieties

Mice

The domestic mouse (*Mus musculus*) has been used for research in Europe since the 17th century. Mice are mainly nocturnal. They make good children's pets but are not long lived. In general females are less odorous than males.

The standard laboratory mouse is white, but there are many colour varieties of pet mice available. In the United Kingdom there is a National Mouse Club that sets standards for these varieties. In America the American Fancy Rat and Mouse Association (AFRMA) has a similar function. Varieties are classed according to their coat type, fur colour and body markings. There are seven main varieties in the USA. In the UK there are five main varieties, as follows:

- **Self**: solid body colour. Includes: black; blue; champagne; chocolate; cream; dove; fawn; lilac; red; silver and white
- **Tan**: one colour on upper body and tan underside
- **Marked**: with specified markings. Includes Dutch, Himalayan, tricolours, etc.
- **Satins**: with fur of high gloss sheen
- **Any Other Variety** (AOV): mice of all other standardized varieties (e.g. long-haired, chinchilla, Siamese).

Rats

The domestic rat (*Rattus norvegicus*) is thought to have originated in Asia and expanded to America and Europe in the 18th century; it was first used in research in the late 19th century. Rats make good pets and are easier to handle than mice, being larger. They are intelligent and have individual personalities. They too are mainly nocturnal.

Pet rats are available as many different varieties but the most common are the hooded colour varieties (coat colour covering the head and shoulders; Figure 1.7). In the UK the National Fancy Rat Society sets standards of excellence for showing fancy rats. These are again classified according to fur colour, markings and coat type. AFRMA recognizes six varieties according to coat type and each is divided into six sections according to colour and body markings. These include:

- Self
- AOC (any other colour)
- AOCP (any other colour pattern)
- Silvered
- Marked
- Odd eye.

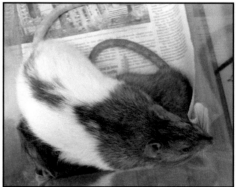

1.7

Hooded rat.

Hamsters

Hamsters belong to the subfamily Cricetinae (Old World hamsters), of which there are 12 species. There are four genera: large hamsters (*Cricetus*); small hamsters (*Mesocricetus*); pygmy hamsters (*Cricetulus*); and short-tailed pygmy hamsters (*Phodopus*). All hamsters have cheek pouches, which are invaginations of the oral mucosa. They can be retracted by the buccinator muscle, which has evolved from the trapezius muscle. The word 'hamster' comes from the German *hamstern*, which means 'to hoard'. The Syrian hamster can hoard in its cheek pouches up to half its body weight in food.

Hamsters are generally nocturnal, but despite this make good children's pets. There are many different colour and coat varieties, but only five species or subspecies are kept commonly as pets (Figure 1.8): the Syrian or Golden hamster (*Mesocricetus auratus*), the Russian Dwarf Campbell (*Phodopus campbelli*), Russian Dwarf Winter White (*Phodopus sungorus*), Roborovski (*Phodopus roborovskii*) and Chinese (*Cricetulus griseus*).

Golden or Syrian hamster

This species is the largest and most commonly kept. It is found in the wild in north-western Syria where it lives in burrows. It is solitary and will fight if kept with others. The Syrian hamster will undergo hibernation if temperatures drop below 5°C. This species was established in captivity in 1930 and has been used extensively for research purposes.

There are many different varieties according to coat colour, pattern and coat type:

- **Golden**: golden brown with white underside and dark cheek flashes (this is the original wild coloration) (Figure 1.9)
- **Self**: includes cinnamon, cream, honey, grey, white, chocolate, mink (name often includes eye or ear colour, e.g. red-eyed cream)
- **Agouti**: multi-coloured coat markings, hair shaft is two-toned
- **Marked**: banded most common (white band across back); also piebald, mosaic, tortoiseshell, roan, etc.
- Satin-coated, long-haired, short-haired, rex-coated.

Russian Dwarf Campbell

In the wild this species inhabits the steppes and semi-deserts of Central Asia. Its adult length is approximately 10–12 cm, with males being larger than females. The body is plump and rounded. Russian hamsters have fur on their feet and are sometimes referred to as the Furry or Hairy Footed Hamster. The normal colouring is brown over the dorsum, dark brown–grey dorsal stripe and a cream underside (Figure 1.10). Other colour varieties and coat patterns are available (e.g. argente, albino, mottled and platinum).

Hamster species	Alternative names	Behavioural characteristics	Housing requirements	Suitability as child's pet
Syrian hamster	Golden hamster Teddy Bear hamster Fancy hamster Standard hamster	Easy to handle. Do not generally bite. Hibernate at <5°C. Nocturnal	Solitary	Excellent
Russian Dwarf Campbell	Djungarian hamster	Most common dwarf species. Do not hibernate. May bite. Move fast and more difficult to handle. Nocturnal	Sociable – keep as single or mixed-sex pairs or group. Able to interbreed with Dwarf Winter White	Not ideal choice
Russian Dwarf Winter White	Siberian hamster Djungarian hamster	More difficult to obtain. Do not hibernate. May bite. Easier to handle than Russian Dwarf Campbell. Nocturnal	Sociable – keep as single or mixed-sex pairs or group. Able to interbreed with Dwarf Campbell	Not ideal choice
Roborovski hamster		Most likely species to be awake during daytime. Entertaining to watch. Less likely to bite. Very fast and difficult to handle	Can be housed on own or as single-sex or mixed-sex pairs or group	Not ideal choice
Chinese hamster		Shy species. Enjoy tunnelling and climbing. Entertaining to watch	Can be housed on own or as single-sex or mixed-sex pairs or group. Mature adults may fight	Not ideal choice

1.8 Differences in behavioural characteristics and housing requirements for the five hamster species.

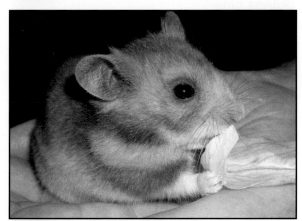

1.9 Golden hamster, wild-type coloration. (© Thomas Kent, National Hamster Council.)

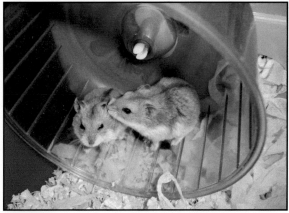

1.10 Russian Dwarf Campbell hamsters. (© Rosie Ray, National Hamster Council.)

Russian Dwarf Winter White

This species originates from the grassy steppe regions of eastern Kazakhstan and south-western Siberia. It is more compact than the Campbell's Russian hamster, with more prominent eyes, a rounded roman nose and a curved spine caudally giving it a bullet-shaped body. Adult length is approximately 8–10 cm, with males being larger than females. The Dwarf Winter White Russian hamster is so named because its coat turns white in the winter. This process is stimulated by shortening day length. The species does not normally breed when white coated. The normal colouring is dark grey with a black dorsal stripe and cream underside. Other colour varieties include sapphire and pearl.

Roborovski hamster

This species originates from western and eastern Mongolia and northern China and was originally imported into the UK in the 1960s by London Zoo. It is now available as pets in many countries, including the USA. It is the smallest of the pet hamster species at only 4–5 cm in length. The natural colour is sandy-gold over the back with a white belly and distinctive white eyebrows (Figure 1.11).

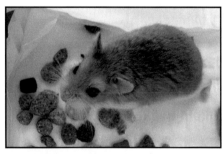

1.11
Roborovski hamster.

Chinese hamster

This species originates from northern China and Mongolia. There are restrictions on keeping these hamsters in some US states, such as California, where a licence is required to keep or transport them within the state. The Chinese hamster is more mouse-like in appearance, with a prominent tail. Adult body length is approximately 10–12 cm, with males being larger than females. The natural coat colour is brown–grey, with a black stripe along the back and light grey underside (Figure 1.12), although other varieties exist.

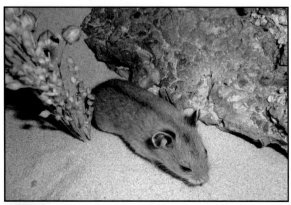

1.12 Chinese hamster. (© Alex Eames, National Hamster Council.)

Gerbils

Gerbils belong to the family Cricetidae (burrowing rodents) in the subfamily Gerbillinae (running mice). There are 15 genera and these include approximately 110 species, all of which have long hind feet adapted for running. The common name for rodents in the gerbil subfamily is 'desert rats' and these rodents are all adapted to desert environments in Africa, India and Asia. The gerbil subfamily includes jirds (genus *Meriones*), of which the Mongolian gerbil or clawed jird (*Meriones unguiculatus*) is most commonly found in captivity. This species originates from Mongolia and was brought to the UK in the 1960s for research. Gerbils are active during the day and therefore make excellent children's pets. They are agile and enjoy burrowing and climbing, being entertaining to watch.

The natural colour variety of the Mongolian gerbil is agouti (Figure 1.13). Other varieties exist according to coat colour and pattern:

- **Agouti**: sandy coat with black guard hairs and black tip to tail; pale underside
- **Self**: albino, cinnamon, black, grey, dove, chinchilla
- **Marked**.

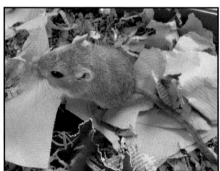

1.13
Agouti or wild-type colour variety of gerbil.

Other species that are less commonly kept as pets, but may occasionally be encountered, include: duprasi, or fat-tailed gerbil (*Pachyuromys duprasis*) (see Chapter 9); Shaw's jird (*Meriones shawi*); Sundevall's jird (*Meriones crassus*); Libyan jird (*Meriones libycus*); and bushy-tailed jird (*Sekeetamys calurus*).

Guinea pigs

The domestic guinea pig (*Cavia aperea f.porcellus*) belongs to the family Caviidae in the rodent suborder Hystricomorpha. This family contains 18 species, including Patagonian hares (or maras) and capybara. Guinea pigs were domesticated approximately 3,000–6,000 years ago, probably from their wild ancestor the cavy (*Cavia aperea*). They were introduced to Europe by the Spaniards in the mid 16th century.

Wild cavies are commonly found in South America and inhabit variable terrains such as savanna, brushland and mountainous regions of the Andes. They are crepuscular/nocturnal and live in colonies of 20–50 animals. They will inhabit burrows made by other animals and grass tunnels. They feed exclusively off plant material.

Domesticated guinea pigs are still farmed for meat in Peru. The origin of their name is obscure and is much speculated. They are excellent children's pets since they are easy to handle, rarely bite, have little odour and are sociable. Guinea pigs have extremely sensitive hearing with large tympanic bullae and four cochlear coils. They are highly vocal and communicate via a range of sounds.

There are many breeds and varieties of guinea pig, with much interbreeding resulting in many coat colours and hair types. Coat colour genetics are complicated with at least six loci.

- **Self**: solid coat colour, e.g. cream, lilac, saffron, chocolate
- **Non-Self**: describes coated breeds, marked breeds and agouti breeds
    - **Coated** breeds include Abyssinian, Rex, long-haired varieties (such as Shelties, Peruvians, Silkies), Crested, Teddy and Satin
    - **Marked** breeds include Dalmatian, Tortoiseshell, Himalayan
    - **Agouti** breeds include gold, silver, lemon, salmon, cinnamon.

Breed standards in the UK are set by the National Cavy Club, which also registers stud names. In the United States the American Cavy Breeders Association has a similar function. The three most common breeds encountered are the English (or American in the United States) which has a short coat, the Abyssinian which has a rosetted coat and the Peruvian, which is long-haired (Figures 1.14 to 1.16).

Chinchillas

Chinchillas are hystricomorph rodents, closely related to guinea pigs, in the family Chinchillidae, genus *Chinchilla*. They originate from the Andes in South America where they inhabit mountainous regions of Chile, Peru, Bolivia and Argentina at altitudes of 3,000–4,000 m. The genus contains three species, one of which, the King chinchilla (*Chinchilla chinchilla*) is now extinct, having been excessively hunted for its fur. Two other species of chinchilla, the short-tailed chinchilla (*Ch. brevicaudata*) and the long-tailed chinchilla (*Ch. lanigera*) are endangered but may still be found in the wild, where they live in colonies in burrows or rock crevices. The two species are similar except that the former has a shorter tail, a thicker neck and shoulders, and shorter ears. Domestic chinchillas are thought to have originated from 13 animals transported in the 1920s to the United States for fur farming. Chinchillas are still farmed for their fur in North America and northern Europe and since the mid 1960s they have become increasingly popular as pets. Chinchillas are primarily nocturnal. They often resent handling and may bite, particularly if frightened or threatened. Because of this they are not considered to be good pets for small children. Chinchilla fur is very dense and soft and there are many colour varieties:

- **Natural** colour is a bluish-grey with white underneath
- **Mutations** of white, brown velvet, black velvet (Figure 1.17), charcoal and pastels now exist.

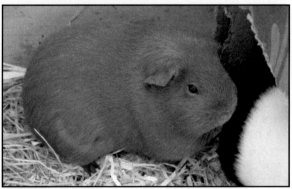

1.14 English or American guinea pig. Note the short hair coat. (Courtesy of BA Innes, Oatridge College.)

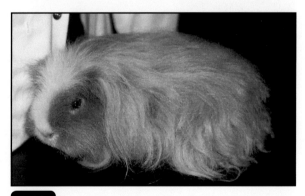

1.16 Peruvian guinea pig. Note the long hair coat.

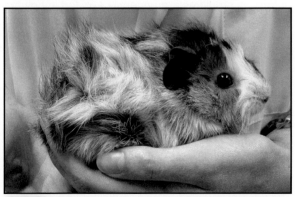

1.15 Abyssinian guinea pig. Note the rosetted hair coat.

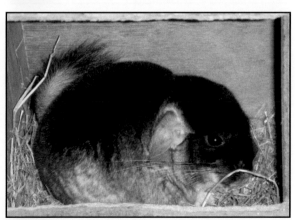

1.17 Black velvet colour variety of chinchilla. (Courtesy of BA Innes, Oatridge College.)

Degus

Degus (*Octodon degus*) are closely related to chinchillas and guinea pigs, belonging to the same rodent suborder Hystricomorpha. They are also known as brush-tailed rats. They are classified in a separate family, Octodontidae, meaning 'eight-toothed rodent'. This refers to the anatomy of the masticatory surface of their molar teeth, which is in a figure-of-eight pattern. They originate from South America and are commonly found in Chile, where they have a wide range of habitats including coastal, urban and the mountainous terrain of the Andes. They are diurnal and live in small groups of 5–10 adults in extensive burrow systems in grassland areas. Territories are fiercely disputed and are marked by large mounds of collected wood, rocks and plants. They have five digits on both fore and hind feet. They have acutely sensitive hearing and are highly vocal, emitting alarm calls when in danger.

Degus were brought to Europe and North America in the 1950s to be used in research on diabetes (see earlier under physiology). They do not make ideal pets for small children since they often resent handling and may bite. Injuries to the tail are common (see under husbandry-related problems later).

The natural coloration is brown over the dorsum with cream underside and lighter coloured circles around the eyes (Figure 1.18).

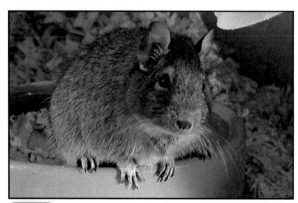

1.18 Degu showing natural coloration. (Courtesy of BA Innes, Oatridge College.)

Husbandry

Mice and rats

Husbandry-related problems are common in these species, particularly in rats. These are often directly due to poor cage hygiene and diet. If cages are not cleaned regularly, ammonia levels rise and will predispose the animals to respiratory disease (see Chapter 12). Urine-soaked bedding can lead to ventral dermatitis and predispose to pododermatitis and tail lesions (see Chapter 10). Inappropriate diet or selective feeding is commonly associated with obesity in rats, which may also predispose to pododermatitis.

Housing

Housing requirements are similar for mice and rats. Cages should be escape proof and easily cleaned. Cage material should be indestructible – ideally comprised of metal, since these species will gnaw through wood or plastic. Cage surfaces should not be coated with any paint or sealant that could be toxic if ingested. It is very important that the cage is well ventilated since respiratory disease is common, particularly in rats (see Chapter 12). Edges should be smooth to avoid injury when climbing. Traditional glass vivaria are not recommended since these are poorly ventilated (predisposing to the development of respiratory disease) and are difficult to clean, leading to the build-up of ammonia, which is irritant to the mucous membranes. When wire or plastic mesh is used the mesh size must be small enough to prevent the escape of young if animals are being bred from (one wire per centimetre for mice; one wire/1.5 cm for rats).

Bedding should be replaced two or three times a week to avoid odours. Wood chips, shavings or sawdust are best since these materials are absorbent and prevent the development of urine scald and dermatitis. However, these materials may be dusty and should be avoided in animals with respiratory disease. Various alternative commercial 'dust-free' bedding materials are now available and are specifically marketed for this situation. Newspaper is not very absorbent on its own; corncob bedding may become mouldy and contain mycotoxins; and cedar, pine and aromatic wood chips may contain aromatic hydrocarbons, which have been shown to have adverse effects on the liver even though no associated clinical signs are noted. These bedding materials are generally not to be recommended.

Rats and mice are inquisitive and highly social animals and it is important that some environmental enrichment is provided. Cage 'furniture' should be provided, such as branches to climb along, ropes, tubes, ladders, exercise wheels (solid rather than open, to prevent tail injuries), cardboard rolls and boxes. It is important to provide hide areas, since rats and mice prefer to sleep under shelter. Bedding material should be provided for animals to nest in.

Being social, mice and rats are best kept as single-sex groups (two females together are best, since males may fight), breeding pairs or harems.

Feeding

Rats and mice are opportunistic omnivores. Their nutritional requirements are well researched and nutritional problems are generally avoided if they are fed a commercial balanced pelleted diet. It is common practice to feed commercial seed-based mixes, which consist of carbohydrate cereals such as wheat, maize, oats and barley, high-fat low-calcium sunflower seeds, peanuts, biscuit and dried rolled peas. Selective feeding is common, particularly in rats, and often leads to obesity (Figure 1.19). A typical pelleted diet should contain approximately 16% protein (increasing to 20% if breeding) and 5% fat. Commercial diets may be supplemented with small amounts of fruit and vegetables, household scraps and dog biscuits. Sugary treats and chocolate, though very much liked, should be avoided. Food may be scattered to encourage foraging behaviour, provide environmental

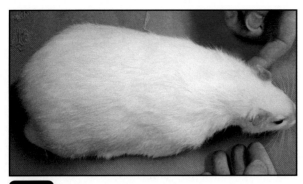

1.19 Obesity is common in rats.

enrichment and increase exercise, reducing obesity. Treat items may be hidden inside toys such as plastic kongs. Feeding is generally *ad libitum*, but dietary restriction may be necessary in obese animals.

Fresh water should be provided daily in drinking bottles with metal sipper tubes. These should be checked regularly for leaks and blockages, which are common. Average daily water consumption for adult mice is 15 ml/100 g body weight and for adult rats 10 ml/100 g body weight.

Hamsters

Housing
Many different varieties of commercial hamster cages exist, from simple single or multi-storey wire cages with a plastic base, to clear plastic or glass aquarium-style tanks, to systems of stacked or linking plastic tunnels and living/nesting 'rooms' (Figure 1.20). Whatever cage type is used, it should be escape proof and safe. Wire cages are not ideal for the dwarf species since they may be able to squeeze through the bars and escape. Plastic tunnel systems have poor ventilation, are difficult to clean and may be too narrow for pregnant animals. Aquarium-style cages also have poor ventilation and do not provide climbing apparatus.

Cages should be large (at least 75 cm × 30 cm × 30 cm) with separate areas for toileting, sleeping, eating and exercise. In addition a nest box should be provided, with nesting material. Paper or cloth-based

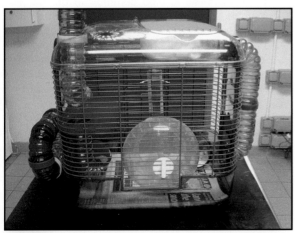

1.20 Plastic cage housing with linking-tube systems for hamsters.

materials should be used for nesting, not cotton wool or synthetic fibres since these may become impacted in cheek pouches and can become wrapped around limbs, causing constrictions

Hamsters require a lot of exercise (they may travel up to 5 miles a night in the wild) so space and cage furniture are important. Solid exercise wheels should be provided, as well as areas for climbing. Exercise balls are popular and are good for environmental enrichment as well as providing exercise.

Hamsters create burrows in the wild and so require a deep layer of shavings or a mixture of peat and shavings as a substrate. They are meticulous about their toilet habits and usually use the same place as a latrine. A small jar turned on its side containing soiled bedding should encourage toilet training and facilitate cage cleaning.

Feeding
Hamsters are omnivores and Syrian hamsters on average consume 5–7 g of feed each day. Wild hamsters live mainly on grains, plant seeds, plant parts (leaves, stems, tubers and roots), earthworms, snails and insects, depending on seasonal availability.

Commercial rodent mixes (seed, grain and nuts) are typically fed. As with rats and mice, pelleted feeds are also available and are less likely to lead to selective feeding, nutritional deficiencies and obesity problems. On average 10 g twice daily of the commercial rodent mix should be fed to Syrian hamsters. This should be supplemented with small amounts of fresh fruit and vegetables such as apple, carrot, broccoli, pear, parsley and cabbage. In the wild, hamsters do take occasional insects and animal protein and this may be added to the diet once or twice a week in the form of hard-boiled egg, cottage cheese or live foods such as mealworms and crickets. Dietary protein requirements are lower in the hamster than in rats and mice (13.7–16.7%). Small amounts of Timothy hay may also be provided to increase fibre content of the diet. Commercially available sugar-based treats should be kept to a minimum, especially since some species are prone to diabetes. It is important to provide substances for the hamster to gnaw on, such as commercial wooden hamster chews, dog biscuits or branches from untreated fruit trees.

Hamsters have basic hoarding instincts and will collect food in their cheek pouches to store in the nest box. Perishable items should be removed regularly as they rapidly become mouldy.

Fresh water should be provided daily from a drinking bottle (as for rats and mice). Average daily water consumption is 10 ml/100 g body weight.

Gerbils
Husbandry-related problems that may be encountered in gerbils include: degloving injuries to the tail associated with improper handling (see Chapter 2); rough hair coat associated with malnutrition, excess humidity, dehydration, poor ventilation and stress; gastric and anal impaction associated with inappropriate nesting materials; nasal dermatitis associated with porphyrin secretion from the Harderian glands secondary to stressors such as overcrowding and

increased humidity; and obesity associated with inappropriate diet, in particular excessive ingestion of sunflower seeds.

Housing

Gerbils are social animals and live in colonies in the wild. They are highly territorial and have a social hierarchy within each colony. Larger males are usually more dominant. They should be kept as single sex pairs or groups (introduced before puberty) or a breeding pair. Gerbils introduced over 10 weeks old are likely to fight.

They are best housed in a 'gerbilarium' – a glass or plastic tank with a close-fitting wire mesh lid or plastic cover and deep substrate (Figure 1.21). Alternatively a modular unit with chambers and plastic tunnels may be used; the main chamber should contain deep substrate.

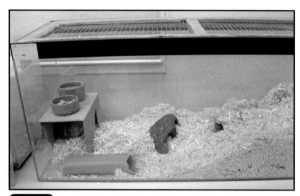

1.21 'Gerbilarium'.

Gerbils will often rest standing on their hind limbs and therefore require housing with some height. The minimum height recommended is 15 cm (Brain, 1999). They are also prolific burrowers and it is essential to provide deep substrate to enable them to build tunnels and chambers. This should be at least 3 cm in depth, but preferably much deeper. Common substrates used include paper by-products, sawdust and peat. Gerbils will spend considerable time creating a system of burrows that they will constantly rearrange. Cardboard rolls and boxes provide good environmental enrichment and are rapidly destroyed. Other items that may be added to the gerbilarium include paper, hay, plastic tubing, flower pots and glass jars. Wood for gnawing should also be provided, along with bedding material (see under hamsters, above). This system only needs to be cleaned out every few weeks as very little urine is produced and faeces are very dry and odourless to conserve water. The only disadvantage is the animals can be difficult to catch.

The tank should be kept out of direct sunlight and away from radiators to avoid heat stress. Being desert species a sand or dust bath should be provided (products marketed for chinchillas may be used). This is important for maintaining coat quality and has a role in thermoregulation. Gerbils can withstand a wide temperature range in the wild, but in captivity the recommended range is 20–22°C. Humidity is also important, since levels above 50% may cause matted hair, leading to excessive grooming and nasal dermatitis.

Feeding

Wild gerbils have a variable and seasonally based diet consisting of leaves, seeds and insects. Commercial pelleted diets or rodent seed-based mixes may be fed, but should be supplemented with small amounts of fresh fruit and vegetables such as apples and carrots. Occasional treats such as dried pumpkin seeds may be offered, but excessive sunflower seeds should be avoided since they lead to obesity and are nutritionally deficient. Pelleted diets alone do not contain sufficient dietary moisture and this may result in problems with dehydration, particularly in juvenile animals around the time of weaning. This problem is avoided by soaking the pellets first in water. Food should be scattered or hidden in tubes to encourage foraging behaviour. Average food intake is 4–10 g per day for adult gerbils. Recommended dietary protein content is high (22%) but fat content should be low (4%) (Brain, 1999), because gerbils rapidly develop high serum and liver cholesterol levels when fed diets with moderate fat content (see earlier under physiology).

Water consumption varies according to diet and environmental humidity, but may be between 2 ml and 4 ml per 100 g body weight per day. Water must be provided at all times in a drinking bottle and changed daily.

Guinea pigs

Husbandry-related problems in guinea pigs include chronic pododermatitis, often associated with *Staphylococcus aureus* skin infection and secondary to obesity, urine scalding of the skin, poor cage hygiene or abrasive/wire cage flooring (see Chapter 10). Immunosuppression and subsequent disease may occur secondary to stress associated with husbandry problems such as poor hygiene, overcrowding, extremes of temperature and humidity and changes in housing and diet. Respiratory problems are common in guinea pigs and may be predisposed by poor husbandry such as build-up of ammonia, poor ventilation, excess humidity and low temperatures. Dietary problems that have been reported in guinea pigs include metastatic calcification in animals over 12 months old possibly related to diets high in calcium or vitamin D, or low in magnesium and high in phosphorus. Urolithiasis is also common in guinea pigs and may be, amongst other factors, diet related. High calcium:phosphate ratios have been implicated, particularly if feeding alfalfa hay or legumes. Calculi may be composed of calcium carbonate, calcium phosphate or calcium oxalate crystals (see Chapter 13).

Housing

Guinea pigs are highly sociable and should be kept in single-sex groups, pairs or harems. Males may live together happily if kept together from a young age, but dominance problems and fighting are still possible. These may be reduced following castration, but can easily become a learned behaviour. Guinea pigs should not be housed with rabbits as rabbits tend to bully them, have different nutritional requirements and can transmit infections such as *Bordetella bronchiseptica*.

Guinea pigs are nervous animals and are easily frightened. They are not hardy and should therefore not be exposed to extremes of temperature or humidity, which may predispose to respiratory disease. Stress-induced inappetence associated with changes in husbandry is common.

A wide range of different systems and materials may be used for housing pet guinea pigs. Typical systems include pens, cages, aquaria and hutches (Figure 1.22). These may be made of wood, plastic, concrete, stainless steel or wire. Unless sealed, wood may become urine soaked, may be gnawed and is difficult to clean. Brick or concrete pens are poorly insulated and deep bedding should be supplied. Glass aquaria are poorly ventilated and should be cleaned regularly to avoid build-up of ammonia and associated respiratory problems (see Mice and rats).

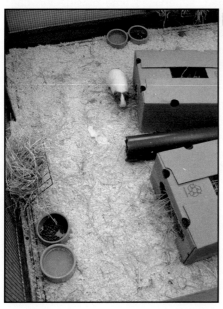

1.22

Typical guinea pig housing.

Whichever system is used, it should be well insulated and draught free. Surfaces should be easy to clean and disinfect and should be smooth to avoid injury. Minimum floor space recommendations are 700 cm^2 per adult animal and the cage sides should be at least 40 cm high (North, 1999). Solid flooring should always be used since wire flooring is often associated with husbandry problems. Hutches and cages should be raised off the ground to avoid damp and draughts.

The ideal environmental temperature range is 20–22°C and relative humidity 40–70%. Guinea pigs should be kept out of direct sunlight and if housed outdoors should have access to shade at all times. Heat stress and sterility may occur at temperatures over 27°C. Guinea pigs may withstand cooler temperatures if adequate bedding and shelter are supplied and there is an acclimatization period. In temperate climates they should be housed indoors (for example in a garage or shed) during the winter months. Day length should be 10–12 hours per day if housed indoors and access to an exercise area is essential to avoid problems such as obesity and osteoporosis.

Regular daily opportunities to exercise and graze should be provided in the form of a moveable run or ark, or permanent outdoor pen. This should be covered to prevent predation and should have a shelter (the hutch, box or a piece of drain pipe) to give a bolt hole if the animal is startled.

A suitable substrate, such as wood shavings, shredded paper or paper by-products, peat or corncob granules, should be provided to a depth of 2–5 cm. Bedding material should also be provided, such as hay, straw or shredded paper. Ideally these materials should be dust free and absorbent. Hay and straw are commonly associated with corneal ulceration due to direct trauma or ocular foreign bodies.

Environmental enrichment may be provided in the form of cardboard boxes and tubes or plastic piping, with wooden blocks or branches (fruit trees, willow or poplar) to gnaw on. Branches from poisonous trees such as cherry, plum, cedar and oleander should be avoided.

Feeding

Guinea pigs are herbivores and their diet should be high in fibre, consisting of plant materials such as hay and grasses. The ideal guinea pig diet comprises a mixture of commercial pelleted diet plus *ad libitum* good quality hay and fresh leafy green foods such as grass, dandelion, groundsel, cow parsley and broccoli. The diet should contain approximately 18–20% crude protein, 12–16% fibre, 3–4% fat and 8–30 mg vitamin C/kg (higher levels being required during pregnancy and lactation). High dietary fibre is essential to prolong chewing activity and promote tooth wear as well as maintaining gastrointestinal health. Commercial dry mixes are not recommended, since these are often low in fibre and lead to selective feeding.

Compared with rabbits, guinea pigs are able to digest fibre more efficiently and tend to eat hay more slowly, only consuming half the amount of hay per unit of body weight (Cheeke, 1987). A solely hay-based diet is therefore inadequate for the pet guinea pig. If pelleted diet and hay are both offered *ad libitum*, guinea pigs will tend to eat more of the pelleted diet. Food is primarily consumed in the late afternoon and evening. Average food intake in adult animals is 60–70 g/kg per day, rising to two or three times that level in growing animals and pregnancy. Average daily water intake is 100–200 ml/kg.

Levels of food hygiene should be high. Food should be stored carefully away from potential bacterial, parasitic or chemical contamination. Mouldy food stuffs, such as hay or peanuts, may be a source of aflatoxins. Grass clippings should not be fed since this may lead to gastrointestinal upset and gastric tympany. Foodstuffs and treats with a high sugar content should also be avoided since these may predispose to dental caries and diabetes. Guinea pigs, like other rodents, are coprophagic, eating caecotrophs directly from the anus.

Vitamin C: Guinea pigs have an absolute dietary requirement for vitamin C (ascorbic acid) since, like primates, they lack the enzyme L-gluconolactone oxidase, which is involved in the synthesis of vitamin C from glucose. They are also only able to store vitamin C for short periods. The average daily vitamin C requirement for an adult guinea pig is 10 mg/kg, rising to 30 mg/kg during pregnancy. If diets are deficient, hypovitaminosis C (scurvy) will develop (see Chapter 14). Vegetables high in vitamin C include peppers, tomatoes, spinach, asparagus, broccoli and leafy greens such as parsley, kale and chicory.

Commercial guinea pig diets are often supplemented with vitamin C, but stability of this vitamin varies with diet composition and storage conditions. Over 50% of the vitamin C content of a diet will be lost in 90 days due to oxidization if stored above 22°C. It is still therefore possible to see deficiencies in guinea pigs fed a commercial pelleted diet. To avoid potential problems it is advisable to supplement the water with 1g vitamin C/litre daily and provide vegetables and greens high in vitamin C in the diet. Excess vitamin C is harmlessly excreted in the urine. Water should be provided *ad libitum* from a plastic water bottle and changed daily, since the vitamin C content reduces by 50% over a 24-hour period. Oxidization occurs more rapidly in direct sunlight, or with hard water or contact with metal or organic material.

Chinchillas

Husbandry-related problems in chinchillas include pododermatitis (see earlier under guinea pigs), ocular problems associated with irritation from dust bathing and heat stress associated with high temperatures. High humidity may also affect breeding performance. Poor nutrition may lead to reduced lactation in females, congenital abnormalities and infertility. Diets low in fibre and high in carbohydrates may lead to imbalances of the gut flora and fauna and loose faeces or diarrhoea. There is much evidence that diets for captive chinchillas that are low in fibre and silicate levels and high in energy content are poorly abrasive compared with foods eaten in the wild; also, these diets are often presented in pelleted forms which minimize the need for chewing, leading in turn to poor attrition and dental disease. (See also Chapter 8.)

Housing

Chinchillas can be housed with others of the same sex, as long as they do not fight. Conflict can be reduced if the chinchillas are either introduced when young, or, if older, are introduced gradually. However, females are often aggressive to each other and so can be kept singly, or in breeding pairs with a male, or in polygamous units with one male to two to six females. If breeding is not desired animals should be neutered.

Due to their dense fur coat and natural habitat at high altitudes, chinchillas are very prone to overheating and should be kept indoors at temperatures of 10–15°C. At 21°C they start to become agitated and may die if exposed to temperatures over 30°C. Ideal housing should be draught free, dry and moderately cool.

Chinchillas may be housed in a room in the house or alternatively a cage. These animals are very active and so the cage should be large (at least 2 m × 2 m

× 1 m). It should also be indestructible and ideally made of wire since they enjoy chewing. They are shy animals, hiding in rock crevices in the wild, and require a hide or nest box. Plastic items should be avoided: they are usually chewed and may be ingested as foreign bodies. Bedding material should be provided in the nest box, as for guinea pigs. Solid or wire-floored cages may be used; wire mesh size should be no more than 15 mm × 15 mm in order to prevent limb injuries. Solid-floored cages should be used for pregnant animals. Wood shavings are ideal as a substrate.

Wooden toys and branches should be provided for gnawing. Chinchillas are very agile and jump readily across rocky terrain in the wild. It is important to provide height and various levels (such as wooden shelves) within the cage to allow animals to be more active. If caged, supervised time outside the cage should also be provided daily as exercise.

Chinchillas require daily dust baths, without which the fur becomes matted due to oily secretions along the back. There are many different types of chinchilla dust available commercially, the most common being volcanic ash or a mixture of Fuller's earth and silver sand (1:9). The baths should be provided for a set period and not left in the cage. This reduces contamination with urine, faeces and food and also reduces the incidence of conjunctivitis associated with excessive dust bathing and ocular irritation. They should be of sufficient size to allow the animal to roll in and dust should be at least 4–6 cm deep. Neonatal animals should avoid dust bathing since material accumulates around orifices causing irritation.

Feeding

Wild chinchillas feed on a high-fibre diet of grasses and bushes in the mountainous terrain of the Andes. They nibble leaves and twigs grasped between their forepaws. They are nocturnal, feeding mainly at night.

In captivity they should be fed a high-fibre diet consisting of grass-based chinchilla pellets and fresh good quality hay, supplemented with occasional treats such as sunflower seeds, pumpkin seeds, dried fruit (banana, apple, cranberries), grapes, raisins and small amounts of carrot and celery. Sugar-rich items and commercially available treats should be avoided since these predispose to dental caries and gastrointestinal disturbances. Dry commercial mixes should be avoided since these are often low in fibre and lead to selective feeding. The average daily adult intake of pellets is 25–50 g per day. Chinchilla pellets are longer than those manufactured for guinea pigs to enable them to be grasped in the forepaws.

The exact nutritional requirement of the chinchilla has not been researched, but it is generally recognized that the diet should consist of 15–35% fibre, 2–5% fat and 16–20% protein. Nutritional requirements increase during lactation and growth. Additional multivitamins may be beneficial in the last stages of pregnancy. Any changes to the diet should be introduced gradually, to avoid gastrointestinal problems. Leafy greens should be avoided since feeding these may predispose to gastric tympany and bloat. Hay may be provided from an overhead rack to increase environmental enrichment. Salt licks containing trace minerals may also be provided and are enjoyed by chinchillas.

Water should be provided at all times via a drinking bottle and changed daily. Wild chinchillas are reported to rarely drink, obtaining most of their water from plants and by licking up dew drops.

Degus

Husbandry-related problems are similar to those of chinchillas. Dental disease is commonly seen in degus fed inappropriate diets. Degloving of the distal tail is common if incorrectly handled. Wire mesh flooring may predispose to pododermatitis. Ocular problems may be seen associated with dust bathing or dental disease. Obesity, diabetes and secondary liver disease may be seen associated with feeding high-sugar or high-fat diets. Respiratory problems are common and may be linked with poor ventilation and dusty bedding.

Housing

Degus are social animals and should be kept in same-sex pairs, ideally introduced from an early age else fighting may occur. They may also be kept as breeding pairs or as a neutered male and female. They enjoy grooming each other and will sleep side by side.

Housing requirements for degus are similar to those for chinchillas (see earlier). Wire cages are most commonly used, with variable levels to allow the animals to climb. Degus form burrows in the wild and deep substrate such as paper-based products or wood shavings should be provided. Degus may also be housed in glass vivaria, but these may predispose to respiratory disease since they are poorly ventilated. One solution is to provide a glass-based cage with deep substrate and a wire cage on top with areas for climbing. Cages should be cleaned at least once a week. Nesting material such as hay or shredded paper and a hide box should also be provided. Degus are highly active and will use a solid-floored exercise wheel. Materials to gnaw should also be available.

Wild degus use sand baths to maintain coat quality and in which they urinate and then roll to mark the coat. Pet degus should be provided with a daily dust bath (see under Chinchillas).

Feeding

Wild degus are herbivorous. They feed on grass, grains, seeds and fruit and hoard food in their burrows. Degus are coprophagic. In Chile they are seen as a pest species since they cause significant damage to crops and cactus plantations.

Degus are prone to type 2 diabetes and should be fed diets low in sugar and fat and high in fibre. The diet should primarily consist of high quality hay with small amounts of chinchilla pellets (1–2 tablespoonfuls per day) and vegetables, such as carrots, broccoli and green beans. Some sources recommend feeding a mix of 50% guinea pig pellets and 50% chinchilla pellets to degus because the vitamin C requirements of degus are unknown. Care should be taken that guinea pig pellets do not contain molasses, which are high in sugar.

Fresh water should be provided via a drinking bottle.

Reproduction

Reproductive biology

Rodents differ from lagomorphs and most other mammals in that females have separate vaginal and urethral orifices. The vaginal opening is usually non-patent (due to the vaginal membrane) until oestrus or parturition. They are polyoestrous and exhibit spontaneous ovulation. The myomorph rodents (mice, rats, hamsters and gerbils) are prolific breeders. Once mating has occurred a vaginal/copulatory plug is formed (a mixture of sperm and accessory sex gland secretions). All species (except chipmunks) show a postpartum oestrus within about 24 hours of parturition, and females should be separated from the male unless a constant state of pregnancy or lactation is desired. Dystocia is rare in the myomorph rodents. Figure 1.23 gives reproductive biological data for selected rodent species.

Characteristic	Mice	Rats	Hamsters	Gerbils	Guinea pigs	Chinchillas	Degus
Oestrous cycle	4–5 days	4–5 days	4 days	4–7 days	15–17 days	30–50 days	21 days
Duration of oestrous	10–20 hours	10–20 hours	8–26 hours	12–18 hours	6–11 hours	40 hours	3 hours
Ovulation characteristics	Polyoestrous; spontaneous ovulators	Polyoestrous; spontaneous ovulators	Polyoestrous; spontaneous ovulators	Polyoestrous; spontaneous ovulators	Polyoestrous; spontaneous ovulators	Seasonally polyoestrous	Induced ovulators
Gestation	19–21 days	21–23 days	15–18 days	23–26 days	59–72 (av. 63) days	111 days	87–93 days
Postpartum oestrus?	yes	yes	yes	yes	yes	yes	yes
Litters per year	Numerous	Numerous	Numerous	Numerous	Numerous	2	2–3
Young per litter	5–12	8–18	5–10	3–8	1–6 (av. 3–4)	2	1–10 (av. 5–7)

1.23 Reproductive biological data in selected rodent species. (Compiled by La'Toya Latney) (continues) ▶

Characteristic	Mice	Rats	Hamsters	Gerbils	Guinea pigs	Chinchillas	Degus
Weight of neonate	1–1.5 g	4–6 g	1.5–3 g	2.5–3.5 g	60–110 g	30–50 g	14 g
Birth characteristics	Nude; eyes open 12–14 days	Nude; eyes open 12–15 days	Nude; eyes open 12–14 days	Nude; eyes open 16–21 days	Precocial	Precocial	Considered precocial; eyes open day 2–3
Weaning age	21–28 days	17–21 days	20–28 days	20–30 days	14–28 days	36–48 days	28 days
Sexual maturity	6–8 weeks	6–8 weeks	6–8 weeks	6–8 weeks	Female: 4–6 weeks Male: 9–10 weeks	8 months	3–4 months
Recommended breeding times	8 weeks	9 weeks	8 weeks	10–14 weeks	Non-seasonal	Nov–May	Year round
Complications			Cannibalistic if disturbed		>8 months old: dystocia is more common, pregnancy toxaemia	Females are the aggressive sex	

1.23 (continued) Reproductive biological data in selected rodent species. (Compiled by La'Toya Latney)

Mice and rats

Sexing

Males have open inguinal canals, an os penis and accessory sex glands. The anogenital distance is greater in the male than the female (Figure 1.24). Females have visible nipples, whereas males do not. Mammary tissue is extensive in these species, with three pairs of mammary glands in the cervicothoracic region and two in the inguinoabdominal region in mice and a total of six pairs in rats. In males the testes may be visible within the scrotum.

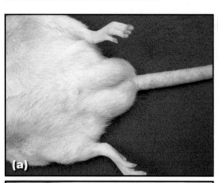
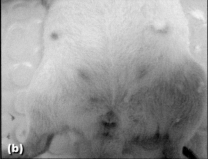

1.24 **(a)** Male rat: note long anogenital distance and obvious testicles. **(b)** Female rat: note short anogenital distance and visible nipples.

Breeding

Females are polyoestrous, with oestrus occurring every 4–5 days. In mice the vaginal plug can persist for up to 2 days, whereas in rats it falls out in 12–24 hours. Young are altricial when born. The male should be separated from the female before parturition to avoid mating at the postpartum oestrus. Disturbance of the mother for the first 2–3 days should be avoided or she may cannibalize the young.

Hamsters

Sexing

Hamsters may be sexed as for rats and mice. In Syrian hamsters the flank gland is larger in adult males than in females, being under androgen control. If viewed from above the male has a rounded perineum and prominent testicular bulges (Figure 1.25). Female hamsters have six or seven pairs of mammary glands.

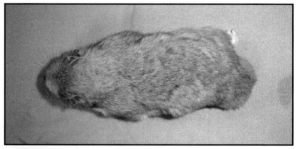

1.25 Male hamster viewed from above, showing rounded perineum and obvious testicular bulges.

Breeding

Mating of Syrian hamsters should be supervised since females can be very aggressive towards the males. Animals should be introduced on neutral territory or alternatively the female should be taken to the male. Females show oestrus every 4 days and are unusual in that they exhibit a characteristic vaginal discharge postovulation (day 2 of the oestrous cycle) (Figure 1.26; see also Chapter 13). The vaginal plug is deep and not obvious after mating. The young are altricial when born. Privacy is essential for the nursing mother.

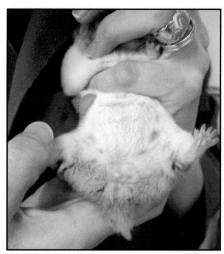

1.26
Female hamster with characteristic post-ovulatory vaginal discharge. Note that this is normal in this species.

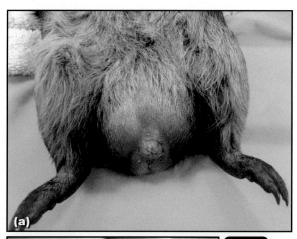

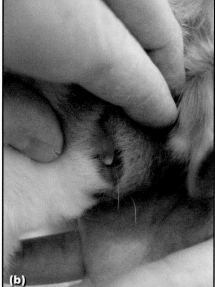

1.27
(a) Male guinea pig: note round preputial orifice and obvious scrotum. **(b)** Female guinea pig: note Y-shaped anogenital area.

Gerbils

Sexing
Gerbils may be sexed as for rats and mice. At weaning, male gerbils have a darkly pigmented scrotal area. Adult male gerbils have larger ventral abdominal scent glands than females. Females have four pairs of mammary glands.

Breeding
Gerbils are unusual in that they form monogamous pairs and the male assists in rearing the young. The female is polyoestrous, every 4–7 days, and the vaginal plug is deep and not easily seen. Young are altricial. The presence of adult males and females within a family group delays the onset of puberty in the offspring.

Guinea pigs

Sexing
In male guinea pigs the preputial orifice is round and the penis can be extruded by gentle pressure cranial to the prepuce. There is an obvious scrotum with palpable testes in intact males (Figure 1.27a). In females the anogenital area is Y-shaped, with the urethral opening forming the branches of the Y and the vagina forming the vertical tail (Figure 1.27b). The anus is at the base of the Y-shape. If gentle pressure is applied to the genital area, the vaginal membrane will be exposed. Both sexes have one pair of inguinal nipples. In female guinea pigs the pelvic symphysis is fibrocartilaginous.

Male guinea pigs have large vesicular glands extending into the abdomen ventral to the urethra. Other accessory sex glands include the prostate gland, bulbourethral glands and coagulating glands. Males have an os penis. Females have paired uterine horns, a short uterine body and a single cervix.

Breeding
The female is polyoestrous, with oestrus occurring every 15–17 days. Ovulation is spontaneous. A female in oestrus will arch her back if stroked (lordosis) and raise her hind quarters and the vulva becomes dilated. Once mated an obvious vaginal plug is formed, which falls out several hours post mating. The young are born after a long gestation period (average of 63 days) and are precocious. Females will synchronize litters if kept together.

It is essential to breed female guinea pigs at a young age, ideally at about 4–5 months old (minimum 500 g body weight) and definitely before 6–8 months old. After approximately 8 months old the pubic symphysis fuses and if they are bred for the first time after this dystocia will occur. Dystocia is relatively common in guinea pigs and is associated with fetal oversize, obesity or failure to breed before 8 months old (see Chapters 7 and 13). Pregnancy toxaemia, eclampsia and ketosis may all occur in gravid animals (see Chapter 13). Pseudopregnancy is rare in guinea pigs but may occur, lasting approximately 17 days.

Chinchillas

Sexing
The anogenital distance is greater in the male than in the female (Figure 1.28). The penis may easily be everted by applying pressure to the genital area. Males do not have a true scrotum and testes are in or near the inguinal canal. Males possess an os penis. Females have a large urethral process cranial to the slit-like vagina, which may easily be confused with a

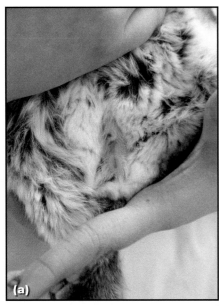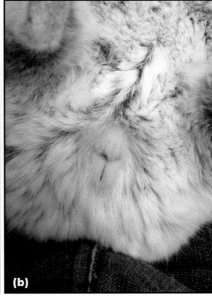

1.28 **(a)** Male chinchilla: note large anogenital distance and lack of obvious scrotum. **(b)** Female chinchilla: note short anogenital distance.

penis. This lies close to the anus in the female, whereas in the male there is a distinct separation and increased distance. Between the urethral papilla and the anus is the vaginal orifice, which is closed and therefore easily overlooked. Females have three pairs of mammary glands: two pairs laterally on the thorax and one pair in the inguinal region. Female chinchillas have paired uterine horns, and two cervices.

Breeding
Chinchillas are seasonally polyoestrous, with oestrus occurring every 30–50 days, shown by an open vulva and mucoid vaginal discharge. Postpartum oestrus occurs 12 hours after giving birth. During oestrus the perineum becomes reddened and the vagina is open. The onset of oestrus is marked by expelling of wax-like oestrous plugs. These should not be confused with copulatory plugs, which form after mating and remain in the vagina for several hours before falling out.

When breeding, chinchillas will form monogamous pairs, or can be kept in harems with one male for every two to six females. The male should be given free-choice access to each separate female. The gestation period is long (111 days) and the young are precocious (fully furred and eyes open). The average litter size is two. Dystocia is rare.

Degus

Sexing
Sexing of degus is as for chinchillas, with males having a greater anogenital distance. Males do not have an obvious scrotum and testes lie within the abdomen or inguinal canal. Females have a prominent urinary (urethral) process or papilla, similar to female chinchillas. The vagina is closed except during oestrus. Females have four pairs of nipples.

Breeding
Like chinchillas, degus can breed at any time of the year. They also have a very long gestation period

(90 days) compared with other rodents. Due to this long pregnancy, degu pups are born fully furred. Litters are usually four to seven in number (average five). Males will assist in rearing the young. Neonates are less precocious than chinchilla or guinea pig offspring and are born with their eyes closed; these open around day 2–3. Fur is initially sparse. The young stay in the nest or are carried by adults. They will eat small amounts of grass from an early age. Weaning occurs by 8 weeks of age. Sexual maturity can be as early as a few months old, but is on average from 6 months of age. A postpartum oestrus is seen.

Hand-rearing
As myomorphs have altricial young, hand-rearing is less successful (in the author's experience) than with hystricomorphs, whose young are precocious.

Myomorphs
Gloves should be worn when handling young animals since the smell of humans may lead to cannibalism or abandonment of the young. Milk substitutes used are the same as for hystricomorphs (see below) but volumes taken are smaller (1–2 drops in mice to 1 ml in rats initially) and feeds should be more frequent. Solid food will be eaten by about 2 weeks for all species. Moistened food should be provided to encourage self-feeding. Cross-fostering is rarely successful.

Hystricomorphs
Young hystricomorphs will start to take some solid food from a few days old. Supplementation with hand-feeding via a dropper, syringe or small nursing bottle and teat is necessary for the first 2–3 weeks of life. Cross-fostering is possible on to other lactating females and is more likely to be successful if the young are first rubbed in the foster mother's bedding or against her kits to transfer the scent.

Milk substitutes used include: evaporated milk, diluted 50:50 with pre-boiled water; goat's milk; or commercially available feeds such as 'Esbilac'

(Pet-Ag). The volume of milk per feed will vary according to the age of the kit, the size and whether there is supplemental feeding from the mother, but on average 1–2 ml is taken each feed. Feeds should be given every 2–3 hours and stimulation of urination and defecation using wet cotton wool gently rubbed on the anogenital area should be performed following each feed for the first 7 days. Solid food should be offered from birth. Supplementary heating using a heat pad should also be provided.

Preventive health care

Routine health checks

Rodents are rarely presented to the veterinary surgeon for routine health checks since there are no annual vaccination programmes. Post-purchase and annual examinations are advisable, particularly in aged or breeding animals, since potential problems may be detected at an early stage. General advice may also be offered at this time on disease prevention practices such as isolation of new or sick animals, cage hygiene, environmental enrichment and diet. Husbandry and diet should be reviewed annually. Annual examination will also allow oral examination for clinical signs of dental disease, which is common in the hystricomorph rodents.

Obesity is common in pet rodents and measures to reduce the incidence should be discussed, such as increased exercise opportunities (exercise wheels, vertical tunnel systems and supervised free access outside the cage) and dietary restrictions.

Respiratory disease is also common in rodents and the animal may be predisposed by husbandry practices (poor ventilation, increased humidity or dust in the environment). Contact with new animals (e.g. at pet shows) should be avoided.

Nail overgrowth is common, particularly in guinea pigs housed indoors. Animals may require regular presentation for nail trimming. Particular care should be taken in guinea pigs to clip the medial claw on the forefeet, which is often overlooked and may become ingrowing. Guinea pigs are also prone to developing large keratinized horns on the feet, which may also require regular trimming.

Neutering should be discussed during the post-purchase or annual examination. This may be desired due to behavioural issues, such as aggression, or to prevent pregnancy, or in clinical cases with reproductive problems such as pyometra, ovarian cysts or uterine neoplasia. (See also Chapter 7.)

Zoonoses

Pet rodents are not routinely treated for ecto- or endo-parasites, unless a clinical problem arises. Although transfer of zoonotic diseases from wild rodents to humans is common, zoonotic diseases from pet rodents are rare. However, owners should be warned of the potential for disease transfer, particularly in immunocompromised humans. For example, the tapeworm *Rodentolepis* (previously *Hymenolepis*) *nana* is often found in myomorphs and may cause infections in humans. Other potential zoonoses from rodents include leptospirosis, salmonellosis, yersiniosis, campylobacteriosis, lymphocytic choriomeningitis, monkeypox, *Trixacarus caviae* infection and ringworm.

Allergic reactions in humans are relatively commonly associated with contact with pet rodents, in particular rats and guinea pigs. Common allergens include rodent dander and urine. Aerosolized rat urine may lead to acute respiratory compromise in owners with allergies.

Geriatric animals

Common problems in geriatric animals include renal disease (particularly in rats, hamsters and guinea pigs), diabetes in hamsters, faecal impactions in male guinea pigs and mammary neoplasia in female rats.

References and further reading

Brain P (1999) The laboratory gerbil. In: *The UFAW Handbook on the Care and Management of Laboratory Animals, 7th edn, Vol. 1: Terrestrial Vertebrates*, ed. T Poole, pp. 345–355. Blackwell Science, Oxford

Brown C and Donnelly T (2004) Rodent husbandry and care. *Veterinary Clinics of North America: Exotic Animal Practice* **7**(2), 201–225

Cheeke PR (1987) Nutrition of guinea pigs. In: *Rabbit Feeding and Nutrition*, pp. 344–353. Academic Press, Orlando

Crossley DA (2001) Dental disease in chinchillas in the UK. *Journal of Small Animal Practice* **42**, 12–19

Daviau J (1999) Clinical evaluation of rodents. *Veterinary Clinics of North America: Exotic Animal Practice* **2**(2), 429–445

Niethammer J (1990) Burrowing rodents, Rodentia. In: *Grzimek's Encyclopedia of Mammals, Vol. 3*, pp. 206–257. McGraw-Hill, New York

Nishi M and Steiner DF (1990) Cloning of complementary DNAs encoding islet amyloid polypeptide, insulin and glucagon precursors from a New World rodent, the degu, *Octodon degus*. *Molecular Endocrinology* **4**, 1192–1198

North D (1999) The guinea pig. In: *The UFAW Handbook on the Care and Management of Laboratory Animals, 7th edn, Vol. 1: Terrestrial Vertebrates*, ed. T Poole, pp. 367–388. Blackwell Science, Oxford

Sainsbury A (2003) Rodentia (Rodents). In: *Zoo and Wild Animal Medicine, 5th edn*, ed ME Fowler and RE Miller, pp. 420–441. WB Saunders, Philadelphia

Stahnke A and Hendrichs H (1990) Chinchillas, Rodentia. In: *Grzimek's Encyclopedia of Mammals, Vol. 3*, pp. 317–324. McGraw-Hill, New York

Strike C (1996) Hand-rearing and supplementation of small mammals. http://www.priory.com/vet/smamam2.htm

Wilson D and Reeder D (2005) Introduction. In: *Mammal Species of the World: A Taxonomic and Geographic Reference, 3rd edn*, ed. D Wilson and D Reeder, p. xxxviii. John Hopkins University Press, Baltimore

2

Rodents: physical examination and emergency care

Marla Lichtenberger and Michelle G. Hawkins

Introduction

In recent years, the number of rodent species kept as pets has grown considerably and demand for appropriate veterinary care for these species has also increased. Unfortunately, as rodents are prey species, clinical signs are often masked until the course of the disease is far advanced and the pet is presented on an emergency basis. For some of the pet rodent species, little information regarding unique medical conditions and their appropriate care is available.

The principles of emergency and critical care apply equally to rodents, but the anatomical, physiological and behavioural differences of these species require careful consideration when developing an initial plan of emergency therapy. Many rodents are highly predisposed to stress and so rapid evaluation and patient stabilization are often required before complete evaluation for a definitive diagnosis can be performed.

Patient handling and restraint

In an emergency situation, the stability of the animal dictates the type of restraint allowable to minimize patient stress. General anaesthesia or deep sedation can minimize stress for a fractious or painful patient and can allow for complete physical examination, diagnostic sampling, intravenous catheter placement and the initiation of therapy, but the risk of adverse effects under anaesthesia must be carefully weighed before anaesthesia for restraint is considered. The animal may need to be placed in a warm and oxygenated cage prior to initiation of any restraint. Pre-oxygenation should be performed whenever possible and always when signs of respiratory distress are present. The benefits of pre-oxygenation sometimes take 5 minutes or longer in a rodent with a compromised respiratory system.

Handling and restraint of rodents varies with the species.

Smaller rodents

The smaller rodents can be challenging to handle in a way that minimizes patient stress. Wearing examination gloves during restraint of some small rodents may decrease the chance of a bite if the animal bites the glove rather than the hand; however, all rodents are capable of inflicting serious bites.

While gerbils can be very docile and held in a cupped hand, they may require scruff-of-the-neck or

over-the-back technique for complete restraint, taking care not to damage their delicate skin (Figure 2.1). Degloving injuries to the tail are commonly associated with incorrect handling technique in gerbils and degus.

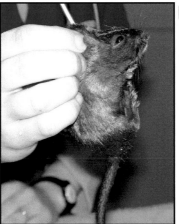

2.1 Restraint of a gerbil using the scruff-of-the-neck technique.

Hamsters are prone to bite, especially if startled; the abundant loose skin over the back and shoulders can be grasped in a full-handed grip for complete immobilization (Figure 2.2).

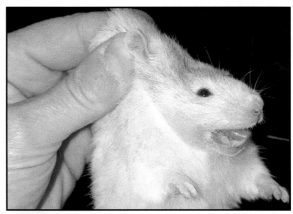

2.2 Restraint of a hamster by grasping the abundant skin over the back and shoulders.

Mice can be captured by gently grasping the base of the tail with one hand and then using a scruff-of-the-neck technique with the other hand (Figure 2.3).

Most pet rats are friendly and amenable to handling; if needed, whole body restraint can be achieved by placing a forefinger below the mandible

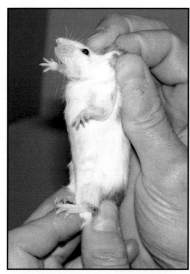

2.3 Restraint of a mouse by grasping the base of the tail with one hand and the scruff of the neck with the other hand.

on one side of the head and a thumb on the opposite side, above or below the forelimb, with the tail and hind limbs held with the opposite hand (Figure 2.4).

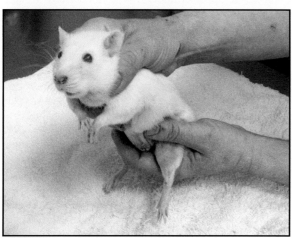

2.4 Restraint of a rat by placing a forefinger below the mandible on one side of the head and a thumb on the opposite side, above or below the forelimb, with the tail and hind limbs held with the opposite hand. (Courtesy of Angela Lennox.)

Chinchillas and guinea pigs

Chinchillas are best supported with one hand under the thorax and a second hand around the rump (Figure 2.5). The examiner must avoid holding the chinchilla by the scruff of the neck, because fur slip is common in chinchillas when exuberant restraint is used.

In general, guinea pigs require minimal restraint but care should be taken to avoid injury from a fall when they are examined on a table.

Restraint devices

Restraint devices are commercially available for all sizes of rodents but these are used mainly in the laboratory setting. Small towels are most commonly used as restraint devices to partially 'burrito' (wrap) the companion animal, allowing for examination of individual limbs. Paper towels, syringe cases and polyethylene or plastic bags with a corner removed have all been used to facilitate restraint of the small rodent.

2.5 Proper restraint of a chinchilla, supported with one hand under the thorax and a second hand around the rump. (Courtesy of Emma Keeble)

Any restraint device used with emergency rodent patients should allow for quick release in the event that the rodent becomes severely stressed.

History and physical examination

History

A comprehensive signalment and history is critical in the determination of the disease process and often may help to determine the exact aetiology of the presenting complaint. Often the history can be obtained while the patient is being stabilized.

The age of the rodent patient is very important. Many rodents have short life spans, sometimes only 1–3 years of age, and the owner may not be aware that their pet is geriatric. The dietary history is of utmost concern in the rodent patient. High fibre is necessary for proper hindgut fermentation. Patients that receive diets containing seed and dried fruit should be assumed to be consuming large amounts of carbohydrates, which can result in overall malnutrition and gastrointestinal abnormalities, including diarrhoea, and dental disease.

Physical examination

Physical examination of the rodent is similar to that of other mammalian species. If the animal is very debilitated the examination should proceed in a stepwise fashion, with the most important sections of the examination being prioritized in advance, and there should be small breaks from handling between examination sections. Oxygen supplementation may be required during physical examination. All equipment needed for the physical examination should be prepared prior to handling the patient and all efforts should be made towards minimizing patient stress by limiting the time the animal is handled.

Observation before handling

In addition to the respiratory rate and effort, a significant amount of physical examination information can be obtained prior to any handling or physical restraint. Symmetry of the eyes, ears and limbs as well as posture and awareness can be evaluated. Ocular or nasal discharge may alert the emergency clinician to diseases of the eyes or upper respiratory tract. In healthy rodents, porphyrin ocular discharge is a normal physiological finding but the discharge is usually not observed if the animal is healthy and grooming properly. In some cases rats are presented as an emergency for 'bleeding from the eyes' when in fact the 'porphyrin tears' are simply a sign of other underlying diseases or stress (see Chapter 15). Musculoskeletal or neurological abnormalities should also be evaluated prior to handling. If the animal's caging is present, note should be taken of the diet provided and the water containers. It is also important to evaluate the substrate and bedding in the cage and to note the volume and consistency of urine or faeces and whether any odours are present.

Body weight and temperature

The body weight should be obtained as soon as possible, using a gram scale for the most accurate weight of small rodents.

The body temperature should be obtained at the onset of examination. Many clinicians avoid taking the body temperature of small rodents but it can be taken if the procedure is performed carefully. It is preferable to use a flexible plastic thermometer instead of glass to minimize the potential for injury.

Eyes, ears, nostrils, integument and abdomen

The eyes, oral cavity, ears, nostrils and integument should be examined closely for any evidence of blood, which may indicate trauma. Because of the pronounced globes of many rodents, trauma of any sort may cause secondary ophthalmic injury and so a thorough ocular examination should always be performed (see Chapter 15). Also, ocular abnormalities as well as nasal discharge can be seen secondary to dental disease of the maxillary teeth in guinea pigs, chinchillas and degus (see Chapter 8). The hair coat and skin should be closely examined, as emergency presentation for dermatological conditions is surprisingly common. Neoplasia and abscesses associated with the integument are also frequently seen in rodents. Abdominal palpation should be performed in all rodents to evaluate for masses, excessive gas ('bloat'), organomegaly or other abnormalities.

Oral examination

The oral examination should be performed last as it is often the most stressful part of the procedure. A complete oral examination is vital, especially in the rodents with continuously growing premolars and molars, such as the guinea pig, chinchilla and degu, as dental disease can be the underlying cause of a wide variety of abnormal clinical signs and emergency presentations. The external oral examination involves visualization of the incisors in all species and thorough palpation of the ventral mandibles of guinea pigs, chinchillas and degus, because apical elongation of the cheek teeth is common with dental disease in these species. An endoscopic oral examination can also be performed, but requires anaesthesia or deep sedation to minimize the potential for equipment damage. For a more detailed description of oral examination in rodents, see Chapter 8.

Clinical techniques

Stabilization of the patient is mandatory prior to extensive diagnostic sampling.

Blood collection

If blood can be safely obtained, it is ideal to collect baseline samples for haematology and biochemistry analysis prior to institution of any treatment. For normal values and reference ranges in rodents, see Chapter 4. Venipuncture can be very stressful even in healthy rodents, as significant restraint is often required to obtain access to appropriate sampling sites. Possible venipuncture sites vary depending on the species and patient stability. Anaesthesia or sedation may be required to facilitate blood collection from any site, but the risk of this must be carefully weighed in the critically ill rodent.

While total blood volume varies according to species, as a rule the total blood volume for most rodents is approximately 6–8% of the body weight. In general, a blood sample of no more than 7–10% of the blood volume, or approximately 1% of total body weight, can be safely collected in healthy rodent patients. In sick patients presenting as an emergency, the general rule of thumb is that no more than 0.5% of total body weight should be collected for blood sampling.

Many techniques have been described for blood sampling in rodents. The lateral saphenous and cephalic veins are often the most accessible vessels and restraint can often be minimized to facilitate collection from these sites. These vessels may yield minimal blood volumes and collapse even with minimal aspiration pressure in very small patients. Alternatively, a 0.3 ml insulin syringe with a swaged-on small-gauge (27 or 29 gauge) needle and the plunger removed can be introduced into the vein and the blood collected from the hub of needle inside the syringe barrel into heparinized haematocrit tubes (Figure 2.6). A small-gauge hypodermic needle can also be introduced into the vessel and blood collected in the same manner (Figure 2.7), but the use of the syringe barrel technique often provides greater stability of the needle in the vessel during blood collection.

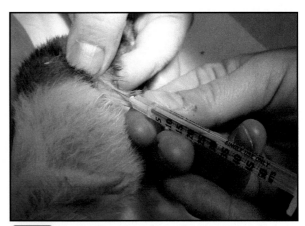

2.6 An insulin syringe (0.3 ml) with a swaged small-gauge needle and the plunger removed can be introduced into the vein. The blood is then collected from the hub of the needle inside the syringe barrel into heparinized haematocrit tubes.

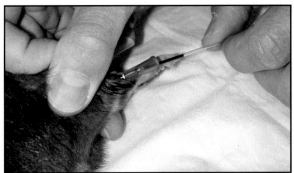

2.7 A small-gauge hypodermic needle can be introduced into the vessel and blood collected in the same manner; however, the use of the syringe barrel technique often provides greater stability of the needle in the vessel during blood collection.

The lateral tail veins can be used to collect small to moderate amounts of blood in gerbils, mice and rats (Figure 2.8). The rat has a ventral tail artery that can yield an adequate blood sample but this technique requires practice (Bober, 1998).

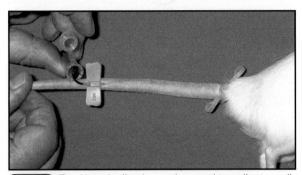

2.8 The lateral tail vein can be used to collect small to moderate amounts of blood from a rat. A tourniquet may be applied to the tail base. The needle is inserted on the lateral surface of the tail to the level of the vertebrae. Gentle negative pressure may be applied to the syringe, or the sample may be collected by free flow into a suitable container. (Courtesy of The Comparative Biology Centre, Newcastle University.)

Jugular venipuncture can be challenging as many rodents have short, thick necks with large fat-bodies covering the jugular groove. Restraint for this can be very stressful; anaesthesia is often necessary to facilitate sample collection from this site.

Cranial vena cava venipuncture under anaesthesia is also possible in some rodents. The potential risks of this technique include haemorrhage into the thoracic cavity and/or pericardial sac and penetration of the heart. To minimize these potential complications, use of a 25–27 gauge hypodermic needle and a ½–1 ml syringe is recommended. In guinea pigs and chinchillas (which have an underdeveloped clavicle), a 25 gauge 5/8 inch (16 mm) length needle is inserted cranial to the manubrium and first rib (Figure 2.9). Other rodents (rat, mouse, hamster, gerbil) have a well developed clavicle and placement of a 27 gauge ½ inch (12mm) needle dorsal to the clavicle will result in easier blood collection (Figure 2.10a). Incorrect placement of the needle between the clavicle and the first rib forces the needle laterally and makes blood collection more difficult (Figure 2.10b).

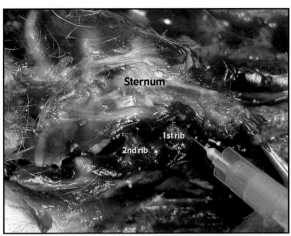

2.9 Correct positioning of the needle for vena cava puncture in a guinea pig cadaver. Larger rodents such as the guinea pig and chinchilla do not have a well developed clavicle. A 25 or 27 gauge 5/8 inch needle is inserted cranial to the first rib, lateral to the notch of the sternum and directed at an angle of 45 degrees towards the opposite hip. The cranial part of the mammal is where the needle and syringe are located in the photograph. (© Vittorio Capello.)

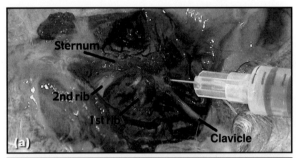
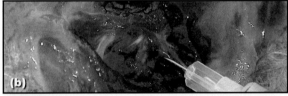

2.10 **(a)** Correct positioning of the needle for vena cava puncture in a golden hamster cadaver. Most smaller rodent species have a well developed clavicle and placement of the needle cranial to the clavicle makes blood collection easier. **(b)** Incorrect placement of the needle between the clavicle and first rib makes blood collection more difficult in all of the smaller rodent species (mouse, rat, gerbil, hamster) since the needle is forced laterally. The head of the animal is to the right of the photographs. (© Vittorio Capello.)

The femoral vein is frequently used for venipuncture in anaesthetized rodents in one author's practice (MGH) and often yields an adequate blood sample (Figure 2.11a). With the rodent in dorsal recumbency, the femoral artery is palpated deep in the inguinal region and the needle is inserted parallel to this site. The venipuncture site should be held off for several minutes after collection if the femoral artery is sampled inadvertently (Figure 2.11b).

Orbital venous plexus collection and cardiac venipuncture are only recommended as terminal procedures in the anaesthetized companion rodent patient.

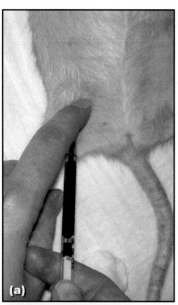

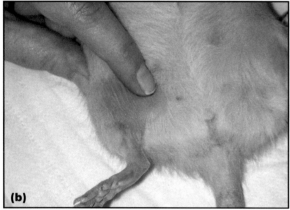

2.11 The femoral vein can be used for venipuncture in sedated or anaesthetized patients and often yields an adequate blood sample. **(a)** The site is identified by palpation of the femoral artery and the needle is inserted and directed parallel and medial to this. **(b)** The venipuncture site should be held off for several minutes after collection if the femoral artery is sampled inadvertently.

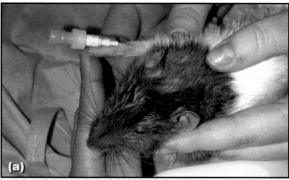

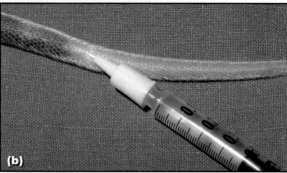

2.12 Intravenous catheters can be placed in the cephalic, lateral saphenous or femoral veins in larger rodents such as chinchilla, guinea pig and rat. Correct placement of an intravenous catheter in **(a)** the cephalic vein and **(b)** the lateral tail vein of a rat. (b, courtesy of The Comparative Biology Centre, Newcastle University.)

Intravenous catheterization

In an emergency situation, intravenous (or intraosseous) catheterization may be required to provide replacement fluids. Sedation or inhalant anaesthesia may be necessary for intravenous catheter placement in the stressed rodent patient. The catheters can be placed in the cephalic, lateral saphenous or femoral veins in larger rodents such as chinchillas, guinea pigs and rats (Figure 2.12a). The authors prefer the cephalic vein for intravenous catheterization in most cases. The superficial lateral tail veins can also be used for short-term catheter placement in the rat (Figure 2.12b).

Peripheral catheterization is difficult in very small rodents due to small vessel size (Antinoff, 1998). While jugular catheterization can be performed in rodents, a surgical cut-down procedure under anaesthesia is necessary. Small-bore over-the-needle catheters (24 gauge or smaller) are most often necessary for small rodent patients. However, catheter maintenance may be hindered by vessel fragility and patient temperament. The catheter site should be aseptically prepared. Catheters should be secured with a bandage tape butterfly and sutured in place. Jugular catheters, if left indwelling, require 24-hour monitoring because fatal haemorrhage can occur if the rodent pulls or chews on the catheter and damages the vessel.

It should be noted that rats, mice and hamsters are generally intolerant of bandaging material and other equipment, such as indwelling catheters, and will attempt to chew and remove the materials, even when they are severely compromised. Careful monitoring of the intravenous catheter is essential.

Intraosseous catheterization

Intraosseous catheterization can be useful in smaller patients or during cardiovascular collapse (Otto and Crowe, 1992) (Figure 2.13). Catheter maintenance is easier to achieve due to stability in the medullary cavity.

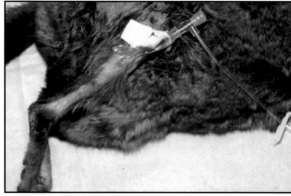

2.13 Common sites for intraosseous catheter placement in the rodent include the femur through the trochanteric fossa, or the tibia (as shown here) through the tibial crest. Placement is similar to normograde insertion of an intramedullary pin and requires strict aseptic technique during placement and maintenance.

Products that can be utilized as intraosseous catheters include 18–24 gauge 1–1½ inch (40 mm) spinal needles, or 18–25 gauge 1 inch (25 mm) hypodermic needles, depending upon the size of the species. The catheter should be long enough to extend one-third to one-half of the length of the medullary cavity. A wire stylet is commonly used to reduce the potential for a bone core to clog the catheter. The authors prepare several hypodermic needles (25 to 18 gauge) with wire stylets (stainless steel suture material) and sterilize them for use as intraosseous catheters.

Common sites for intraosseous catheter placement in the rodent include the femur through the trochanteric fossa, or the tibia through the tibial crest. Placement is similar to that of a normograde insertion of an intramedullary pin and requires strict aseptic technique during placement and maintenance. The procedure is generally performed under anaesthesia since it is painful. One small drop of a local anaesthetic such as bupivacaine (0.5%) or lidocaine (1%) can be injected through the skin down to the periosteal bone before placement of the catheter. Once the cortex is penetrated, the catheter should advance easily with little resistance. If there is further resistance, most likely the opposite cortex has been penetrated. The cannula should be flushed with heparinized saline immediately as the bone marrow quickly clots. The insertion site should be covered with an antibiotic ointment and the cannula secured with a bandage tape butterfly and suture. A bandage can be placed over the cannula site for additional security and to prevent possible trauma or damage to the catheter.

Intraosseous catheters have been reported to remain patent for 72 hours without flushing. However, if fluid therapy is not continuous, it is recommended to flush the catheter gently with heparinized saline twice daily.

Complications associated with intraosseous catheterization include penetration of both cortices, failure to enter the medullary cavity properly and extravasation of fluids, with associated pain. Intraosseous catheterization is contraindicated in patients that are septic or have metabolic bone disease. Administration of alkaline or hypertonic solutions can cause pain and so these solutions should be diluted prior to delivery through an intraosseous catheter and the catheter should be flushed with heparinized saline after any drug injection.

Intraosseous catheters should be used primarily for short-term vascular volume expansion, until an intravenous catheter site can be obtained. Many rodents appear to become uncomfortable on limbs supporting intraosseous catheters even after short-term placement.

Endotracheal wash and bronchoalveolar lavage

An endotracheal wash or a bronchoalveolar lavage may be useful to determine the cause and extent of respiratory disease. Both procedures should be performed under general anaesthesia in rodents, but this will also depress the cough reflex and reduce the volume yield of the wash.

These procedures are performed as in the dog or cat, using either endoscopic or endotracheal tube methods for collection of airway fluid. Fluid volumes of no more than 0.5% body weight are commonly used in pet rodents. Sterile samples can be submitted for cytology and/or bacterial or fungal culture and sensitivity (see also Chapter 12).

Urine collection

Urine samples can be collected via cystocentesis, catheterization or free catch after either natural voiding or gentle manual expression of the bladder. The techniques for manually expressing the bladder are the same as those used in dogs and cats. Expression of urine specimens for collection should not be attempted if the rodent has partial or complete urethral obstruction or recent bladder trauma, or if a cystotomy has recently been performed (see Chapter 7). Rupture of a normal bladder can occur if too much digital pressure is applied; rupture of a diseased bladder may occur more readily.

Urinary catheterization is rarely performed in rodents, due to their small size and the need for general anaesthesia for the procedure. This technique is most commonly employed in female rodents, as they have larger urethral openings. A small tomcat (3.5 F) rigid or red rubber catheter is inserted directly into the urethral orifice using sterile technique.

Cystocentesis is the technique of choice for urine collection when a urine culture is desired. Blind cystocentesis can be performed but the authors recommend ultrasound-guided cystocentesis under general anaesthesia or heavy sedation using a 25 gauge needle and 3 ml syringe. A potential complication of cystocentesis is caecal penetration.

Euthanasia

In most situations an intravenous catheter may be placed. The rodent can be euthanased using a pentobarbital euthanasia solution at the same dose recommended for dogs and cats. When it is not possible to place a catheter, euthanasia can best be accomplished by first inducing general anaesthesia with a facemask or in an induction chamber (see Chapter 6). Euthanasia solution can subsequently be administered via intravenous, intraosseous or intraperitoneal routes.

Triage of the emergency rodent patient

The ABC (Airway, Breathing, Circulation) of small animal emergency medicine and the principles of cardiopulmonary–cerebral resuscitation (CPCR) are universal and apply equally to the small rodent patient. The principles of CPCR and their application to small rodents will be discussed.

If a rodent is showing extreme respiratory difficulty or open-mouthed breathing, or if the rodent is collapsed or exhibiting weakness, emergency respiratory care should be provided prior to undertaking a complete physical examination. The rodent is given oxygen support, with immediate assessment for respiratory rate and effort.

Shock and fluid therapy are important when dealing with the critical care rodent patient and are presented below with application to these small mammals. Nutritional and environmental supportive care for the rodent patient will also be discussed.

Cardiopulmonary–cerebral resuscitation

The goal of cardiopulmonary resuscitation (CPR) is the restoration of spontaneous circulation. The American Heart Association changed the guidelines to include the preservation of neurological function as a goal of successful resuscitation, and the term cardiopulmonary–cerebral resuscitation (CPCR) was adopted.

The International Heart Association guidelines for CPCR and emergency cardiac care in humans (American Heart Association Guidelines, 2005) have been modified and reviewed for use in small mammals (Costello, 2004). Basic life support consists of the ABC approach. Advanced life support consists of electrocardiographic identification of the arrest rhythm, defibrillation, fluid and drug administration, and post-resuscitative care. A crash cart should be readily available with supplies (Figure 2.14) to maximize the chances of a successful outcome.

CPCR in rodents

In the authors' experience, rodents become bradycardic prior to respiratory arrest while under inhalant anaesthesia. The authors always recommend the use of Doppler blood pressure or ECG monitoring during any short procedures or longer surgeries. The bradycardia can be heard on the Doppler monitor or seen on the ECG. When respiratory arrest occurs, the inhalant anaesthesia should be turned off. Intubation is covered in more detail below.

Anaesthesia-related arrests represent one of the more treatable causes of arrest in veterinary patients. Doxapram is given as a respiratory stimulant with respiratory arrest. Intubation with an endotracheal tube and supplementation with 100% oxygen is ideal, but most rodents are difficult to intubate and therefore the authors recommend the following considerations:

- If it is not possible to intubate, forced high-flow oxygen ventilation using a tight-fitting mask over the nose and mouth should be considered. Positive-pressure ventilation should be provided using 100% oxygen at a rate of 20–30 breaths per minute. The disadvantage of this technique is accumulation of gastric air and bloating, which can limit diaphragm movement. However, ventilation is more important initially and gastric air can be eliminated with the use of an orogastric tube.
- The second technique is tracheostomy. This procedure is similar to that in dogs and cats and is described below.

Cardiac arrest involves cessation of effective circulation and is recognized by the loss of consciousness and collapse. No palpable pulse is felt, the mucous membranes are pale or cyanotic, and respirations commonly cease (i.e. cardiopulmonary arrest). Immediate basic life-support principles (ABC) should be initiated. The animal is intubated and ventilated with 100% oxygen or an alternative method using forced high flow oxygen, as given above. The chest compressions of 80–100 times per minute directly compress the myocardium, which leads to increased cardiac output. It is important that both hands be used, placing one on each side of the chest, with compressions done at the widest portion of the chest. The duration of the compression should take up half of the total compression–release cycle.

The team should continually assess their efforts at CPCR, checking to see whether the efforts are generating a palpable pulse. If no pulse is felt, the force of chest compressions should be increased and the electrocardiogram assessed. Different cardiac arrhythmias (bradycardia, ventricular fibrillation, pulseless

Drug and concentration	Dose rate (mg/kg)	Body wt = 25 g (ml/25 g)	Body wt = 50 g (ml/50 g)	Body wt = 100 g (ml/100 g)	Body wt = 1 kg (ml/kg)	Body wt = 2 kg (ml/2 kg)
Adrenaline low (1:10,000) (0.1 mg/ml)	0.01	0.0025	0.005	0.01	0.1	0.2
Adrenaline high (1:1000) (1 mg/ml)	0.1	0.0025	0.005	0.01	0.1	0.2
Atropine (0.54 mg/ml)	0.02	0.001	0.002	0.004	0.037	0.074
Glycopyrrolate (0.2 mg/ml)	0.01	0.0025	0.005	0.01	0.1	0.2
Glucose (50%)	1 ml/kg diluted 50% with saline	0.025	0.05	0.1	1	2
Calcium (100 mg/ml)	50	0.01	0.025	0.05	0.5	1
Doxapram (20 mg/ml)	2	0.0025	0.005	0.01	0.1	0.2
Vasopressin (20 units/ml)	0.8	0.001	0.002	0.004	0.04	0.08

2.14 Quick reference chart for CPCR drugs for rodents.

electrical activity (PEA), asystole) may require specific treatments as given in the CPCR chart (Figure 2.15). Intraosseous or intravenous access should be considered at this time.

Effectiveness of CPCR

The presence of palpable pulses is not an indication of adequate blood flow. Although palpable pulses may be used to evaluate the response to CPR, they do not indicate the adequacy of organ perfusion during CPR. Two other measurements, end-tidal CO_2 and blood gas measurement, can provide a more accurate assessment of organ perfusion (American Heart Association Guidelines, 2005). End-tidal CO_2 measurements are only practical in the intubated patient weighing more than 350 g. Blood gas measurements are only possible when arterial or venous access is available, but normal values have not been established in rodents.

Respiratory evaluation and support

During the physical examination, care should be taken to hold the patient upright and oxygen support should be provided if there are signs of respiratory distress or if any fluid or masses are palpated in the abdominal cavity. Clinical signs of respiratory disease may be subtle, but can include discharge from the eyes or nares, tachypnoea, abnormal respiratory sounds and open-mouthed breathing. Because of the small size of the rodent thorax, it is sometimes difficult to auscultate the normal breathing patterns; the use of a neonatal or paediatric stethoscope often facilitates this part of the examination.

The respiratory rate and effort should always be evaluated in rodents prior to handling. Immediate assessment of a patent airway is critical (see Chapter 12). When an airway obstruction is present, or if the patient is in respiratory arrest, tracheal intubation is a necessity (see also Chapter 6).

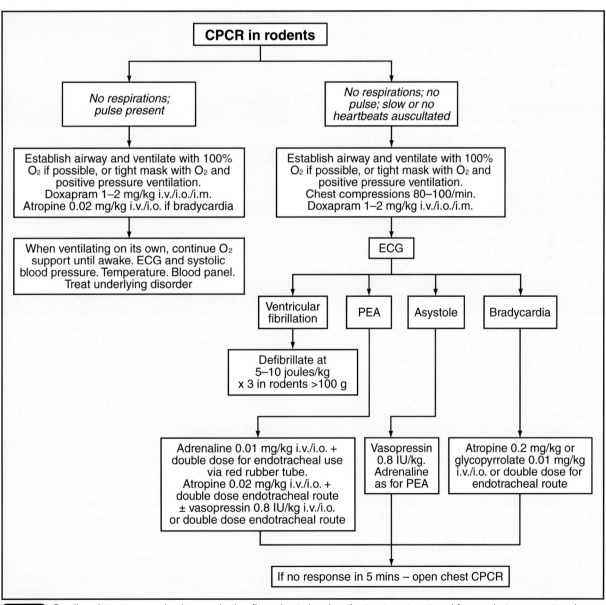

2.15 Cardiopulmonary–cerebral resuscitation flow chart showing the treatment protocol for respiratory arrest and treatment of common arrhythmias during cardiac arrest. PEA = pulseless electrical activity.

Tracheal intubation

Tracheal intubation can be challenging in rodents as most are obligate or dependent nasal breathers with limited oral access, so the clinician should be prepared to perform an emergency tracheostomy procedure if necessary to provide ventilation. In the guinea pig, orotracheal intubation is also complicated by the fusion of the soft palate to the base of the tongue creating only a small opening called the palatal ostium (Blouin and Cormier, 1987; Timm *et al.*, 1987). Small endotracheal tubes of 1.0–2.5 mm internal diameter (ID) are most often needed for small rodent species. The smallest commercially available tubes have an ID of 1 mm, but tubes less than 2 mm ID are often highly flexible and kink easily during use. Very small rodents may be intubated with Teflon intravenous catheters (14 and 16 gauge), red rubber or urinary catheters, but occlusion with mucous plugs due to the small ID of these tubes occurs frequently. Care must be taken to ensure that no sharp edges are present on the end of the tubes.

Cole tubes are uncuffed endotracheal tubes with a narrow distal insertion tip to allow facilitation of placement into the airway and a broader shoulder to fit snugly at the larynx. In the authors' experience, these tubes tend to slip from the airway easily. The smallest diameter cuffed tube is 3 mm, which is too large for many rodents. Non-cuffed tubes do not provide a sealed airway and so airway protection from aspiration of secretions or gastrointestinal contents is reduced; therefore it is imperative that the oral cavity is clean before performing intubation, as many rodents store food in their cheek pouches. Elevating the head and neck of the patient may reduce the potential for regurgitation of gastrointestinal contents into the oral cavity.

An otoscopic cone, modified paediatric blade or endoscope can help to facilitate intubation. Otoscopic cones that have been modified by removing a section laterally can facilitate both visualization of the epiglottis and direct placement of the endotracheal tube (Figure 2.16a). In smaller rodents as well as in guinea pigs (to minimize trauma to the palatal ostium), a stylet may be placed first to facilitate endotracheal tube placement (Figure 2.16b). Endoscopy may provide the best visualization of the epiglottis and minimize trauma during tube placement. One drop of a 2% lidocaine solution applied directly to the larynx usually reduces laryngospasm and eases tube placement.

Tracheostomy: If an endotracheal tube cannot be placed, a temporary tracheostomy can be performed. A 2–3 cm skin incision is made on the ventral midline parallel to the trachea, just caudal to the larynx. The subcutaneous fat and fascia are bluntly dissected, which will minimize the potential to cut through blood vessels (which can bleed excessively) imbedded in the fat. Blunt dissection is continued through the paired strap muscles to isolate the trachea. A transverse incision, which should not exceed 50% of the circumference of the trachea, is made between the tracheal rings. Stay sutures are placed in the trachea cranial and caudal to the tracheostomy site. An endotracheal tube is inserted into the trachea and secured in place.

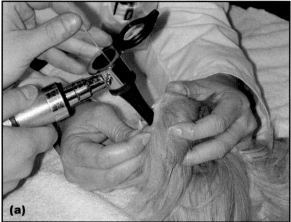

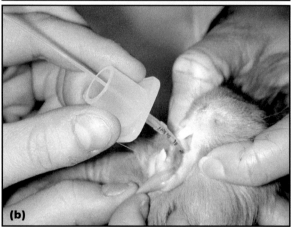

2.16 Guinea pigs have a palatal ostium that can easily be traumatized during intubation. To minimize trauma: **(a)** an otoscopic cone can enhance visualization of the larynx; **(b)** a stylet is then placed into the larynx, allowing the endotracheal tube to be manipulated gently past the palatal ostium.

IPPV: Intermittent positive pressure ventilation (IPPV) should be administered with 100% oxygen at a rate of 20–30 breaths per minute at 8–10 cmH$_2$O airway pressure if respiratory arrest is present. If the patient is not intubated, positive pressure ventilation via a tight-fitting mask can provide indirect ventilation, but this must be monitored carefully as aerophagia can occur and may lead to severe gastrointestinal dilatation and tympany. Nasal intubation is not generally practical in rodents, due to the small size of the nasal cavity.

Oxygen enrichment

If a rodent is showing signs of respiratory distress but does not require intubation, the patient should immediately be placed into a quiet oxygen-enriched environment (Figure 2.17) (see also Chapter 12). If a commercial oxygen cage is not available, one can be fashioned from an induction chamber, or a small pet carrier covered with a plastic bag, or, if the patient is small enough, the rodent can be placed inside a large anaesthetic facemask to provide an oxygen-enriched environment. The use of oxygen delivered via an anaesthetic mask over the nose or by nasal insufflation is feasible but can be very stressful for the rodent patient. The authors recommend the use of

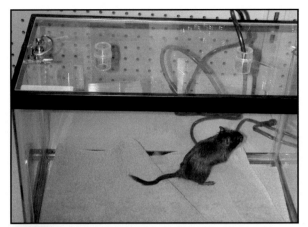

2.17 If a rodent is showing signs of respiratory distress but does not require intubation, the patient should immediately be placed in a quiet oxygen-enriched environment. If a commercial oxygen cage is not available, one can be fashioned from a small pet carrier covered with a plastic bag or, if the animal is small enough, the patient can be placed inside a large anaesthetic facemask to provide an oxygen-enriched environment.

sedation and oxygen delivery in a quiet environment to minimize stress if this is necessary. Humidification of oxygenated air by bubbling through an isotonic fluid solution is recommended, to assist with clearance of respiratory secretions and foreign material within the trachea and bronchi. Commercially manufactured intensive care units can provide oxygen, heat, and humidity.

Shock, cardiovascular monitoring and fluid therapy

Shock is defined as poor tissue perfusion from either low blood flow or unevenly distributed flow (Lichtenberger, 2004). This results in an inadequate delivery of oxygen to the tissues. This definition applies to all species of animals. Although there are many types of shock (e.g. cardiogenic, distributive or septic), this chapter will concentrate on the pathophysiological characteristics of hypovolaemic shock.

Shock pathophysiology

Hypovolaemic shock is caused by either an absolute or a relative inadequate blood volume. Absolute hypovolaemia occurs as a result of actual loss of blood by arterial bleeding, gastrointestinal ulcers or coagulopathies. In relative hypovolaemia, there is no direct blood loss (haemorrhage) from the intravascular space. Examples of relative hypovolaemia would include severe dehydration from gastrointestinal tract loss, significant loss of plasma (burns), or extensive loss of intravascular fluids into a third-body space such as the peritoneal cavity. Continued loss of blood volume results in hypovolaemic shock and hypotension. Fluid therapy is required to optimize patient outcome.

Cardiovascular evaluation

Electrocardiogram evaluation: The heart should be auscultated and the heart rate as well as any abnormal rhythm should be recorded using an electrocardiograph. This can be used to evaluate

cardiac rhythm, but because of the rapid heart rate of many small rodents the ECG complexes can be difficult to assess at standard speeds of 50 mm/s. A number of ECG devices are now available that can provide speeds of 100 and 200 mm/s that can allow for accurate evaluation of the small complexes. Atraumatic ECG leads or leads attached to hypodermic needles placed in the skin (Figure 2.18) are ideal for small rodents as they provide excellent conduction without the use of gels or alcohol (which can cool the body temperature of the patient). Alternatively, metal alligator clips attached to a hypodermic needle or to an alcohol-soaked cotton ball can be used. It is important not to saturate the patient with alcohol as this can cause rapid reduction in body temperature.

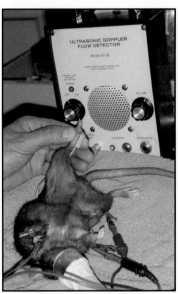

2.18 An electrocardiograph can be used to evaluate cardiac rhythm. Atraumatic alligator clips or clips attached to hypodermic needles placed in the skin can provide appropriate signal conduction while minimizing trauma.

Indirect blood pressure monitoring: Indirect blood pressure monitoring can be performed using a Doppler ultrasonic probe to detect the arterial flow, a pressure cuff to occlude arterial blood flow and a sphygmomanometer to measure pressures. An oscillometric device can be used that will measure pressures automatically by detecting the pressure changes in the cuff as it is deflated, but these devices can be unreliable in the small hypotensive or hypothermic patient.

The general rule for size of blood pressure cuffs is the same as for other mammals in that the size of the cuff should approximate 40% of the circumference of the limb on which it is used. Cuffs that are too large can give falsely decreased pressures. Small human infant, newborn or digital cuffs are available for the small rodent.

The cuff can be placed above the carpus or tarsus or the base of the tail. The Doppler ultrasonic probe (Figure 2.19) can then be placed distal to the cuff. Shaving of the areas beneath the probe is necessary. The pressures determined with use of a sphygmomanometer are thought to correlate with systolic pressures, though to the authors' knowledge no studies have correlated indirect Doppler blood pressures with direct blood pressures in rodents. The clinician should evaluate the patient carefully and

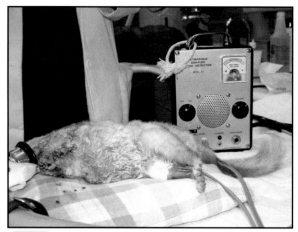

2.19 Pulse rate and subjective changes in pulse quality by evaluating loudness of signal can be assessed using a Doppler ultrasonic probe placed over an artery. Indirect blood pressure monitoring can be performed using a Doppler ultrasonic probe to detect the arterial flow, a pneumatic pressure cuff to occlude arterial blood flow and a sphygmomanometer to measure pressures.

respond to trends in the Doppler measurements rather than rely on the absolute number generated. In the authors' experience, normal blood pressure measurements obtained with Doppler flow detection in rodent patients range from 90 to 120 mmHg.

Fluid resuscitation plan

A fluid therapy plan involves the type, quantity and rate of fluid to be administered. Fluid therapy is used to correct life-threatening abnormalities in volume, electrolyte and acid–base status. The primary goal is to give the least amount of fluids possible to reach the desired endpoints of resuscitation. Clinical markers are the most frequently used endpoints of resuscitation. The markers used are those parts of the initial survey that suggest a patient is in shock and include the following: altered mentation; prolonged capillary refill time; weak and thready pulse/hypotension; tachycardia/bradycardia; tachypnoea; cold extremities; weakness; reduced urine output; and pale mucous membranes.

The fluid therapy plan typically has a resuscitation phase (correction of perfusion deficits), a rehydration phase (correction of interstitial deficits) and a maintenance phase. Maintenance requirements are higher in rodents, due to their high metabolic rate, and are typically double those used in cats and dogs.

Types of fluids: Individual characteristics of fluids influence the type and volume of fluid administered. Isotonic crystalloid solutions are commonly used together with colloids in the resuscitation phase. The four basic groups of fluids are crystalloids, synthetic colloids, haemoglobin-based oxygen carriers and blood products, which are commonly used in rodents for shock, rehydration and maintenance therapy (Lichtenberger, 2004). Oxyglobin® is a colloid, as is hetastarch, but the latter has the added advantage of carrying oxygen on the haemoglobin molecule.

Fluid therapy for rodents: In the authors' experience, rodents with hypovolaemia commonly present in the early decompensatory stage of shock, which is similar to cats and small mammals. The earlier compensatory stages of shock commonly seen in the dog and bird are not seen in the rodent (or cat or small mammal) patient. Signs of early decompensatory shock in the rodent (as in the cat and small mammals) are bradycardia, hypothermia and hypotension. When intravascular volume deficits result in poor perfusion, it has been recommended in the past that crystalloids be administered quickly in volumes equivalent to the animal's blood volume. However, resuscitation with crystalloids alone can result in significant pulmonary and pleural fluid accumulation. The resultant hypoxaemia contributes to the shock pathophysiology. Rodents are difficult to resuscitate from hypotensive episodes and aggressive intravenous or intraosseous fluid therapy is recommended early.

In the rabbit, when baroreceptors have detected inadequate arterial stretch, it has been found that vagal fibres are stimulated simultaneously with sympathetic fibres (Lichtenberger, 2004). As a result, the heart rate may be normal or slow, instead of the typical tachycardia in the dog with a compensatory stage of shock. This baroreceptor response may be similar in rodents. In the authors' experience, normal rodents have heart rates between 180 and 350 beats per minute (bpm), systolic blood pressure between 90 and 120 mmHg, and body temperatures between 36 and 38.8°C (97–102°F) (see also Chapter 1). Most rodents presenting with hypovolaemic shock demonstrate heart rates less than 200 bpm, hypotension (systolic blood pressure less than 90 mmHg), and hypothermia (temperature <36°C), which are the classic decompensatory signs of shock. The bradycardia and low cardiac output contribute to hypothermia, and hypothermia accentuates the bradycardia. Because cardiac output is a function of contractility and rate, the compensatory response to shock normally seen in dogs and birds is most likely blunted in rodents, small mammals and cats (Rudloff and Kirby, 2001; Lichtenberger, 2004) and so the hyperdynamic signs of shock seen in the dog and birds are not typically seen in the rodent.

Resuscitation from hypovolaemic shock can be safely accomplished with a combination of crystalloids, colloids and rewarming procedures. In the hypovolaemic rodent, a bolus infusion of isotonic crystalloids is administered at 10–15 ml/kg. Intravenous or intraosseous administration of hetastarch (HES) is given at 5 ml/kg over 5–10 minutes. The blood pressure is checked; once it is above 40 mmHg systolic, only maintenance isotonic crystalloids are given, while the patient is aggressively warmed. The warming should be done within 1–2 hours with warm-water bottles, forced-air heating blankets and warming the intravenous fluids. Intravenous fluid warmers (or running the intravenous fluid line through a pan of hot water) facilitate core temperature warming. Once the rectal temperature approaches 36.6°C, it appears that the adrenergic receptors begin to respond to catecholamines and fluid therapy. Temperatures during this rewarming phase must be checked frequently in all rodents to prevent hyperthermia. Blood pressure is rechecked when the temperature is >36.6°C and isotonic crystalloid (10 ml/kg) with HES at 5 ml/kg increments can be repeated over 15 minutes until the systolic blood pressure rises above 90 mmHg. The rectal temperature must be maintained as needed by a warm incubator and warmed fluids. When the systolic blood pressure is >90 mmHg, the rehydration phase of fluid resuscitation begins. A constant-rate infusion (CRI) of HES at 0.8 ml/kg per hour is continued during the rehydration phase (e.g. perfusion deficits persist or hypoproteinaemic).

If endpoint parameters (normal blood pressure, heart rate, mucous membrane colour and CRT) are still not obtained, the animal is evaluated and treated for causes of non-responsive shock (excessive vasodilation or vasoconstriction, hypoglycaemia, electrolyte imbalances, acid–base disorder, cardiac dysfunction, hypoxaemia).

If cardiac function is normal, and glucose, acid–base and electrolyte abnormalities have been corrected, treatment for nonresponsive shock is continued. Oxyglobin® has not been approved for use in the cat, small mammal or rodent, but has been used successfully at the authors' hospital when given in small-volume (2 ml/kg) boluses over 10–15 minutes until normal heart rate and blood pressure (systolic blood pressure greater than 90 mmHg) are obtained. This is followed by a continuous-rate infusion of Oxyglobin® at 0.2–0.4 ml/kg/h. When Oxyglobin® is not available for treatment of refractory hypotension the authors have used 7.5% hypertonic saline at 2–3 ml/kg bolus with HES at 3 ml/kg bolus given slowly over 10–15 minutes. Vasopressors such as dopamine or noradrenaline can be used to treat refractory hypotension, but when using the above protocol the authors have never had to use these drugs in rodents.

Dehydration deficits are assessed when perfusion parameters are normal. Replacement of dehydration deficits is done with the use of isotonic crystalloids. This will be discussed in the rehydration section below.

To summarize the guidelines for fluid administration for hypovolaemia:

1. Establish intravenous or intraosseous catheterization.
2. Begin warming in case of hypovolaemia.
3. Measure indirect systolic blood pressure.
4. Administer warmed isotonic crystalloids at 10–15 ml/kg and hetastarch (6%) at 5 ml/kg over 5–10 minutes, until systolic Doppler blood pressure reads greater than 40 mmHg.
5. Continue external and core body temperature warming until rectal body temperature is greater than 36.6°C.
6. Administer bolus crystalloids (10–15 ml/kg) and colloids such as hetastarch (5 ml/kg), until systolic Doppler blood pressure reads greater than 90 mmHg.

Blood transfusions

Blood products are administered when albumin, antithrombin, coagulation factors, platelets or red blood cells are required. Most fluid-responsive shock patients will tolerate acute haemodilution to a haematocrit of 20%. Also, most animals can tolerate an acute blood loss of 10–15% of their blood volume without requiring a blood transfusion. Acute haemorrhage exceeding 20% of the blood volume often requires transfusion therapy in addition to initial fluid resuscitation (Lichtenberger, 2004). If promoting cardiac output is the first priority in the management of acute haemorrhage, blood is not the ideal resuscitation fluid for acute blood loss because blood products do not promote blood flow as well as the acellular fluids (e.g. hetastarch) do. Blood is rarely used for initial resuscitation unless the patient is exsanguinating or there is excessive loss of clotting factors secondary to rodenticide toxicity. The density of erythrocytes impedes the ability of blood products to promote blood flow (a viscosity effect).

As in other species, continued blood loss, non-regenerative anaemia with PCV 12–15% or below, and clotting disorders (such as rodenticide toxicosis) are indicators used to determine the potential need for a whole-blood transfusion. In animals with acute blood loss requiring transfusion therapy, fresh whole blood or packed red blood cells should be used in an attempt to stabilize the clinical signs of shock, maintain the haematocrit above 25% and sustain the clotting times within the normal range. Whole blood can be administered at 10–20 ml/kg intravenously or intraosseously.

The availability of blood products in sufficient quantities to meet the needs of exotic patients is often the limiting factor in survival.

Blood groups have not been identified in rodents. Information on blood transfusion medicine for rodents is lacking and the authors therefore recommend that a major cross-match be performed for all blood transfusions in rodents. A simplified cross-match can be performed in these small patients by mixing two drops of plasma of the recipient with one drop of whole blood from the donor on a slide at room temperature. The development of macroscopic agglutination within 1 minute would suggest incompatibility (Lichtenberger, 2004). This does not eliminate the occurrence of reactions, but it can minimize the other potential complications of agglutination. Homologous transfusions with species-specific blood is recommended.

To prevent hypothermia, blood should be warmed for at least 15 minutes before administration. Warming can be done in a warm-water bath (42°C). The blood-administration set must include a filter to remove most of the aggregated debris. The donor blood should be administered by slow bolus or by infusion with a syringe pump into a catheter placed in the jugular, saphenous or cephalic vein, or into an intraosseous catheter. Blood transfusions should be administered within 4 hours to prevent the growth of bacteria, according to standards set by the American Association of Blood Banks (Stark *et al.*, 1981). In cases of massive haemorrhage, blood can be given within minutes.

Glucocorticoids in shock

The use of glucocorticoids in the treatment of shock is controversial. These drugs have been extensively investigated in the shock syndrome. Although they have repeatedly shown promise in some experimental studies, they have not shown consistent efficacy in clinical shock syndromes. The side effects of immuno-suppression, increased risk of infection, hyperglycae-mia and gastric ulceration may outweigh their benefits. Use of corticosteroids in rodents with haemorrhage and hypovolaemia is not currently recommended.

Sodium bicarbonate in shock

The most important method of correction of severe metabolic acidosis is aimed at increasing the pH through increasing the extracellular fluid pH.

Crystalloid fluids containing lactate, acetate and gluconate (e.g. lactated Ringer's solution) are consid-ered an important means of increasing the alkalinity of the extracellular fluid. In most cases, the acidaemia is corrected with fluids used to correct the rodent's per-fusion and dehydration deficits. When faced with severe acidaemia resulting from lactic acidosis, and when aggressive measures to improve oxygen deliv-ery and reverse tissue hypoxia have already been initiated without improvement (i.e. optimal fluid resus-citation), sodium bicarbonate may be employed cau-tiously. Blood gas parameters should be monitored carefully if bicarbonate therapy is deemed necessary.

Fluids for rehydration

The percentage of dehydration can be subjectively estimated based upon body weight, mucous mem-brane dryness, decreased skin turgor, sunken eyes and altered mentation, but these parameters can also be affected by decreased body fat and increased age. Dehydration deficits >5% ideally require intravenous fluid replacement and a constant-rate infusion of a crystalloid fluid to support patients that are dehy-drated and have ongoing losses. Fluid requirements for dehydration are calculated as follows:

% dehydration × kg × 1000 ml/l = fluid deficit (l).

Dehydration requirements should be added to fluids provided for daily maintenance fluid require-ments and ongoing losses. Fifty to 75% of the calculated fluid deficit can be replaced in the first 24 hours. An objective way to assess whether the fluid volume is adequate is to evaluate body weight regularly throughout the day. Acute weight loss is commonly associated with fluid loss and can be used to determine the patient at risk of becoming further dehydrated. Maintenance fluids are added to the dehydration deficit requirements. The maintenance requirements for the rodent are 3–4 ml/kg per hour for most species (Lichtenberger, 2004).

All fluids should be warmed to the body temperature of the patient, regardless of the route of administration. Fluids can be warmed to 38–39°C without affecting their composition (Harkness, 1994). Fluid line warmers are available commercially; alternatively, the fluid line may be passed though a bowl of warm water to maintain the fluid temperature. The protocol for fluid therapy should be based upon PCV, total protein, urine output and ideally blood pressure and acid–base status. While urinary catheterization of rodents can be used to determine urinary output objectively, this is not usually practical in small rodents. Alternatively,

urine output can be subjectively evaluated by weighing dry bedding before placing it into the rodent's cage and then weighing the bedding after removal. Hospital pads are often pre-weighed and placed into the cage for urine collection.

Oral fluids should only be given if the rodent is stable, less than 5% dehydrated and standing. Care must be taken when administering oral fluids to ensure that the gastrointestinal tract is functioning properly and that fluid is not aspirated. Subcutaneous fluids are only used when venous access cannot be obtained.

An ideal site for administration of subcutaneous fluids in most rodents is the subcutaneous space over the neck or the back. Intraperitoneal fluids can be given in the lower left quadrant, with the head of the patient lower than the abdomen to allow the viscera to slide forward (Figure 2.20).

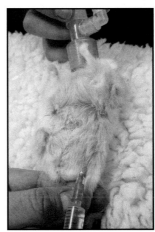

2.20 Administration of intraperitoneal fluids in a rodent. The needle is inserted in the left lower quadrant with the head of the patient lower than the abdomen to allow the viscera to slide forward. Sterile technique is recommended, to avoid peritonitis. (Courtesy of Emma Keeble.)

Dextrose solutions may be added to crystalloid solutions for the treatment of hypoglycaemia only when this has been documented by a blood glucose measurement. An initial bolus of 50% dextrose at 0.25 ml/kg can be given as a 1:1 dilution with saline intravenously. The parenteral use of dextrose should be conservative as it may induce compartmental shifts in electrolytes and water, which could ultimately lead to further hypovolaemia.

Nutritional support

As in any species of animal, the goal is to provide enteral nutrition as soon as possible to sick rodents. Anorexia for long periods of time allows breakdown in the tight junctions between the gastric and intestinal cells (Astiz, 2005). Bacterial overgrowth and trans-location occur early through these tight junctions. This will lead to sepsis. Nutritional support is a vital compo-nent of treatment and is crucial to resolve or prevent gastric stasis and ileus in rodents. Replacement fluid therapy must also play a role in nutritional support as the gastrointestinal tract must be hydrated to facilitate motility and function during nutritional therapy.

In general, sick rodents tolerate hand-feeding via syringe extremely well. Uncommonly a nasogastric tube is required for enteral nutrition. Nasogastric tube placement is more difficult in the small rodent patient and there is no nutritionally complete fibre diet that will pass through these small lumen tubes. Attempts can be made to mix these formulations with other formulas, such as isotonic feeding formulas or baby food, to reduce the particle size, but the nutritional value of the food will be reduced as well. Patience is often required to feed small boluses of food with a 1 mm syringe directed into the interdental space, with breaks given to the patient as needed. In the authors' experience, rodent patients respond positively with minimal stress to this type of enteral support.

Currently a Timothy hay-based critical care feeding formula for herbivores is commercially available (Oxbow Critical Care, Oxbow Pet Products, Murdock, Nebraska); when mixed with water it provides a homogenous and palatable high-fibre mixture for anorectic herbivores. The amount fed and frequency of feeding should be according to the manufacturer's guidelines. Although blending pellets and greens with water is an alternative to the commercial diet, it is more time consuming and generally results in a less homogenous mixture.

Total parenteral nutrition or partial enteral nutrition is not commonly used in small exotic animal medicine, due to catheter-related complications, patient intolerance and the lack of appropriate formulations for herbivorous species.

It should be remembered that guinea pigs require an exogenous source of vitamin C and in some cases will present on emergency with clinical signs of hypovitaminosis C (scurvy) such as hindlimb weakness or lameness, anorexia and diarrhoea (O'Rourke, 2004). Vitamin C supplementation should be provided routinely to the hospitalized critically ill guinea pig at 50–100 mg/kg per day (Harkness, 1994).

Analgesia

Analgesia is recommended for all patients that are critically ill (see Chapter 6 for anaesthesia and analgesia).

Environmental support

Rodents should always be hospitalized away from noise and any predator species (e.g. ferrets, cats) to minimize stress. Noise should also be minimized during the physical examination and diagnostic procedures. Appropriate diets, suitable bedding and hide areas should be provided based upon the needs of the individual species. Dust baths should be provided for chinchillas at least every 72 hours during hospitalization.

Thermal support is often necessary for the emergency rodent patient. Normal body temperatures of rodents vary and can be as low as 35.5°C (95.7°F) in prairie dogs (see Chapter 9). Caution should be exercised if providing thermal support because many of the small rodents are susceptible to heat stress; chinchillas are particularly prone at temperatures above about 24°C (75°F). An obtunded patient may be unable to move away from a heat source when becoming overheated. Careful monitoring is essential when supplemental heat is being provided and body temperature should be taken frequently. The exception to this rule is head trauma, where heat support may cause vasodilation of intracranial vessels and exacerbate haemorrhage.

References and further reading

Adams R (2002) Techniques of experimentation. In: *Laboratory Animal Medicine, 2nd edn*, ed. J Fox *et al.*, pp. 1005–1045. Elsevier, San Diego

American Heart Association (2005) Guidelines for Cardiopulmonary Resuscitation and Emergency Cardiovascular Care. *Circulation* **112**, IV-1–IV-5

Antinoff N (1998) Small mammal critical care. *Veterinary Clinics of North America: Exotic Animal Practice* **1**, 153–175

Astiz ME (2005) Pathophysiology and classification of shock states. In: *Textbook of Critical Care*, ed. MP Fink *et al.*, pp. 897–997. Elsevier/Saunders, Philadelphia

Bihun C and Bauck L (2004) Basic anatomy, physiology, husbandry, and clinical techniques. In: *Ferrets, Rabbits, and Rodents: Clinical Medicine and Surgery, 2nd edn*, ed. K Quesenberry and J Carpenter, pp. 286–298. WB Saunders, St Louis

Blouin A and Cormier Y (1987) Endotracheal intubation in guinea pigs by direct laryngoscopy. *Laboratory Animal Science* **37**, 244–245

Bober R (1988) Technical review: drawing blood from the tail artery of a rat. *Laboratory Animals* **17**, 33–34

Cambron H, Latulippe JF, Nguyen T *et al.* (1995) Orotracheal intubation of rats by transillumination. *Laboratory Animal Science* **45**, 303–304

Costello M (2004) Principles of cardiopulmonary cerebral resuscitation in special species. *Seminars in Avian and Exotic Pet Medicine* **13**, 132–141

Daviau J (1999) Clinical evaluation of rodents. *Veterinary Clinics of North America: Exotic Animal Practice* **2**, 429–445

Donnelly T (2004a) Disease problems of chinchillas. In: *Ferrets, Rabbits, and Rodents: Clinical Medicine and Surgery*, ed. K Quesenberry and J Carpenter, pp. 255–265. WB Saunders, St Louis

Donnelly T (2004b) Disease problems of small rodents. In: *Ferrets, Rabbits, and Rodents: Clinical Medicine and Surgery*, ed. K Quesenberry and J Carpenter, pp. 299–315. WB Saunders, St Louis

Fallon M (1996) Rats and mice. In: *Handbook of Rodent and Rabbit Medicine*, ed. K Laber-Laird *et al.*, pp. 1–38. BPC Wheatons, Exeter

Harkness J (1994) Small rodents. *Veterinary Clinics of North America: Small Animal Practice* **24**, 89–102

Haskins S (1990) Fluid therapy. In: *Handbook of Veterinary Procedures and Emergency Treatment*, ed. R Kirk *et al.*, pp. 574–600. WB Saunders, Philadelphia

Heard D (2004) Anesthesia, analgesia, and sedation of small mammals. In: *Ferrets, Rabbits, and Rodents: Clinical Medicine and Surgery*, ed. K Quesenberry and J Carpenter, pp. 356–369. WB Saunders, St Louis

Hem A, Smith A and Solberg P (1998) Saphenous vein puncture for blood sampling of the mouse, rat, hamster, gerbil, guinea pig, ferret, and mink. *Laboratory Animals* **32**, 364–368

Kujime K and Natelson B (1981) A method for endotracheal intubation of guinea pigs (*Cavis porcellus*). *Laboratory Animal Science* **31**, 715–716

Laber-Laird K (1996) Gerbils. In: *Handbook of Rodent and Rabbit Medicine*, ed. K Laber-Laird *et al.*, pp. 39–58. BPC Wheatons, Exeter

Lichtenberger M (2004) Principles of shock and fluid therapy in special species. *Seminars in Avian and Exotic Pet Medicine* **13**, 142–153

O'Rourke D (2004) Disease problems of guinea pigs. In: *Ferrets, Rabbits, and Rodents: Clinical Medicine and Surgery*, ed. K Quesenberry and J Carpenter, pp. 245–254. WB Saunders, St Louis

Otto C and Crowe D (1992) Intraosseous resuscitation techniques and applications. In: *Current Veterinary Therapy XI: Small Animal Practice*, ed. R Kirk and J Bonagura, pp. 107–112. WB Saunders, Philadelphia

Quesenberry K, Donnelly T and Hillyer E (2004) Biology, husbandry, and clinical techniques of guinea pigs and chinchillas. In: *Ferrets, Rabbits, and Rodents: Clinical Medicine and Surgery, 2nd edn*, ed. K Quesenberry and J Carpenter, pp. 232–244. WB Saunders, St Louis

Reuter R (1987) Venipuncture in the guinea pig. *Laboratory Animal Science* **37**, 245–246

Rudloff E and Kirby R (2001) Colloid and crystalloid resuscitation. *Veterinary Clinics of North America Small Animal Practice: Critical Care* **31**(6), 1207–1229

Stark R, Nahrwold M and Cohen P (1981) Blind oral tracheal intubation of rats. *Journal of Applied Physiology* **51**, 1355–1356

Strake J, Davis L, LaRegina M *et al.* (1996) Chinchillas. In: *Handbook of Rodent and Rabbit Medicine*, ed. K Laber-Laird *et al.*, pp. 151–181. Elsevier, Oxford

Timm KI, Jahn SE and Sedgwick CJ (1987) The palatal ostium of the guinea pig. *Laboratory Animal Science* **37**, 801–802

Tran D and Lawson D (1986) Endotracheal intubation and manual ventilation of the rat. *Laboratory Animal Science* **36**, 540–541

Yasaki S and Dyck P (1991) A simple method for rat endotracheal intubation. *Laboratory Animal Science* **35**, 596–599

3

Rodents: diagnostic imaging

Allison Zwingenberger and Sam Silverman

Introduction

Diagnostic imaging of rodents presents several technical challenges related to their small body size, rapid respiratory rate, reluctance to accept mechanical restraint and unusual conformation. None of these factors is insurmountable but they do necessitate modification of the radiographic imaging techniques and principles of interpretation used for dogs and cats.

Radiographic technique and instrumentation

Normal radiographic anatomy and examples of radiographic special procedures have been recently published for rodents (Silverman and Tell, 2005) and an excellent gross anatomical reference is also available (Popesko *et al.*, 1992). Normal radiographic anatomy and examples of the radiographic features of common disease entities in these species are also documented (Rubel *et al.*, 1991).

Anaesthesia and sedation

General anaesthesia or sedation is highly recommended since many of these patients are uncooperative and have rapid respiratory rates (Figure 3.1). Short-acting inhalation anaesthesia is preferred by the authors. Although proper patient positioning is facilitated by anaesthesia or sedation, this can have deleterious effects and often results in misdiagnosis if certain factors are not considered during radiographic interpretation. For example, the respiratory tidal volume is commonly decreased by sedation and anaesthesia. This results in increased

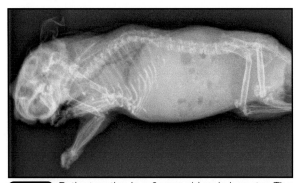

3.1 Patient motion in a 2-year-old male hamster. The skull and forelimbs in this lateral radiograph are blurred from patient motion during the exposure.

pulmonary radiographic opacity, decreased distinctness of bronchovascular markings and an artefactual increase in the cardiothoracic ratio (cardiac width/thoracic width) on the frontal (dorsoventral or ventrodorsal) projections. Erroneous diagnoses of pulmonary disease, i.e. pneumonia, oedema or haemorrhage, is possible if this factor is not considered.

Positioning

Principles used for patient positioning are identical to those used for cats and dogs. Dorsoventral (DV) radiographs are preferred to ventrodorsal (VD) radiographs for abdomen and thoracic studies in the smaller rodents since it is easier to obtain symmetrical positioning. Paper bandage tape is recommended for restraining the patient in position for radiography.

Instrumentation

The small patient size imposes unique restrictions on radiographic technique formulation. High-detail film screen systems are recommended if digital radiography is not used. The challenge involves providing sufficient mAs to produce radiographic density while maintaining a low kVp (40–60 kVp). Selection of mA and exposure times often requires compromise. Exposure times must be minimized (0.017 seconds or shorter) to counteract the effects of patient motion, including respiration. The smaller focal spot should be selected if it allows short exposure time and sufficient mA. The smaller focal spot usually limits mA selection to the lower settings. If this results in exposure times greater than 0.017 seconds, the larger focal spot should be used. The low kVp and mAs radiographic technique may result in a grey appearance to the background and poor image contrast. Most radiographic units will not allow for the relatively minor adjustments of mAs required to optimize exposure factors without adversely affecting exposure time or kVp settings. This can be circumvented by decreasing the focal film distance (FFD) slightly to increase effective mAs, and therefore image density. A reduction of the FFD from the standard 100 cm to 60–80 cm will allow use of the short exposure times while increasing image density (radiopacity). Excessive reduction of the FFD, however, will produce geometric image distortion. Alterations in line voltage or X-ray output due to a damaged anode may therefore be much more apparent than when using higher kVp and mAs. Poor processing technique can also be a significant cause of poor radiographic contrast.

Digital radiographic systems

Digital radiographic systems (direct radiography and computed radiography) have distinct advantages over film screen systems in the ability to post process images for optimal detail and contrast, but they have the same limitations associated with induced artefacts, small patient size, and a lack of inherent tissue contrast. One major advantage is the ability to display good detail for bone and soft tissue at the same time. In conventional radiography, different kVp and mAs settings are necessary for optimal detail of different tissues.

Computed tomography and magnetic resonance imaging

Cross-sectional imaging methods do have applications in rodents but the small patient size is a limiting factor. Diagnostic studies can be obtained in the larger rodents such as rats and chinchillas, but mice are too small for adequate image detail in most clinical scanners. In a clinical CT scanner with 0.2–0.3 mm resolution, or a 1.5–3 T MRI scanner, the lower limit of body weight for diagnostic quality studies is about 200 g. Research scanners are available that provide much higher spatial resolution in CT, MRI and advanced imaging modalities such as positron emission tomography (PET) and single photon emission computed tomography (SPECT). These machines have limited availability in a clinical setting, and images take much longer to acquire.

Many clinical CT scanners are capable of helical scanning protocols. Since the table travels continuously while the scanner is acquiring images, the scan time is shortened compared with axial scanning protocols where the table halts for each 360 degree rotation of the X-ray tube. This is an advantage where patient motion is a factor (e.g. the thorax), but helical scanning can introduce image artefacts that are very prominent in small patients. The objective of the scan should be weighed against detail and motion artefacts during the planning phase.

Ultrasonography

Although limited by small patient size, ultrasonography is frequently utilized. High frequency (8 MHz or greater) micro convex transducers with a small footprint are essential. Sector angle should be decreased to obtain the maximum possible frame rate and therefore minimize the effects of patient motion.

Radiographic interpretation

Although the sizes of these species are often similar, there are considerable differences in internal anatomy. The shape of the thorax, the cardiothoracic ratio and the location of the heart can differ significantly. Obesity is common in captive raised rodents. Fat deposition will increase thoracic opacity and decrease visualization of the internal thoracic and abdominal organs (Figure 3.2). Abdominal variables include the size, shape and position of the internal organs, especially the stomach, and digestive tract physiology.

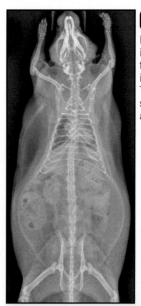
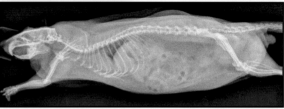

3.2 Obesity in a 2-year-old male rat: DV and lateral whole body views. There is increased opacity in the thorax due to fat accumulation in the cranial mediastinum. There are also fat deposits subcutaneously and within the abdomen.

Thorax

The principles of radiographic interpretation for larger mammals cannot be directly extrapolated to the smaller rodent species. Most imaging systems are not capable of accurately documenting thoracic structures and patterns in the smaller patients. The interstitial pattern is consequently the most commonly identified pulmonary pattern but this may be a summation of other patterns that result in pulmonary opacification, erroneously identified to be interstitial in origin. Even if the bronchovascular patterns are identified in smaller rodents, it is often difficult (or sometimes impossible) to identify the alveolar pattern, i.e. air bronchograms, and to quantify alterations in bronchial diameter or wall thickness accurately. The shape of the heart, its location in the thorax and internal fat may limit distinct cardiac visualization. This limits use of the cardiothoracic ratio as an indicator of heart size. There is also considerable species difference in the width and length of the cranial mediastinum. This affects visualization of the cranial thoracic border and the heart base vessels. It is difficult to document cranial mediastinal masses on radiographs.

The limitations imposed by the previously mentioned factors mandate the use of optimal radiographic technique and patient positioning. Asymmetrical positioning is a particularly treacherous factor. Patient rotation on the frontal projections (DV or VD) results in artefactual alterations in lung opacity. One hemithorax will be hyperlucent and the contralateral thorax will be hypolucent as compared with a well positioned study. Full extension of the neck on the lateral view will improve visualization of the cranial thoracic structures. Complete evaluation of the thorax requires a lateral and frontal projection.

The DV projection is preferred to the VD projection because it is easier to produce radiographs with proper positioning. The forelegs should be extended symmetrically cranially for both projections. Evaluation of the thoracic skeletal structures requires evaluation of both projections, due to the small size of the patient and relatively large amount of surrounding soft tissues. Figure 3.3 demonstrates how a clavicular fracture can be identified well on one projection.

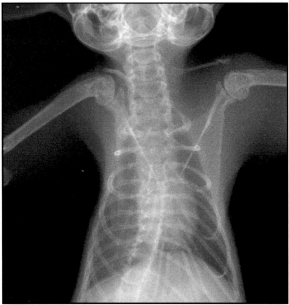

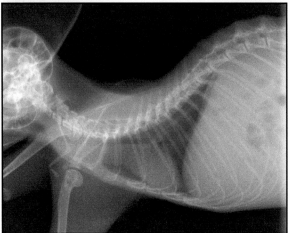

3.3 Fractured clavicle in an immature chinchilla: VD and lateral thoracic views. The left clavicle was acutely fractured and the fracture is best seen on the lateral view.

Pneumonia

Pneumonia is common in pet rodents and the principal radiographic change is increased pulmonary opacity (Figure 3.4). As explained above, this is most likely due to a mixed pattern, but image detail restrictions result in the diagnosis of interstitial lung disease. The diagnostic accuracy is increased if ancillary signs such as pleural thickening, free pleural fluid or air bronchograms are present. Enhanced visualization of interlobar fissure lines on the lateral view is a common finding in rodents with chronic pneumonia and it is often a permanent alteration. It is therefore difficult

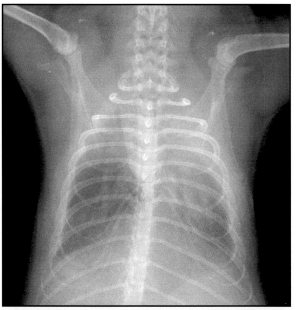

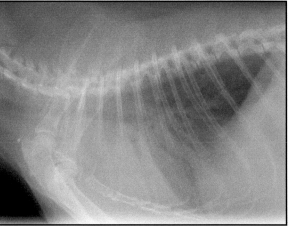

3.4 Pneumonia in a 1-year-old female guinea pig: VD and lateral thoracic views. Bacterial pneumonia produced severe consolidation of the right cranial and middle lung lobes and there is compensatory hyperinflation of the left lung. Therapy was partially successful and the changes persisted for over one year, until the patient was eventually euthanased.

to differentiate between chronic active pneumonia and chronic fibrotic changes solely on radiographs. Variations in pulmonary inflation at the time of radiographic exposure can be significant. Expiratory radiographs can simulate the appearance of atelectasis and consolidation.

It is important to recognize differences in radiographic technique when deciding on the significance of interval changes. In the smaller rodents it is impractical to identify 'complete' resolution of previously documented changes attributed to pneumonia. Small foci of consolidation may not be seen and persistent consolidation or pleural thickening may not be indicative of active infection. An additional factor in anaesthetized patients is that subtle increases in pulmonary radiopacity may be minimized or completely obliterated by positive pressure ventilation. Atelectasis and air bronchograms can be undetected in patients who are positively ventilated.

Thoracic neoplasia

Thoracic neoplasia in rodents is most often multifocal and associated with free pleural fluid. It is difficult to distinguish chronic fibrotic changes secondary to pneumonia from neoplasia, but as a general rule the more distinct the nodularity the more likely it is to be neoplastic. Progression of radiographic findings is helpful, but interpretation is often difficult if there is free pleural fluid present.

Cranial mediastinal masses in rodents, especially those that are obese, are often difficult to diagnose radiographically. They have a radiographic appearance similar to that described in dogs and cats, causing caudal displacement of the cardiac silhouette with a relatively midline distribution (Figure 3.5).

Ultrasonography is essential in formulating a differential diagnosis of thoracic disease when pleural fluid is present. It will allow for differentiation of mass lesions and free fluid. Large amounts of intrathoracic fat can simulate the appearance of free pleural fluid. Ultrasonography is also essential to rule out cranial thoracic masses and can be used to guide needle aspiration for cytology.

Cardiac disease

Cardiac disease is not unusual in rodents, especially guinea pigs. Hypertrophic and dilated cardiomyopathies are more common than valvular heart disease. An ancillary sign of heart failure commonly seen in guinea pigs is sternal and cervical subcutaneous oedema ('brisket disease'). This may further increase radiographic opacity of the cranial thorax. Oedema is most commonly identified in guinea pigs (Figure 3.6). Heart disease is usually very severe at the time of initial presentation and so the radiographic signs include enlargement of the cardiac silhouette, pulmonary oedema and pleural fluid. Radiographs do

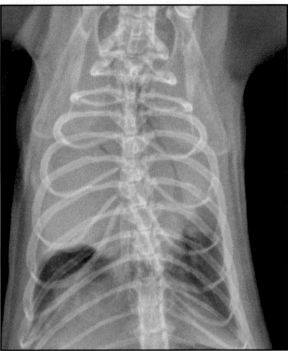

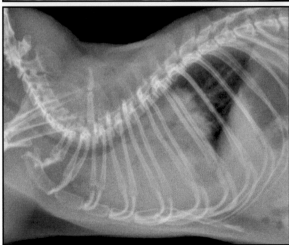

3.5 Mediastinal lymphoma in a 1½-year-old male neutered rat. DV and lateral thoracic radiographs show a large mediastinal mass that is displacing the cardiac silhouette caudally and the trachea to the left. This mass was diagnosed as a T-cell lymphoma by ultrasound-guided fine-needle aspirate.

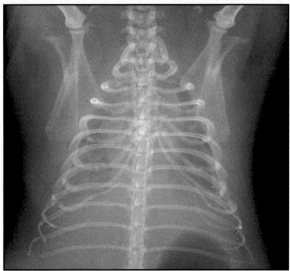

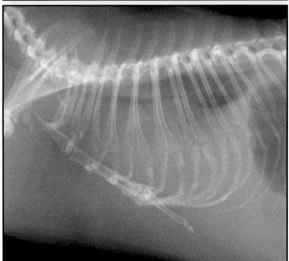

3.6 Dilated cardiomyopathy in a 2½-year-old male guinea pig: VD and lateral thoracic views. Dilated cardiomyopathy was diagnosed on an echocardiogram. The enlargement of the cervical and sternal soft tissues is due to oedema. The cardiac silhouette is best evaluated on the ventrodorsal radiograph.

demonstrate an enlarged cardiac silhouette, but ultrasound is required for a definitive diagnosis. In contrast to dogs and cats, the DV view may be superior to the lateral view for evaluation of heart size.

Echocardiographic techniques in rodents are similar to those described in dogs (Thomas *et al.*, 1993), with the subcostal window being commonly used. The transducer is placed just caudal to the sternum and angulated through the liver into the heart. This does limit short axis measurement of cardiac parameters, but the subcostal window provides excellent qualitative information about cardiac chamber size and contractility.

Abdomen

Radiographic evaluation of the abdomen in rodent species also suffers from the limitations of small patient size and patient motion. Digestive tract contents often preclude full visualization of abdominal organs (Figure 3.7). It is rare to differentiate distinctly the entire demarcation between the liver and the stomach on the lateral projection, but an indirect evaluation of liver size and shape can be made by identifying the gastric gas (Figure 3.8). When the kidneys are visualized, their entire outline is usually not seen, or they are superimposed on other organs (Figure 3.9). In guinea pigs it is somewhat more difficult to identify right- and left-sided hepatomegaly using the gastric gas pattern because of the rounded shape of the stomach. In other species caudal displacement of the stomach is characteristic of hepatomegaly.

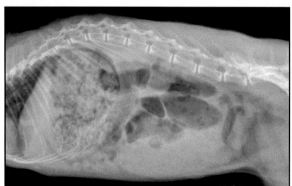

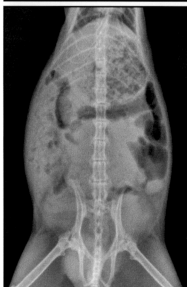

3.7
Normal abdomen in a 4-year-old male chinchilla: lateral and VD views. The full stomach and caecum obscure the rest of the abdominal organs.

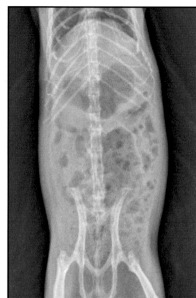

3.8
Normal abdomen in a 4-year-old male guinea pig: VD and lateral views. The liver occupies the space between the stomach and the diaphragm, but the borders are not visible.

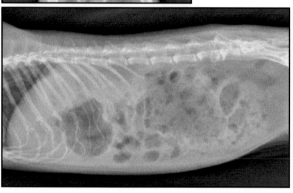

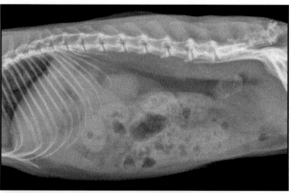

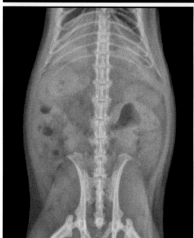

3.9
Normal abdomen in a 1-year-old male rat: lateral and VD views. The kidneys are superimposed on portions of the gastrointestinal tract.

Abdominal ultrasonography utilizes similar principles of interpretation as for dogs and cats, but the differences in organ anatomy and digestive tract gas patterns must be recognized. Small organ size and the renal anatomy decrease the sensitivity of ultrasonography for diagnosis of renal parenchyma and collecting system pathology.

Calculi

Urinary tract calculi and calcification can be identified with survey radiographs, but anatomical variation in these species, including the size and shape of the os penis (especially in guinea pigs), must be considered prior to diagnosis. Rodents can harbour distinct calculi as well as large amounts of amorphous debris and sand in the urinary bladder. The calculi are often very small but are visible on radiographs. Vaginal calculi can also be present in rodents, especially guinea pigs (Figure 3.10). Radiography is helpful in documenting the location and number of the calculi as well as their spontaneous passage (Figure 3.11).

Gastric tympany

Gastric tympany is much more common than gastric torsion in rodents. It can produce severe respiratory and cardiovascular compromise. Radiographs are important to document the response to treatment and secondary cardiopulmonary complications. It is

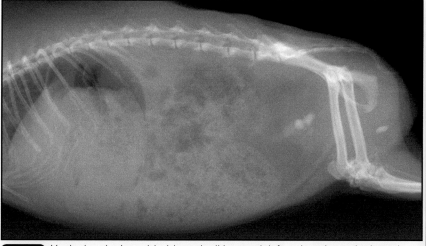
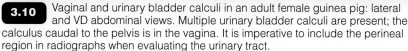
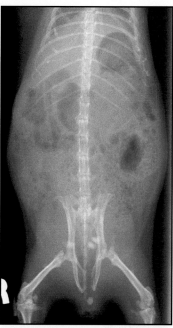

3.10 Vaginal and urinary bladder calculi in an adult female guinea pig: lateral and VD abdominal views. Multiple urinary bladder calculi are present; the calculus caudal to the pelvis is in the vagina. It is imperative to include the perineal region in radiographs when evaluating the urinary tract.

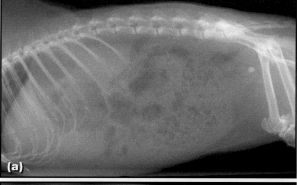
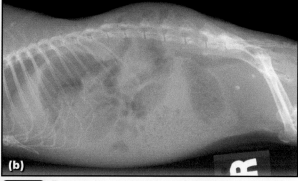
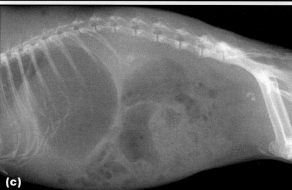

(a)

(b)

(c)

3.11 Progressive development of urinary calculi in an adult male guinea pig. Three lateral views demonstrate: **(a)** a single cystic calculus on admission; **(b)** two calculi present 3 months later; and **(c)** 8 months later there are renal and ureteral calculi, but the urinary bladder calculi previously seen had been passed spontaneously.

sometimes difficult to differentiate primary gastric tympany from ileus associated with systemic disease, and aerophagia-induced tympany. Accurate identification and quantification of the severity of enteritis are impractical.

Obstructive bowel disease

Radiographic signs used to diagnose obstructive bowel disease in rodents are similar to those described in dogs and cats, but there are variations in intestinal length and caecal development (Silverman and Tell, 2005). Radiolucent gastric and high small intestinal foreign bodies can produce obstruction with minimal distortion of the digestive tract gas pattern.

Reproductive tract

Survey radiographs are recommended for verification of pregnancy, identification of the number of fetuses and evaluation of fetal viability. They are recommended in all cases of dystocia (Figure 3.12). Ultrasonography is more sensitive than radiology for identifying fetal demise, though intrauterine gas and collapse of the skeleton are definitive radiographic signs (Figure 3.13).

Female reproductive tract disorders, including cystic ovaries and pyometra, do occur (see Chapter 13) and may be diagnosed with imaging techniques. The mass effects produced by the enlargement of the female organs are often identified as poorly marginated mass effects. Ultrasonography is required for a more definitive diagnosis than can be obtained with radiography alone. Figure 3.14 demonstrates a large ovarian cyst in a guinea pig, which was definitively identified and drained percutaneously under ultrasound guidance. The origin of the mass effect could not be determined radiographically.

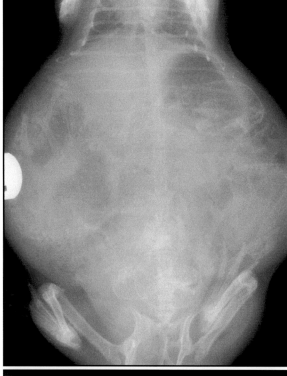

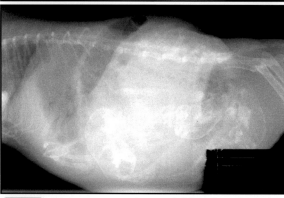

3.12 Triple pregnancy in an adult female guinea pig: VD and lateral abdominal views. The patient was presented for dystocia. The large size of the fetuses indicated that a Caesarean operation was required. Three viable fetuses were delivered.

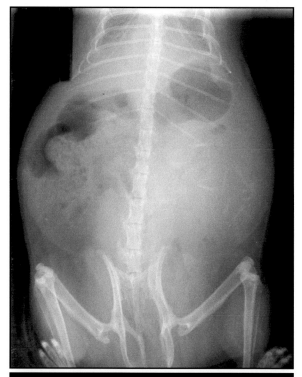

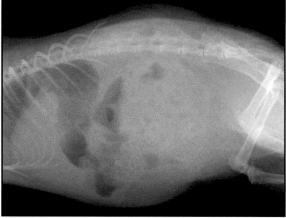

3.13 Fetal demise in an adult female guinea pig: VD and lateral abdominal views. The partially ossified and distorted fetus is not viable.

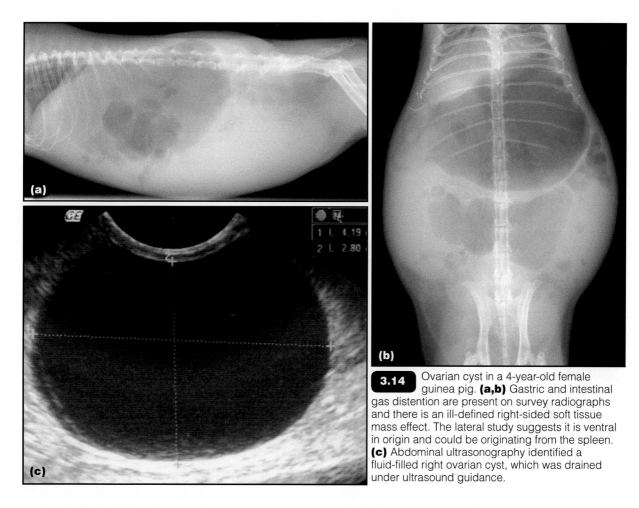

3.14 Ovarian cyst in a 4-year-old female guinea pig. **(a,b)** Gastric and intestinal gas distention are present on survey radiographs and there is an ill-defined right-sided soft tissue mass effect. The lateral study suggests it is ventral in origin and could be originating from the spleen. **(c)** Abdominal ultrasonography identified a fluid-filled right ovarian cyst, which was drained under ultrasound guidance.

Musculoskeletal radiology

Skeletal interpretation of rodent radiographs is very similar to interpretation of canine and feline radiographs except for the small patient size. This may limit identification of minor changes in bone opacity. Low kVp techniques (40–50 kVp) are recommended for extremity studies. Digital magnification and electronic manipulation of contrast and brightness can increase the accuracy of diagnosis. Traumatic fractures are common injuries in rodents (Figure 3.15).

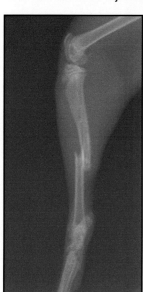

3.15 Acute fracture in a 17-week-old female chinchilla. There is a comminuted fracture of the tibia with cranial displacement. Small patient size requires low kVp technique for optimal evaluation. The small calcific opacities superimposed on the stifles are normal. Their origin has not been documented.

Dental disease

Radiography is essential for evaluation of dental disease. Lateral skull radiographs should be made with the mouth slightly open, to minimize dental superimposition. Additional views can include dorsoventral and oblique projections, as well as a rostrocaudal projection to examine the curvature of the cheek teeth and angle of the occlusal table (Figure 3.16). Dental film, or non-screen film, gives excellent spatial resolution and ability to detect very small dental lesions. The limiting factor is the ability to place the film within the oral cavity. Axial CT and three-dimensional reconstruction CT are also helpful for documentation of dental disease and therapy planning.

The crown length, root length, alignment of occlusal surfaces and incisors, as well as curvature of the incisors, should be evaluated. The roots of the incisors and cheek teeth should not distort the mandibular cortex. Common abnormalities include overgrowth, malocclusion (Figure 3.17), enamel points, trauma, caries and periodontal disease. (See also Chapter 8.)

Otitis media

Radiography is often the primary method of diagnosis of otitis media. Thickening of the os bullae and opacification of the tympanic cavities can often be identified on survey radiographs, but CT studies are required for full evaluation (Figure 3.18). The changes are usually asymptomatic and present in middle-aged and older patients.

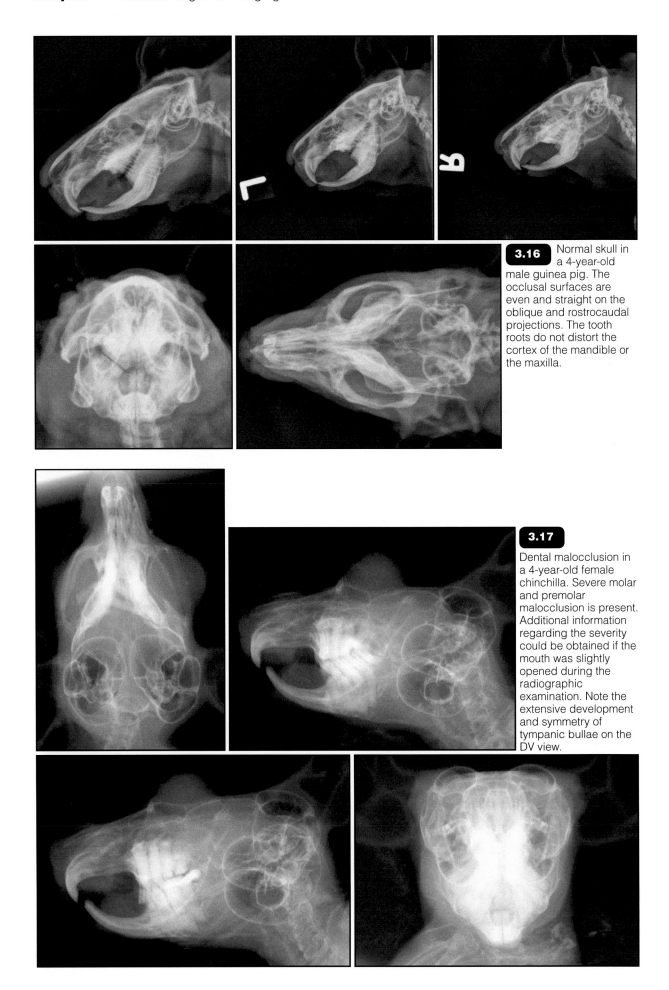

3.16 Normal skull in a 4-year-old male guinea pig. The occlusal surfaces are even and straight on the oblique and rostrocaudal projections. The tooth roots do not distort the cortex of the mandible or the maxilla.

3.17 Dental malocclusion in a 4-year-old female chinchilla. Severe molar and premolar malocclusion is present. Additional information regarding the severity could be obtained if the mouth was slightly opened during the radiographic examination. Note the extensive development and symmetry of tympanic bullae on the DV view.

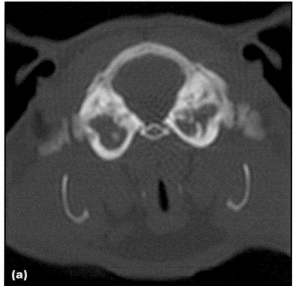

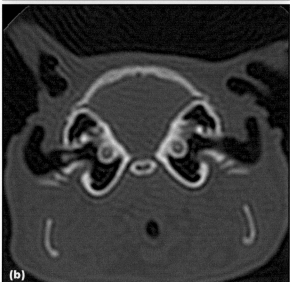

3.18 Otitis media in a 1-year-old male guinea pig. On these 1 mm CT images viewed with bone window and edge enhancement: **(a)** both tympanic bullae are thickened and filled with soft tissue and mineral attenuating material; the ear canals are also mineralized. Compare these to the normal bullae **(b)**.

Bone disease

Mineralization of the intracapsular and extracapsular tissues of the stifle is commonly seen in rodents. Dystrophic soft tissue calcification and osteophyte/

syndesmophyte formation are common, but usually asymptomatic in the authors' experience (see Figure 3.15).

Spondylosis is commonly identified in the spine of middle-aged and older rodents. It is rare to see signs of infection, e.g. vertebral end-plate lysis. The flaccid nature of the abdominal wall allows the intestines to be superimposed on the lateral view of the spine. The lucencies associated with the intestinal gas pattern can be misinterpreted as osteolytic spinal disease (Figure 3.19).

Bone tumours are seen in rodents and have similar characteristics to those seen in dogs and cats. The periosteal new bone production in osteosarcomas is often very intense.

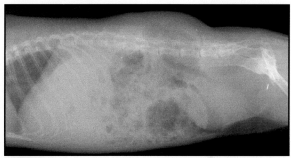

3.19 Increased intestinal gas in an adult female guinea pig: lateral abdominal view. Intestinal gas is superimposed on the spine and can simulate lytic spinal lesions. The left femur was previously amputated because of trauma.

References and further reading

Crossley DA (2000) Rodent and rabbit radiology. In: *An Atlas of Veterinary Dental Radiology*, ed. DH Deforge and BH Colmery. Iowa State University Press, Ames

Legendre LF (2003) Oral disorders of exotic rodents. *Veterinary Clinics of North America: Exotic Animal Practice* **6**, 601–628

Morgan J (1993) *Techniques of Veterinary Radiography*. Iowa State University Press, Ames

Popesko P, Rajitova V and Horak J (1992) *A Color Atlas of Anatomy of Small Laboratory Animals I and II*. WB Saunders, St Louis

Rubel GE, Isenbugel E and Wolvekamp P (1991) *Atlas of Diagnostic Radiology of Exotic Pets*. WB Saunders, Philadelphia

Silverman S and Tell L (2005) *Radiology of Rodents, Rabbits, and Ferrets*. Elsevier Saunders, St Louis

Thomas WP, Gaber CE, Jacobs GJ *et al.* (1993) Recommendations for standards in transthoracic two-dimensional echocardiography in the dog and cat. Echocardiography Committee of the Specialty of Cardiology, American College of Veterinary Internal Medicine. *Journal of Veterinary Internal Medicine* **7**, 247–252

Wiggs RB and Lobprise HB (1990) Dental diseases in rodents. *Journal of Veterinary Dentistry* **7**, 6–8

4

Rodents: clinical pathology

Petra Wesche

Blood sampling

The rodent species discussed here have a similar vascular configuration. Blood collection should be swift and preferably without sedation to minimize artefacts, though in many cases it may be necessary to anaesthetize the animal or use small restraint devices such as plastic syringe cases or small boxes.

Ideally the animals should have been fasted for a few hours. However, this is often not possible and is contraindicated in sick animals.

The total blood volume in normal healthy animals is approximately 7% of the body weight and 10% of this can safely be withdrawn for examination. Adjustments have to be made for anaemic or otherwise compromised animals and also for repeated withdrawals within short periods of time.

The jugular vein is the most accessible vessel for withdrawing larger blood samples but can be difficult to access in many species, whereas peripheral veins can be used for smaller samples. The cranial vena cava is a good alternative but requires more experience (see Chapter 2). Where blood is withdrawn from the tail veins it is advisable to warm the tail in warm water first for vasodilatation and easier access.

An insulin syringe with a small 23–25 gauge needle can be used successfully to obtain the blood sample, as large syringes and needles cause the vein to collapse. Very small vessels can be easily cannulated with a small needle and the blood collected directly in the appropriate sampling container or microhaematocrit tube (see Chapter 2). Cardiocentesis should only take place under anaesthesia and for terminal procedures.

A fresh blood smear should always be made at the time of venipuncture. This will enable the haematologist to estimate at least the white blood cell count, perform a differential count and make comments on the morphology of individual cell populations and differentiate pathology from transport artefacts. It is also the method of choice in many cases where only a very small sample can be obtained. Here it is often recommended that biochemistry from the blood sample should be requested and that the blood smear should be used for haematology.

Suitable anticoagulants for haematology are EDTA or heparin, but the latter occasionally causes clumping of leucocytes. Samples for biochemistry should be collected in heparin or plain tubes and ideally spun immediately after collection. The serum should then be separated into a tube without further additives and labelled correctly. Unsuitable or excessive quantities of anticoagulants can cause various haematological and biochemical artefacts and invalidate results.

Depending on the collection site, sample results can vary. Peripheral samples or lymph dilution will cause variations and best practice is to make the pathology laboratories aware of the sampling site.

Guinea pigs have a prolonged prothrombin time (Sisk, 1976), which makes clotting of samples less of an issue. There is no stress leucogram in this species.

Reference ranges for coagulation tests are given in Figure 4.1.

Parameter	Mice	Rats	Hamsters	Guinea pigs
Prothrombin time (PT) (seconds)	7–19	8–14	9.9 ± 1.2 ♂ 9.3 ± 1.8 ♀	26 ± 2.5
Activated prothrombin time (APTT) (seconds)				28.7 ± 3.8

4.1 Coagulation values in adult rodent species.

Haematology and biochemistry

Values for haematology and biochemistry have often been derived from laboratory animals and should be used as a guide only. In general, values vary according to individual physiology, sampling technique, strains and breeds and laboratory procedures. Most laboratories will have established their own reference ranges for many species. Wherever possible a reliable laboratory with known expertise in exotic animal diagnostics should examine the samples. Suggested haematology and biochemistry reference values are given in Figures 4.2 and 4.3.

The haemogram may vary with age, sex, diet and husbandry conditions. A stress leucogram, associated with transport and handling, is likely in most species (apart from guinea pigs). It takes approximately 2 weeks for haematology parameters to return to baseline from the time of sampling and this should be taken into consideration when repeated withdrawals are necessary. Erythrocytes in general have a shorter lifespan in the species described here than those of larger mammals such as cats and dogs. The predominant leucocyte in all species is the lymphocyte.

Parameter	Mice	Rats	Hamsters	Gerbils	Guinea pigs	Chinchillas	Degus
PVC (%)	35–40	37.6–50.6	45–50	35–45	35–45	27–54	26–54
RBC (10⁶/µl)	7–11	6.76–50.6	7–8	7–8	4–7	5.6–8.4	4.2–13.8
Hb (g/dl)	10–20	14.5–16.1	45–50	14–16	11–17	8–15.4	7.2–15.0
MCV	45.5–60.3	50–77.8	64–77	46.6–60	77.5–88.5	39–58	37.5–54.7
MCH	14.1–19.3	16–23.1	20–26	16.1–19.4	22–28	14–29	13.6–17.2
MCHC	30.2–34.2	28.2–34.1	28–37	30.6–33.3	28.9–32	32–35	286–422
WBC (10⁹/l)	2–12	5–23	5–10	6.5–21.6	6–14	5.4–15.6	3.2–19.9
Segmented neutrophils %	5–40	10–50	17–35	2–23	13–60	39–54	11–91
Banded neutrophils %		0–1			0–1	0–2	0–5
Lymphocytes %	30–90	50–93	56–80	73–97	30–83	45–60	9–86
Monocytes %	0–10	0–10	0.4–4.4	0–4	2–20	0–6	0–8
Eosinophils %	0–5	0–5	0–1	0–4	0–5	0–5	0–6 ♂ 0–18 ♀
Basophils %	0–2	0–1	0–1	0–1	0–1	0–1	0–10 ♂ 0–2 ♀
Platelets (10⁹/l)	592–2972	685–1436	300–573	400–600	380–650	200–482	53–475
Reticulocytes	1–3	2–4	1–4	3.2	2–3	0–2.8	

4.2 Haematological data for selected rodent species.

Parameter	Mice	Rats	Hamsters	Gerbils	Guinea pigs	Chinchillas	Degus
Total protein (g/l)	35–72	56–76	52–70	43–125	44.4–65.8	38–56	56–61
Albumin (g/l)	25–48	38–48	35–49	18–55	25.4–41.1	23–41	31–33
Globulin (g/l)	6–24	18–30	27–42	12–60	13.1–38.6	9–22	25–28
Glucose (mmol/l)	3.3–12.7	4.7–7.3	3.6–7.0	2.8–7.5	3.3–6.9	3.3–6.1	4.12–4.56
Calcium (mmol/l)	0.8–2.0	1.3–3.2	5.3–12	0.93–1.55	2.4–3.1	1.4–3.02	2.55
Phosphorus (mmol/l)	1.94–3.56	1–3.6	0.96–3.19	1.20–2.26	1.03–6.98	1.29–2.58	2.00
Sodium (mmol/l)	112–193	62.2–67.9	128–144	61–75	130–150	142–166	151
Potassium (mmol/l)	5.1–10.4	1.38–1.79	3.9–5.5	3.3–6.3	4.5–8.8	3.3–5.7	3.9–9
Chloride (mmol/l)	82–114	28.2–31.0	95–110	93–118	94–111	108–129	116
Magnesium (mmol/l)			0.95–1.75		0.99–2.56		
Iron (µmol/l)					26–76		
Urea (mmol/l)	6.1–10.0	2.4–3.4	4.28–9.28	6.1–9.6	3.34–10.33	6.06–16.06	4.1–8.3
Creatinine (µmol/l)	27–88	17.6–70.1	35.4–88.4	53–124	0–77	35.4–114.9	18–44
ALP (IU/l)	45–222	16–125	99–186	12–37	0–418	6–72	113
ALT (IU/l)	26–77	17.5–30.2	22–128		0–61	10–35	3–12
AST (IU/l)	54–269	45.7–80.8	28–122		0–90	96	33–56
Bilirubin (µmol/l)	2–15	3.4–9.4	1.7–15.4	3–10	0–1.59	5.13–15.4	
Cholesterol (mmol/l)	0.68–2.13	1.04–3.38	1.43–4.7	2.34–3.9	0.31–1.67	1.3–7.85	
Triglycerides (mmol/l)			0.79–2.49		0.33–2.35		
Bile acid (µmol/l)					0.0–84.5		
Fructosamine (µmol/l)					134–271		
γ-GT (IU/l)					0–13		

4.3 Biochemical data for selected rodent species. (continues) ▶

Parameter	Mice	Rats	Hamsters	Gerbils	Guinea pigs	Chinchillas	Degus
CK (IU/l)			0.5–190		0–2143		
LDH (IU/l)			148–412		0–515		
GLDH (IU/l)					0–17		
Lipase (IU/l)					0–152		
Amylase (IU/l)		128–313	160–210		0–3159		
T4 (mmol/l)					7.8–15.6		
Cortisol (mmol/l)			13.8–27.6				

4.3   (continued) Biochemical data for selected rodent species.

Infectious processes in rodents often result in toxic granulation, formation of Döhle bodies and the presence of immature white blood cells rather than an overall increase of leucocytes. Neutrophils respond with a left shift and increased numbers. A left shift with concurrent neutropenia is often due to overwhelming infection and subsequent consumption of this cell population. More chronic inflammatory processes, such as abscesses, may be associated with marked leucocytosis and neutrophilia. In guinea pigs, lymphocytic leukaemia of the circulating blood or bone marrow manifests itself with markedly increased numbers of frequently abnormal lymphocytes with prominent nucleoli or increased cytoplasm and sometimes vacuolization if spotted on smears made at venipuncture.

Low platelet numbers on machine readings should always be confirmed manually by screening the feathered edge of blood films for clumps. These may be due to rapid clotting or inadequate mixing of samples immediately after venipuncture. Pathological conditions that may cause thrombocytopenia include infection, toxins, immune-mediated conditions or neoplasia.

Degeneration of cells and vacuolization due to prolonged storage prior to analysis will severely hamper interpretation.

In general, biochemical values respond in a similar fashion to those in cats and dogs. Stress due to transport or handling will elevate alkaline phosphatase (ALP), cortisol and glucose values to a degree and is almost always unavoidable. Haemolysis and lipaemia will interfere with results and should be avoided by using appropriate equipment and taking a fasted sample where possible.

Mice

Slight rouleaux formation is frequently observed in this species. The short erythrocyte lifespan causes polychromasia and anisocytosis in normal blood samples. Small numbers of Howell–Jolly bodies can be found in healthy animals. White blood cell counts are highly variable and samples drawn in the morning often have higher leucocyte counts than samples taken later in the day. Normal lymphocytes occasionally contain azurophilic granules. Stress directly decreases lymphocyte numbers. Mature males have more granulocytes than females. Nuclei lack distinct lobes and are doughnut (Figure 4.4) or horseshoe shaped. Drumstick formation can be found, especially

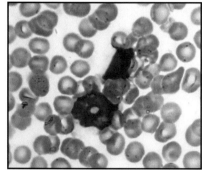

4.4   Mouse granulocyte with typical doughnut-shaped nucleus. (Courtesy of M. Hart)

in blood samples taken from female mice. The cytoplasm is colourless but sometimes contains reddish granules that stain pink with Romanowsky-based stains. Basophils are very rare. Mice are prone to lymphoma and leukaemia.

Rats

A circadian rhythm, just like in mice, has been reported for total leucocyte numbers in rats. Erythrocytes display considerable anisocytosis. At birth erythrocyte numbers are about half of adult values. Small numbers of Howell–Jolly bodies can be found in healthy animals. The lymphocyte population consists of more small than large cells and often shows azurophilic granules (Figure 4.5). Mature males have more lymphocytes and granulocytes than females. Rat neutrophils may contain small eosinophilic granules that stain pink with Romanowsky-based stains, otherwise the cytoplasm is colourless. The nuclei are doughnut, drumstick or horseshoe shaped. Eosinophils often have a rope-like nucleus and small round strongly acidophilic granules. Basophils are only rarely observed.

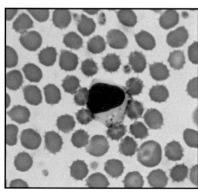

4.5   Rat lymphocyte with azurophilic granules. (Courtesy of M. Hart)

Hamsters

The lifespan of erythrocytes is about 10 days. It is normal to see occasional spherocytes, target cells, normoblasts and ovalocytes. Juveniles younger than 9 weeks have fewer erythrocytes and lower haemoglobin and haematocrit values than adults, as well as larger numbers of reticulocytes and basophilic stippling in erythrocytes. Lipaemia and hypercholesterolaemia are reported even when animals are fed on normal rodent diets. Hamsters that suffer from diabetes mellitus show elevated blood glucose levels. Hyperadrenocorticism may be suspected with elevated cortisol and ALP levels (see also Chapter 16). Glucose values rise in non-fasted samples and show seasonal variations.

Gerbils

The lifespan of the typical erythrocyte is approximately 10 days and, due to the rapid turnover, pronounced basophilic stippling, polychromasia and anisocytosis are often observed.

Neonates show erythrocyte macrocytosis and panleucocytosis. Erythrocyte numbers can be up to half of the adult range. Males have significantly higher total erythrocyte numbers and haemoglobin values; the lymphocyte to neutrophil ratio is 6:1 in males and 3:1 in females. Neutrophils often contain a ring-shaped nucleus (doughnut cell). Frequent lipaemia and hypercholesterolaemia are reported even from animals fed on normal rodent diets (see also Chapter 1). This may lead to obesity and diabetes. The latter is associated with glucose intolerance, hyperglycaemia and hyperinsulinaemia. Hyperadrenocortism, although rare, is only seen in breeding animals and often linked to myocardial necrosis/fibrosis, diabetes and obesity. With this condition, as well as diabetes, elevated triglycerides and hepatic lipidosis may be seen (see also Chapter 16). Gerbils older than 1 year also often suffer from hepatitis, chronic nephropathy and amyloidosis and corresponding biochemical values are often subsequently altered.

Guinea pigs

Erythrocytes are proportionally larger than in the other species discussed here, but compared with other rodents the PCV, haemoglobin levels and erythrocyte levels are relatively low.

Leucocytes incorporate a unique population of 'Kurloff' cells, recognizable by their oval or round inclusions (Figure 4.6). These particular cells are influenced by oestrogens and therefore are most commonly found in females and increase with pregnancy. They are rare in males and juveniles and are believed to have a cytotoxic effect on leukaemic cells. Acanthocytes may be seen with diets high in cholesterol.

Haematology and biochemistry are not affected by steroid response. The neutrophils often contain red-staining granules that are smaller and less abundant than in eosinophils. Granules in basophils often stain purple or black.

Peripheral lymphadenopathy may be caused by lymphosarcoma. Affected animals are typically leukaemic with total white cell counts > 25,000/µl, although aleukaemic forms can occur (see also Chapter 16).

Alanine aminotransferase (ALT) is not sensitive or specific for determining hepatocellular pathology as it is present at low levels in hepatocytes. Albumin, aspartate aminotransferase (AST), creatine kinase (CK) and glucose are normally higher than in other species. Hypercholesterolaemia is common, especially associated with hepatic lipidosis. Amylase is generally high, due to the high carbohydrate turnover, whereas lipase activity is low.

Spontaneous diabetes mellitus may occur in guinea pigs and in young animals it can be due to infection. Animals may have a history of hyperglycaemia, glucosuria and possible ketonuria (see also Chapter 16). Soft tissue mineralization is common in animals over 1 year of age and is associated with mineral imbalances (high phosphorus, low magnesium) (see also Chapter 14). Hyperthyroidism due to hyperplasia, adenoma or carcinoma and hypothyroidism due to thyroidal, pituitary and hypothalamic dysfunction have been reported (Ewringmann, 2006) and can be evaluated with T4 measurements (see Figure 4.3 for normal values).

Chinchillas

Neutrophils are often hyposegmented and contain polymorphic nuclei. Frequently bright red-staining granules are observed, but these are fewer and smaller than the ones found in eosinophils. Wild chinchillas have been reported to show seasonal variations in erythrocytes and haemoglobin values that are higher in winter. Leucocyte numbers are higher in winter and spring, when the reproductive season starts. Diabetes is the most common endocrine disease in chinchillas. See above under Guinea pigs for biochemical changes associated with this condition.

Degus

Hepatic lipidosis and subsequently elevated hepatic enzymes are often associated with diabetes and pregnancy.

Electrophoresis

Individual species have a very distinct normal pattern. The γ-globulin fraction in particular is characteristic and alters between species but also with age. A monoclonal gammopathy is often observed in cases of lymphocytic leukaemia and lymphoma.

Normal reference ranges are given in Figure 4.7.

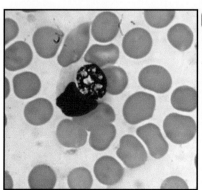

4.6

Guinea pig 'Kurloff' cell. Note the normal round intracytoplasmic inclusion. (Courtesy of M. Hart)

Parameter	Rats	Gerbils	Guinea pigs	Chinchillas	Degus
Total protein	100%	100%	44.6–65.8 g/l 100%	100%	♂ 44–47 g/l ♀ 32–74 g/l
Albumin	24–45	62.8–63.5	25.5–41.1 g/l (53–69.7%)	54.3–67.9	♂ 32.5–59.6 g/l ♀ 16–57.4 g/l
α_1-globulin	21–29	4.8	1.0–3.6 g/l (2.0–6.3%)	6.0–11.1	♂ 0–4.1 g/l ♀ 1.1–3.3 g/l
α_2-globulin	5–18	9.4–10.0	7.9–14.8 g/l (16.3–27.1%)	7.1–8.3	♂ 0–4.1 g/l ♀ 0–3.3 g/l
β-globulin	18–29	9.9–10.0	2.5–6.8 g/l (4.8–11.4%)	β_1-globulin 9.4–13.5 β_2-globulin 4.3–9.1	♂ 4.6–12.1 g/l ♀ 5.2–10.8 g/l
γ-globulin	3–7	11.6–12.2 (including fibrinogen)	1.7–7.8 g/l (3.3–13.4%)	3.2–10.2	♂ 0–8.8 g/l ♀ 0.9–8.5 g/l
	Highly strain specific				

4.7   Electrophoresis data for adult rodent species.

Cytology and microbiology

As with all other species, cytology can be a useful and very quick diagnostic tool that enables the practitioner to make informed choices about further testing, treatment or surgery. It is generally a very safe procedure that is ideal for animals where size, anaesthetic risk and cost matter, and may complement histology. Figure 4.8 lists selected neoplasms that may be diagnosed by cytology in rodents.

Fine-needle aspirates, punches and impression smears can be obtained from cutaneous, subcutaneous and internal masses or organs. Ultrasonographic guidance aids the sampling procedure. Hypodermic needles with a gauge of 20–25 can be used, with the preferred size being a 22 gauge. Syringes should be coated with EDTA rather than heparin to prevent clotting. Where multiple animals are at risk (e.g. rescue centre, pet shop), cytology can also be performed on impression smears made post mortem or from lesions, scrapings, swabs, urine and faeces to aid with the diagnosis.

If possible, more than one slide should be prepared. This enables the pathologist to compare several slides and use special stains. Quick stains can be used for staining in practice, but should be changed frequently to prevent artefacts.

Where enough of a sample can be obtained (e.g. from fluids), the surplus should be submitted in EDTA for cytology and plain tubes for protein evaluation. Some air-dried smears should always be prepared.

Bone marrow cytology may be a useful tool where the haematology indicates non-regenerative anaemia, neutropenia and thrombocytopenia of unknown origin, or leukaemia. Bone marrow films are made immediately after collection by spreading a drop of aspirate between two slides and pulling them apart without pressure. Core marrow biopsies should be

Tumour/neoplasia	Species
Adenoma	Guinea pig
Adenocarcinoma	Mouse
Adrenal tumours	Gerbil
Fibroadenoma	Rat
Haematopoetic tumours	Mouse, rat, guinea pig
Hepatocellular carcinoma	Mouse
Lipoma	Rat, guinea pig, chinchilla
Lymphoma [a]	Mouse, rat, hamster, gerbil, chinchilla
Mammary tumour [b]	Mouse, rat, hamster, guinea pig
Melanoma	Hamster
Ovarian tumour	Guinea pig, gerbil
Papilloma	Hamster
Renal tumours	Mouse, degu
Skin tumours	Mouse, rat, guinea pig, gerbil
Squamous cell carcinoma	Mouse
Thymoma	Mouse
Thyroid tumours	Mouse, guinea pig
Trichoepithelioma	Hamster, guinea pig
Zymbal's gland tumour	Rat

4.8   Selected neoplasms that may be diagnosed by cytology in rodents (see also Chapter 16). [a] Often multicentric. [b] Only very malignant ones – otherwise histology better. In guinea pigs, males are more often affected than females.

performed without negative pressure and the samples rolled over the slide surface. Normal bone marrow is highly cellular (Figure 4.9).

Parameter	Mice	Rats	Hamsters	Gerbils	Guinea pigs	Chinchillas
TNC [a]						1.14–1.16
Myeloid %	54.7–56.6	49.2–53.5	61.41	69.4	63.3	
Erythroid %	26.7–28.4	23.8–25.0	36.18	26.1 ± 7.6	26.7	
Lymphoid %	13.3–14.9	21.7–23.8	2.52	8.4 ± 4.2	4.6	
Reticulocytes %					5.4	
M:E	0.8:1 to 2.4:1	1.9:1 to 2.3:1	1.7:1	0.75:1 to 2.35:1	1.5:1 to 1.9:1	0.9:1 to 1.1:1
Comment				Higher amount of stippled RBCs than circulating blood	Occasional 'Kurloff' bodies	

4.9 Bone marrow analysis for adult rodent species. [a] TNC = total nucleated cells.

A variety of masses and tumours have been described in the species discussed here (see also Chapter 16), many of which can be investigated by cytology. Certain organs, masses or areas (e.g. renal, hepatic, mammary) do not exfoliate well, or they provide only limited information, and this hampers a cytological diagnosis. In these cases histological evaluation is recommended.

Bacterial infections and inflammatory or hyperplastic conditions may also be diagnosed.

Bacteriology

The success and ultimate value of examining clinical specimens is influenced by the care exercised in the selection, collection and shipment of the specimens. Samples should reach the laboratory without delay and in adequate storage medium. For most bacteria, charcoal swabs are sufficient for transport to the laboratory. A number of bacterial infections may also be diagnosed by PCR techniques.

Bacteriological samples often contain numerous non-pathogenic bacteria. This requires plating on selective media and non-selective media, as well as anaerobic culture in some cases. Laboratories with experience in exotic species should be chosen as they will be able to advise on transport media, significance of results and suitable antibiotics. Clinical history will enable the laboratory to make informed decisions and aid the pathologist in giving appropriate advice. See also Figure 4.10 for selected bacterial infections in rodents.

Bacterium	Host	Comment
Bordetella bronchiseptica	Guinea pig, chinchilla	ZOONOSIS, pneumonia
Clostridium piliforme	Guinea pig, gerbil	Enteritis (Tyzzer's disease)
Corynebacterium kutscheri	Mouse, rat	Polyarthritis
Eschericha coli	Guinea pig, hamster, chinchilla	Enteritis
Helicobacter	Hamster	Chronic gastritis
Klebsiella pneumoniae	Guinea pig, chinchilla	Pneumonia
Leptospira	Rat, gerbil	ZOONOSIS. Infections are often without clinical signs
Listeria monocytogenes	Mouse, gerbil, chinchilla	ZOONOSIS. Visceral and encephalitic forms, especially in chinchillas
Mycoplasma pulmonis	Mouse, rat	Pneumonia
Pasteurella multocida	Guinea pig, chinchilla	Pneumonia
Pasteurella pneumotropica	Hamster, rat	Pneumonia, abscessation
Pseudomonas aeruginosa	Mouse, chinchilla	Pneumonia
Salmonella typhimurium, enteritidis	Guinea pig, hamster, mouse, gerbil, chinchilla	ZOONOSIS, enteritis
Staphylococcus aureus	Guinea pig, hamster, chinchilla	Dermatitis, abscessation, pneumonia, septicaemia
Streptobacillus moniliformis	Mouse, rat	ZOONOSIS ('Rat bite fever' in humans), polyarthritis in mice and rats
Streptococcus pneumoniae	Guinea pig, hamster, rat	Pneumonia
Streptococcus zooepidemicus	Guinea pig, hamster, chinchilla	Dermatitis, abscessation
Yersinia pseudotuberculosis	Guinea pig, mouse, chinchilla	ZOONOSIS, septicaemia, abscessation
Yersinia enterocolitica	Chinchilla	Enteritis

4.10 Selected bacterial infections in rodents.

Many rodents are highly susceptible to antibiotic-associated clostridial enterotoxaemia and enteritis. Incidences occur, especially in hamsters, guinea pigs and chinchillas, when antibiotics with a primarily Gram-positive spectrum are given, or when application is via the oral route. Toxicity has been reported in guinea pigs that received streptomycin and dihydro-streptomycin, and some penicillin preparations including procaine. Gerbils are susceptible to streptomycin and mice, hamsters and chinchillas to some penicillin preparations. Chloramphenicol and aminoglycosides above the recommended dosage may cause ototoxic effects in chinchillas and guinea pigs. (See Chapter 5 for more details.)

Potentially zoonotic diseases in rodents include infections with *Salmonella*, *Pasteurella*, *Bordetella*, *Yersinia pseudotuberculosis*, *Y. pestis*, *Y. enterocolitica*, *Listeria* spp., lymphocytic choriomeningitis virus, *Leptospira* and dermatophytes. (See also Chapter 1.)

Chlamydophila

Microscopic demonstration of the organism consists of visualizing the inclusion bodies with, for example, modified Ziehl–Neelsen stains. The elementary bodies may be extra- or intracellular and are usually arranged in groups, staining red. Fluorescence microscopy, serology and PCR are alternative diagnostic techniques. The organism can only be grown on suitable cell cultures.

Leptospira

Leptospirosis, mainly caused by *Leptospira ictero-haemorrhagiae*, usually runs an asymptomatic course, but rats serve as a reservoir for human infection. If clinical signs are present they are usually characterized by haemolytic anaemia and icterus. Leptospires are very difficult to isolate on culture and grow best in fluid or semi-solid media between 28 and 30°C. Dark-field or phase contrast microscopy of fresh material reveals coiled organisms. They do not stain with the general bacterial dyes, but require silver staining techniques. Most laboratories will not offer this service. Leptospirosis can be serologically diagnosed (e.g. Leptospira Reference Unit (LRU), Department of Microbiology and Immunology, County Hospital, Hereford, HR1 2ER).

Listeria

Listeria monocytogenes produces a trypsin-sensitive and antigenic haemolysin that lyses erythrocytes of various animal species. The bacteria grow better under anaerobic conditions. Carrier material often contains only a few organisms and needs to be enriched prior to culture.

Mycoplasma

Mycoplasmas have no cell wall and require a special transport medium. The organisms are very demanding in their cultural requirements and the mere isolation of a *Mycoplasma* sp. without strain determination is of little clinical value. Specialist laboratories should be contacted. Serology (ELISA) is the test of choice to identify mycoplasmal infections, particularly in older animals. PCR is also available for certain strains. (See also Chapter 12.)

Pasteurella

Pasteurella multocida is the most frequent isolated strain. The bacterium causes mainly respiratory disease in rodents. Diagnosis from tracheal or nasal swabs can be obtained via culture, serology or PCR. (See also Chapter 12.)

Streptococcus

Streptococcus moniliformis is fastidious and difficult to culture. Synovial cytology aids diagnosis.

Yersinia

Yersinia spp. will readily grow on blood agar and selective agars. Most rapid growth occurs between 28 and 30°C. Cold enrichment between 2 and 4°C may be helpful.

Dermatophytes

Suspicious lesions may be touched with sticky tape, creating an imprint of the surface, and stained for cytological investigation. Hair plucks are best taken by pulling in the direction of hair growth with rubber-coated forceps in order to prevent damage to hairs. Skin scrapings are used to detect hyphae and spores of some dermatophytes, such as *Microsporum* and *Trichophyton* spp. Irrespective of depth, a no.10 scalpel blade (or no.15, for areas that are difficult to reach) should be used. The specimen should be stained and initially examined under low power (X40). Any details are usually best viewed at X100 using oil immersion.

Wood's lamps are useful to investigate *Microsporum canis*. This dermatophyte fluoresces with an apple-green colour. *Trichophyton* and other species do not show fluorescence. False negatives are possible and suspicious lesions, broken hairs and scales should be further examined by microscopy and culture. (See also Chapter 10.)

Material for fungal culture

Hair plucks (broken hairs from the centre and intact hairs from the margins) or a toothbrush, using the Mackenzie technique whereby the entire body is brushed down, should be used to isolate most dermatophytes. Some are only found in the stratum corneum and require dry skin scrapings. Hairs should be removed along the direction of hair growth with rubber-tipped tweezers and placed in a sterile container. The most commonly encountered dermatophytes of rodents are *Trichophyton* spp. and *Microsporum* spp.

Yeasts can be sampled by using a moist, sterile swab submitted in appropriate transport medium.

Culture is best carried out on Sabouraud medium (contact plates are available). Alternatively a dermatophyte test medium (DTM) can be used in practice for quicker results but this yields occasional false negatives. Samples from cultures are placed on slides and air-dried. They are then stained and examined under the microscope.

Deep fungal infections may only be diagnosed by culturing a biopsy sample. Swabbing the site with alcohol prior to sampling will reduce bacterial contamination. Ideally treatment success should be determined by two negative cultures.

Serology

Immunoassays for serology in exotic animal practice are offered by specialist laboratories, such as university laboratories (e.g. Acarus), laboratory animal specialists, or those with special expertise (e.g. Biobest, Greendales, Surrey Diagnostics, The Microbiology Laboratories in the UK). They offer a distinct advantage in cases where the infectious agent is difficult to culture or isolate or dangerous to handle. Moreover, serology generally offers faster results than culture. As with any test, accuracy and reliability are of utmost importance. Further important test characteristics to assess the diagnostic probabilities are sensitivity and specificity.

As a rule of thumb it can be said that screening tests need to detect the rate of infection (e.g. in a colony) and must therefore produce a very high sensitivity. Diagnostic tests, on the other hand, are more concerned with the individual animal and must have a high sensitivity (true positive) and specificity (true negative). Unfortunately this ideal scenario is non-existent and the clinician must often resort to a combination of tests and methods to determine the likelihood of infection. In order to diagnose a condition, tests with a high specificity should be chosen; and in order to rule out a particular diagnosis, a test with a high sensitivity should be requested. Reliability is the most important feature for monitoring disease processes.

Culture is used for most bacterial agents. Serological tests, mainly enzyme-linked immunosorbent assays (ELISAs) and immunofluoresence assays (IFAs), are available for a number of bacteria. However, tests have a higher risk of false positive reactions when compared with those for viruses, due to the more complex antigenic structure. In recent times PCR has become available for a number of bacterial and viral agents.

Viral infections

Pet rodents may be affected by viral infections, which are often facilitated by poor husbandry. For the general practice it is usually not practical to purchase test kits. Specialist laboratories with particular experience should be sought to receive appropriate samples. Figure 4.11 describes selected viral infections in rodents.

Virus	Host	Comments
Adenovirus	Mouse, rat, guinea pig	Renal problems, kidney lesions (mouse), fatal pneumonia in guinea pigs, stunted growth
Cavian leukaemia virus (oncorna virus)	Guinea pig	Diagnosis with haematology, bone marrow and lymph node aspirate/biopsy
Cytomegalovirus (herpes virus)	Mouse, guinea pig, degu	Immunosuppression, intranuclear inclusion bodies
Ectromelia virus (orthopoxvirus)	Mouse	High mortality (> 90%), eosinophilic inclusion bodies in skin and intestinal mucosa
Herpesvirus (Human herpes simplex virus)	Chinchilla	Acute lymphocytic meningoencephalitis with intranuclear inclusions, hepatic necrosis, ulcerative keratitis, uveitis
Lymphatic leucosis	Mouse	Enlarged lymph nodes
Lymphocytic choriomeningitis virus (LCM)	Mouse, rat, hamster, guinea pig	ZOONOSIS, immunosuppression, latent asymptomatic carriers are common, infections of tear and salivary glands
Mouse hepatitis virus (coronavirus)	Mouse, rat	Immunosuppression, elevation in hepatic enzymes, enteric and respiratory problems
Mouse mammary virus	Mouse	Often metastasis to liver and lung
Murine norovirus	Mouse	Often lethal, encephalitis, meningitis, pneumonia, hepatitis
Parvovirus	Mouse, rat, hamster	Immunosuppression
Pneumonia virus of mice	Mouse, rat, hamster, guinea pig, gerbil	Reaches chronic stages in immunocompromised animals
Polyomavirus	Mouse	Shed mainly via urine; can induce tumours, paralysis and wasting in nude (immunocompromised) mice
Reovirus-3	Mouse, rat, hamster, guinea pig	Multisystemic disease, steatorrhoea, produces 'oily skin'
Rotavirus	Mouse, rat	Severe epizootic diarrhoea especially in juveniles, stunted growth
Sendai virus (RNS-paramyxovirus)	Mouse, rat, hamster, guinea pig	Immunosuppression, delayed wound healing, respiratory problems, often weanlings affected
Sialodacryoadenitis virus (coronavirus)	Rat	Stunted growth, red tears, swelling of salivary glands, affects mainly juveniles
Theiler's murine encephalomyelitis virus	Mouse, rat	Neuropathic, latent infection common
Toolan's and Kilham's rat virus (H-1) (KRH)	Rat	Immunosuppression, hepatic necrosis, skeletal defects in neonates

4.11 Selected viral infections in rodents.

In most cases an ELISA is the method of choice test for detecting viruses. Indirect IFAs are also used in laboratories with appropriate equipment since they are usually more sensitive.

Due to the fact that seroconversion occurs over a period of time post infection, acute illness may produce false negative results. Single results are not able to determine the current infection status; they only give information about exposure and subsequent antibody levels.

PCR assays, where available, are extremely sensitive and offer information about the current status of infection. However, the technique has its limitations with viruses that are only circulating for short periods of time (e.g. herpesvirus).

Lymphocytic choriomeningitis (LCM)

This zoonotic disease is caused by an Arenavirus. Human infections from hamsters may occur. The virus is only shed for the first 3 months of a hamster's life, via urine, faeces and saliva. Main transmission is through bite wounds. Lehmann-Grube (1979) reported no difference in infection rates in humans regardless of contact with hamsters. Diagnosis is via ELISA, virus isolation or IFA in specialist laboratories.

Urinalysis

In order to obtain urine, animals can be placed on a cold surface or in a cooled plastic bag or, where available, into a metabolic cage. Urine may also be collected by applying slight pressure on the urinary bladder, by cystocentesis or by careful catheterization in some of the larger species (see also Chapters 2 and 13). Anaesthesia may be necessary for restraint and in order to minimize stress.

In general, the colour of the urine is affected by the diet and can change dramatically, so has to be put in context with the clinical signs. Species prone to diabetes may produce up to 10 times the normal urine output. Alkaline urine may give false positive protein readings. Apart from diabetes, glucosuria may be due to stress, transport and handling, anorexia and subsequent hepatic lipidosis and ketosis and this must be taken into consideration. Urine reference values in rodents are given in Figure 4.12.

Mice

Urine is constantly voided in small drops and so obtaining a meaningful sample can be a challenge. Handling stress usually causes mice to urinate. Males in particular are proteinuric and the urine in general is highly concentrated. Taurine and creatinine are excreted in the urine. Urethral plugs have been reported.

Rats

Juvenile proteinuria is normal. There is also a progressive non-pathological albuminuria in rats over 1 year of age. Rats excrete only small amounts of calcium, even when fed on high-calcium diets.

Hamsters

Urine frequently contains calcium and phosphate-based crystals. Urolithiasis, possibly related to feeding dry food, has been reported. Degenerative renal problems with clinical signs of uraemia, proteinuria and polyuria as well as a high incidence of amyloidosis have been reported. However, proteinuria can be a normal finding.

Gerbils

Gerbils frequently produce small quantities of highly concentrated urine during the day and so obtaining a meaningful sample can be a challenge. Handling stress usually causes gerbils to urinate. Pyelonephritis, urethral obstruction, hydronephrosis, nephrocalcin-

Parameter	Mice	Rats	Hamsters	Gerbils	Guinea pigs	Chinchillas	Degus
Description	Turbid yellow to milky urine	Turbid yellow to milky urine	Turbid yellow to milky urine	Clear yellowish	Opaque creamy white to yellow	Turbid, yellow to slightly amber	Yellow to orange
Glucose	Negative	Negative	Negative	Negative	Negative	Negative	Negative
Bilirubin	Negative	Negative	Negative	Negative		Negative	
Urobilinogen						0.1–1.0 ng/dl	
Erythrocytes	Negative	Negative	Rare	Negative	Negative	Negative	Negative
pH	7.3–8.5	7.3–8.5	5.1–8.4	6.5–7.5	8–9	8.5	
Protein	Proteinuria normal	Proteinuria can be normal finding in older rats	Proteinuria can be normal finding	Negative		Negative to trace	
Nitrates						Negative	
Ketones	Small amounts normal		Small amounts normal	Negative		Negative	
Leucocytes	Negative	Negative	Rare	Negative	Negative	Negative	Negative
Specific gravity (g/l)	1.034–1.058	1.022–1.070	1.014–1.060	Highly concentrated	<1.050	>1.045	1.123

4.12 Urinalysis data for selected rodent species.

osis, cystitis and urethritis have been reported in aged gerbils. (See also Chapter 13.)

Guinea pigs

In female guinea pigs the urethra ends outside the vestibulum and so catheterization is possible in both genders via small probes. Older females more than 2½ years of age are particularly prone to urolithiasis. Diets high in calcium will facilitate hypercalciuria. Older males are prone to proteinaceous plugs. Normal urine contains calcium oxalate, calcium carbonate and ammonium phosphate crystals. Glucosuria and rarely ketonuria can be found with diabetes mellitus. Vitamin C, which must be supplemented in guinea pigs, can interfere with urinary glucose levels and falsely elevate them.

Chinchillas

Male chinchillas are prone to urinary calculi and urolithiasis and present with haematuria, dysuria or anuria.

Degus

Because these animals are desert species, they are capable of significantly concentrating their urine.

References and further reading

Boot R (2001) Development and validation of ELISAs for monitoring bacterial and parasitic infections in laboratory rodents and rabbits. *Scandinavian Journal of Laboratory Animal Science* **28**, 2–8

Campbell T and Ellis C (2007) *Avian and Exotic Animal Hematology and Cytology, 3rd edn.* Blackwell Publishing, Ames, Iowa

Capello V (2001a) Pet hamsters: clinical evaluation and therapeutics. *Exotic DVM* **3**(2), 33–39

Capello V (2001b) Pet hamsters: infectious, parasitic and metabolic diseases. *Exotic DVM* **3**(6), 27–32

Deeb B (2005) Respiratory disease in pet rats. *Exotic DVM* **7**(2), 31–33

Dineen JK and Adams DB (1970) The effect of long-term lymphatic drainage on the lympho-myeloid system in the guinea pig. *Immunology* **19**, 11–30

Donelly TM (2006) Application of laboratory animal immunoassays to exotic pet practice. *Exotic DVM* **8**(4), 19–26

Ewringmann A (2006) Erkrankungen der Schilddruese bei Meerschweinchen. *VI Berliner Symposium, Berlin* 21–22

Gabrisch K and Zwart P (2008) Fehr M (2008) *Krankheiten der Heimtiere, 7th edn*, Sclütersche, Hannover

Garner M (2007) Cytologic diagnosis of diseases of rabbits, guinea pigs and rodents. *Veterinary Clinics of North America: Exotic Animal Practice* **10**, 25–49

Handler AH, Magalini SI and Pav D (1966) Oncogenic studies on the Mongolian gerbil. *Cancer Research* **26**, 844–847

Harris RS, Herdan G, Ancill RJ *et al.* (1954) A quantitative comparison of the nucleated cells in the right and left humeral bone marrow of the guinea pig. *Blood* **9**, 374–378

Hein J and Hartmann K (2003) Reference ranges for laboratory parameters in guinea pigs. *Tierärztliche Praxis Kleintiere* **30**, 383–389

Hrapkiewicz K and Medina L (2007) *Clinical Laboratory Animal Medicine: an Introduction, 3rd edn.* Blackwell Publishing, Ames, Iowa

Johnson-Delaney C (1996) *Exotic Animal Companion Medicine Handbook for Veterinarians.* Zoological Education Network, Greenacres, Florida

Johnson-Delaney C (2002) Exotic pet care: degus. *Exotic DVM* **7**(4), 39–42

Jones RD (1970) Age and sex differences in the serum proteins of the chinchilla. *Journal of Mammology* **51**, 425–429

Keeble E (2001) Endocrine diseases in small mammals. *In Practice*, 570–585

Lehmann-Grube (1979) Untersuchungen über die Rolle des Goldhamsters (*Mesocricetus auratus*) bei der Übertragung des Virus der Lymphozytären Choriomeningitis auf den Menschen. *Medical Microbiology and Immunology* **167**, 205–210

Manning PJ, Wagner JE and Harkness JE (1984) Biology and diseases of guinea pigs. In: *Laboratory Animal Medicine*, ed. JC Fox, BJ Cohen and FM Loew, pp. 149–181. Academic Press, Orlando

Martin RA, Brott DA, Zandee JC *et al.* (1992) Differential analysis of animal bone marrow by flow cytometry. *Cytometry* **13**, 638–643

Merry CJ (1990) An introduction to chinchillas. *Veterinary Technician* **11**, 315–331

Murphy JC, Niemi SM, Hewes KM, Zink M and Fox JG (1978) Hematologic and serum protein reference values of the *Octodon degus*. *American Journal of Veterinary Research* **39**, 713–715

Ness RD (1999) Clinical pathology and sample collection of exotic small mammals. *Veterinary Clinics of North America: Exotic Animal Practice* **2**, 591–620

Ness RD (2001) Rodents. In: *Exotic Animal Formulary, 3rd edn*, ed. JW Carpenter, pp. 377–410. Elsevier Saunders, Philadelphia

O'Malley B (2005) Small mammals. In: *Clinical Anatomy and Physiology of Exotic Species*, pp. 197–236. Elsevier Saunders, Philadelphia

Percy DH and Barthold SW (2001) Guinea pig. In: *Pathology of Laboratory Animals, 2nd edn*, pp. 209–244. Iowa State University Press, Ames

Quesenberry K, Donelly T and Hillyer E (2004) Biology, husbandry and clinical techniques of guinea pigs and chinchillas. In: *Ferrets, Rabbits and Rodents, 2nd edn*, ed. K Quesenberry and J Carpenter, pp. 232–244. WB Saunders, Philadelphia

Robinson DJ (1968) Age changes in plasma proteins of the Mongolian gerbil. *American Journal of Physiology* **204**, 275–278

Sisk DB (1976) Physiology. In: *The Biology of the Guinea Pig*, ed. JE Wagner and PJ Manning, pp. 63–92. Academic Press, New York

Strike TA (1970) Hemogram and bone marrow differential of the chinchilla. *Laboratory Animal Care* **20**, 33–38

White EJ and Lang CM (1989) The guinea pig. In: *The Clinical Chemistry of Laboratory Animals*, ed. WF Loeb and FW Quimby, pp. 27–30. Pergamon Press, New York

5

Rodents: therapeutics

Ricardo de Matos

Introduction

The administration of drugs to pet rodents poses some unique challenges to the veterinary surgeon. Rodents are routinely used as research laboratory animals and a significant amount of information has been gathered on drug use in different species. Much of this information is not readily available to the general clinician and applies to specific laboratory conditions that do not necessarily correspond to clinical situations in pets.

There are no drugs approved for use in domestic rodents in the USA, whereas in the UK a limited number of licensed products are available. For this reason, the veterinary surgeon is encouraged to investigate local government policies and guidelines regarding the extra-label use of medications in these species. Many of the dosages of medications used in pet rodents are based on anecdotal reports or empirical dose ranges available for other species of mammal, with very few dosages based on pharmacological studies. Allometric scaling may be used to obtain more correct dosages, but this applies only to drugs with simple absorption and excretion. The owners of domestic rodents should be aware of these facts and the inherent risks associated with treating their pets. Where possible, signed consent should be sought.

In order to maximize safety and efficacy of the drugs, species-specific characteristics and pharmacological properties of the drug(s) being used must be taken into consideration when implementing a therapeutic plan. For example, antibiotics that specifically target Gram-positive organisms can cause a fatal enterotoxaemia in hindgut-fermenter rodents, such as guinea pigs and chinchillas. Other factors such as age, body condition, surface area, metabolic rate, glomerular filtration, diet and behaviour (nocturnal vs. diurnal) can affect drug absorption and metabolism, influencing general effects and the incidence of toxicity. To the advantage of the veterinary surgeon, the small size of most pet rodents can make even the most expensive pharmaceuticals usually affordable.

The dosages presented in this chapter are based on the review of the literature available (see References).

Routes of drug administration

Oral medications

Most clients prefer medications that can be given orally. Pet rodents accept oral medications best if they are administered in a palatable liquid form, such as paediatric syrups or compounded oral suspensions. Tuberculin and insulin syringes allow accurate measurement of the often small volume needed and facilitate insertion in the diastema. The client should always be shown how to give oral medications before prescribing a drug, to ensure that they are comfortable with the procedure.

Medications can also be mixed with favourite foods and treats, such as fruit juice, honey, vegetable baby food or given in fruits. Chinchillas, being naturally inquisitive, normally take tablets hidden in raisins. Care should be taken for some medications as some of these 'vehicles' can inactivate the drug or affect its absorption. In a hospital or research setting, intragastric gavage with a bulbed metal feeding needle or a flexible feeding tube can also be used.

The use of medicated feed or water can result in erratic drug intake, making it difficult to achieve effective blood levels of medication. Sick animals tend to eat and drink less. Some rodents are very selective in their dietary habits and they may stop eating or drinking if the taste of their food or water is altered with the medication. If medicated food or water needs to be used, such as for treating many animals at the same time, it is important to know daily food and water intake for the species to be treated (Figure 5.1) for dosing purposes.

	Mice	Rats	Hamsters	Gerbils	Guinea pigs	Chinchillas
Food (g)	12–18	5–6	8–12	5–8	6	3–6
Water (ml)	15	10–12	8–10	4–7	10	4–6

5.1 Food and water intake for different species of rodent per 100 g body weight per day (Ness, 2005).

Parenteral injections

The recommended maximum volumes of administration for subcutaneous, intramuscular, intraperitoneal and intravenous injections in small rodents are presented in Figure 5.2.

Route	Mice	Rats	Hamsters, gerbils
Subcutaneous	Scruff, 2–3 ml	Scruff, flank, 5–10 ml	Scruff, 3–4 ml
Intramuscular	Quadriceps, 0.05 ml	Quadriceps, 0.3 ml	Quadriceps, 0.1 ml
Intraperitoneal	2–3 ml	10–15 ml	3–4 ml
Intravenous	Lateral tail vein, 0.2 ml	Lateral tail vein, 0.5 ml	Femoral vein (hamster), lateral tail vein (gerbil), 0.3 ml

5.2 Drug/fluid administration routes and maximum recommended volume at any one site in small rodents.

Subcutaneous injection

Subcutaneous injection is the preferred method of parenteral drug administration in rodents, because it allows for easy and safe delivery of small or relatively large volumes. Most injectable medications used in rodents can be given subcutaneously at the scruff of the neck or over the caudal flank. The skin on the dorsum of guinea pigs is thick, especially in intact males, making it difficult to penetrate with a 25 gauge or smaller needle. Care should be taken in chinchillas, where fur slip may occur following restraint for subcutaneous injection (see also Chapter 2). Some drugs (e.g. enrofloxacin) may cause local skin reactions when administered via this route.

Intramuscular injection

Intramuscular injection in rodents can be challenging because of the small muscle masses. In guinea pigs and chinchillas, intramuscular injections are normally given in the paralumbar muscles but may be given into the quadriceps. In the smaller rodents, the recommended site is the quadriceps muscle group, which covers the anterior aspect of the thigh (Figure 5.3). This site can also be used for intramuscular

injections in less common pet rodents, such as degus, duprasi and prairie dogs. Injections in the posterior thigh muscles should be avoided, because injection of an irritating substance close to the sciatic nerve may result in lameness or local self-mutilation. In general, intramuscular injections should be avoided where possible as even apparently small volumes are relatively large compared with the muscle mass and can cause pain and muscle damage.

Intravenous adminstration

Intravenous administration is required for certain antimicrobials, chemotherapeutics and blood replacement products and for treatment of moderate to severe dehydration or shock (see also Chapter 2). Single injections can be given using a small-gauge needle in the cephalic vein (guinea pigs and chinchillas), femoral vein (hamsters) or lateral tail vein (gerbils, mice, rats). A small-gauge (24–26) over-the-needle intravenous catheter can be placed in the same sites for multiple or continuous intravenous administration. A 'jugular cut-down' can be done in guinea pigs and chinchillas for placement of jugular catheters if a peripheral catheter cannot be placed. Vascular access devices are used in many laboratory animals and are an alternative if long-term intravenous therapy is anticipated. Clinical use has been described in a chinchilla (Orcutt, 2000).

Intraosseous administration

An alternative to intravenous catheterization is the placement of an intraosseous catheter in larger rodents. The proximal femur is the site most commonly used. The proximal humerus and tibia can also be used (see also Chapter 2). Most drugs that are given intravenously can be administered intraosseously, except hypertonic or alkaline solutions, which should be avoided or diluted before infusion (Powers, 2006).

Intraperitoneal injection

Intraperitoneal injection allows easy administration of small or large volumes of drugs or fluids (Figure 5.4). Although commonly used in laboratory rodents, intraperitoneal injections are not routinely performed in pet rodents, because administered drugs must first pass through the portal circulation, with potential for metabolism or biotransformation to occur before the

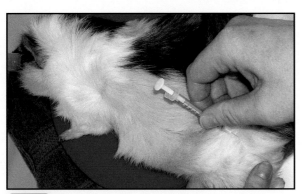

5.3 One of the recommended intramuscular injection sites in guinea pigs is the quadriceps muscle group on the anterior aspect of the thigh. (Courtesy of Lesa Longley.)

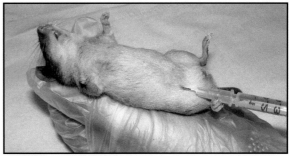

5.4 Intraperitoneal injection technique in a mouse. This route allows easy administration of small or large volumes of drugs or fluids. Although commonly used in laboratory rodents, intraperitoneal injections are not routinely performed in pet rodents. (Courtesy of Hannah Orr.)

drug reaches general circulation. Other drawbacks of this technique are related to the risk of organ damage/ perforation and the fact that administration is not 100% reliable, with the drug potentially being injected into the subcutaneous space, intramuscularly or within the lumen of abdominal organs.

Alternative routes of drug administration

Nebulization

Nebulization allows delivery of drugs such as antibiotics, antifungals and mucolytic agents to the upper and lower airways and to the lung parenchyma (see also Chapter 12). This will result in direct application of high concentrations of the medication to the targeted tissue, reducing the risk of systemic toxicity associated with parenteral administration. Nebulization is a complement to, not a substitute for, systemic antimicrobial therapy. Different types of nebulizer will create different size particles, with very small particle size being required for the drug to reach the lung parenchyma. For example, in humans, particles of 1–5 µm are deposited in the trachea and proximal bronchi, while particles less than 0.5 µm reach the alveoli. The success of therapy is more dependent on adequate drug delivery rather than being a function of drug efficacy. For this reason, the small size of some species of rodents may limit the use of nebulization for treating pulmonary disease.

A compressor unit or ultrasonic nebulizer can be used to deliver medications within an anaesthesia chamber or sealed cage (Figure 5.5). The animal

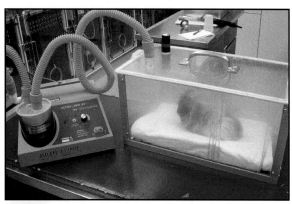

5.5 Nebulization in a guinea pig using an ultrasonic nebulizer and an anaesthesia induction chamber.

should be monitored during nebulization as excessive fluid deposition in the respiratory airways or aerosolized mucolytic drug-induced airway spasm may cause worsening of the respiratory clinical signs.

In general, antimicrobials used for aerosol treatment should be effective topically and have poor systemic absorption (i.e. aminoglycosides, nystatin and amphotericin B). Not all antimicrobials have the physiochemical properties required to be aerosolized. Drugs with high surface tension, such as beta-lactam antibiotics, are refractory to aerosolization, while antibiotics with low surface tension tend to foam excessively, reducing aerosolization.

Intranasal administration

The intranasal administration of sedatives and analgesics has been investigated and used as an alternative for delivery of drugs usually administered intravenously, particularly when rapid sedation is necessary. Dosages of common sedatives in mice and rats have been published and are often slightly higher than parenteral dosages (Johnson-Delaney *et al.*, 2001).

Localized antibiotic treatment

As has been described for rabbits, antibiotic-impregnated umbilical tape or polymethylmethacrylate beads can be applied to infected sites (such as tooth root abscesses). These techniques provide high local tissue levels with minimal or no systemic absorption, which will result in higher efficacy and reduced toxicity, and allow the use of certain antibiotics normally contraindicated for systemic use in some species of rodent.

Antibiotics

Antibiotics are the most commonly prescribed class of drugs in veterinary medicine. They should be selected based on culture and sensitivity results whenever possible. Special characteristics of the gastrointestinal physiology and anatomy of the rodent species must be taken into account when choosing a drug (see below). Antibiotics considered safe for all species of rodent include enrofloxacin, ciprofloxacin and trimethoprim/sulphonamide combinations (Figure 5.6).

Drug	Dosage						Comments
	Mice	*Rats*	*Hamsters*	*Gerbils*	*Guinea pigs*	*Chinchillas*	
Amikacin	10 mg/kg s.c., i.m. q12h	10 mg/kg s.c., i.m. q12h	10 mg/kg s.c., i.m. q12h	10 mg/kg s.c., i.m. q12h	10–15 mg/kg s.c., i.m., i.v., divided q8–24h	10–15 mg/kg s.c., i.m., i.v., divided q8–24h	
Amoxicillin	100–150 mg/kg s.c., i.m. q12h	100–150 mg/kg s.c., i.m. q12h	–	–	–	–	
Amoxicillin / clavulanate	2 ml/kg orally (Synulox®)	2 ml/kg orally (Synulox®)	–	–	–	–	

5.6 Rodent antibiotic dose rates. (Data from Rossoff, 1994; Antinoff *et al.*, 1999; Adamcak and Otten, 2000; Burgmann, 2000; Hoefer and Crossley, 2002; Keeble, 2002; Orr, 2002; Morrisey and Carpenter, 2004; O'Rourke, 2004; Ness, 2005; Hrapkiewicz and Medina, 2007) (continues) ▶

Drug	Dosage						Comments
	Mice	**Rats**	**Hamsters**	**Gerbils**	**Guinea pigs**	**Chinchillas**	
Ampicillin	20–50 mg/kg orally, s.c., i.m. q12h 0.5 mg/ml drinking water	20–50 mg/kg orally, s.c., i.m. q12h	Do not use	6–30 mg/kg orally q8h	Do not use	Do not use	
Carbenicillin	100 mg/kg orally q12h	100 mg/kg orally q12h	–	–	–	–	
Cefalexin	60 mg/kg orally q12h 30 mg/kg s.c. q12h	15 mg/kg s.c. q12h	–	25 mg/kg s.c. q24h	50 mg/kg orally, i.m. q12–24h	–	
Cefaloridine	10–25 mg/kg s.c., i.m. q24h	–	10–25 mg/kg s.c., i.m. q24h	30 mg/kg i.m. q12h	10–25 mg/kg i.m. q8–24h	–	
Cefaxolin	–	–	–	–	15 mg/kg i.m. q12h	–	
Ceftiofur	–	–	–	–	1 mg/kg i.m. q24h	–	
Chloramphenicol	30–50 mg/kg orally, s.c., i.m. q8–12h 0.5mg/ml drinking water	30–50 mg/kg orally, s.c., i.m. q8–12h	30–50 mg/kg orally, s.c., i.m. q8–12h	30–50 mg/kg orally, s.c., i.m. q8–12h 0.83 mg/ml drinking water	30–50 mg/kg orally, s.c., i.m. q8–12h 1 mg/ml drinking water	30–50 mg/kg orally, s.c., i.m. q8–12h	
Chlortetracycline	25 mg/kg orally, s.c. q12h	10 mg/kg orally, s.c. q12h	20 mg/kg orally, s.c. q12h	–	–	50 mg/kg orally q12h	
Ciprofloxacin	10 mg/kg orally q12h	10 mg/kg orally q12h	10 mg/kg orally q12h	10 mg/kg orally q12h	5–15 mg/kg orally q12–24h	5–15 mg/kg orally q12–24h	May cause arthropathies in young animals
Doxycycline	2.5–5 mg/kg orally q12h 100 mg/kg s.c. q7d	2.5–5 mg/kg orally q12h 100 mg/kg s.c. q7d	2.5–5 mg/kg orally q12h	2.5–5 mg/kg orally q12h	2.5–5 mg/kg orally q12h	2.5–5 mg/kg orally q12h	Do not use in young or pregnant animals
Enrofloxacin	5–10 mg/kg orally, s.c., i.m. q12h 0.05–0.2 mg/ml drinking water	5–10 mg/kg orally, s.c., i.m. q12h 0.05–0.2 mg/ml drinking water	5–10 mg/kg orally, s.c., i.m. q12h 0.05–0.2 mg/ml drinking water	5–10 mg/kg orally, s.c., i.m. q12h 0.05–0.2 mg/ml drinking water	5–10 mg/kg orally, s.c., i.m. q12h 0.05–0.2 mg/ml drinking water	5–10 mg/kg orally, s.c., i.m. q12h 0.05–0.2 mg/ml drinking water	Local tissue reactions may occur at the site of injection
Erythromycin	20 mg/kg orally q12h 18–25 mg/kg s.c. q12h	20 mg/kg orally q12h	Do not use	–	Do not use	Do not use	
Furazolidone	–	–	30 mg/kg orally q24h	–	5.5 mg/ml drinking water	–	
Gentamicin	5–8 mg/kg s.c., i.m., divided q8–24h	5-8 mg/kg s.c., i.m. divided q8–24h	5–8 mg/kg s.c., i.m., divided q8–24h	5–8 mg/kg s.c., i.m., divided q8–24h	5–8 mg/kg s.c., i.m., divided q8–24h	5–8 mg/kg s.c., i.m., divided q8–24h	
Metronidazole	20 mg/kg orally q12h 2.5 mg/ml drinking water	10–40 mg/kg orally q24h	20 mg/kg orally q12h	20 mg/kg orally q12h	20 mg/kg orally q12h	10–20 mg/kg orally q12h	Use with caution in chinchillas
Neomycin	25 mg/kg orally q12h 2.6 mg/ml drinking water	25 mg/kg orally q12h 2.6 mg/mL drinking water	30 mg/kg orally q12h 0.5 mg/mLl drinking water	100 mg/kg orally q24h 2.6 mg/ml drinking water	15 mg/kg orally q12h	15 mg/kg orally q12h	
Netilmicin	–	–	–	–	6–8 mg/kg s.c., i.m., i.v., divided q8–24h	6–8 mg/kg s.c., i.m., i.v., divided q8–24h	

5.6 (continued) Rodent antibiotic dose rates. (Data from Rossoff, 1994; Antinoff *et al.*, 1999; Adamcak and Otten, 2000; Burgmann, 2000; Hoefer and Crossley, 2002; Keeble, 2002; Orr, 2002; Morrisey and Carpenter, 2004; O'Rourke, 2004; Ness, 2005; Hrapkiewicz and Medina, 2007) (continues) ▶

Drug	Dosage						Comments
	Mice	*Rats*	*Hamsters*	*Gerbils*	*Guinea pigs*	*Chinchillas*	
Oxytetracycline	10–20 mg/kg orally q8h 60 mg/kg s.c., i.m. q3d (long-acting injection) 0.4 mg/ml drinking water	10–20 mg/kg orally q8h 60 mg/kg s.c., i.m. q3d (long-acting injection) 0.4 mg/ml drinking water	16 mg/kg s.c. q24h 0.25–1 mg/ml drinking water	10 mg/kg orally q8h 20 mg/kg s.c. q24h 0.8 mg/ml drinking water	5 mg/kg i.m. q12h 50 mg/kg orally q12h 1 mg/ml drinking water	50 mg/kg orally q12h 1 mg/ml drinking water	Toxicity in guinea pigs reported
Penicillin G	Do not use	22,000 IU/kg s.c., i.m. q24h	Do not use	–	Do not use	Do not use	
Sulfadimethoxine	10–15 mg/kg orally q12h	10–15 mg/kg orally q12h	10–15 mg/kg orally q12h	10–15 mg/kg orally q12h	10–15 mg/kg orally q12h	10–15 mg/kg orally q12h	
Sulfamerazine	1 mg/ml drinking water	1 mg/ml drinking water 1 mg/4 g feed	1 mg/ml drinking water	0.8 mg/ml drinking water	1 mg/ml drinking water	1 mg/ml drinking water	
Sulfamethazine	1 mg/ml drinking water	1 mg/ml drinking water	1 mg/ml drinking water	0.8 mg/ml drinking water	1 mg/ml drinking water	1 mg/ml drinking water	
Sulfaquinoxaline	1 mg/ml drinking water	1 mg/ml drinking water 0.05% feed	1 mg/ml drinking water	1 mg/ml drinking water	1 mg/ml drinking water	1 mg/ml drinking water	
Tetracycline	10–20 mg/kg orally q8–12h 2–5 mg/ml drinking water	10–20 mg/kg orally q8–12h 2–5 mg/ml drinking water 0.1–0.5% feed	10–20 mg/kg orally q8–12h 0.4 mg/ml drinking water	10–20 mg/kg orally q8–12h (20 mg/kg i.m. q12h) 2–5 mg/ml drinking water	10 mg/kg orally q8–12h 0.7 mg/ml drinking water	10–20 mg/kg orally q8–12h 0.3–2 mg/ml drinking water	Toxicity in guinea pigs reported
Trimethoprim/sulphonamide	15–30 mg/kg orally, s.c., i.m. q12h	15–30 mg/kg orally, s.c., i.m. q12h	15–30 mg/kg orally, s.c., i.m. q12h	15–30 mg/kg orally, s.c., i.m. q12h	15–30 mg/kg orally, s.c., i.m. q12h	15–30 mg/kg orally, s.c., i.m. q12h	Tissue necrosis may occur when given s.c.
Tylosin	10 mg/kg orally, s.c., i.m. q12–24h 0.5 mg/ml drinking water	10 mg/kg orally, s.c., i.m. q12–24h 0.5 mg/ml drinking water	2–8 mg/kg orally, s.c., i.m. q12h 0.5 mg/ml drinking water	10 mg/kg orally, s.c., i.m. q24h 0.5 mg/ml drinking water	10 mg/kg orally, s.c., i.m.	10 mg/kg orally, s.c., i.m. q12–24h	Toxicity reported in guinea pigs and hamsters

5.6 (continued) Rodent antibiotic dose rates. (Data from Rossoff, 1994; Antinoff *et al.*, 1999; Adamcak and Otten, 2000; Burgmann, 2000; Hoefer and Crossley, 2002; Keeble, 2002; Orr, 2002; Morrisey and Carpenter, 2004; O'Rourke, 2004; Ness, 2005; Hrapkiewicz and Medina, 2007)

Adverse effects of antibiotic treatment in rodents

Antibiotic-related toxicity in rodents can result from direct or indirect effects of the drug. As in rabbits, the most important mechanism of antibiotic toxicity in rodents results from disruption of the normal enteric flora. Species with predominantly Gram-positive intestinal flora, such as chinchillas, guinea pigs and hamsters, are at higher risk. Mice, gerbils and rats are less susceptible to antibiotic-associated enterotoxaemia. Although oral administration of the antibiotic is associated with a higher incidence of complications, toxic effects can also occur with parenteral administration of drugs that are excreted in an active form in the bile.

In susceptible species, antibiotics with limited spectrum targeting Gram-positive bacteria disrupt the normal enteric flora and create conditions for Gram-negative bacteria and clostridial species to proliferate. The most common species of bacteria that proliferate and cause problems include *Clostridium difficile*, *C. spiroforme*, *C. perfringens* and *Escherichia coli*,

with their incidence depending on the rodent species and antibiotic used. The proliferation of these bacteria causes a change in the intestinal lumen pH and increases the production of volatile fatty acids. The volatile fatty acids inhibit further growth of normal intestinal bacteria and create conditions for production of toxins by *Clostridium* spp. These toxins destroy the mucosal epithelium, resulting in inflammation, diarrhoea and possible systemic disease (Rosenthal, 2004). *Clostridium* spp. enterotoxaemia can occur as early as 3 days after the administration of one dose of an antibiotic (Collins, 1995).

Classes of antibiotics that have caused mortality when given to hamsters, guinea pigs and chinchillas include beta-lactams (amoxicillin, ampicillin and penicillin), macrolides (erythromycin, tylosin and spiramycin), lincosamides (clindamycin and lincomycin), and the specific antibiotics bacitracin and vancomycin. Tetracyclines (tetracycline, chlortetracycline, oxytetracycline) and cephalosporins have also been associated with enterotoxaemia in these species (Collins, 1995; Adamcak and Otten, 2000;

Ellis and Mori, 2001; Hoefer and Crossley, 2002; Ness, 2005). Chloramphenicol, a generally 'safe' antibiotic for rodents, can cause enterotoxaemia in hamsters when given at a higher dosage (300 mg/kg) (Collins, 1995).

Treatment of antibiotic-associated enterotoxaemia includes supportive care, suppression of abnormal bacterial overgrowth (with antibiotics), and re-establishment of normal intestinal flora (with probiotics and/or feeding fresh faeces from a healthy animal). The use of colestyramine, an ion-exchange resin that absorbs toxins, has been shown to alleviate clinical signs in rabbits and appears to have a similar effect in rodents (Lipman *et al.*, 1992).

Antibiotic-associated enterotoxaemia is best prevented by careful antibiotic selection. Although guinea pigs, chinchillas and hamsters are more susceptible, all species of rodent can potentially develop antibiotic-associated diarrhoea. The owners must be aware of this complication, monitor their pet closely and discontinue the antibiotic if diarrhoea develops during treatment. Even when 'safe' antibiotics are used, the author recommends the use of a *Lactobacillus*

probiotic supplement during treatment and for 5–7 days beyond termination of antibiotic administration (see Figure 5.12).

Antibiotics (and associated drugs in some preparations) can also have direct toxic effects in rodents. For example, streptomycin and procaine are toxic to mice, hamsters and guinea pigs; nitrofurantoin causes neuropathology in rats; and gerbils do not tolerate streptomycin and dihydrostreptomycin (Morris, 1995; Burgmann, 2000; Donnelly, 2004b). There are also anecdotal reports of metronidazole toxicity in chinchillas, causing vestibular disease or liver failure. Guinea pigs and chinchillas are highly susceptible to the ototoxic effects of chloramphenicol and aminoglycosides at dosages above those recommended.

Figure 5.7 lists the antibiotics that are toxic for each species of rodent.

Antifungal agents

Antifungal agents commonly used in rodents are listed in Figure 5.8.

Mice	Rats	Hamsters	Gerbils	Guinea pigs	Chinchillas
Streptomycin	Nitrofurantoin	Penicillins (penicillin, ampicillin, carbenicillin, ticarcillin) Cephalosporins Macrolides (erythromycin, tylosin) Tetracyclines Lincosamides (clindamycin, lincomycin) Aminoglycosides (gentamicin, neomycin, streptomycin) Bacitracin Vancomycin	Streptomycin, dihydrostreptomycin	Penicillins (penicillin, ampicillin, amoxicillin) Cephalosporins Macrolides (erythromycin, spiramycin, tylosin) Tetracyclines Lincosamides (clindamycin, lincomycin) Aminoglycosides (streptomycin) Bacitracin Vancomycin	Penicillins (penicillin, ampicillin, amoxicillin) Cephalosporins Macrolides (erythromycin) Lincosamides (clindamycin, lincomycin)

5.7 Antibiotics toxic to rodents.

Drug	Dosage						Comments
	Mice	*Rats*	*Hamsters*	*Gerbils*	*Guinea pigs*	*Chinchillas*	
Amphotericin B	0.11 mg/kg s.c. 0.43 mg/kg orally	–	1 mg/animal s.c. q12h 5d/ week for 3 weeks	–	–	–	Mice: use with caution; renal toxicity
Fluconazole	–	–	–	–	16 mg/kg orally q24h for 14d	–	Effective against *Trichophyton mentagrophytes*
Griseofulvin	25 mg/kg orally q12–24h 4–6 weeks	25 mg/kg orally q12–24h 2–4 weeks	25 mg/kg orally q12–24h 3–4 weeks	25 mg/kg orally q12–24h 2–4 weeks	25 mg/kg orally q12–24h 2–4 weeks	25 mg/kg orally q12–24h 4–8 weeks	Potentially teratogenic
Itraconazole	50–150 mg/kg q24h (blastomycosis)	2.5–10 mg/kg q24h	–	–	5 mg/kg q24h	–	
Ketoconazole	10–40 mg/kg orally q24h	10–40 mg/kg orally q24h	10–40 mg/kg orally q24h	10–40 mg/kg orally q24h	10–40 mg/kg orally q24h	10–40 mg/kg orally q24h	
Terbinafine	–	–	–	–	10–30 mg/kg orally q24h	8–20 mg/kg orally q24h	

5.8 Antifungal agents used in rodents. (Data from Antinoff *et al.*, 1999; Adamcack and Otten, 2000; Ellis and Mori, 2001; Hoefer and Crossley, 2002; Keeble, 2002; Orr, 2002; Pollock, 2003; Morrisey and Carpenter, 2004; O'Rourke, 2004; Ness, 2005; Hrapkiewicz and Medina, 2007)

Antiparasitic agents

Figure 5.9 lists antiparasitic agents and dosages used in rodents. Although ivermectin is considered an overall safe drug, rodents are significantly more sensitive to ivermectin toxicity than other species.

Despite this, ivermectin toxic doses are much higher than the recommended doses (for example, the LD_{50} in mice and rats is 25 mg/kg and 50 mg/kg, respectively) (Lankas and Gordon, 1989).

Drug	Dosage						Comments
	Mice	*Rats*	*Hamsters*	*Gerbils*	*Guinea pigs*	*Chinchillas*	
Albendazole	–	–	–	–	–	25 mg/kg orally q12h for 2 days	Giardiasis
Dimetridazole	1 mg/ml drinking water	1 mg/ml drinking water	0.5 mg/ml drinking water	–	20 mg/kg orally, s.c. q24h	–	GI protozoa
Fenbendazole	20 mg/kg orally q24h for 5 days	20 mg/kg orally q24h for 5 days	20 mg/kg orally q24h for 5 days	20 mg/kg orally q24h for 5 days	20 mg/kg orally q24h for 5 days	20 mg/kg orally q24h for 5 days	
Ivermectin	0.2–0.4 mg/kg orally, s.c. q7–14d 2 mg/kg orally, repeat 10d (pinworms) 8 mg/l drinking water for 4 days on, 3 days off, for 4 treatments (pinworms)	0.2–0.4 mg/kg orally, s.c. q7–14d 25 mg/l drinking water for 4 days on, 3 days off, for 4 treatments (pinworms)	0.2–0.4 mg/kg orally, s.c. q7–14d	0.2–0.4 mg/kg s.c. q7–14d	0.2–0.4 mg/kg orally, s.c. q7–14d	0.2–0.4 mg/kg orally, s.c. q7–14d	
Mebendazole	40 mg/kg orally q7d for 3 weeks	40 mg/kg orally q7d for 3 weeks	–	2.2 mg/ml drinking water for 5 days	–	–	Pinworms
Metronidazole	20 mg/kg orally q12h 2.5 mg/ml drinking water for 5 days	10–40 mg/rat orally q24h 0.05–0.2 mg/ml drinking water	70 mg/kg orally q8h	–	25 mg/kg orally q12h	50 mg/kg orally q12h for 5 days	Use with caution in chinchillas
Niclosamide	–	–	–	100 mg/kg orally, repeat 7 days	–	–	Cestodes
Piperazine adipate	200–600 mg/kg orally q24h for 7 days, off 7 days, repeat 4–7 mg/ml drinking water for 3–10 days	200 mg/kg orally q24h for 7 days, repeat 4–7 mg/ml drinking water for 3–10 days	3–5 mg/ml drinking water for 7 days, off 7 days, repeat	200–600 mg/kg orally q24h for 7 days, off 7 days, repeat	4–7 mg/ml drinking water for 3–10 days	500 mg/kg orally q24h	Pinworms
Piperazine citrate	2–5 mg/ml drinking water for 7 days, off 7 days, on 7 days	2–5 mg/ml drinking water for 7 days, off 7 days, on 7 days	2–5 mg/ml drinking water for 7 days, off 7 days, on 7 days	2–5 mg/ml drinking water for 7 days, off 7 days, on 7 days	2–5 mg/ml drinking water for 7 days, off 7 days, on 7 days	2–5 mg/ml drinking water for 7 days, off 7 days, on 7 days	Pinworms
Praziquantel	6–10 mg/kg orally, s.c., repeat 10d 140 ppm in feed for 7 days	6–10 mg/kg orally, s.c., repeat 10d	6–10 mg/kg orally, s.c., repeat 10d	6–10 mg/kg orally, s.c., repeat 10d	6–10 mg/kg orally, s.c., repeat 10d	6–10 mg/kg orally, s.c., repeat 10d	Cestodes
Pyrantel pamoate	–	–	50 mg/kg orally	50 mg/kg orally	–	–	Nematodes. Repeat dose may be necessary in 1–3 weeks depending on the lifecycle of the parasite

5.9 Antiparasitic agents used in rodents. (Data from Antinoff *et al.*, 1999; Adamcack and Otten, 2000; Ellis and Mori, 2001; Hoefer and Crossley, 2002; Keeble, 2002; Orr, 2002; Donnelly, 2004; Morrisey and Carpenter, 2004; Ness, 2005; Hrapkiewicz and Medina, 2007) (continues) ▶

Drug	Dosage						Comments
	Mice	*Rats*	*Hamsters*	*Gerbils*	*Guinea pigs*	*Chinchillas*	
Quinacrine	75 mg/kg q8h	75 mg/kg q8h	75 mg/kg q8h	75 mg/kg q8h	75 mg/kg q8h	75 mg/kg q8h	Giardiasis. Treatment length depends on parasite species being treated, parasite load and age of animal
Sulfadimethoxine	10–15 mg/kg orally q12h 50 mg/kg orally once, then 25 mg/kg orally q24h for 10–20 days	10–15 mg/kg orally q12h 50 mg/kg orally once, then 25 mg/kg orally q24h for 10–20 days	10–15 mg/kg orally q12h 50 mg/kg orally once, then 25 mg/kg orally q24h for 10–20 days	10–15 mg/kg orally q12h 50 mg/kg orally once, then 25 mg/kg orally q24h for 10–20 days	10–15 mg/kg orally q12h 50 mg/kg orally once, then 25 mg/kg orally q24h for 10–20 days	10–15 mg/kg orally q12h 50 mg/kg orally once, then 25 mg/kg orally q24h for 10–20 days	Coccidiosis
Sulfamerazine	1 mg/ml drinking water	1 mg/ml drinking water	1 mg/ml drinking water	0.8 mg/ml drinking water	1 mg/ml drinking water	1 mg/ml drinking water	Coccidiosis
Sulfamethazine	1 mg/ml drinking water	1 mg/ml drinking water	1 mg/ml drinking water	0.8 mg/ml drinking water	1 mg/ml drinking water	1 mg/ml drinking water	Coccidiosis
Sulfaquinoxaline	1 mg/ml drinking water	1 mg/ml drinking water	1 mg/ml drinking water	1 mg/ml drinking water	1 mg/ml drinking water	1 mg/ml drinking water	Coccidiosis
Tiabendazole	100 mg/kg orally q24h for 5 days	100 mg/kg orally q24h for 5 days	100 mg/kg orally q24h for 5 days	100 mg/kg orally q24h for 5 days	100 mg/kg orally q24h for 5 days	50–100 mg/kg orally q24h for 5 days	Chinchillas: ascaridiasis

5.9 (continued) Antiparasitic agents used in rodents. (Data from Antinoff *et al.*, 1999; Adamcack and Otten, 2000; Ellis and Mori, 2001; Hoefer and Crossley, 2002; Keeble, 2002; Orr, 2002; Donnelly, 2004; Morrisey and Carpenter, 2004; Ness, 2005; Hrapkiewicz and Medina, 2007)

Topical agents

Topical agents available for use in rodents are presented in Figure 5.10 (ophthalmic therapeutics) and Figure 5.11 (topical medications). When topical agents are used, the potential of toxicity by ingestion should be considered as a result of self- or companion grooming. Topical creams and ointments are generally considered ineffective in smaller rodents because of their fastidious grooming habits.

Drug	Application recommendation	Comments
Atropine (1%)/phenylephrine (10%)	Topical	Mydriasis for non-albino eyes
Chloramphenicol	Topical q6–12h	
Ciprofloxacin drops	Topical q8–12h	
Flurbiprofen	Topical q6–12h	Topical anti-inflammatory
Gentamicin ophthalmic solution	Topical q8h	
Neomycin, dexamethasone, polymyxin B ophthalmic solution	Topical q8–12h	May cause gastrointestinal stasis from steroids
Tropicamide 1%	Topical 1–2 times before eye exam or q8–12 hours following cataract surgery	Mydriasis for albino eyes

5.10 Ophthalmic therapeutics used in rodents. (Data from Antinoff *et al.*, 1999; Adamcak and Otten, 2000; Ness, 2005)

Drug	Application recommendation	Comments
Amitraz	*Guinea pigs*: 0.3% solution topically q7d *Hamsters, rats, mice*: 1.4 ml/l topically q7d *Gerbils*: 1.4 ml/l topically q14d for 3–6 treatments	Apply with cotton ball, brush Use with caution Not recommended in young
Butenafine 1% cream	*Guinea pigs*: apply topically q24h for 10–20 days	Dermatophytosis

5.11 Topical medications used in rodents. (Data from Antinoff *et al.*, 1999; Adamcack and Otten, 2000; Ellis and Mori, 2001; Hoefer and Crossley, 2002; Keeble, 2002; Orr, 2002; Pollock, 2003; Morrisey and Carpenter, 2004; O'Rourke, 2004; Ness, 2005; Hrapkiewicz and Medina, 2007) (continues)

Drug	Application recommendation	Comments
Carbaryl powder 5%	Dust lightly q7d	Carbamate insecticide
Chlorpyrifos	6 g per 29 × 12 cm cage added to bedding material, q7d for 2 weeks	Organophosphate insecticide
Clotrimazole ointment	*Guinea pigs* and *chinchillas*: apply topically	
Dichlorvos strip (5 cm long)	Suspend 15 cm above cage for 24h, twice a week for 3 weeks	Organophosphate insecticide. Useful for treating groups of rodents. Studies indicate non-toxic to mice (http://www.inchem.org/documents/ehc/ehc/ehc79.htm)
Dimethylsulfoxide (DMSO)	Apply small amount to affected area q12–24h for 3–5 days	Topical anti-inflammatory and analgesic effect; wear gloves during application. Teratogenic to hamsters in high dosages
Enilconazole 0.2%	*Chinchillas, mice, rats*: dip q7d	
Fipronil	*Hamsters, rats, mice*: 7.5 mg/kg topically q30–60d	Flea adulticide
Griseofulvin	1.5% in DMSO topically for 5–7 days	Potentially teratogenic
Ivermectin	*Mice*: 2 mg/kg topically behind ear	Use 1% ivermectin diluted 1:100 with 1:1 propylene glycol/water (0.1 mg/ml)
Lime sulphur dip (2.5%)	Dip q7d	
Malathion powder (3–5%)	Topically three times a week for 3 weeks. *Mice*: 0.37% powder in bedding	Caution with using powder in younger animals
Malathion spray 0.5% or dip 2%	Topically q7d for 3 weeks	
Miconazole ointment or cream 1% or 2%	*Guinea pigs*: apply q24h for 2–4 weeks	
Moxidectin	*Mice*: 0.5 mg/kg of 0.5% pour-on solution topically on dorsum	
Permethrin	0.25% dust in cage or 5% solution soaked cotton ball in cage 4–5 weeks	
Pyrethrin powder	*Guinea pigs* and *chinchillas*: topically q7d for 3 weeks (0.1%). *Hamsters, mice, rats, gerbils*: topically three times a week for 3 weeks (0.5%)	
Pyrethrin 0.05% shampoo	Shampoo q7d for 4 weeks	Fleas
Selamectin	*Guinea pigs*: 6 mg/kg topically. *Rats and mice*: 6 mg/kg topically	Rats and mice – the editors have used this dose successfully with no noted side effects
Silver sulfadiazine ointment	Apply topically to skin wounds q12–24h	Topical antibacterial and antifungal
Terbinafine cream 0.25%	*Guinea pigs*: apply q24h for 4 weeks	

5.11 (continued) Topical medications used in rodents. (Data from Antinoff *et al.*, 1999; Adamcack and Otten, 2000; Ellis and Mori, 2001; Hoefer and Crossley, 2002; Keeble, 2002; Orr, 2002; Pollock, 2003; Morrisey and Carpenter, 2004; O'Rourke, 2004; Ness, 2005; Hrapkiewicz and Medina, 2007)

Miscellaneous agents

Figure 5.12 lists dosages for miscellaneous drugs.

Drug	Dosage	Comments
Adrenaline	*Guinea pigs*: 0.003 mg/kg i.v. prn. *All species*: 0.01mg/kg (see Chapter 2)	Cardiac arrest
Aluminium hydroxide	20-40 mg/animal orally as needed	Hyperphosphataemia caused by renal disease
Aminophylline	*Guinea pigs*: 50 mg/kg	Bronchodilator

5.12 Miscellaneous drugs used in rodents. (Data from Vannevel, 1998; Antinoff *et al.*, 1999; Adamcack and Otten, 2000; Boothe, 2000; Ellis and Mori, 2001; Hoefer and Crossley, 2002; Keeble, 2002; Orr, 2002; Kottwitz and Kelleher, 2003; Donnelly, 2004; Morrisey and Carpenter, 2004; Ness, 2005; Hrapkiewicz and Medina, 2007) (continues) ▶

Drug	Dosage	Comments
Atropine	0.05–0.1 mg/kg s.c., i.m.	Preanaesthetic
	10 mg/kg s.c. q20min	Organophosphate toxicity; may cause cardiovascular abnormalities in guinea pigs
Betamethasone	*Rats, mice*: 0.1 mg/kg s.c.	Anti-inflammatory dose
Calcium gluconate	*Chinchillas*: 100 mg/kg i.p. *Guinea pigs*: 100 mg/kg i.m.	Hypocalcaemic tetany and eclampsia
Chlorphenamine	*Guinea pigs*: 0.6 mg/kg orally q24h	Antihistamine
Cimetidine	5–10 mg/kg orally, s.c., i.m., i.v. q6–12h	Oesophagitis, gastroesophageal reflux, gastric and/or duodenal ulceration
Cisapride	0.1–0.5 mg/kg orally q8–12h	Gastrointestinal prokinetic agent
Cyclophosphamide	*Guinea pigs*: 300 mg/kg i.p. q24h	Antineoplastic
Derm Caps® (essential fatty acid supplement; IVX Animal Health Inc, St Joseph, Missouri, USA)	*Mice*: 0.1 ml/animal q24h	Idiopathic skin disease
Dexamethasone	0.5–2 mg/kg s.c., i.m., i.v.	Anti-inflammatory
Digoxin	*Hamsters*: 0.05–0.1 mg/kg orally q12–24h	Dilated cardiomyopathy
Diphenhydramine	*Guinea pigs*: 7.5 mg/kg orally, 5 mg/kg s.c. prn *Chinchillas, hamsters, mice, rats*: 1–2 mg/kg orally, s.c. q12h	Antihistamine, anaphylaxis
Diphenylhydantoin	*Gerbils*: 25–50 mg/kg orally q12h	Anticonvulsant
Dopamine	*Guinea pigs*: 0.08 mg/kg i.v. prn	Hypotension, especially during anaesthesia
Doxapram	5 mg/kg i.v.	Respiratory stimulant
Edetate calcium disodium	*Guinea pigs, chinchillas, gerbils*: 30 mg/kg s.c. q12h for 5 days	Lead chelation
Ephedrine	*Guinea pigs*: 1 mg/kg orally, i.v. prn	Antihistamine, anaphylaxis
Fluoxetine	*Chinchillas*: 5–10 mg kg orally q24h	Fur chewing behaviour
Furosemide	*Guinea pigs, chinchillas*: 2–5 mg/kg orally, s.c. q12h *Hamsters, rats, mice, gerbils*: 2–10 mg/kg orally, s.c. q12h	
Glycopyrrolate	0.01–0.02 mg/kg s.c.	Bradycardia
Heparin	*Guinea pigs*: 5 mg/kg i.v. prn	DIC
Human chorionic gonadotrophin (hCG)	*Guinea pigs*: 1000 USP units/animal i.m., repeat 7–10d (100 IU/animal i.m.)	Cystic ovaries
Hydralazine	*Guinea pigs*: 1 mg/kg i.v. prn	Antihistamine
Insulin	*Guinea pigs*: 1–2 IU/animal q12h s.c. (NPH insulin) *Hamsters*: 2 U/animal s.c. *Rats*: 3 U or less/animal s.c.	
Kaolin pectin	*Guinea pigs*: 0.2 ml orally q6–8h	Antidiarrhoeal
Lactobacilli	Orally 2 hours prior to or following antibiotic administration	
Loperamide	0.1 mg/kg orally q8h for 3 days, then q24h for 2 days	Antidiarrhoeal; give in 1 ml water
Metoclopramide	0.2–1 mg/kg orally, s.c., i.m. q12h	Gastrointestinal prokinetic agent
Metyrapone	*Hamsters*: 8 mg/animal orally q24h for 30 days	Hyperadrenocorticism
Oxytocin	0.2–3 IU/kg s.c., i.m., i.v.	Induction or enhancement of uterine contractions and milk letdown
D-Penicillamine	*Gerbils*: 50 mg/kg orally q12h	Heavy metal chelator
Phenobarbital	*Guinea pigs*: 10–20 mg/kg i.v., i.p. *Gerbils*: 10–20 mg/kg orally	Seizures
Potassium citrate	*Guinea pigs*: 10–30 mg/kg orally q12h	Urinary alkalinizer

5.12 (continued) Miscellaneous drugs used in rodents. (Data from Vannevel, 1998; Antinoff *et al.*, 1999; Adamcack and Otten, 2000; Boothe, 2000; Ellis and Mori, 2001; Hoefer and Crossley, 2002; Keeble, 2002; Orr, 2002; Kottwitz and Kelleher, 2003; Donnelly, 2004; Morrisey and Carpenter, 2004; Ness, 2005; Hrapkiewicz and Medina, 2007) (continues) ▶

Drug	Dosage	Comments
Prednisone/prednisolone	0.5–2.2 mg/kg orally, s.c., i.m.	Anti-inflammatory
Primidone	*Gerbils*: 2.5–5 mg/animal orally q12h	Anticonvulsant
Pseudoephedrine	*Chinchillas*: 1.2 mg/animal orally q12h	Antihistamine
Sucralfate	25–50 mg/kg orally q8–12h	Treatment of oral, oesophageal, gastric and duodenal ulcers
Verapamil	*Hamsters*: 0.25–0.5 mg/kg s.c. q8h for 30 days	Cardiomyopathy
Vitamin A	*Guinea pigs, hamsters*: 500–5000 IU/kg i.m.	
Vitamin B complex	0.02–0.2 ml/kg s.c., i.m.	Dose based on small animal injectable formulation
Vitamin C	*Guinea pigs*: 10–30 mg/kg , orally, s.c., i.m. 0.2–0.4 mg/ml drinking water 50–100 mg/kg orally, s.c., i.m. q24h	Maintenance Treatment of deficiency
Vitamin D	200–400 IU/kg s.c., i.m.	May help with hamster cage paralysis
Vitamin E/selenium	0.1 ml/100–250 g body weight s.c.	Dose based on Bo-Se, Schering® formulation
Vitamin K	1–10 mg/kg i.m. q24h for 4–6 days 2.5–5 mg/kg i.m. q24h for 21–28 days	Warfarin poisoning Brodifacoum poisoning

5.12 (continued) Miscellaneous drugs used in rodents. (Data from Vannevel, 1998; Antinoff *et al.*, 1999; Adamcack and Otten, 2000; Boothe, 2000; Ellis and Mori, 2001; Hoefer and Crossley, 2002; Keeble, 2002; Orr, 2002; Kottwitz and Kelleher, 2003; Donnelly, 2004; Morrisey and Carpenter, 2004; Ness, 2005; Hrapkiewicz and Medina, 2007)

References and further reading

Adamcak A and Otten (2000) Rodent therapeutics. *Veterinary Clinics of North America: Exotic Animal Practice* **3(1)**, 221–237

Antinoff N, Boyer TH, Brown SA, Harkness JE and Sakas PS (1999) Rodent drug dosages. In: *Exotic Animal Formulary, 2nd edn*, pp. 113–132. AAHP Press, Lakewood, Colorado

Bihun C and Bauck L (2004) Rodents: basic anatomy, physiology, husbandry and clinical techniques. In: *Ferrets, Rabbits and Rodents Clinical Medicine and Surgery, 2nd edn*, ed. KE Quesenberry and JW Carpenter, pp. 286–298. WB Saunders, St Louis

Boothe DM (2000) Drugs affecting the respiratory system. *Veterinary Clinics of North America: Exotic Animal Practice* **3(2)**, 371–394

Burgmann (2000) Antimicrobial drug use in rodents, rabbits and ferrets. In: *Antimicrobial Therapy in Veterinary Medicine, 3rd edn*, ed. JF Prescott *et al.*, pp. 656–677. Veterinary Learning Systems, Trenton, New Jersey

Collins BR (1995) Antimicrobial drug use in rabbits, rodents, and other small mammals. In: *Antibiotic Therapy in Caged Birds and Exotic Pets*, pp 3–10. Iowa State University Press, Ames

Donnelly TM (2004a) Disease problems of chinchillas. In: *Ferrets, Rabbits and Rodents Clinical Medicine and Surgery, 2nd edn*, ed. KE Quesenberry and JW Carpenter, pp. 255–265. WB Saunders, St Louis

Donnelly TM (2004b) Disease problems of small rodents. In: *Ferrets, Rabbits and Rodents Clinical Medicine and Surgery, 2nd edn*, ed. KE Quesenberry and JW Carpenter, pp. 299–315. WB Saunders, St Louis

Ellis C and Mori M (2001) Skin diseases of rodents and small exotic mammals. *Veterinary Clinics of North America: Exotic Animal Practice* **4(2)**, 493–542

Harkness JE (1994) Small rodents. *Veterinary Clinics of North America: Small Animal Practice* **24(1)**, 89–102

Harkness JE and Wagner JE (1995) *Biology and Medicine of Rabbits and Rodents, 4th edn*. Williams and Wilkins, Media, Pennsylvania

Hoefer HL (1994) Chinchillas. *Veterinary Clinics of North America: Small Animal Practice* **24(1)**, 103–111

Hoefer HL and Crossley DA (2002) Chinchillas. In: *BSAVA Manual of Exotic Pets, 4th edn*, ed. A Meredith and S Redrobe, pp. 65–75. BSAVA Publications, Gloucester

Hrapkiewicz K and Medina M (2007) *Clinical Laboratory Animal Medicine: an Introduction, 3rd edn*. Blackwell Publishing Professional, Ames, Iowa

Johnson-Delaney CA, Carpenter J, Penner J *et al.* (2001) Nasal administration of sedatives to mice and rats. *Contemporary Topics in Laboratory Animal Science* **40(4)**, 83

Keeble E (2002) Gerbils. In: *BSAVA Manual of Exotic Pets, 4th edn*, ed. A Meredith and S Redrobe, pp 34–46. BSAVA Publications, Gloucester

Kottwitz J and Kelleher S (2003) Emergency drugs: quick reference chart for exotic animals. *Exotic DVM* **5(5)**, 23–25

Lankas GR and Gordon LR (1989) Toxicology. In: *Ivermectin and Abamactin*, ed. WC Campbell, pp. 89–112. Springer-Verlag, New York

Lipman NS, Weischedel AK, Connors MJ *et al.* (1992) Utilization of cholestyramine resin as a preventive treatment for antibiotic (clindamycin) induced enterotoxaemia in the rabbit. *Laboratory Animals* **26**, 1–8

Morris TH (1995) Antibiotic therapeutics in laboratory animals. *Laboratory Animals* **29**, 16–36

Morrisey JK and Carpenter JW (2004) Formulary. In: *Ferrets, Rabbits and Rodents Clinical Medicine and Surgery, 2nd edn*, ed. KE Quesenberry and JW Carpenter, pp. 436–444. WB Saunders, St Louis

Ness RD (2005) Rodents. In: *Exotic Animal Formulary, 3rd edn*, ed. JW Carpenter, pp. 377–408. Elsevier Saunders, St Louis

O'Rourke DP (2004) Disease problems of guinea pigs. In: *Ferrets, Rabbits and Rodents Clinical Medicine and Surgery, 2nd edn*, ed. KE Quesenberry and JW Carpenter, pp. 299–315. WB Saunders, St Louis

Orcutt C (2000) Use of vascular access ports in exotic animals. *Exotic DVM* **2(3)**, 34–38

Orr HE (2002) Rats and mice. In: *BSAVA Manual of Exotic Pets, 4th edn*, ed. A Meredith and S Redrobe, pp 13–25. BSAVA Publications, Gloucester

Pollock C (2003) Fungal diseases of laboratory rodents. *Veterinary Clinics of North America: Exotic Animal Practice* **6(2)**, 401–413

Powers LV (2006) Techniques for drug delivery in small mammals. *Journal of Exotic Pet Medicine* **15(3)**, 201–209

Quesenberry KE (1994) Guinea pigs. *Veterinary Clinics of North America: Small Animal Practice* **24(1)**, 67–87

Ramsey I (2008) *BSAVA Small Animal Formulary, 6th edn*. BSAVA Publications, Gloucester

Rosenthal KL (2004) Therapeutic contraindications in exotic pets. *Seminars in Avian and Exotic Pet Medicine* **13(1)**, 44–48

Rossoff IS (1994) *Handbook of Veterinary Drugs and Chemicals, 2nd edn*. Pharmatox Publishing, Taylorville, Illinois

Vannevel J (1998) Diabetes mellitus in a 3-year-old intact female guinea pig. *The Canadian Veterinary Journal* **39**, 503–504

6

Rodents: anaesthesia and analgesia

Claire Richardson and Paul Flecknell

Introduction

Veterinary surgeons may be wary of anaesthetizing rodents as they are often less familiar with these small species. Rodent anaesthesia can be challenging because, although the various species of rodent tend to be physically similar, they often differ in their response to anaesthetics. Similarly, drug effects vary with the age, sex and strain of the animal. The relatively short life span of these species can also result in a high proportion of aged patients being anaesthetized. For example, a 30-month-old rat presented for removal of a mammary tumour should be considered geriatric. These factors may explain why anaesthetic mortality in rodents has been higher than for other small animals such as dogs and cats (Brodbelt, 2006).

Fortunately rodents can be anaesthetized safely and reliably provided that the anaesthetic regimens are chosen with care and that attention is given to all stages of the procedure. There has also been a growth in resources available on the subject of the veterinary care of rodents and an increase in the number of veterinary surgeons with a special interest in 'exotic' species, including rodents. This has led to practices becoming better equipped to treat small mammals. The increased demand for appropriate anaesthetic equipment and monitoring devices has resulted in these becoming more affordable and hence more widely available. The results of research into pain assessment and alleviation, aimed at improving the welfare of laboratory animals, can also be applied to pet rodents. This has provided information on the safe and effective use of a range of different analgesics.

General considerations

Four main factors are critical for improving the outcome of anaesthetic protocols: reduction of risk factors by improving the clinical condition of the patient; prevention of hypothermia; prevention of hypoxia; and provision of safe and effective analgesia.

Risk factor reduction

Clearly the risk of anaesthetic complications is higher if an animal's health is compromised. Although sometimes it is necessary to anaesthetize animals with pre-existing clinical problems, these should be corrected prior to anaesthesia whenever possible.

Carrying out a complete physical examination prior to anaesthesia is therefore particularly important. Dental diseases are common in rodents (see Chapter 8) and these conditions may lead to other problems, such as dehydration. Fluid deficits may also arise from numerous other conditions and so the state of hydration should be assessed and fluid deficits should be corrected prior to induction of anaesthesia (see Chapter 2). Small mammals are prone to obesity and overweight patients are higher anaesthetic risks. Prevention of obesity is therefore critical and clients should be educated about appropriate diets when pets are first presented for examination or treatment (see Chapter 1).

Prevention of hypothermia

One of the most common complications to occur when anaesthetizing rodents is hypothermia. All animals are susceptible to hypothermia when anaesthetized since most anaesthetics depress thermoregulatory mechanisms. Rodents are particularly prone to losing heat quickly because of their high ratios of surface area to volume. Hypothermia can result in increased anaesthetic recovery times and other complications (such as cardiovascular depression) and so measures to minimize heat loss must be employed.

There are numerous methods that can used to help to maintain body temperature (for review see Murison, 2001) and typically several of these methods are combined during anaesthesia. Insulation should be provided from blankets (e.g. Drybed®, William Daniels, UK), bubble wrap (Figure 6.1) or foil 'space blankets'. If the rodent is wrapped, this should be done carefully so as not to impede respiration. The area of fur clipped prior to surgery should also be minimized as fur provides natural insulation for the animal. The administration of warmed fluids intraoperatively can help to keep the animal warm

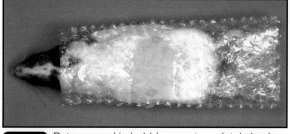

6.1 Rat wrapped in bubble wrap to maintain body temperature, with hole cut over surgical site.

and whenever possible the environmental temperature of the room should be raised. To minimize heat loss through evaporative losses, surgical scrub should be warmed prior to application and it should be used sparingly. Warming devices include electric heating blankets and circulating water-warming blankets, but the blanket temperature should be monitored to avoid burns. It is advisable to place a temperature probe between the heat pad and the animal, in addition to monitoring rectal or oesophageal temperature. A warm environment is also important in the recovery period (see postoperative care).

Respiratory depression

Most anaesthetics depress respiratory function, resulting in hypercapnia and hypoxia. During the relatively brief periods of anaesthesia needed for most surgical procedures in rodents, hypercapnia is usually well tolerated. Hypoxia, however, can be life-threatening. Small rodents often have an increased risk of respiratory failure because of the high incidence of chronic respiratory disease in some species (e.g. rats and mice). To minimize the risk of hypoxia, oxygen should be administered as a routine. Intubation where possible is also recommended.

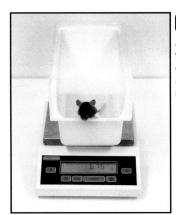

6.2 Rat on scale. Determining an accurate weight to within 0.1–0.5 g allows effective dosing and aids postoperative monitoring.

Analgesia

Analgesics should be administered to all patients undergoing potentially painful procedures. Unalleviated pain increases the likelihood of postanaesthetic complications, including increased recovery times, postoperative anorexia and gastrointestinal disturbances.

Preanaesthetic preparations

Rodents should be weighed accurately (Figure 6.2) prior to induction of anaesthesia. This will allow a safe and effective dose of anaesthetic to be administered and also enables effective postoperative monitoring. Suitable scales, which are widely available and inexpensive, should weigh to an accuracy of 0.1–0.5 g, to allow monitoring of blood and fluid loss in the smallest animals. Because rodents do not vomit, it is unnecessary to withhold food and water prior to anaesthesia. Guinea pigs often retain food at the back of their mouth and so food and water can be removed 1 hour prior to the induction of anaesthesia. Food and water should not be withheld from guinea pigs and chinchillas for any longer than this, since fasting increases the likelihood of them developing postoperative gastrointestinal disturbances.

Every effort should be made to minimize stress prior to the induction of anaesthesia as anaesthetic complications are less likely when the animal is calm during induction. To minimize stress, careful thought should be given as to where rodents are housed prior to anaesthesia. Small mammals should be housed away from the sight and smells of potential predators, including dogs, cats and ferrets, but housed with cage mates if possible. Stress can be minimized during the preanaesthetic physical examination by the use of humane and effective handling techniques (see Chapter 2). Sedation should be considered for fractious animals and those that are not routinely handled (Figure 6.3).

Sedative/ tranquillizer	Mice	Rats	Hamsters	Gerbils	Guinea pigs	Chinchillas	Degus
Acepromazine	2–5 mg/kg s.c., i.p.[a]	2.5 mg/kg i.m., i.p.[a]	5 mg/kg i.p.[b]	*	0.5–1 mg/kg i.m.[c]	0.5–1 mg/kg i.m.[d]	–
Diazepam	5 mg/kg i.m., i.p.[a]	2.5–5 mg/kg i.m., i.p.[a]	5 mg/kg i.m., i.p.[b]	5 mg/kg i.m., i.p.[a]	2.5 mg/kg i.m., i.p.[c]	1–5 mg/kg i.m.[d]	–
Fentanyl/ fluanisone	0.1–0.3 ml/kg i.p.[a]	0.2–0.5 ml/kg i.m.[a]	0.5 ml/kg i.m.[b]	0.5–1 ml/kg i.m., i.p.[a]	0.5. ml/kg i.m.[b]	–	–
Medetomidine	30–100 µg/kg s.c.[a]	30–100 µg/kg s.c.[a]	100 µg/kg s.c., i.p.[a]	100–200 µg/kg i.p.[a]	–	–	300 µg/kg s.c.[e]
Midazolam	5 mg/kg i.m.[a]	2.5 mg/kg i.p.[b]	5 mg/kg i.m., i.p.[a]	5 mg/kg i.m., i.p.[a]	5 mg/kg i.m.[b]	1–2 mg/kg s.c., i.m.[d]	–
Xylazine	5–10 mg/kg i.p.[a]	1–5 mg/kg i.m., i.p.[a]	5 mg/kg i.m., i.p.[a]	2 mg/kg i.m., i.p.[a]	–	2–10 mg/kg i.m.[d]	–

6.3 Sedatives and tranquillizers for rodents. Doses at the lower end of the range should be used for old and overweight animals and for animals in poor health. Data adapted from: [a] Flecknell (1996); [b] Flecknell (2007); [c] Flecknell (2002); [d] Hoefer and Crossley (2002); [e] Johnson-Delaney (2005). * Acepromazine is contraindicated in gerbils as it may lower the seizure threshold (Heard, 2004).

The routine administration of preanaesthetic medication/sedation is recommended for many species due to its anaesthetic-sparing effect and because the use of preanaesthetic medication often results in smoother anaesthetic induction and recoveries (Penderis and Franklin, 2005). In rodents, however, their use is less common due to the techniques generally used for anaesthesia.

In some rodents, an anticholinergic premedication may be necessary to reduce bronchial and salivary secretions and to inhibit vagal responses, including bradycardia. Atropine (0.004 mg/kg s.c or i.m; Flecknell *et al.*, 2007) or glycopyrrolate (0.01–0.02 mg/kg s.c or i.m; Heard, 2004) may be administered.

Choice of anaesthetic

A variety of inhaled and injectable anaesthetic agents are suitable for use in rodents. It is always preferable to select an agent that allows the anaesthetist to adjust the depth of anaesthesia quickly; therefore inhaled anaesthetic agents are preferred by the authors. If injectable anaesthetic agents are used, it is safer to use a drug that can be administered intravenously rather than by subcutaneous, intramuscular or intraperitoneal routes. With intravenous administration, drug effects are seen quickly and the dose can be

adjusted and given to effect, but the small size of rodents often makes intravenous administration difficult. To minimize the risk of anaesthetic complications, it is preferable to use an anaesthetic with a wide safety margin and one with a specific antagonist that allows the drug effects to be reversed quickly (e.g. medetomidine, which can be reversed with atipamezole).

The use of two or more anaesthetic agents in combination ('balanced anaesthesia') is also recommended as the undesirable side effects of individual drugs can be reduced by giving lower doses of each. Balanced anaesthesia can be achieved by combining two or more systemic anaesthetic or analgesic agents or by combining systemic anaesthetics with local anaesthetics. Local anaesthetics such as lidocaine or bupivacaine may be infiltrated on to the surgical field (Figure 6.4) and they will reduce the general anaesthesia requirement. Lidocaine is a shorter-acting anaesthetic than bupivacaine (60–120 vs. 180–480 minutes) (Skarda and Tranquilli, 2007). Compared with other small animals, such as dogs and cats, rodents do not have an increased susceptibility to the toxic effects from local anaesthetics, but it is much easier to overdose rodents because of their small size. Therefore, it is advisable to draw up the maximum safe volume for infiltration in advance (e.g. lidocaine at up to 5 mg/kg, equivalent to 0.05 ml of a 2% solution for a 200 g rat) and then to ensure that this safe volume is not exceeded. Lidocaine can be diluted to 0.25% by the addition of saline to allow more effective tissue infiltration. The maximum safe volume for infiltration of bupivacaine is 2 mg/kg (Hawkins, 2006).

Use of injectable anaesthetics

A variety of injectable anaesthetic agents are available for use in rodents (Figure 6.5). These drugs, with the exception of fentanyl/fluanisone, do not have a veterinary product licence and therefore in the UK the veterinary prescribing cascade should be adhered to. Oxygen supplementation should be provided throughout the anaesthetic and can be administered through a facemask, an endotracheal tube or an intranasal catheter.

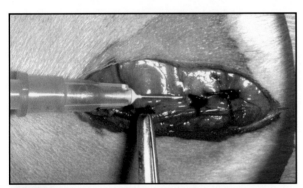

6.4 Infiltration of the surgical field with a local anaesthetic such as lidocaine or bupivacaine.

Anaesthetic	Mice	Rats	Hamsters	Gerbils	Guinea pigs	Chinchillas
Fentanyl/fluanisone and diazepam	0.3 ml/kg i.m. + 5 mg/kg i.p.[a]	0.3 ml/kg i.m. + 2.5 mg/kg i.p.[a]	1 ml/kg i.m. or i.p. + 5 mg/kg i.p.[b]	0.3 ml/kg i.m. or i.p. + 5 mg/kg i.p.[b]	1 ml/kg i.m. + 2.5 mg/kg i.p.[b]	–
Fentanyl/fluanisone and midazolam	10 ml/kg i.p.[b]*	2.7 ml/kg i.p.[b]*	4 ml/kg i.p.[b]*	8 ml/kg i.p.[b]*	8 ml/kg i.p.[b]	–
Ketamine and medetomidine	75 mg/kg + 1 mg/kg i.p.[b]	75 mg/kg + 0.5 mg/kg i.p.[b]	100 mg/kg + 0.25 mg/kg i.p.	75 mg/kg + 0.5 mg/kg i.p., s.c., i.m.[d]	40 mg/kg + 0.5 mg/kg i.p.[b]	5 mg/kg + 0.06 mg/kg i.m.[e]
Ketamine and xylazine	80–100 mg/kg + 10 mg/kg i.p.[b]	75–100 mg/kg + 10 mg/kg i.p.[b]	50–200 ml/kg + 5–10 mg/kg i.p.[c]	50 mg/kg + 2 mg/kg i.p.[b]	40 mg/kg + 5 mg/mg i.p.[b]	20–40 mg/kg + 3–5 mg/kg i.p., i.v.[c]
Propofol	26 mg/kg i.v.[b]	10 mg/kg i.v.[b]	–	–	10 mg/kg i.v.[c]	10 mg/kg i.v.[c]

6.5 Injectable anaesthetics for rodents. Note that most drugs do not have a product licence for use in rodents. Variations in individual responses may occur, so dose rates should be taken only as a general guide. Data adapted from: [a] Flecknell (2007); [b] Flecknell (1996); [c] Heard (2004); [d] Keeble (2002); [e] Henke *et al.* (2004). * Dose rates of fentanyl/fluanisone and midazolam are given as ml/kg of a mixture of one part fentanyl/fluanisone (Hypnorm®, VetaPharma, Leeds), one part midazolam (initial concentration 5 mg/ml) and two parts water for injection. Add the active components to the water for injection and mix well.

Although intravenous anaesthetic administration is usually preferable, intravenous access can be difficult in rodents and it is often necessary to use alternative routes of administration. Subcutaneous, intraperitoneal and intramuscular injection techniques are straightforward (see Chapters 2 and 5) but drug absorption and therefore drug effects by these routes are variable. As previously discussed, there is also often a large variation in response to anaesthetics between different strains and ages and between male and female rodents. Due to these factors, it is not uncommon for an injectable anaesthetic to be used at the recommended dose rate but for the rodent to remain insufficiently anaesthetized for surgery. If this occurs, the injectable anaesthetic can be supplemented with a low concentration of volatile anaesthetics and/or the surgical site can be infiltrated with local anaesthetic. It is also possible to administer a 'top-up' dose of injectable anaesthetic at approximately one-third of the original dose rate, though this should be used as a last resort due to the risk of overdosing the animal and because additional doses of injectable anaesthetics tend to result in a prolonged recovery period.

Recommended injectable anaesthetic regimens for rodents

Neuroleptanalgesia: fentanyl/fluanisone (Hypnorm®) with a benzodiazepine (diazepam or midazolam): Neuroleptanalgesia is the state of profound sedation and analgesia produced by the administration of an opioid analgesic combined with a sedative. For surgical anaesthesia, it is preferable to use fentanyl/fluanisone in combination with other agents since, on its own, muscle relaxation is generally poor and because the high doses of fentanyl/fluanisone required for surgical anaesthesia result in respiratory depression. Fentanyl/fluanisone may be combined with a benzodiazepine such as diazepam or midazolam. The agents can be mixed with water for injection and given as a single intraperitoneal injection (for dose rates see Figure 6.5). The dose of fentanyl/fluanisone mix by subcutaneous injection is variable as there is significant first-pass extraction of the fentanyl by the liver. The authors therefore do not recommend its use subcutaneously without further dose-ranging studies. To prolong anaesthesia, diazepam or midazolam may be administered intravenously to effect (fentanyl/fluanisone produces vasodilation so subsequent intravenous access is easier).

An advantage of using this neuroleptanalgesic combination is that recovery can be enhanced by the administration of a mixed opioid agonist/antagonist such as butorphanol or a partial agonist such as buprenorphine. Butorphanol and buprenorphine will both reverse the respiratory depression caused by fentanyl but maintain postoperative analgesia. Although antagonists of benzodiazepines can be administered (e.g. flumazenil) to speed recovery, their duration of action is short and resedation may occur. These antagonists are also expensive and often available only in large-dose single-use vials.

Ketamine combinations: ketamine with an alpha₂ agonist (medetomidine or xylazine): Ketamine is a dissociative anaesthetic agent and when used alone in rodents it produces immobility rather than surgical anaesthesia. The combination of ketamine with an alpha₂ agonist such as medetomidine or xylazine, however, results in surgical anaesthesia with good muscle relaxation. The ketamine and medetomidine or xylazine can be combined and given by a single injection, usually by the intraperitoneal route (see Figure 6.5). Subcutaneous injection of these drugs is not recommended by the authors, due to the lack of controlled studies using this route. There is a significant risk of cutaneous reactions or muscle necrosis following subcutaneous or intramuscular ketamine injection. Compared with smaller rodents, the effects of ketamine and medetomidine or xylazine in guinea pigs are less uniform and some guinea pigs may not be sufficiently deeply anaesthetized for surgery to be carried out humanely. It is not known whether the same is true for chinchillas and degus, but anecdotal reports suggest that these combinations do provide a uniform plane of anaesthesia in these species.

Propofol: Propofol produces short-term general anaesthesia that can be prolonged by the use of 'top-up' doses. Its use is limited in rodents since it needs to be administered intravenously (if given by the intraperitoneal route the effects are less predictable) and, as discussed, intravenous access can be difficult in rodents. Apnoea may be a problem when administering the drug intravenously since it is difficult to give a sufficiently slow injection, because of the low volume of injectate required in these small animals.

Use of volatile anaesthetics
Isoflurane and sevoflurane are the most commonly used inhaled/volatile anaesthetics. Although sevoflurane is more expensive, it is sometimes preferred to isoflurane in other species since induction and recovery tend to be faster and smoother. In small rodents, the difference in induction and recovery times between the two agents is not large, but the recovery from sevoflurane is often smoother. Induction of anaesthesia can be via a facemask, but induction chambers are usually preferable as they are associated with less handling stress. Use of an appropriately small chamber for smaller rodents increases the speed of induction and allows some reduction of fresh gas flow rates. It is possible to induce anaesthesia with sevoflurane and then maintain anaesthesia with isoflurane if economic considerations are important.

Anaesthetic induction chambers
Anaesthetic induction chambers can be manufactured from transparent polypropylene boxes (Figure 6.6). Chambers should be filled from the bottom and waste gases scavenged from the top. Commercially available anaesthetic induction boxes that incorporate a scavenging system are also available (Figure 6.7).

When an anaesthetic induction chamber is used, the animal should initially be placed into the clean empty chamber. The chamber may be preoxygenated and should then be filled rapidly with the safe induction

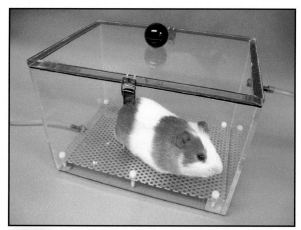

6.6 Guinea pig in a simple anaesthetic induction chamber. The chamber is filled from the bottom and waste gases are scavenged from the top.

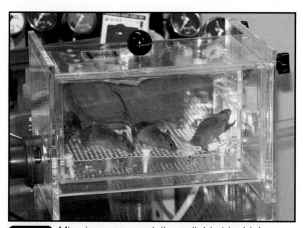

6.7 Mice in a commercially available 'double' induction box which incorporates gas scavenging. (Courtesy of Harvard Apparatus, IMS, Kent)

concentration of the anaesthetic agent (e.g. 5% isoflurane, 8% sevoflurane). This minimizes any involuntary excitement during induction. After the animal has lost its righting reflex, it can be removed from the chamber and anaesthesia maintained on a facemask (e.g. 1.5–2% isoflurane, 3–5% sevoflurane).

In guinea pigs, induction with isoflurane often results in salivation and lacrimation, probably due to irritation of mucous membranes (Flecknell, 2002). Although sevoflurane appears to be less irritating, lacrimation and salivation still occur and so preanaesthetic sedation should be administered to guinea pigs prior to anaesthetic induction with an inhaled anaesthetic agent.

Endotracheal intubation
Although endotracheal intubation in small mammals is possible, it can be technically difficult due to the small diameter of the rodent trachea. Plastic intravenous catheters (e.g. 14 gauge catheter for use in rats) or infusion-set tubing may be used as endotracheal tubes, though they are often associated with kinks or occlusions. Techniques described for intubation of rodents include the blind technique (Redrobe and Meredith, 1999) and the use of a flexible videoendoscope (Fuentes *et al.*, 2004; Lichtenberger and Ko, 2007). Mouse and rat intubation is also possible using

commercially available rodent workstands and intubation packs (Halowell Instruments). (This technique is illustrated on a CD available from www.digires. co.uk; see also Chapter 2 for a description.)

Facemasks
A variety of facemasks suitable for use with small mammals is available commercially, or masks can be constructed from materials such as plastic syringe barrels. A convenient system that ensures effective gas scavenging is also available (Figure 6.8) and, to provide more effective gas scavenging, it can be used in combination with a heated mini downdraft table (Fluovac masks and heated mini downdraft table, VetTech Solutions Ltd, Cheshire).

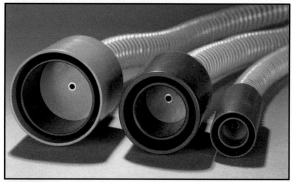

6.8 Rodent facemasks of various sizes that incorporate a gas-scavenging system. Anaesthetics are delivered through the inner ring and scavenged from the outer ring.

Intranasal catheters
Although use of inhalational agents is a safe and effective method of anaesthetizing all small rodents, maintenance using a facemask can make access to the head and neck difficult. This is a particular problem when undertaking dental procedures. As an alternative to endotracheal intubation, delivery of anaesthetic vapour using a nasal catheter can provide a convenient method of maintaining anaesthesia. This technique is effective as many rodents are nasal breathers. In guinea pigs, small nasogastric feeding tubes, or urinary catheters, can be used. In rats and mice, plastic intravenous catheters can be used (Figure 6.9).

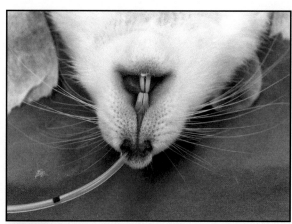

6.9 Rat with an intranasal catheter that can be used for oxygen supplementation or inhaled anaesthetic administration.

In most rodents the external nares have a muscular sphincter and the nasal passage has a larger diameter. Gentle pressure is applied to introduce the catheter, directing it medially and ventrally. If the animal is too lightly anaesthetized it will sneeze, and anaesthesia should be deepened in the induction chamber. Slight epistaxis occasionally occurs at this stage but is easily resolved by applying direct pressure to the side of the nose. This technique is also useful for delivering oxygen to animals anaesthetized using injectable agents. The gas flow rates needed to maintain anaesthesia are similar to those needed to prevent rebreathing when using a facemask (3 times minute volume). However, lower flows will be sufficient to prevent hypoxia. Unfortunately, waste gas scavenging may be difficult using this technique, unless a small downdraft table is used (see above), but due to the low flow rates required with this system, the concentration of waste gases at the level of the operator is typically very low.

Intraoperative care and anaesthetic monitoring

As with larger species, small rodents should be monitored during anaesthesia and in the postoperative period. Whichever method of anaesthesia is used, the eyes should be protected to prevent corneal desiccation and ulceration, either by covering them with damp gauze or by applying a topical ophthalmic ointment (Figure 6.10).

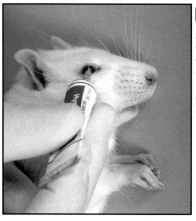

6.10 Application of ophthalmic ointment to cover corneas and prevent corneal desiccation during anaesthesia.

As discussed earlier, hypothermia is a common complication of rodent anaesthesia; therefore body temperature should be monitored carefully and sufficient warmth should be provided throughout the anaesthetic. Fluid therapy should also be considered (see also Chapter 2).

Clinical monitoring

Simple observation of the animal's vital signs should not be neglected. The depth of anaesthesia can be assessed using the pedal withdrawal or tail pinch reflex. The tail pinch is assessed by firmly pinching the tip of the tail using the operator's fingernails. It is important to pinch hard enough to produce a painful stimulus, but not so hard as to damage the tail. If the animal is too lightly anaesthetized for surgery, it will flick its tail and may vocalize. The tail pinch response is usually lost at light to medium planes of anaesthesia, and this is followed by a loss of the pedal withdrawal response at medium to deep planes of anaesthesia. Most surgical procedures can be carried out when the pedal withdrawal reflex is absent or barely detectable. In guinea pigs, the ear pinch reflex can also be used to measure anaesthetic depth.

Ocular reflexes are not as useful in small mammals as in the dog and cat. With most anaesthetic regimens, the position of the eye remains fixed in rodents, and the palpebral (blink) reflex may still be present at surgical planes of anaesthesia.

Although a peripheral pulse cannot usually be felt, the heart rate can be monitored by gentle palpation (so as not to restrict respiratory movements) of the thorax. The heart rate will be too rapid to count in a normal animal, but may slow dramatically during cardiovascular failure. This can be monitored by use of an ECG, but a device that can record rapid heart rates (e.g. >400 bpm) is required. Commercially available oesophageal stethoscopes are too large for use in the majority of rodents.

The rate and pattern of respiration can be monitored, but the animal may be obscured by surgical drapes. This problem can be avoided by use of transparent plastic drapes, which are also lighter than their cloth counterparts. The colour of the toes, ears, nose and mucous membranes allows some assessment of oxygen saturation, but visible cyanosis only occurs when the saturation has fallen to 50–60%, so should be regarded as an emergency.

Although both the pattern and rate of respiration will change during anaesthesia, this varies greatly depending upon the anaesthetic regimen used. Becoming familiar with one or two regularly used regimens allows changes to be interpreted more reliably. In general, once anaesthesia has been induced, respiratory rate decreases markedly, especially as most of these animals will show tachypnoea prior to induction. Typical respiratory rates for rodents during anaesthesia are 50–100 breaths per minutes. A reduction to less than 50% of the estimated normal respiratory rate should give cause for concern.

As with dogs and cats, it is more common to see gradual changes in rate, rather than a sudden reduction. For this reason, it is helpful to keep a written anaesthetic record when assessing the state of the animal during anaesthesia.

It is also important to monitor the activities of the surgeon, since traction during surgery, placing instruments across the animal's chest or steadying the surgeon's hand on the animal can seriously compromise respiratory movements and must be avoided.

Electronic monitoring devices

When using electronic monitoring devices, a number of practical problems will be encountered, particularly when anaesthetizing the smallest rodents. The small size of these animals results in low signal strength that may not be detected by some monitors. These species also have high heart rates that can exceed the upper limits of some pulse oximeters. The low tidal volumes can restrict the use of capnographs, and (in the authors' experience) non-invasive blood pressure monitors do not function effectively. Despite these limitations, some degree of monitoring should always be possible (see also Chapter 2 for a more detailed description of these techniques in rodents).

Probably the most useful electronic monitoring devices are pulse oximeters and electronic thermometers. Pulse oximeters that can detect high heart rates and low signal strengths are now available (Figure 6.11). Probes can be placed on the paws or in the mouth of larger species (>200 g). Electronic thermometers with a probe size suitable for placement in the rectum of animals of 200 g or larger are readily available. It is important to check that the model selected will read temperatures lower than 35°C, since animals may have cooled to this temperature or lower during preparation for surgery.

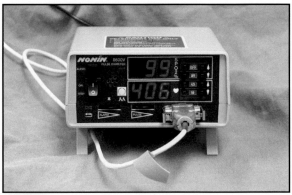

6.11 Pulse oximeter. (Courtesy of Nonin, Kruuse, North Yorkshire)

Respiratory monitors that are triggered by heating of a thermistor by the animal's breath function well in larger rodents (>500 g), but often fail to detect expiration in smaller mammals. Mainstream capnographs have too large a deadspace and usually require intubation to monitor end-tidal carbon dioxide effectively. Side-stream capnographs often have relatively high sampling rates, so accurate measurements may not be provided. However, trends in carbon dioxide concentrations can be of value. Instruments with a sample rate of 50 ml/min are available (e.g. Capnovet 10, Vet-Tech Solutions Ltd, Cheshire) and these provide more accurate measures.

Monitoring blood loss

Blood loss should be monitored by weighing swabs. As in other species, loss of more than 15% of circulating volume should be a cause for concern, and fluid therapy should be provided (see Chapter 2). Ideally, this should be by the intravenous route, but this is difficult to achieve. An alternative is to place an interosseous catheter (Chapter 2) and this can remain in place to allow continued therapy in the postoperative period. If neither of these options is considered practicable, warmed fluid should be given intraperitoneally or subcutaneously, though absorption will be considerably slower. Since most small mammals will either lose fluid, or have reduced intake postoperatively, routine use of fluids is advisable.

Dealing with anaesthetic emergencies

If respiratory failure occurs, oxygen should be provided immediately if it is not already being administered. The animal's head and neck should be extended, and respiration assisted by gently squeezing the thorax. Alternatively, a mask can be placed over the animal's nose and the chest inflated by gently blowing into a tube attached to the other end. This should only be done in emergencies, as gastric dilatation and bloat are potential complications associated with this technique in some species. If surgery has been completed, the anaesthetic should be discontinued, or reversed using a specific antagonist. Respiration can also be stimulated using doxapram at 5–10 mg/kg, which may be administered by the intravenous, intramuscular or intraperitoneal route (see Chapter 2 for more details).

Cardiovascular failure can be managed in a similar way as in larger species. External cardiac massage can provide effective circulatory support, but practical problems of venous access limit the use of fluid therapy and emergency drugs. It is best to prevent problems by careful adjustment of the anaesthetic depth to avoid anaesthetic overdose and by meticulous surgical technique to avoid blood loss (see also Chapter 2).

Postoperative care

Monitoring and supportive measures should be continued into the postoperative period. In particular, body temperature must be maintained, initially by providing a temperature of approximately 35°C. This can be lowered to 26–28°C as the animal recovers consciousness. Provision of a suitable recovery area (e.g. an incubator) should be established as part of the *pre*operative preparations, so that it can be stabilized at an appropriate temperature. Animals should be provided with warm, comfortable bedding. Sawdust is not suitable; a layer of bedding such as Drybed® (William Daniels, UK) should be provided for the initial recovery period, and once the animal has regained activity it can be transferred to a cage or pen containing either shredded paper (small rodents) or good quality hay or straw (chinchillas and guinea pigs). This type of bedding allows the animal to surround itself with insulating material, which provides both warmth and a sense of security (Figure 6.12). Chinchilla dust baths should be removed until the animal is fully recovered, else ocular trauma and inhalation of dust may occur.

Animals should be provided with water, but care must be taken that they do not spill water bowls (if the animal becomes wet it will lose heat rapidly). Small rodents are usually accustomed to using water bottles, so this is rarely a problem, but it can present difficulties with guinea pigs. With all species it is usually advisable to administer warmed (37°C) subcutaneous or intraperitoneal dextrose/saline at the end of surgery to provide some fluid supplementation in the immediate postoperative period.

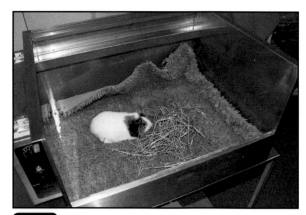

6.12 Guinea pig in a warm incubator with hay.

Animals should be encouraged to eat as soon as possible after recovery from anaesthesia. Rats and mice may prefer a softened diet and other species should be given their preferred foods. Prokinetic drugs should also be administered to guinea pigs and chinchillas, to avoid postanaesthetic ileus. Metoclopramide (0.2–1 mg/kg) may be administered orally, subcutaneously or intramuscularly every 12 hours. In rats, NSAIDs are effective at preventing postsurgical ileus.

One final point to note is that small mammals should ideally be allowed to recover away from the sight, sound and smell of predators such as dogs and cats. It should be noted that handling a cat or dog and then handling a small rodent can result in the animal experiencing considerable stress, so wearing a clean laboratory coat or gown and washing hands between patients is advisable.

Analgesia

As previously discussed, it is particularly important that good pre- and postoperative analgesia is provided to small rodents; pain can cause inappetence and prolong the effects of surgery. A major obstacle to achieving this goal is the relative lack of information relating to signs of pain in small mammals and a consequent uncertainty about effective dose rates of analgesic agents.

As a general guide, two principles can be adopted:

1. Changes in the normal behaviour of an animal, in circumstances that would be expected to cause pain in more familiar species (and in humans), should be considered as possible indicators of pain. Administering an analgesic and noting the animal's response can help to determine whether the changes in behaviour were pain related.
2. Small mammals have the same mechanisms for detecting and transmitting painful stimuli as larger species (for review see Livingston and Chambers, 2000). It is reasonable to assume, even in the absence of behavioural changes, that pain will be present after procedures such as surgery and so analgesics should be administered.

Pain-related behaviours

Studies in rats and mice have shown that both species display some specific behavioural changes after abdominal surgery, including orchidectomy. Rats show characteristic back arching, belly pressing and contractions of the abdominal muscles (Roughan and Flecknell, 2001, 2003). Mice show similar abdominal contractions and belly pressing but no back arching (Wright-Williams et al., 2007). Both species may show a twitching of the skin of the back and may stagger when moving. All of these behaviours are typically interspersed with normal activities such as grooming, rearing, walking and so on. Similar studies have not been undertaken in other species of small mammals, but additional analgesia should be provided if behaviours such as these are noticed.

In rats, mice and guinea pigs, food and water consumption are reduced following surgery, and this reduction can be minimized by administration of analgesics. Direct monitoring of food and water consumption can be difficult but reductions in intake are reflected in a fall in body weight, which is easy to monitor.

In addition to these more specific signs of pain, it is believed that rodents in pain may be less active, show guarding behaviour and may become more aggressive or, conversely, relatively apathetic. Other signs may include a ruffled coat or hunched posture. In rats the build-up of a red/brown discharge around the eyes and nose (porphyrin staining) is a non-specific response to pain or other stress (Figure 6.13). One problem that will be encountered when trying to detect behavioural signs of pain is that some animals (including most guinea pigs) may become completely immobile when observed.

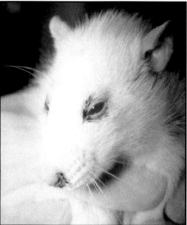

6.13
Porphyrin staining around the eyes and nose of a rat.

Analgesic administration

Safe dose rates for a wide range of analgesics have been established for rats and mice when the various drugs were developed and their efficacy assessed before being marketed for use in humans. Dose rates that are effective for postoperative pain relief have been established for some laboratory strains of rats and mice. There is much less information for small mammals such as guinea pigs and hamsters, and no controlled studies have been undertaken in chinchillas, degus and less familiar rodents. The dose rates listed in Figure 6.14 have been developed using these data,

Analgesic	Mice	Rats	Hamsters	Gerbils	Guinea pigs	Chinchillas	Degus
Buprenorphine	0.1 mg/kg s.c., q8–12h[a]	0.05 mg/kg s.c., q8–12h[a]	0.1 mg/kg s.c.[f], ?q6–8h	0.1 mg/kg s.c.[f], ?q6–8h	0.05 mg/kg s.c., q8–12h[a]	0.01–0.05 mg/kg s.c., q6–12h[g]	0.05 mg/kg s.c., q8–12h[d]
Butorphanol	1–5 mg/kg s.c., q4h[f]	2 mg/kg s.c., q2–4h[a]	?	1–5 mg/kg s.c., q2–4h[h]	1 mg/kg s.c.[e]	0.2–2 mg/kg s.c., q2–4h[g]	?
Carprofen	5 mg/kg s.c. or orally[a] q12–24h	5 mg/kg s.c.[b] q12–24h or 1.5 mg/kg orally q12h[i]	?	5 mg/kg s.c., q8–12h[h]	5 mg/kg s.c., q12–24h[e]	4 mg/kg s.c., q24h[d]	4 mg/kg s.c., q24h[d]
Flunixin	2.5 mg/kg s.c., ?q12–24h[a]	2.5 mg/kg s.c., ?q12–24h[a]	?	2.5 mg/kg s.c., ?q12–24h[h]	?	?	?
Ketoprofen	5 mg/kg s.c.[b] q12–24h	5 mg/kg s.c.[b] q12–24h	?	?	1 mg/kg s.c., q12–24h[g]	1 mg/kg s.c., q12–24h[g]	?
Meloxicam	5 mg/kg s.c. q24h[j]	1 mg/kg s.c.[c] or orally, ?q12–24h	?	?	0.1–0.3 mg/kg s.c. or orally, q24h[g]	0.1–0.3 mg/kg s.c. or orally, q24h[g]	?
Morphine	2–5 mg/kg s.c., q4h[a]	2–5 mg/kg s.c., q4h[a]	?	?	5 mg/kg s.c., q4h[e]	?	?

6.14 Analgesics for use in rodents. "?" indicates that information is insufficient to make a firm recommendation of an appropriate dose. Data adapted from: [a] Dobromylskyj *et al.* (2000); [b] Roughan and Flecknell (2001); [c] Roughan and Flecknell (2003); [d] Richardson (2003); [e] Flecknell (2002); [f] Flecknell (2007); [g] Hawkins (2006); [h] Keeble (2002); [i] Longley (2008); [j] Wright-williams *et al.*, 2007.

from clinical experience and by extrapolation from information in related species. Fortunately, the most widely used analgesics (buprenorphine, carprofen, meloxicam and ketoprofen) appear to have a relatively wide safety margin in most small mammals. There also have been no reports of problems associated with use of NSAIDs in patients with chronic renal problems. Nevertheless, care should be taken when using these agents: a single dose of an NSAID analgesic, or of an NSAID in combination with an opioid, is likely to be well tolerated, but prolonged use (e.g. to manage arthritis or dental disease) could lead to adverse reactions. Small rodents should therefore be monitored during treatment, as would be done with larger patients. In the editors' experience, long-term NSAID therapy, particularly with oral meloxicam, is well tolerated in rodents and no side effects have been documented.

Administration protocols

As in larger species, pre-emptive analgesia and multimodal analgesic approaches should be adopted whenever possible. Preoperative use of NSAIDs such as meloxicam and carprofen (which have product licences for this indication in larger species) has, in the authors' experience, proved safe and effective. The administration of NSAIDS preoperatively has no effect on anaesthetic dose rates. In contrast the administration of buprenorphine preoperatively potentiates the actions of all anaesthetics; for example, the concentration of isoflurane required can often be reduced by 0.5% (Criado *et al.*, 2000). Administration with injectable agents has similar effects (e.g. Roughan *et al.*, 1999; Penderis and Franklin, 2005) but the degree of potentiation has not been established for most drug combinations. For this

reason it is best to delay administration until the recovery period when injectable anaesthetics are given, but to give buprenorphine preoperatively when using volatile agents.

If it is considered that prolonged therapy is needed, oral dosing with meloxicam is particularly well accepted by many small mammals (Figure 6.15). Once-daily dosing for up to 3 days appears to be safe and effective in most species.

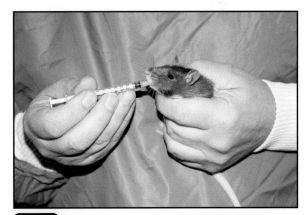

6.15 Oral administration of meloxicam to a rat.

References and further reading

Brodbelt DC (2006) *The Confidential Enquiry into Perioperative Small Animal Fatalities.* Royal Veterinary College, London

Criado AB, de Segura IA Gomez, Tendillo FJ and Marsico F (2000) Reduction of isoflurane MAC with buprenorphine and morphine in rats. *Laboratory Animals* **34**, 252–259

Dobromylskyj P, Flecknell PA, Lascelles BD *et al.* (2000) Management of postoperative and other acute pain. In: *Pain Management in Animals*, ed. PA Flecknell and A Waterman-Pearson, pp. 53–79. WB Saunders, London

Flecknell PA (1996) *Laboratory Animal Anaesthesia, 2nd edn.* Academic Press, London

Flecknell PA (2002) Guinea pigs. In: *BSAVA Manual of Exotic Pets, 4th edn*, ed. A Meredith and S Redrobe, pp. 52–64. BSAVA Publications, Gloucester

Flecknell PA (2007) Anaesthesia and perioperative care. In: *Manual of Animal Technology*, ed. SW Barnett, pp. 382–401. Blackwell, Oxford

Flecknell PA, Richardson CA and Poponic A (2007) Laboratory animals. In: *Lumb and Jones' Veterinary Anaesthesia and Analgesia, 4th edition*, ed. WJ Tranquilli *et al.*, pp. 765–784. Blackwell, Oxford

Fuentes JM, Hanly EJ, Bachman SL *et al.* (2004) Videoendoscopic endotracheal intubation in the rat: a comprehensive rodent model of laparoscopic surgery. *Journal of Surgical Research* **122**, 240–248

Hawkins MG (2006) The use of analgesics in birds, reptiles, and small exotic mammals. *Journal of Exotic Pet Medicine* **3**, 177–192

Heard DJ (2004) Anesthesia, analgesia, and sedation of small mammals. In: *Ferrets, Rabbits and Rodents, Clinical Medicine and Surgery*, ed. KE Quesenberry and JW Carpenter, pp. 356–369. WB Saunders, St Louis

Henke J, Baumgartner C, Röltgen I, Eberspächer E and Erhardt W (2004) Anaesthesia with midazolam/medetomidine/fentanyl in chinchillas (*Chinchilla lanigera*) compared to anesthesia with xylazine/ketamine and medetomidine/ketamine. *Journal of Veterinary Medicine* **51**, 259–264

Hoefer HL and Crossley DA (2002) Chinchillas. In: *BSAVA Manual of Exotic Pets, 4th edn*, ed. A Meredith and S Redrobe, pp. 65–75. BSAVA Publications, Gloucester

Johnson-Delaney CA (2005) Practical rabbit and rodent anesthesia and analgesia. *Association of Exotic Animal Veterinarians Conference, Fort Lauderdale, Florida*

Keeble E (2002) Gerbils. In: *BSAVA Manual of Exotic Pets, 4th edn*, ed. A Meredith and S Redrobe, pp. 34–46. BSAVA Publications, Gloucester

Lichtenburger M and Ko J (2007) Anesthesia and analgesia for small mammals and birds. *Veterinary Clinics of North America: Exotic Animal Practice* **10**, 293–315

Livingston A and Chambers P (2000) The physiology of pain. *Pain Management in Animals*, ed. PA Flecknell and A Waterman-Pearson, pp. 9–19. WB Saunders, London

Longley L (2008) Anaesthesia and analgesia in rabbits and rodents. *In Practice* **30**, 92–97

Murison P (2001) Prevention and treatment of perioperative hypothermia in animals under 5 kg bodyweight. *In Practice* **23**, 412–418

Penderis J and Franklin RJM (2005) Effects of pre- *versus* post-anaesthetic buprenorphine on propofol-anaesthetised rats. *Veterinary Anaesthesia and Analgesia* **32**, 256–260

Redrobe S and Meredith A (1999) Small mammal, exotic animal and wildlife nursing. In: *BSAVA Manual of Advanced Veterinary Nursing*, ed. A Hotston Moore, pp. 171–198. BSAVA Publications, Gloucester

Richardson VCG (2003) *Diseases of Small Domestic Rodents, 2nd edn.* Blackwell Publishing, Oxford

Roughan JV and Flecknell PA (2001) Behavioural effects of laparotomy and analgesic effects of ketoprofen and carprofen in rats. *Pain* **90**, 65–74

Roughan JV and Flecknell PA (2003) Evaluation of a short duration behaviour-based post-operative pain scoring system in rats. *European Journal of Pain* **7**, 397–406

Roughan JV, Burzaco Ojeda O and Flecknell PA (1999) The influence of pre-anaesthetic administration of buprenorphine on the anaesthetic effects of ketamine/medetomidine and pentobarbitone in rats and the consequences of repeated anaesthesia. *Laboratory Animals* **33**, 234–242

Skarda RT and Tranquilli WJ (2007) Local anaesthetics. In: *Lumb and Jones' Veterinary Anesthesia and Analgesia, 4th edn*, ed. WJ Tranquilli *et al.*, pp. 561–593. Blackwell Publishing, Oxford

Wright-Williams SL, Courade J-P, Richardson CA, Roughan JV and Flecknell PA (2007) Effects of vasectomy surgery and meloxicam treatment on faecal corticosteroid levels and behaviour in two strains of laboratory mouse. *Pain* **130**, 108–118

7

Rodents: soft tissue surgery

R. Avery Bennett

Introduction

In recent years, small mammals have increased in popularity as pets. While it would be inexpensive to 'just buy a new one', many rodent pet owners develop a strong emotional attachment to their pet and are willing to spend money for high quality medical care for their beloved companion.

The rodents' small size, susceptibility to stress-related problems and short natural life expectancy present unique challenges to the veterinary surgeon, compared with traditional companion animals. Surgical magnification is very important because of the small patient size. Loss of relatively small volumes of blood can have serious consequences, including death. It is often not feasible to intubate them for anaesthesia and vital signs routinely monitored in larger patients (such as blood pressure and oxygen tension) often cannot be evaluated accurately in these small pets (see also Chapters 2 and 6). Being prey species, pain and stress must be minimized both pre- and postoperatively. There are several common geriatric conditions that should be identified preoperatively, such as amyloidosis in hamsters, which can affect the prognosis and surgical outcome (see also Chapter 1).

Many challenging surgical procedures can be performed on rodent pets with a positive outcome and good prognosis. Magnification, gentle tissue handling, strict attention to haemostasis and appropriate postoperative pain management improve the chances for a positive end result.

Equipment

Magnification

Because of the small size of rodent pets, magnification is strongly recommended for performing surgical procedures. When structures are magnified 2–3 times normal, the surgeon can be more precise during tissue dissection and is able to identify small vessels that might go unnoticed without magnification. When small volumes of blood loss are potentially life-threatening, being able to visualize small vessels can make a significant difference. Additionally, the surgeon is likely to be more gentle when handling tissues, causing less tissue damage and local irritation and decreasing the risks of postoperative infection.

There are many systems available for magnification surgery, ranging from hobby loupes to operating microscopes. Operating microscopes are expensive and difficult to use effectively without specialized training, and the degree of magnification (10X or more) is generally not necessary for surgery in rodent pets. Hobby loupes, marketed for building models, are inexpensive and readily available at hobby shops. They have significant limitations because the optics are inexpensive. They have a set focal distance and anything other than this distance from the lenses is not in focus; the higher the magnification, the shorter the focal distance. Often this means that the surgeon's face is unacceptably close to the sterile field. Objects go out of focus whenever the surgeon moves their head, causing the surgeon to feel dizzy. While this happens to varying degrees with any magnification system, those with a focal *range* and those that function like bifocals allowing the surgeon to look over the lenses when magnification is not required are less nauseating.

More expensive loupe systems often have the lenses mounted securely on the lenses of a pair of glasses. This type is tailor-made for a specific individual and, generally, will not function well for someone else. Additionally, they are usually mounted so that the magnification is directly in front of the eyes. This is a disadvantage, because the surgeon cannot look over the lenses but is committed to looking through them at all times. Tasks that do not require magnification, such as loading suture material, will be more difficult. They also force the surgeon to bend the neck to look at the operating field. This will rapidly cause neck fatigue and can have serious consequences. The Surgitel® loupe (Figure 7.1) alleviates many of these problems. The lenses are in front of the glasses or on a head-band. They have an interpupillary adjustment so they can be altered to fit anyone's eyes. The lenses function as bifocals and are adjusted so that the surgeon looks *over* the lenses when magnification is not needed and looks down *through* the lenses when performing the surgery. They are available in strengths from 2.5X to 5.5X and a focal light source that clips on to the lens cross-piece is available.

Magnification surgery initially induces motion sickness. With time and practice, this will go away and does not return. An exercise that is very useful to train the brain to adapt is writing while wearing the loupes. When feeling queasy, the exercise should be discontinued and done again another time. The next step in the exercise is training the brain to go between magnification and normal vision. To do this, it is

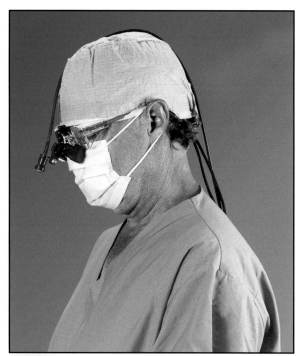

necessary to look over the lenses at something and then redirect the eyes through the lenses to write something down. Within a few days the brain will learn to adapt to these visual changes and the nausea factor will subside.

Light

A focal light source is important when doing surgery on small patients. Overhead surgical lights are inadequate as they are not intense in a small area and do not illuminate within the body cavity. Appropriate light is necessary for identifying structures and controlling haemorrhage.

Many light sources are available, but the most convenient are those that attach to the loupes or headband, since they are designed and manufactured to function together. Digital video cameras that mount on the loupes have recently become available, allowing the surgeon to document the surgery digitally.

Microsurgical instruments

Microsurgical instruments are specifically designed for multiplanar magnification surgery. Ophthalmic instruments are not ideal for rodent surgery. Microsurgical instruments should be of a standard length (ophthalmic instruments are short), have rounded handles (ophthalmic instruments have flat handles), and have a miniaturized tip.

Standard length is important so that the instrument rests in the hand without being actively held, else muscles will fatigue and tremors will occur. When instruments are longer they are held like a pen, balanced and resting supported within the surgeon's hand so that the surgeon does not have to grip them (Figure 7.2).

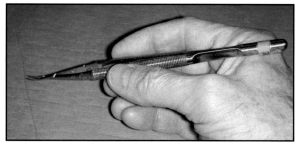

7.2 Microsurgical instruments should balance in the surgeon's hand much like a pen does. If they must be gripped, the hand will fatigue and tremor will result.

Rounded handles are ideal (though not essential) since they are easier to roll between the thumb and index finger (Figure 7.3). Rounded handles are most useful in needle holders, allowing the needle to pass into tissues by rolling the instrument. Many microsurgeons use jeweller's forceps for tissue handling. They have fine tips but are inexpensive. They do not have rounded handles but are available in a standard length.

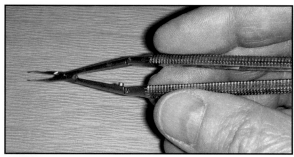

7.3 Movement of instruments during magnification surgery is through rolling the instrument between the thumb and forefinger. The hand should rest firmly on the table.

Only three microinstruments are needed to get started: micro-scissors, a micro-needle holder and micro-tissue or jeweller's forceps (Figure 7.4). These are used along with a standard soft tissue pack. Other microinstruments such as micro-mosquito haemostats are added as desired.

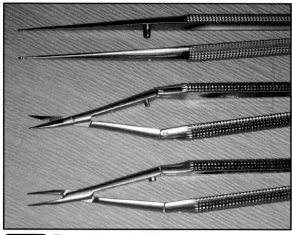

7.4 Three microsurgical instruments are recommended for a basic set: (from top) micro-forceps, micro-scissors and micro-needle holders.

Retractors

A variety of small self-retaining retractors are available for surgery in rodent pets. The Bennett Avian Cross Action retractor (Sontec Instruments, Centennial, CO 80112, USA) has a ratchet mechanism, while the Alm retractor has a thumbscrew mechanism to separate the jaws and maintain retraction (Figure 7.5). These two instruments are preferred over spring-loaded retractors such as eyelid retractors, because the tension can be adjusted to maintain retraction without causing undue pressure on the tissues.

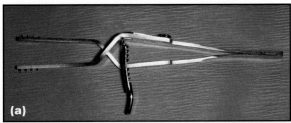

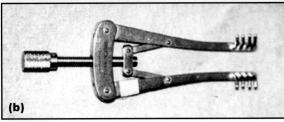

7.5 **(a)** The Bennett Avian Cross Action retractor is small and is opened and held open by a ratchet mechanism. **(b)** The Alm retractor opens and is held open by a thumbscrew.

The Lone Star Retractor (Lone Star Medical Products, Inc., Stafford, TX 77477, USA) is composed of an autoclavable plastic frame and autoclavable hook and elastic band 'stays' (Figure 7.6). The stays are placed in the tissue and the elastic band part is secured into notches in the plastic frame with only the required amount of tension. This retractor is versatile and inexpensive. It works well as an abdominal wall retractor or for retracting skin or muscle during soft tissue dissection.

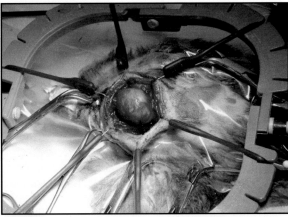

7.6 The Lone Star Retractor is completely autoclavable and consists of a plastic ring with slots into which the elastic bands of the stay hooks are inserted as shown. It is useful for patients of any size as the tension is adjusted before the bands are inserted into the slots.

Irrigation and suction

An ophthalmic irrigation bulb with a nasolacrimal cannula or small avian gavage tube attached is ideal for rodent surgery (Figure 7.7). The bulb and tip are small, delivering appropriate volumes of irrigation solution under appropriate pressure. Alternatively, a syringe can be used. A fine Baron suction tip is useful in rodent surgery. This tip has a hole that can be occluded with the index finger. The hole is not occluded for most applications because the suction will pull tissues against the tip, making it non-functional and, potentially, damaging the tissue. The degree of suction is less with the finger hole open, but still enough to aspirate fluid and blood. Large pockets of fluid are aspirated with the finger hole occluded.

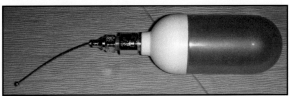

7.7 Ophthalmic bulb syringes are very useful for irrigation in small rodent patients. A nasolacrimal cannula or, as shown, an avian gavage feeding tube is attached to direct the irrigation solution.

Patient and surgeon preparation and considerations

Minimum database

A preoperative minimum database is indicated to determine the general health status of the patient and identify any anaesthetic risks. Most rodent patients cannot afford to lose much blood; however, many chemistry analysers are capable of providing a complete blood count and biochemistry panel from a very small volume of blood. At a minimum, a preoperative haematocrit, total solids and urine specific gravity should be determined. Unless a urine culture is needed, a clean voided sample is acceptable (see Chapters 2 and 4). The specific gravity is determined and there is usually enough volume to do a urine dipstick test as well, checking for proteinuria.

Whole-body radiographs are indicated as part of the data base (see Chapter 3). The chest is evaluated for cardiac and/or pulmonary disease such as mycoplasmosis. The abdomen is evaluated for masses, urinary calculi, and other abnormalities.

Fasting

Rodents cannot vomit, making a preanaesthetic fast of little importance (see also Chapter 6). A prolonged fast is contraindicated because they are small animals with a high metabolic rate and relatively little stored hepatic glycogen. For oral surgery, a short fast of 1–2 hours may be beneficial in reducing the amount of food material in the mouth. If the patient is to be intubated, a brief fast reduces the risk of carrying food down the trachea during intubation. While some sources recommend a fast prior to coeliotomy to decrease the gastrointestinal volume, there is no objective data that this is helpful. Most patients in need of gastrointestinal surgery are anorectic anyway.

Pre-emptive analgesia

Various studies document the benefit of pre-emptive analgesia, i.e. administering analgesics *before* injuring tissues. Administration of preanaesthetic analgesics will also reduce the amount of inhalant anaesthetics needed to maintain a surgical plane (see Chapter 6 for further details). Appropriate analgesics should be administered postoperatively for at least 3 days (longer for some procedures).

Because rodent pets are phylogenetically prey species, they do not tolerate pain and stress as well as predators. Hystricomorph rodents seem especially fragile in this regard. It is not uncommon for them to succumb a few days after surgery, often with no apparent premonitory signs or gross post-mortem abnormalities. Postoperative pain management can reduce the risk of stress and pain-related death.

Patient positioning

Rodents have a relatively small lung volume compared with their body size. Some advocate positioning rodents with the head elevated so that the abdominal contents do not push against the diaphragm, compromising ventilation; however, the surgeon must also take into account what procedure is being performed. If a cystotomy is being performed, placing the patient tilted with the head up will displace viscera caudally, making it more difficult to perform the procedure.

A patient restraint board allows the patient's position to be changed as needed during the anaesthetic event.

Patient preparation

Proper aseptic technique is indicated for surgery in rodents as in other species. Chlorhexidine scrub has an advantage over povidone–iodine because of its residual bacteriocidal effects. Warm sterile saline is preferred over isopropyl alcohol, because evaporative cooling with alcohol can lower the patient's body temperature. Additionally, if electrosurgery or laser surgery is planned, the alcohol can ignite – resulting in the patient catching fire. If saline (not flammable) is used, the risk of fire is minimal. Also note that anaesthetic gases and oxygen are not flammable.

The fur of some rodents (e.g. chinchillas and teddy bear hamsters) is very fine and difficult to clip. In patients with fine fur and delicate skin, a size 50 clipper blade works well. The teeth are closer together, preventing the skin from being cut and preventing larger clumps of fur from binding between the teeth, rendering the clippers ineffective.

Because of the small patient size and difficulty monitoring the patients, quarter draping around the whole patient rather than quarter draping only the incision site will minimize the potential for contamination from the table while allowing the patient to be monitored through a clear plastic patient drape placed on top. Thick clear plastic drapes are available in small sizes and are mainly used for minor procedures where the risk of infection is low. Larger sizes are designed to cover the entire surgical table, creating a large sterile field and minimizing the risk of surgical site contamination.

Rodents are prone to rapidly developing hypothermia, because they are small with a relatively large surface-to-volume ratio. It is important to monitor the patient's body temperature and provide external thermal support. It is best to use more than one patient warming device. The ideal is to use a circulating warm-water blanket under the patient, a forced warm-air blanket around the patient and a radiant heat source or lamp above the patient. A plastic drape will trap in heat, minimizing patient heat loss. If an abdominal procedure is being performed, filling the abdomen with warm saline (39°C) and letting it dwell for several minutes will raise the patient's body temperature. While this is often done prior to closure, this can be of benefit at any time if the patient's body temperature decreases significantly intraoperatively (see also Chapter 6).

Perioperative antibiotics are indicated with many surgical procedures. In rodents, a short course of a broad-spectrum antibiotic (3–7 days) may be appropriate, because pain and stress can suppress their immune system. Stressors include being in a strange environment, anaesthesia, surgery and being treated or syringe fed, and can make the patient less able to eliminate minor bacterial contamination associated with aseptic surgery. Rats and mice often have subclinical mycoplasmosis, which can progress to life-threatening pneumonia when they are stressed.

Haemostasis

Because of their small blood volume, strict attention must be paid to intraoperative haemostasis (Figure 7.8). It is important to monitor the estimated amount of blood loss and use crystalloids, colloids or whole blood as needed to support the cardiovascular system (see Chapter 2). Subcutaneously administered fluids are not appropriate for fluid resuscitation during haemorrhage, especially in an anaesthetized patient. Fluids must be administered intravenously or intraosseously.

Species	Safe volume	Number of cotton-tipped applicators [a]
Mouse	0.5 ml	5
Rat	4.0 ml	40
Hamster	1.4 ml	14
Gerbil	1.2 ml	12

7.8 Safe volumes of acute blood loss in rodent species (Harkness, 1993). [a] Each cotton-tipped applicator holds 0.1 ml of blood, i.e. 0.5 ml = 5 CTAs full of blood.

Standard techniques for haemostasis, haemostats and ligatures, are effective but time-consuming. Topical adrenaline can be useful but care must be taken not to overdose the patient. Topical thrombin provides thrombin but requires the patient's fibrin to form clots, thereby controlling haemorrhage. Surgicel™ (Ethicon, Inc., Johnson & Johnson, Sommerville, NJ, USA) is composed of oxidized regenerated cellulose. It is cloth-like, biologically inert, absorbable and conforming. It provides scaffolding for clot formation. Gelatin sponges are also inert and absorbable and provide scaffolding for clot formation; however, they are thick pads that have more absorptive capacity but do not conform to surfaces well.

Haemostatic clips are available in several sizes. They are quick and easy to apply, providing haemostasis even to very small vessels. Small and medium clips are most applicable to rodent surgery.

In **electrocautery** electricity is used to heat a metal tip to red-hot. The red-hot tip is touched to the bleeding vessel and the heat coagulates the blood and tissue. Ophthalmic heat cautery pencils have some application in rodent surgery but are not preferred, because of the large amount of collateral heat damage they produce. **Electrosurgery** (monopolar) refers to the use of electrical current passing from the tip of the cautery pencil and through the patient to the ground plate. The electrical current heats intracellular water to its boiling point, causing cells to rupture (cutting mode) or causing blood and tissues to coagulate (coagulation mode). When set to cut, it is not efficient at haemostasis; and when set to coagulate, it does not cut well and causes more collateral heat damage. With bipolar electrosurgery, the current only passes between the tips of the forceps, not through the patient. Bipolar electrosurgery is mainly used when it is not desirable for the current to pass through nearby tissues and the entire patient, such as during neurosurgery. Monopolar electrosurgery can cause patient burns as the current exits the body if only a small area is in contact with the ground plate, making it important to maximize the surface area of the patient in contact with the ground plate.

The Surgitron Dual Frequency 120 radiosurgery unit (Figure 7.9) emits high-frequency current in the radiofrequency range (4.0 MHz). With this high-frequency unit, the patient does not need to be in contact with the ground plate. It acts as an antenna and can even be wrapped in plastic. There is little risk of burning the patient from the current exiting the body. Most studies agree that, if used properly, this unit causes the least amount of collateral heat when compared with CO_2 laser, ND-YAG laser and lower-frequency electrosurgery units (Olivar, 1999; Bennett and Mullen, 2004a). Another useful feature of this unit is that both monopolar and bipolar hand pieces can be connected at the same time and the mode changed by pushing a button.

CO_2 lasers have become popular in veterinary practice. The CO_2 laser produces a beam of light at a wavelength of 10,600 nm, which is highly absorbed by water. It heats intracellular water, causing cells to rupture, cutting the tissue. To cut, a higher power is used and a fine tip held as close to the tissue as possible without touching it. For coagulation, the beam is diffused (tip held farther from the tissue) or a larger tip and lower power setting are used. When used for coagulation, the tissue is heated, resulting in coagulation of blood and tissue; however, there is more collateral heat produced in this mode. This can result in postoperative necrosis and incisional dehiscence, which is an indication that the unit is not being used properly. The CO_2 laser seals vessels less than 0.6 mm in diameter and so, when used properly, bloodless incisions can be made. The CO_2 laser reportedly causes less pain, because it seals nerves, and less swelling, because it seals blood and lymphatic vessels.

The amount of heat produced by the laser is a function of the power setting, the spot size (smaller spots produce less collateral heat) and the amount of time the beam is in contact with the tissue. The beam must not stay in one place or it will cause significant collateral heat and risk of tissue necrosis. The unit can be set in pulse mode or super pulse mode, which will allow the tissue to cool before it is hit by the laser beam again. These modes are especially recommended for beginners.

Sutures and closure

The needle and suture sizes in the average small animal practice are too large for rodent patients. In general, there is no need for suture material larger than 1.5 metric (4/0 USP). The smallest atraumatic swaged-on needle available is best, since it will create the smallest hole and least amount of tissue damage and will be less likely to tear through tissue. Polyglactin 910, polydioxanone and poliglecaprone 25 suture materials are now available coated with triclosan, a broad-spectrum antibacterial. These are safe and efficacious and no bacterial resistance has been reported. It is best to avoid catgut, which induces a profound inflammatory reaction, in favour of synthetic materials absorbed by hydrolysis.

Many rodent patients will chew out skin sutures. If time permits, an intradermal skin closure is preferred. As an alternative, skin staples seem to be well tolerated by rodents. Some rodents will tolerate skin sutures and will groom them, but this is difficult to predict. If skin sutures are used and the patient removes them, skin staples are easily applied to replace them (see also later under postoperative care).

7.9 The Surgitron Dual Frequency radiosurgical unit emits radiofrequency electromagnetic radiation that cuts tissues and coagulates vessels. It causes very little collateral heat damage. (Photograph reproduced with kind permission of Ellman International, Inc., Oceanside, NY, USA.)

Common conditions and techniques

Gonadectomy/neutering

It is important to know the anatomy of the species being neutered in order to perform the procedure efficiently. One of the main reasons for neutering rodent pets is to control reproduction. Castration is generally considered easier to perform and is associated with less morbidity and mortality than ovariohysterectomy. In most species, castration makes male mammals less aggressive both to other animals and to their owners. Behaviour can often be modified by neutering; however, it is considered best to neuter before the animal develops bad behaviours. In some species (e.g. rats), mammary neoplasia is influenced by the presence of prolactin and ovariectomy can decrease the development of mammary masses. Pyometra and other uterine diseases are effectively prevented or treated by performing ovariohysterectomy. Atrial thrombosis occurs at a younger age in female hamsters (13.5 months) than in male hamsters (21.5 months), confirming a hormonal influence (Sichuk *et al.*, 1965). In one study, spaying females resulted in a decreased lifespan, as did castrating males, indicating that androgens may have a protective effect.

Because most uterine diseases are influenced by ovarian hormones, ovariectomy is expected to be nearly as effective at preventing female reproductive diseases as is ovariohysterectomy. In many countries it is routine to perform ovariectomy, not ovariohysterectomy, in dogs and cats. Recent reports comparing ovariectomy and ovariohysterectomy have shown no increase in incidence of uterine disease in dogs with ovariectomy (van Goethem *et al.*, 2006). Ovariectomy is often easier to perform in rodent pets, with less morbidity than ovariohysterectomy.

Orchidectomy

There are three basic groups of rodents: myomorphs (e.g. mice, rats, hamsters, gerbils), sciuromorphs (e.g. squirrels, prairie dogs) and hystricomorphs (e.g. guinea pigs, chinchillas, degus). Anatomically, the hystricomorphs are unique. The males do not have a distinct scrotum and the testicles are located in the inguinal region, one on each side of the penis (see also Chapter 1). The testicles of the rodents are large in comparison with body size and descend in the first week or two of life. The inguinal canals remain open and a functional cremaster muscle allows the testicle to migrate into and out of the abdominal cavity. Rodents have a large epididymal fat pad and a fat pad in the caudal abdomen on each side that prevent intestinal herniation. The large seminal vesicles (especially in guinea pigs) also partially occlude the internal inguinal ring, preventing visceral herniation (see Chapter 1).

When neutering rodents the goal is to remove the gonads, which are responsible for hormone production. In a laboratory animal setting, it is common not to ligate the vessels supplying the gonads, because the vessels are small and haemorrhage from the severed vessels is usually minimal. However, in pet rodents, ligation of the blood supply is recommended. It is not necessary to pull the testicle far from the body, risking accidentally tearing the vessels. The surgeon only needs the entire testicle exposed. The vessels can be ligated close to the testicle. Once transected (or torn) the vascular pedicle retracts into the retroperitoneal space, since the testicular vessels are branches of the renal vessels. Haemorrhage from these vessels, therefore, occurs in the region of the kidney and does not come out via the incision or cause scrotal haematomas. Inadequate control of subcutaneous vessels and vessels within the tunics are the likely causes of incisional haemorrhage or scrotal haematomas.

In general, the testicles are easier to exteriorize using an open castration technique, because the only attachment to other tissues is to the tunic at the epididymis (ligament of the tail of the epididymis) (Evans, 1993). With a closed castration, the spermatic fascia surrounding the tunic is attached to the subcutaneous tissues. All of these attachments must be broken down to exteriorize the testicle. The main advantage to a closed technique is that the tunic is ligated near the external inguinal ring, minimizing the potential for an inguinal hernia to develop. Inguinal hernias are rare in rodent pets, affording the surgeon a choice between open or closed castration.

Some surgeons feel that guinea pigs are more likely to herniate the seminal vesicles through the inguinal ring and recommend closure of the inguinal ring to prevent this. However, reports of this complication are so uncommon that it is not likely to be necessary. Hystricomorph rodents also seem to be more prone to the development of incisional infections than other species. The reason for this is undetermined. To try to minimize the risk of infection, proper aseptic technique, gentle tissue handling and perioperative antibiotics are recommended. Because of the location of the incisions, it is feasible that the incisions are dragged along a dirty substrate, soaked in urine and contaminated with food and faeces, predisposing to infection. The owners must pay close attention to hygiene, cleaning the substrate frequently (at least daily) postoperatively until the incisions have healed (10–14 days). Fortunately, most of these abscesses respond to local debridement and systemic antibiotics.

The testicles of hystricomorph rodents are located in the inguinal region (Figure 7.10). The fur is clipped on each side of the penis and the skin is prepared for aseptic surgery. A 1 cm skin incision is made on each side of the penis to exteriorize each testicle in turn. An open or a closed technique can be used. To minimize the risk of inguinal herniation of seminal vesicles or intestine, a closed technique or ligating the tunic following an open technique is commonly recommended.

In myomorph and sciuromorph rodents, following routine clipping or plucking of the fur and surgical preparation of the scrotum, a single 1 cm transverse incision is made at the distal (caudal) tip of the scrotum (Figure 7.11). The incision is extended through the tunic on each side of midline to allow exteriorization of each testicle. The tail of the epididymis is prised away from the tunic. Caudal retraction is applied, exposing the spermatic cord. The cord is ligated (or double ligated, depending on surgeon preference) and

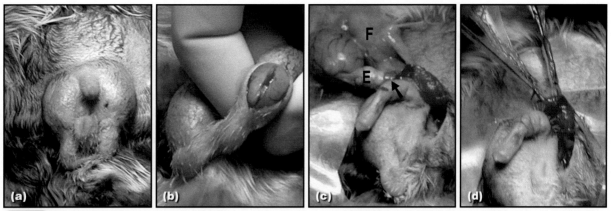

7.10 Orchidectomy in a chinchilla. **(a)** The testicles are located in the inguinal region, one on each side of the penis. **(b)** An incision is made in the scrotum, allowing the testicle to be exteriorized. **(c)** For an open castration, the ligament of the tail of the epididymis (arrowed) must be carefully detached from the tunic. (E = epididymis; F = fat). **(d)** In this patient the ductus deferens and pampiniform plexus were ligated individually.

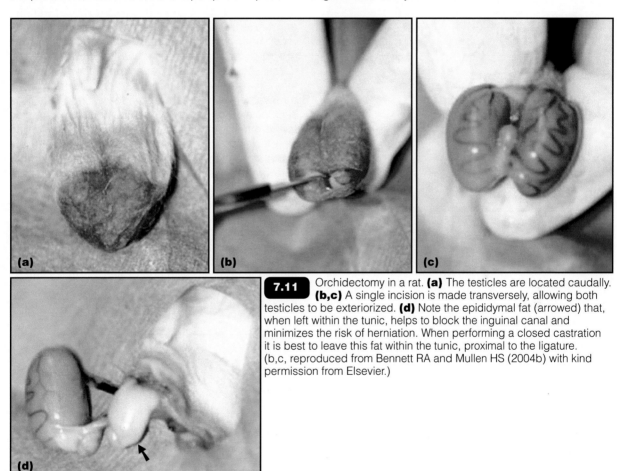

7.11 Orchidectomy in a rat. **(a)** The testicles are located caudally. **(b,c)** A single incision is made transversely, allowing both testicles to be exteriorized. **(d)** Note the epididymal fat (arrowed) that, when left within the tunic, helps to block the inguinal canal and minimizes the risk of herniation. When performing a closed castration it is best to leave this fat within the tunic, proximal to the ligature. (b,c, reproduced from Bennett RA and Mullen HS (2004b) with kind permission from Elsevier.)

transected distal to the ligatures. The tunic may be closed using a 1.5 to 0.7 metric (4/0 to 6/0 USP) synthetic absorbable material if the surgeon is concerned about visceral herniation through the scrotal incision. The skin incision may be left open to heal by second intention or may be closed using a tissue adhesive.

Because of the open inguinal canals, some prefer an abdominal approach for castration of rodents (Redrobe, 2002). Using this approach a 1–2 cm incision is made in the body wall just cranial to the pubis. The urinary bladder is exteriorized and reflected caudally, exposing the vasa deferentia dorsal to the neck of the bladder. One vas deferens is grasped and pulled on to bring the testicle into the abdomen.

Sexual activity should cease after 1–2 weeks. In rodents that have already had sexual experiences, mounting and intromission may persist following castration. Castrated rodents are considered fertile for up to 8 weeks following castration because viable sperm will be present in the remaining epididymis.

Ovariectomy and ovariohysterectomy

Indications for ovariohysterectomy in rodents include control of reproduction, dystocia, control of mammary and pituitary tumours (rats), pyometra, ovarian disease such as cystic ovaries and, potentially, behavioural alteration.

The ovaries are located at the caudal pole of the kidneys within a large accumulation of fat. The uterus is linear, with a uterine body and a single cervix (Figure 7.12). The ovarian artery and vein are branches of the renal artery and vein. They split into the ovarian branch, which supplies the ovary, and the uterine branches that supply the uterus. Thus, there is a single artery and vein medial to the ovaries and along the uterus, following the uterine horns to the uterine body (Popesko, 1992).

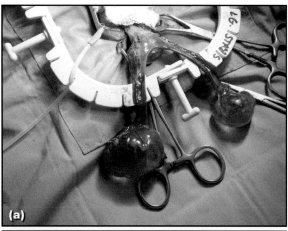

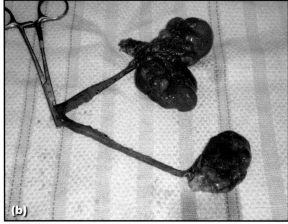

7.12 Ovariohysterectomy in a guinea pig. **(a)** A single or double encircling ligature is generally all that is required on the uterine body due to its small size. **(b)** The uterus has a linear configuration. This animal had cystic ovaries. The uterine and ovarian ligaments show abundant fat. Rodents do have a uterine body. For ovariohysterectomy the broad ligament is torn caudally to the body of the uterus, being careful not to tear the uterine vessels. The procedure is repeated on the contralateral side. (Courtesy of Krystan Grant.)

Ovariohysterectomy: The patient is placed in dorsal recumbency and prepared for aseptic surgery. A 1–3 cm incision (depending on patient size) is made midway between the umbilicus and the pubis. Care must be taken not to damage the urinary bladder and caecum directly under the body wall. The uterine horns are identified dorsally in a position similar to that in dogs and cats. One horn is grasped and exteriorized through the incision. The horn is traced cranially to the ovary. The oviduct circles around the ovary. It is only necessary to exteriorize the ovary enough to expose the vessels in order to effectively ligate them. A window is made in the mesovarium and a ligature or haemostatic clip is placed through the window to ligate the ovarian vessels. The broad ligament is torn caudally to the body of the uterus, being careful not to tear the uterine vessels. The procedure is repeated on the contralateral side. A single or double encircling ligature is generally all that is required on the uterine body due to its small size (Figure 7.12). Abdominal closure is routine.

Ovariectomy: In myomorph rodents, ovariectomy (without removing the uterus) is commonly performed through a lumbar approach (Jenkins, 2000; Bennett and Mullen, 2004a). The patient is placed in ventral recumbency and the dorsal lumbar and flank areas are clipped and prepared for aseptic surgery. A single dorsal incision is made approximately at the third lumbar vertebra (Figure 7.13) or, alternatively, a transverse incision can be made on each side. The skin incision on the dorsum is shifted from one side to the other to gain access to each ovary. Following skin incision, blunt dissection is used caudal to the last rib approximately at the level of the third lumbar vertebra to penetrate the muscles and enter the peritoneal cavity. The ovary is located within the fat at the caudal pole of the kidney and it is carefully exteriorized. Especially in young animals, no ligation is required and haemorrhage is generally minimal; however, the risk of haemorrhage can be reduced by applying a ligature to the ovarian vessels. The muscle is apposed with one or two 1.5 to 0.7 metric (4/0 or 6/0 USP) synthetic, absorbable sutures and the skin is closed routinely.

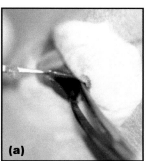 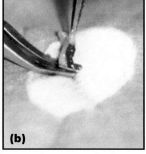

7.13 To perform an ovariectomy in a rat, a single incision is made across the back at the third lumbar vertebra. **(a)** The incision is shifted from side to side and a haemostat is used to bluntly enter the abdomen to retrieve the ovary. **(b)** The ovarian pedicle can be ligated or a Hemoclip® applied as shown.

In hystricomorph rodents, ovariectomy is performed in a similar manner (Redrobe, 2002). A skin incision is made on each side ventral to the erector spinae muscle and about 1 cm caudal to the last rib. A haemostat is used to bluntly penetrate the muscle, allowing the ovary to be exteriorized for excision.

Uterine diseases

Dystocia

Dystocia is rare in myomorph and sciuromorph rodents, because they are born small and altricious. If dystocia is diagnosed in small rodent pets and the pups are not naturally delivered with medical treatments including oxytocin and calcium, a Caesarean section or ovariohysterectomy can be performed using standard techniques.

In hystricomorph rodents, the offspring are delivered looking like miniature versions of the adults and precocious. It is well known that guinea pigs are prone to dystocia if they have not been bred by 6 months of age because, to deliver the large neonates, the pubic symphysis must separate to widen the birth canal. The symphysis of unbred females can fuse at 6–9 months of age, predisposing them to dystocia. It should be noted that the symphysis does not always fuse. Many times, even females bred later in life will deliver naturally. Normally, 10 days prior to parturition, the symphysis begins to separate and a 1.5 cm gap should be present 48 hours prior to parturition. At parturition a 2–2.5 cm gap should be present. Unfortunately, the breeding date is often unknown, making it difficult to decide whether surgical intervention is needed.

If the symphysis is open, fetuses are palpated or radiographs confirm the presence of a fetus, and the sow has been in non-productive labour for 60 minutes, 0.5–1.0 IU oxytocin should be administered. If she still does not deliver in 20–30 minutes, surgical intervention is indicated. Caesarean section is performed if there is a chance the babies are still viable. If not, ovariohysterectomy is performed. For Caesarean section, a coeliotomy is made from the xiphoid to the pubis to allow the uterus to be exteriorized. The uterus is isolated with warm saline-moistened gauze. An incision is made on the ventral aspect of the uterine body if there is more than one fetus to allow them all to be delivered through one incision. If there is only one fetus, an incision is made in the ventral uterus over the fetus, care being taken not to incise the fetus. The fetus should be delivered as quickly as possible and passed to a non-sterile assistant assigned to stimulate it and remove fetal fluids from the mouth. If the reproductive viability of the uterus is to be maintained, the incision is closed with a single-layer simple continuous monofilament absorbable material. If the sow is to be spayed, the blood supply should not be ligated until all viable fetuses are removed. Ligating the uterine vessels will cut off the oxygen supply to the fetuses, resulting in fetal death.

Uterine torsion

Uterine torsion has been reported as a post-mortem finding in both guinea pigs (after 30 days' gestation) and chinchillas (Wallach and Boever, 1983). There are no reports of the dam surviving uterine torsion. If it is suspected, it must be considered an emergency and ovariohysterectomy should be performed as soon as the patient is stable enough to be anaesthetized.

Uterine prolapse

In rodents, uterine prolapse is usually associated with dystocia. The patient presents with a mass of tissue protruding from the vulva (Figure 7.14). Some rodents will eat the exposed tissue. Ovariohysterectomy is the treatment of choice and is performed only after the patient is stabilized. In some patients, it may be necessary to delay surgery because of metabolic compromise and it is best to replace the prolapsed tissue until definitive surgery can be performed. Application of hypertonic sugar solutions will usually reduce the oedema, allowing the prolapse to be reduced. This is done under a very brief anaesthesia using isoflurane or sevoflurane gas to stop any straining. A blunt probang appropriate to the patient's size is used to push the tissue back into the abdomen. It is important to reduce the uterus back into the abdomen by advancing the probang to the mid-abdominal region. One or two sutures are placed across the vulvar opening to avoid entrapping the urethral papilla as could happen with a purse-string suture.

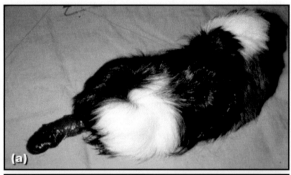

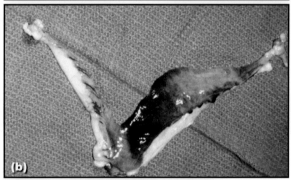

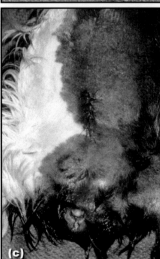

7.14
(a) This guinea pig presented the morning after parturition for uterine prolapse.
(b) The prolapse was reduced and an ovariohysterectomy was performed.
(c) Postoperative incision following ovariohysterectomy.

Pyometra

Pyometra is rare in myomorph and sciuromorph rodents and is uncommon in hystricomorph rodents (Bennett, 2000; Bennett and Mullen, 2004a). The patient is stabilized with intravenous or intraosseous fluids and broad-spectrum intravenous antibiotics are administered preoperatively. Ovariohysterectomy is the treatment of choice and care is taken not to spill uterine contents into the abdomen. A portion of the uterine wall is submitted for aerobic and anaerobic cultures. The abdomen is irrigated with warm saline prior to closure. It is best to continue intravenous or intraosseous fluids and antibiotics for at least 24 hours after surgery, or until the patient is eating and drinking adequately.

Cystic ovaries

Cystic ovarian disease has been reported in commonly kept species of pet rodents but occurs most often in hamsters and gerbils (Toft, 1991). Ovariectomy or ovariohysterectomy is the treatment of choice. It is best to drain as much fluid as possible from the cyst prior to anaesthesia, to improve the patient's ability to ventilate, especially since intubation is difficult.

Uterine adenocarcinoma is fairly common in Syrian hamsters and has been shown to spread by seeding of malignant cells (see also Chapter 16). In hamsters with uterine adenocarcinoma it is contraindicated to drain the fluid from the lesion as this can result in metastasis. Ultrasonography is helpful to determine if the swelling is due to an ovarian cyst or uterine neoplasia. Ovariohysterectomy is the treatment of choice for hamsters with uterine cancer.

Mammary glands

Tumours

Benign and malignant mammary gland tumours occur commonly in various species of rodent pets. In rats and hamsters, mammary tumours are usually benign; in mice and gerbils they are more commonly malignant (Toft, 1991; Cooper, 1994). Mammary tumours in chinchillas are rare (Bennett and Mullen, 2004b). In guinea pigs, 70% are reportedly benign fibroadenomas and 30% are malignant adenocarcinomas (Collins, 1988). Interestingly, it is not uncommon for male guinea pigs to develop mammary tumours and clinically it seems that most are malignant.

A preoperative diagnosis by cytology or biopsy is very helpful for surgical planning and prognostication because mammary gland tumours, in any species and either sex, can be malignant. Complete staging is recommended to rule out concomitant disease processes as well as tumour metastasis. Staging includes a CBC, biochemistry panel, chest or whole-body radiographs and abdominal ultrasonography.

Surgical removal along with ovariectomy or ovariohysterectomy is recommended for rats with benign fibroadenomatous mammary tumours. Tumour removal has been shown to prolong survival (Goya *et al.*, 1990) and it is believed that ovariectomy at or near the time of tumour removal can help to prevent the development of new tumours. Ovariectomy at an early age (90 days) is recommended to minimize the risk of developing both mammary tumours and pituitary tumours (Hotchkiss, 1995). Mammary tumour development occurs due to the influence of prolactin, not oestrogen; however, ovariectomy prior to tumour development has been shown to reduce significantly the risk of rats developing benign mammary tumours. Rats ovariectomized at 90 days of age had a significantly lower incidence of mammary tumour development (4% in ovariectomized rats, compared with 47% in intact females) and pituitary chromophobe adenomas (4% in ovariectomized rats and 66% in intact rats).

Mammary tissue in rats and mice is extensive and occurs from the neck to the inguinal area and dorsally to the level of the shoulders and ilium. In hamsters and gerbils it is only along the ventral thorax and abdomen. Guinea pigs have only two mammary glands, located (one on each side) in the inguinal region. Chinchillas have three pairs of mammary glands: one pair is located inguinally and the other two are thoracic (see also Chapter 1). Degus have four pairs of mammary glands.

Surgical removal of benign masses carries a good prognosis. With malignant tumours, a surgical cure is difficult because it may not be feasible to remove enough tissue to prevent recurrence. If the surface of the mass is ulcerated or if the mass is malignant, the skin should be removed. With benign masses, it is often best to remove excess skin after the tumour is removed to be sure the defect can be closed. Haemostasis and a short operative time are important factors in a successful outcome. Often, large masses have several large blood vessels supplying them. Haemostatic clips are very useful for speed and haemostasis. Radiosurgery or laser surgery will also aid in haemostasis, but laser is generally not as fast as radiosurgery or a scalpel. After the tumour is removed, excess skin is resected with Mayo or Metzenbaum scissors. Drains are not routinely used and the defect is closed in two layers: subcutaneous tissue with a simple continuous pattern, and skin. Skin staples are fast and effective (Figure 7.15). If the patient is not stable, the subcutaneous tissues should not be closed.

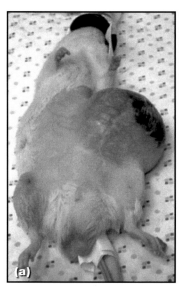

7.15

(a) Mammary tumours in rats are usually benign but can reach large proportions. (continues) ▶

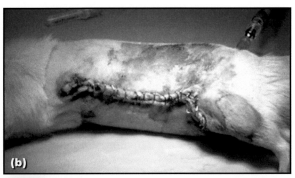

7.15 (continued) **(b)** Skin staples offer a rapid method for closing skin in a single layer, shortening the surgery time.

The blood and lymphatic supply to the mammary glands in guinea pigs is not shared and so cancer does not usually spread from one gland to the other. Because many of these tumours are malignant, obtaining a preoperative diagnosis is very helpful in surgical planning. For benign tumours, only the affected gland needs to be removed. A fusiform incision is made around the teat in a cranial to caudal direction. Blunt and sharp dissection are used to free the mammary gland from surrounding soft tissues, being careful to identify and ligate or clip the caudal superficial epigastric artery and vein. The defect is closed in two layers: subcutaneous tissues and skin.

For malignant mammary tumours in guinea pigs, 1–2 cm of normal tissue around the affected gland is removed. The borders of the mammary gland and mass are marked using a sterile skin marker and ruler 1–2 cm away from the mass. Proper surgical planning is important and the surgery may require reconstructive techniques if the mass is large. The inguinal lymph node is identified and removed for staging. Once the tissue has been removed, it is marked with sutures or ink for orientation. It is submitted for histological evaluation to obtain a definitive diagnosis and determine the completeness of excision.

In guinea pigs with bilateral mammary neoplasia, the larger mass is removed first and the tissues are allowed to heal for 2–4 weeks before the other mass is removed. This allows the tissues to stretch, making it easier to close the defect on the second side. These patients are more likely to need reconstructive procedures such as rotation or advancement flaps.

Enucleation and exenteration

Many species of rodent have prominent globes prone to proptosis, especially hamsters. The problem often goes unnoticed until the globe is desiccated and necrotic. Anatomically, rodents have a large venous sinus surrounding the extraocular muscles and the Harderian gland extending caudal to the globe (see also Chapter 15). The venous sinus is a source for blood collection in laboratory settings. If this sinus is damaged during enucleation, haemorrhage can be significant. A haemostatic gelatin sponge and digital pressure will usually control the haemorrhage. The gelatin sponge is absorbed by fibrous tissue ingrowth, reducing the divot created.

Enucleation refers to the removal of the globe along with the nictitating membrane (in species that have one) and the eyelid margins. There are two variations. In transconjunctival enucleation the bulbar conjunctiva is incised at the limbus and the globe is removed through this incision. In transpalpebral enucleation the eyelids are sutured together and the skin around the eyelid margins is incised to the bulbar conjunctiva. The globe is removed without exposing the tissue to the conjunctiva or cornea; this is indicated if these are infected. A transconjunctival approach is most often used because of the prominent eyes of rodents. Performed correctly, dissecting as close to the globe as possible, it leaves the extraocular muscles and reduces the risk of damaging the venous sinus.

With exenteration, the entire contents of the orbit are removed along with the globe, the nictitans and the eyelid margins. This technique is used in patients with periocular disease such as abscesses and neoplasia. Damage to the venous sinus is more likely to occur.

With either procedure, a prosthetic globe can be made using polymethylmethacrylate (PMMA) to minimize the divoting after enucleation. When treating an infectious process, antibiotic-impregnated PMMA is used as an ocular prosthesis, providing long-term local antibiotic therapy. In either case the eyelids are sutured together over the prosthesis.

Cystotomy

Urinary calculi occur most commonly in guinea pigs but are also reported in chinchillas and other rodent pets (see Chapter 13). Male guinea pigs can present with urethral obstruction due to calculi or concretions of seminal fluids and sperm. The obstruction can usually be alleviated by passing a catheter and irrigating the urethra.

Calculi can be located in any part of the urinary system but appear to be most common in the bladder. Ultrasonography is very helpful in determining the location and significance of urinary calculi. Ureteral calculi can cause obstruction with secondary hydroureter and hydronephrosis. In some patients, a stone visible on radiographs is not causing obstruction, either because urine can pass around the stone or the stone has migrated through the wall of the ureter. An excretory urogram can provide information about whether a stone is causing obstruction and about the functional status of the kidneys. If a kidney is not functioning because of a chronic ureteral obstruction, there is no point in removing the ureterolith. The entire kidney should be removed.

Most stones are located in the bladder and removed through a cystotomy. A ventral midline approach is made to the caudal abdomen. The urinary bladder is isolated with saline-moistened gauze. Stay sutures are placed at the apex of the bladder and on each side of the proposed ventral cystotomy incision. Urine is suctioned as it escapes from the bladder, care being taken not to suction out all of the stones. The stones are removed with a small spoon or blunted curette to minimize damage to the bladder wall. The stones are analysed and cultured. In addition, 1 mm of the bladder mucosa is trimmed from one side of the incision: one piece is submitted for culture and another for histopathology if indicated. After the mucosal samples have been collected, a systemic broad-spectrum antibiotic can be administered.

The bladder wall is usually thick, making it difficult to invert. A single layer of simple continuous sutures is all that is necessary; however, if an inverting oversew is possible, it will result in serosa-to-serosa contact and more rapid sealing of the incision. A monofilament absorbable material 1.5 to 0.7 metric (4/0 to 6/0 USP) on a small needle is used and it is not necessary to avoid the mucosa. Rodents do not hold their urine long and so the risk of the bladder becoming overly distended is low.

In patients with ureteral stones, it is ideal to manipulate them into the urinary bladder and remove them through a cystotomy, but this is usually not possible without causing significant trauma. Because of the small size of rodent ureters, microsurgical techniques and magnification are required. A longitudinal incision is made over the calculus, which is then removed. The incision is closed transversely with 0.5 to 0.4 metric (7/0 to 8/0 USP) monofilament suture material to minimize the risk of lumen narrowing and stricture. Urethral calculi are more common in male rodents and can often be retrohydropulsed into the bladder and removed through cystotomy. If this is not possible, a urethrotomy, usually perineal, is performed to remove the stone. The urethrotomy is *not* closed. Studies in dogs have shown no difference in healing with sutured *versus* non-sutured urethrotomies (Weber *et al.*, 1985).

The patient should be maintained on intravenous or intraosseous fluids for 24–48 hours postoperatively (see Chapter 2). Antibiotics are continued pending culture results. Haematuria may persist for several days and with unsutured urethrotomies the bleeding may continue for a week or more.

Unfortunately, recurrence of urolithiasis is common. In one report, calcium oxalate urolithiasis was reported secondary to *Stretococcus pyogenes* cystitis (O'Rourke 2004). The stones formed around a bacterial nidus, underscoring the need for bacterial culture in guinea pigs with urolithiasis. (See also Chapter 13.)

Tail degloving

Rodents with long tails, especially gerbils and degus, are prone to degloving injury when they are grabbed by the tail or the tail is caught in something (see Chapter 2). Gerbils have thinner skin covering their tail than rats and mice. When owners pick them up by the tail they are at risk of pulling the skin off. The skin is peeled off the tail, leaving tendons and bone exposed. Tail amputation is generally recommended because the skin has lost its blood supply. Left untreated, the exposed tissue will usually undergo dry necrosis and eventually slough. However, surgical amputation is recommended as it will result in faster healing and a reduced risk of developing a systemic infection. It also seems more humane.

The patient is positioned in ventral recumbency with the tail suspended during surgical preparation. The skin is incised 1–2 mm proximal to the location of

skin loss, with the dorsal skin incised more proximal than the ventral skin to allow the ventral skin to be pulled over the bone and sutured along the dorsal aspect, elevating the incision off the substrate. The skin is retracted proximally a few millimetres and the tail is severed between two vertebrae proximal to the skin incision. The ventral coccygeal vessels are ligated or coagulated prior to closure. The ventral flap of skin is apposed to the dorsal skin with subcutaneous sutures followed by an intradermal suture layer or tissue adhesive.

Everted cheek pouch

Hamsters have large storage pouches in their cheeks to accommodate large quantities of food. Occasionally, a cheek pouch will evert spontaneously. When this happens, the pouch separates from the skin of the cheek so the lateral aspect of the face looks normal and the everted cheek pouch looks like a tissue mass protruding from the mouth (see Chapter 8).

Treatment involves a brief anaesthesia to reduce and secure the pouch to the cheek skin. A 1 ml syringe case is used to reposition the pouch within the mouth. One or two mattress sutures are placed through the skin and cheek pouch, bouncing off the syringe case, and exiting the skin again. A non-absorbable 1.5 metric (4/0 USP) suture material is preferred and sutures are removed in 2 weeks. Because these sutures are not tied tightly, there is no need for stents.

If the cheek pouch everts after suture removal, a lateral skin incision is made to create stronger adhesions between the cheek pouch and skin. A small piece of the cheek pouch is taken for culture and histopathological evaluation to rule out other disease processes that might result in recurrent cheek pouch prolapse. The incised cheek pouch is then sutured to the subcutaneous tissues to create stronger adhesions. The skin is closed with fine monofilament sutures, since the animals cannot chew them out.

Postoperative care

It is important to monitor the patient's recovery from surgery and ensure that it is not showing signs of distress (increased heart and respiratory rates), that it begins eating in a timely manner and that it is not bothering its incision site. Analgesia is vital during the recovery period. After the first 12 hours, it is often possible to decrease the amount of narcotics used. Non-steroidal anti-inflammatory drugs (NSAIDs) are safe and efficacious in rodents, with minimal risk of side effects. They are best used postoperatively as they are more likely to have side effects when blood pressure drops during anaesthesia and surgery.

The patient is offered food within an hour after surgery and encouraged to eat. Often novel food items such as fresh greens for hystricomorph rodents and dried fruits and nuts for sciuromorph and myomorph rodents will be accepted before items that are nutritionally complete and should be offered in the early postoperative period along with their normal diet. Once they are eating well, the treat items can be removed or decreased. Stool production is a good indicator of gastrointestinal motility. Because rodents defecate frequently, the absence of stool for 8 hours is cause for concern. Medical management of ileus includes syringe feeding and metoclopramide. It is best to continue fluid therapy until the patient is eating, drinking and defecating. (See also Chapters 2, 6 and 11.)

Depending on the species and the disease process, postoperative antibiotics are often continued for 3–14 days. A combination of enrofloxacin (10 mg/kg orally q12h) and doxycycline (5 mg/kg orally q12h) for 7 days has been recommended for mycoplasmosis in rats. Trimethoprim/sulphonamide (15–30 mg/kg orally or s.c. q12h) is a good broad-spectrum prophylactic antibiotic in rodent pets (see also Chapter 5).

It can be quite challenging to prevent some rodent patients from self-trauma. Many will aggressively chew incisions and bandages. Most do not tolerate Elizabethan collars well either. If an Elizabethan collar is needed, it is best to keep the patient hospitalized until it has been determined that the animal has accepted the collar and is not overly stressed by it. If the patient is unacceptably stressed, a dose of a tranquillizer (midazolam 1–2 mg/kg i.m.) will usually calm the patient and they come to accept the collar as the drug effect wears off. In some patients, it may be necessary to administer a tranquillizer for several days or until the incision has healed. While this may seem extreme, it is preferred to having to repeat the procedure or having the patient cause severe self-trauma such as evisceration. An alternative to an Elizabethan collar is a yoke (Figure 7.16). Most rodents accept a yoke better because it does not obstruct their vision and allows them to eat more readily.

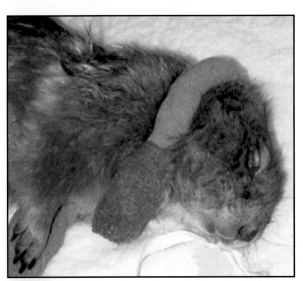

7.16 Many rodents tolerate a yoke (such as the one on this prairie dog) better than an Elizabethan collar.

References and further reading

Bennett RA (2000) Preparation and equipment useful for surgery in small exotic pets. *Veterinary Clinics of North America: Exotic Animal Practice* **3**, 563–585

Bennett RA and Mullen HS (2004a) Soft tissue surgery – small rodents. In: *Ferrets, Rabbits and Rodents: Clinical Medicine and Surgery*, ed. KE Quesenberry and JW Carpenter, pp. 316–328. WB Saunders, Philadelphia

Bennett RA and Mullen HS (2004b) Soft tissue surgery – guinea pigs, chinchillas, and prairie dogs. In: *Ferrets, Rabbits and Rodents: Clinical Medicine and Surgery*, ed. KE Quesenberry and JW Carpenter, pp. 274–284. WB Saunders, Philadelphia

Collins BR (1988) Common disease and medical management of rodents and lagomorphs. In: *Exotic Animals*, ed. ER Jacobson and GV Kollias, pp. 261–316. Churchill Livingstone, New York

Cooper JE (1994) Tips on tumours. *Proceedings of the North American Veterinary Conference*, pp. 897–898

Evans HE and Christensen GC (1993) Urogenital system. In: *Miller's Anatomy of the Dog, 3rd edn*, ed. HE Evans, pp. 494–558. WB Saunders, Philadelphia

Fossum TW (2007) Biomaterials, suturing, and hemostasis. In: *Fossum TW (ed) Small Animal Surgery*, ed. TW Fossum, pp. 57–78. Mosby Elsevier, St Louis

Goya RG, Lu JK and Meites J (1990) Gonadal function in aging rats and its relation to pituitary and mammary pathology. *Mechanisms of Ageing and Development* **56**, 77–88

Harkness JE (1993) Anesthesia, surgery. In: *A Practitioner's Guide to Domestic Rodents*, ed. JE Harkness, pp. 37–50. American Animal Hospital Association, Denver

Hotchkiss CE (1995) Effects of surgical removal of subcutaneous tumors on survival of rats. *Journal of the American Veterinary Medicine Association* **206**, 1575–1579

Jenkins JR (2000) Surgical sterilization of small mammals, spay and castration. *Veterinary Clinics of North America: Exotic Animal Practice* **3**, 617–627

Olivar AC, Forouhar FA, Gillies CG and Servanski DR (1999) Transmission electron microscopy: evaluation of damage in human oviducts caused by different surgical instruments. *Annals of Clinical and Laboratory Science* **29**, 281–284

O'Rourke DP (2004) Disease problems in guinea pigs. In: *Ferrets, Rabbits and Rodents: Clinical Medicine and Surgery*, ed. KE Quesenberry and JW Carpenter, pp. 245–254. WB Saunders, Philadelphia

Popesko P, Rajtova V and Horak J (1992) *A Colour Atlas of Anatomy of Small Laboratory Animals. Vol. 1: Rabbit, Guinea Pig; Vol. 2: Rat, Mouse, Hamster*. Wolfe, London

Redrobe S (2002) Soft tissue surgery in rabbits and rodents. *Seminars in Avian and Exotic Pet Medicine* **11**, 231–245

Sichuk G, Bettigole RE, Der BK and Fortner JG (1965) Influence of sex hormones on thrombosis of the left atrium in Syrian (golden) hamsters. *American Journal of Physiology* **208**, 465–470

Toft JD (1991) Commonly observed spontaneous neoplasms in rabbits, rats, guinea pigs, hamsters, and gerbils. *Seminars in Avian and Exotic Pet Medicine* **1**, 80–92

van Goethem B, Schaefers-Okkens A and Kirpensteijn J (2006) Making a rational choice between ovariectomy and ovariohysterectomy in the dog: a discussion of the benefits of either technique. *Veterinary Surgery* **35**, 136–143

Wallach JD and Boever WJ (1983) *Diseases of Exotic Animals: Medical and Surgical Management*. WB Saunders, Philadelphia

Weber WJ, Boothe HW, Brassard JA and Hobson HP (1985) Comparison of the healing of prescrotal urethrostomy incisions in the dog: sutured versus nonsutured. *American Journal of Veterinary Research* **46**, 1309–1315

8

Rodents: dentistry

Vladimír Jekl

Introduction

As a result of the increasing numbers of guinea pigs, chinchillas and other small rodents being kept as private pets, dental disease is being observed more frequently in veterinary clinics. Incidence of oral cavity diseases is approximately 30–80%. It varies both between species and within a species with age. A wide range of local and systemic conditions that affect the mouth and oral cavity have been described in rodents, including hereditary, infectious and metabolic diseases, trauma, electrical accidents and neoplasia.

The diagnosis of dental disease in small mammals is complicated due to the anatomical structure of the oral cavity and special mechanics of the jaw movements. Being able to recognize variable anatomical and physiological variations, to understand disease pathophysiology and assess even minor changes will help in optimal treatment of many commonly seen conditions.

Anatomy and physiology

Rodent dentition is monophyodont and heterodont: the animals develop one permanent set of teeth (Figure 8.1) and their teeth have different shapes and functions. However, guinea pigs, degus and squirrels have been classified as diphyodont: their deciduous teeth are replaced by permanent dentition *in utero* or early postnatally.

A single pair of well developed incisor teeth is present on each jaw. Incisors are continually growing (open-rooted) in all rodent species, with the enamel thickest on the lingual surface and thinning as it extends to the distal and mesial surfaces. The labial surface is covered with dentine and cementum. This configuration of dental tissues gives a sharp chisel-like occlusion. About one-third of the incisor is erupted,

while two-thirds seats in the alveolus. The maxillary clinical crowns are much shorter than those of mandibular incisors. In rodents, the incisors grow 2–4 mm per week and the elodont (continually growing and erupting) cheek teeth in hystricomorphs and sciuromorphs grow approximately 3–4 mm per month. In general, rodents have reduced tooth numbers with a long diastema between the incisor teeth and the cheek teeth. The cheek folds separate the gnawing apparatus (incisors) from the caudal part of the oral cavity. The mandibles and mandibular cheek tooth arcades are frequently wider in comparison with the maxilla and maxillary tooth arcades. This gives rodents their typical head appearance.

Myomorphs

In mouse-like rodents (myomorphs), the labial surface of the incisors is whitish-yellow or white. The apex of the mandibular incisors extends to the level of, or distally to, the last molar. The mandibular symphysis does not fuse completely in some species (e.g. hamsters), therefore relative independent movement of each jaw is possible. Molars have a limited period of growth and are short-crowned with typical long and narrow tooth roots (brachyodont). Each mandibular cheek tooth is in occlusion with the corresponding maxillary cheek tooth.

- In rats, the apices of the maxillary incisors extend for two-thirds of the diastema. The mandibular molar M1 has four to five roots; M2 has four roots and M3 three roots. Maxillary molars have two roots. The molar crowns are divided into lobes by transverse fissures and possess cusps, which vary among different rat species.
- In mice, the apices of maxillary incisors are longer, reaching up to three-quarters of the diastema. The cheek teeth have three to four roots.

Rodent group	Incisors	Canines	Premolars	Molars
Myomorphs (mice, rats, hamsters, gerbils)	1/1	0/0	0/0	3/3
Hystricomorphs (guinea pigs, chinchillas, degus)	1/1	0/0	1/1	3/3
Sciuromorphs (chipmunks, squirrels, prairie dogs)	1/1	0/0	1–2/1	3/3

8.1 Permanent dental formulae in selected rodents.

- In gerbils, the apices of maxillary incisors reach up to two-thirds of the diastema. The molars are arranged in a straight line. The occlusal surfaces of all molars are almost flat and without cusps or fissures. Each of the first molars has three roots, each of the second molars has two roots and the third molars have one root.
- In hamsters, the apices of maxillary incisors reach to one-half to two-thirds of the diastema. The molar crowns are rectangular and flat with small cusps on the occlusal surface. The mandibular molars have two roots; maxillary M1 has four roots and M2 and M3 have three roots. The cheeks are occupied by the cheek pouches, which are situated between the skin and masticatory muscles.

Rodent incisors are used for slicing food, gnawing hard materials and for social interactions. When the incisors are gnawing, the mandible is pulled forward until the edges of the mandibular incisors approximate the cutting edges of the maxillary incisors. In this case, the maxillary and mandibular molars do not occlude. When food is to be masticated, the mandible assumes its normal position with the tips of the mandibular incisors posterior to the gnawing edges of the maxillary incisors and the cheek teeth in occlusion. In mastication, a rapid vertical movement of the mandible is obvious. Crushing of food occurs when the mandibular molars are moving upwards and forwards over the upper part of the ellipse.

Hystricomorphs

Guinea pigs, chinchillas and degus are true herbivores, with incisors and all cheek teeth continually growing throughout life. Elodont teeth never form true anatomical roots, and the whole tooth is termed 'reserve crown'. Vegetation is tough and fibrous, and its low energy content requires a high intake and thorough chewing. This natural diet results in the proper continual wear of the cheek teeth.

The labial surface of the incisors is yellow in chinchillas and degus, while in guinea pigs it is white. The apices of guinea pig maxillary incisors extend to the mesial aspect of the first premolar and those of the mandibular incisors reach to the level of the first mandibular molar. Chinchillas have maxillary incisor apices that reach to approximately one-half of the diastema, with lower incisor apices that end near the mesial aspect of the premolar. In degus, the maxillary incisor apices extend for two-thirds of the diastema to the apex of the premolar and the apices of the mandibular incisors reach distal to the last molar.

Premolars and molars have similar structure and in each quadrant of the oral cavity they form a uniform functional grinding unit. The cheek teeth in chinchillas and guinea pigs diverge from rostral to caudal. Occlusal surfaces consist of alternating exposures of enamel, dentine and cementum. Deep longitudinal grooves are present on the buccal surface of the cheek teeth, especially in guinea pigs. Each mandibular cheek tooth is in occlusion with the corresponding maxillary cheek tooth. In resting jaw position, their occlusal planes are almost in contact.

The occlusal plane is almost horizontal in chinchillas and degus, while in guinea pigs it is oblique (Figure 8.2). In degus, the cheek teeth are typically octagonal in shape.

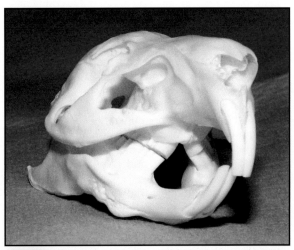

8.2 Oblique occlusal plane of the cheek teeth in a guinea pig.

Guinea pigs have bilateral and unilateral types of jaw movement cycles within mastication. In chinchillas, the mandible is repeatedly moved diagonally forward and to the side opposite to that in use ('propalineal' jaw movement). This slides the occluding surface of the mandibular cheek tooth arcade along that of the maxillary cheek teeth during the power stroke, with the teeth being separated on return to the starting position.

Sciuromorphs

The teeth of squirrel-like rodents are heterodont and the cheek teeth are brachyodont. The lower incisors have a degree of independent movement from each other. This is because the mandibular symphysis is not ossified, and the two hemimandibles are connected by muscle. The apices of the mandibular incisors are situated distal to the last molar roots, while the maxillary ones reach to the apex of the first cheek teeth.

The cheek teeth are quadrate with rounded blunt cone-shaped bunodont marginal cusps and a concave central area on their occlusal surfaces. The prominent inner cusps of the maxillary cheek teeth grind food in the concavity of the opposing mandibular teeth, while the cusps on the outer surface of the maxillary cheek teeth shear food against those of the mandibular cheek teeth.

Clinical signs

Clinical signs of dental disease are mostly non-specific. Different forms of congenital, developmental or acquired dental disease induce hypersalivation, anorexia, progressive weight loss, malfunction of chewing, change of feeding habits and feed preferences and deterioration of fur quality. In some cases, the malocclusion can also be accompanied by the development of facial abscesses, moist dermatitis, epiphora, exophthalmia and damage to the temporomandibular joint.

Coronal elongation of the incisors may be seen in all rodent species. Maxillary incisors twist or curve into the oral cavity, while the mandibular incisors continually grow forward or curl into the nostrils. Incisor fractures may also be seen. If the condition is left untreated, maxillary incisors may lacerate soft tissues of the oral cavity and, in severe cases, penetrate the skull. Any deviation of the incisors in animals with elodont cheek teeth may indicate uneven wear of the premolars and molars. Severe coronal elongation of the elodont cheek teeth may be associated with cheek laceration or perforation.

Skin and fur may appear unkempt if an animal has problems with grooming due to dental pain. Excess salivation is often one of the causes of wet dermatitis and cheilitis in chinchillas and guinea pigs. Epiphora may occur as a result of apical cheek teeth elongation or other apical pathology that causes obstruction of the lacrimal duct. Once infected, the serous discharge may become purulent. Fur chewing in chinchillas is in many cases associated with malocclusion and correlates with excessive salivation (Figure 8.3).

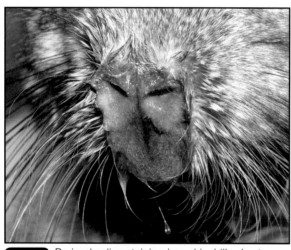

8.3 Perioral saliva staining in a chinchilla due to excessive salivation.

Secondary gastrointestinal disease is often associated with changes in feeding habits and painful stimuli in the oral cavity (see also Chapter 11). Problems in formation and ingestion of caecotrophs are also recorded. Depending on species-specific feeding habits and gastrointestinal physiology, any oral pathology may result in scant and smaller droppings, aerophagy, gastrointestinal hypomotility, meteorism or secondary enteritis.

In degus, a high incidence of dyspnoea is seen associated with malocclusion, particularly in cases with maxillary cheek teeth apical elongation and elodontoma formation (Jekl et al., 2007). Odontoma-like tumours (elodontomas) causing respiratory signs are common in prairie dogs and squirrels.

Oral cavity examination

An accurate history should be obtained from the owner and a routine clinical examination should be performed on all patients presented for dental or other procedures (see also Chapter 2). Animals suffering from systemic disease require special attention and life-threatening conditions should be addressed immediately.

For basic oral examination larger rodents, such as guinea pigs and chinchillas, may be restrained manually. In smaller rodents, and where conscious oral cavity inspection is not possible, the animal should be sedated or anaesthetized (see Chapter 6). An assistant holds the animal's thoracic limbs and supports its back; the practitioner holds the animal's head and retracts its upper lips with one hand, while examining the oral cavity with the laryngoscope in the other. An alternative is to wrap the animal in a towel.

Conscious oral cavity examination starts with an evaluation of facial symmetry and palpation of the jaws. Signs of heat, discharge, crepitus and presence of facial masses should be noted. Lateral and horizontal lower jaw excursion should also be evaluated. Discomfort and pain on manipulating the jaws may be due to a jaw fracture, disease of the temporomandibular joint or because of retrobulbar pathology. If pain is noted, the animal should be monitored closely since it may easily become stressed during examination, leading to possible collapse. Palpation of the ventral border of the mandible and zygomatic area can reveal bony swellings associated with apical teeth elongation.

The oral cavity of herbivorous rodents is long and narrow, making it technically more difficult to examine than the oral cavity of other mammals. An otoscope is often recommended as a tool for oral examination of conscious animals. As an alternative, the use of a nasal or vaginal speculum is described. At the author's practice, the use of a paediatric laryngoscope is recommended. When a pathological process is found during conscious oral cavity examination, the animal should be anaesthetized for a more thorough examination (see Chapter 6).

Endoscopic examination under anaesthesia is the most suitable method for a detailed visualization of pathological changes in the oral cavity and oropharynx (Taylor, 1999; Jekl and Knotek, 2007). For this examination it is necessary to open the oral cavity in both horizontal and vertical directions; special rodent mouth gags are particularly useful for this purpose (Figure 8.4). The use of a specialist rodent mouth table-top or the combined use of the vertical dilator,

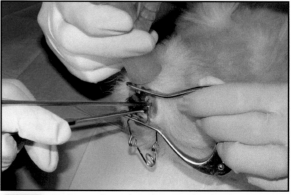

8.4 Endoscopic oral cavity examination in an anaesthetized guinea pig.

cheek dilator and paediatric laryngoscope or dental spatula is suitable when examining rodents with a very narrow oral cavity. Care should be taken to manipulate the oral cavity and associated structures very gently, in particular taking care not to open the oral cavity more than necessary, to prevent temporomandibular joint damage. Rigid endoscopes, 2.7 or 4 mm in diameter with viewing angles of 0, 30 and 70 degrees, are suitable. These optics improve the visualization of the oral cavity, particularly on all visible surfaces of the teeth, and the mucosal surface of the tongue, hard palate and oropharynx. The use of a protective sheath can reduce accessibility and limit manipulation in the oral cavity.

Each tooth and its surface should be examined individually along with its supportive structures. With the help of a periodontal probe, each tooth should be palpated and each gingival sulcus probed circumferentially to monitor tooth movement and depth of the sulcus. Soft tissue pathology, food impaction and presence of purulent discharge should also be recorded. Areas of black (metal-like) staining on the tooth surface suggest the presence of caries lesions.

Conventional radiography is an essential part of a thorough orofacial examination. Due to the small size of rodents, mammography or dental films should be used. Of all skull radiographic views, the lateral view followed by the two oblique views are the most helpful when evaluating dentition. Digital dental radiography is particularly useful, especially in small rodents, because this system produces high resolution and high quality images, with a wide range of post-processing adjustments. Extraoral or intraoral dental images can be performed on anaesthetized rodents (Figure 8.5).

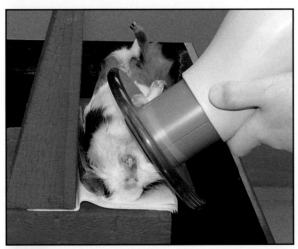

8.5 Extraoral dental radiography with the use of a portable X-ray unit.

Although high quality radiographs offer much information, they are still hindered by superimposition. This problem may be overcome with computed tomography (CT). CT imaging provides better soft tissue imaging and excellent detail of the bone structure. CT scanning is mostly suitable for detection of early evidence of apical teeth elongation, periodontitis and osteoresorptive lesions. (See Chapter 3 for further details.)

Record charts of oral lesions, endoscopic records and X-ray/CT images all serve as essential clinical information for determining further therapy and treatment. Depending on the results of the clinical examination and above-mentioned imaging methods, the examination may be complemented with microbiological analysis and blood sampling.

Dental disease

Malocclusion
Factors that affect tooth positioning, such as abnormalities of jaw width, length and height, may also result in malocclusion, as may variations in tooth arrangement along the jaw, the degree of eruption, tooth rotation and tipping. The following contribute to elongation of premolars and molars in those species with continually growing teeth: traumatic injuries of the orofacial area, lowered frequency of chewing movements, metabolic and infectious diseases, neoplasia, and developmental and genetic factors.

Myomorphs and sciuromorphs
Dental problems are seen in myomorphs because of their continually erupting incisors. Overgrown and fractured incisors with lateral mandibular shifting are seen most frequently. Occasionally, the long incisors penetrate the soft tissues of the upper or lower jaw or the hard palate, and acute or chronic inflammation and abscess formation ensues. Such lesions could lead to inanition through mechanical interference with food intake. The incisors may also break as a result of trauma (e.g. a fall or fighting). If the tooth root is damaged, it fails to erupt and the corresponding incisor on the opposite jaw is not worn down, and will overgrow (Figure 8.6). The highly mobile mandibular symphysis in the myomorphs and squirrel-like rodents permits the abnormal forces created by such malocclusions to rotate the mandibles, so that the mandibular incisors tend to bypass the maxillary teeth laterally, with the maxillary incisors curving into the oral cavity. Spontaneous reversed palatal perforation by upper incisors has been described in species with very high mechanical pressure at the apical sites of the upper incisors (e.g. blind mole-rats) (Zuri and Terkel, 2001).

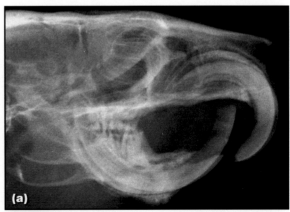

(a)

8.6 Incisor malocclusion due to traumatic fracture and mandibular osteomyelitis in a rat.
(a) Periosteal mandibular reaction is present radiographically. (continues) ▶

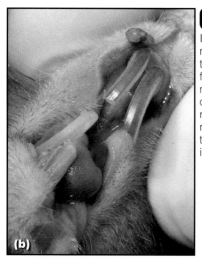

8.6

Incisor malocclusion due to traumatic fracture and mandibular osteomyelitis in a rat. **(b)** The reserve crown of the left mandibular incisor is affected.

occlusal surfaces are common findings at this stage.

In addition, occlusal pressure could prevent eruption of cheek teeth, so that the apices intrude and induce bony remodelling of adjacent tissues (Crossley, 2005). When this painful condition occurs in maxillary cheek teeth, epiphora or respiratory difficulties may be clinically evident. Mandibular cheek teeth apices also elongate and, in more severe cases, penetrate through the ventral mandibular cortex. As the condition progresses, mastication becomes more uncomfortable and only soft foods may be selectively eaten, resulting in further tooth growth due to lack of wear.

Guinea pigs: In guinea pigs, the most commonly affected teeth are the mandibular premolars, first mandibular molars and last maxillary molars. This is because any cheek teeth elongation has a tendency to push the mandible rostrally, so these teeth (or their parts) are not worn adequately and elongate lingually (Figure 8.7) or mesially (Crossley, 2005). As the disease progress, the tongue may become entrapped due to overgrowth of clinical crowns, which interferes with bite formation.

Sharp spur formation on cheek teeth is not as common in guinea pigs as in chinchillas. The normal occlusal surface is almost perpendicular to the longitudinal axis of the clinical crown. Lateral mandibular shifting may be seen when mastication is affected by coronal elongation or unilateral temporomandibular joint damage. This condition is mostly associated with an oblique occlusal incisor surface and changes in coronal height of the cheek teeth.

Hystricomorphs

The incidence of incisor malocclusion is higher in hystricomorphs with elodont cheek teeth. If the cheek teeth are not worn adequately and elongate intraorally (coronally), the mouth is held more open, stretching the masseter muscles and increasing the resting occlusal pressure on the teeth. As a result, the incisors elongate and lose the normal chisel-like wear pattern and animals have problems with bolus formation. Loss of supporting alveolar bone, pathological forces generated during chewing and tooth growth affect the curvature of the cheek teeth. Widening of the interproximal coronal surfaces, presence of sharp spurs, coronal elongation and abnormal cheek teeth

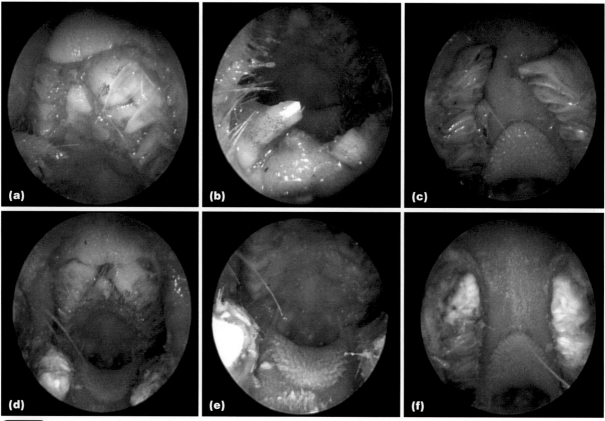

8.7 Endoscopic views showing malocclusion in a guinea pig before **(a–c)** and after **(d–f)** cheek teeth occlusal adjustment. Note that the animal is in dorsal recumbency in (c) and (f).

Chinchillas: Chinchillas have a high incidence of gum erosions and gingivitis. This correlates with the presence of elongated clinical crowns and spur formation, particularly involving the maxillary cheek teeth (Figure 8.8). In chinchillas, the main cause of partial or total obstruction of the lacrimal duct is bony remodelling around elongating maxillary premolar and first molar tooth 'roots'.

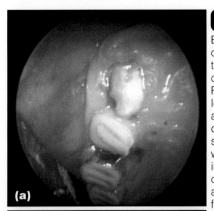

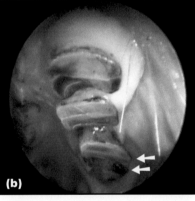

8.8 Endoscopic view of the cheek teeth in a chinchilla. Right **(a)** and left **(b)** maxillary arcades showing different occlusal surfaces, widening of the interproximal coronal spaces and spike formation on last two molars (arrows in (b)).

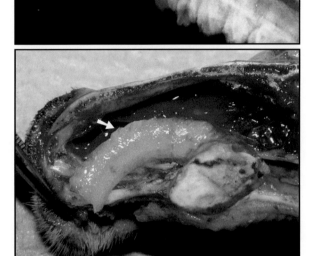

8.10 Elodontoma in a prairie dog (post-mortem specimens). The abnormalities and irregularities of the new dentine and enamel on the incisor labial surface may be seen (arrowed).

Degus: The incidence of dental disease in degus is very high, especially in older animals. In this species the normal curvature of the cheek teeth is straighter than in other rodents with elodont teeth, so that pathological coronal and apical elongation is more prominent (Figure 8.9). Apical cheek teeth elongation and apical incisor damage may result in elodontoma formation and nasal passage obturation (Figure 8.10).

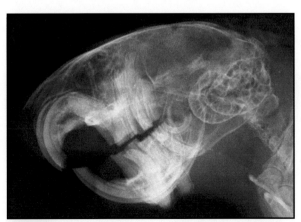

8.9 Slightly oblique lateral radiographic view of a degu skull. Severe cheek teeth malocclusion with apical elongation, particularly of the third maxillary cheek teeth, may be seen.

Caries, periodontitis and osteoresorptive lesions

The development of caries requires multiple interactions involving anatomy, physiology, diet and bacterial flora of the host. Periodontal disease and tooth decay are very common in captive rodents with bunodont cheek teeth (cheek teeth with low, rounded cusps on the occlusal surface of the crown, i.e. myomorphs and sciuromorphs) secondary to high sugar diets. Conversely, caries is rare in healthy animals with elodont dentition. Rodents with dental disease are however prone to dental caries and periodontal disease, due to reduced eruption of the cheek teeth, and/or a natural preference for high-energy and easy palatable food. In many cases, food impaction of the interproximal coronal spaces and between cheek and dental arcades may be seen. Foreign material and impacted hairs introduce bacteria into gingival sulci, resulting in bacterial colonization of the periodontal tissues and a pronounced inflammatory reaction (Figure 8.11). In severe cases, this may result in periodontitis, osteoresorptive lesions and abscess formation. Hypovitaminosis C in guinea pigs may cause loosening of teeth, gingival haemorrhage and periodontal lesions (see also Chapter 14).

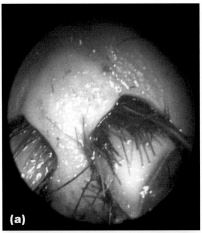

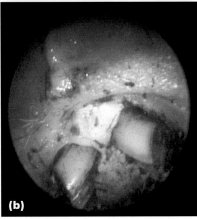

8.11

Impacted hairs around the gingival sulci causing periodontal inflammation in a guinea pig. Endoscopic views **(a)** before and **(b)** after periodontal pocket flushing with chlorhexidine solution.

Pseudoneoplastic and neoplastic lesions

Odontoma-like tumours (elodontomas) are commonly seen in prairie dogs (Phalen *et al.*, 2000). Spontaneous complex odontomas are described in mice and rats. It is postulated that the primary cause of these lesions could be of traumatic, inflammatory or toxic origin or may be associated with ageing and disrupted eruption due to malocclusion. Severe damage of odontogenic germ tissue is thought to result in the continuous development of dental tissue, possibly leading to the formation of tumorous masses. These lesions are mostly associated with the apex of the incisor teeth and result in upper respiratory signs that may be severe enough to cause death. Early changes include abnormalities and irregularities of the new dentine. Skull radiography reveals areas of increased opacity of the nasal cavity with the lost of conchal detail (see Figure 8.10). One or more teeth may be affected. Other spontaneous oral cavity tumours in rodents are rare.

Soft tissue injury

Foreign bodies, such as hay, seeds or grass, may become impacted around the teeth or in the cheeks, causing different stages of inflammation. Spurs on abnormally elongated teeth may damage adjacent soft tissues and cause erosive to ulcerative lesions, which may become secondarily infected.

'Wooden tongue' has been diagnosed by the author in chinchillas and rats due to infection with *Actinobacillus israelii*. The disease has a sudden onset, with the tongue becoming hard, swollen and painful. Affected animals are unable to eat or drink and there is rapid loss of condition. There is excessive salivation and the animal may appear reluctant to chew. The ulcerated tongue is often seen protruding between the lips. Diagnosis is made on histological examination of a tissue biopsy. The disease completely resolves after surgical excision and antibiotic (tetracycline) therapy.

Electrical burns involving the lips are the most common electrical injury in animals with access to power cables. These injuries are common in rodents given free access around the house. The burn most often invades both upper and lower lips, oral commissures and the tongue. Oedema, paraesthesia and tissue destruction contribute to drooling.

Osteoresorptive lesions are also evident in cases of severe malocclusion and apical cheek teeth elongation (Crossley, 2001). The causes are probably periodontitis, redirection of the resorption of alveolar bone towards the tooth itself and loss of blood supply. Dental resorptive lesions are common in chinchillas, guinea pigs and degus (Figure 8.12).

Dentoalveolar abscesses in myomorphs usually involve the incisor teeth. Infection often spreads and results in osteomyelitis, depending on the position of the incisors in relation to the molar teeth and the bone of the jaw.

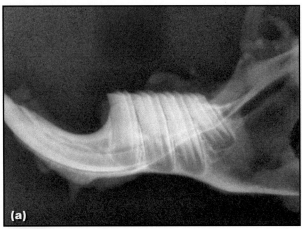
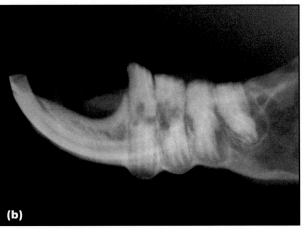

8.12   Lateral radiographic views of the left hemimandible in two chinchillas. Note the healthy cheek teeth **(a)**, compared with **(b)** cheek teeth with osteoresorptive lesions, apical elongation and variable crown size.

Therapy

Detailed examination of the oral cavity and any dental treatment should be carried out under general anaesthesia. Endotracheal intubation is not routinely practised since the endotracheal tube restricts access to the already limited space in the oral cavity. Analgesia is essential in all cases associated with dental pain. Supportive care, fluid therapy and assisted feeding are also often necessary (see Chapter 2).

Tooth extraction

Extraction should be considered only where there will be positive benefits to the animal. Pre-extraction radiographs are necessary to establish tooth morphology, curvature, fractures, or adjacent tissue disease. Dental instruments should be manipulated with careful and controlled force to prevent any iatrogenic injury.

Firstly, adjacent tissue and the tooth itself should be cleaned, and a gingival incision is made, which separates the gingival tissues from the tooth. Fine dental luxators and elevators are used to sever the periodontal ligament, to compress alveolar bone and to loosen the tooth. When the tooth/alveolar bone curvature is considerable or the animal is too small, hypodermic needles may be used to break down periodontal ligaments. Gentle rotational force is used to loosen and dislodge the tooth. In multi-rooted bunodont cheek teeth, the crown is sectioned or amputated to allow whole tooth extraction. Fine extraction forceps are used for tooth or tooth root extraction. The author recommends narrow extraction forceps for tooth roots and fine extraction forceps for upper premolars and upper molars. After extraction, the alveolar socket should be cleaned and flushed with saline. Use of mucoperiosteal or gingival flaps for extraction wound closure is sometimes necessary, especially when removing incisors.

In cases of incisor overgrowth, the author has had good experience with initial coronal height adjustment followed by extraction 5–7 days later. Tooth extraction is performed more easily, because the rate of incisor eruption in hypo-function (out of occlusion) is more rapid due to lack of wear (approximately 5–6 mm per week) and the dentoalveolar junction is more delicate.

A possible complication of elodont tooth extraction (especially the incisors) may be regrowth and eruption of a new tooth. Due to previous alveolar bone remodelling, the incisors mostly erupt in the same anatomical position as before or show various degrees of malpositioning and deformity. For this reason, the recommendation is to damage apical germinative tissue. When the pulp is not evident in extracted teeth, various techniques, or combinations of techniques, for tooth pulp damage may be used: apical curettage; the use of intrusive pressure of the corresponding teeth (the extracted tooth is pushed back into the alveolar socket and any remaining germinative tissue is destroyed); or administration of a cytotoxic agent directly into the germinative tissue with the use of an intravenous cannula. In the latter case, alveolar socket flushing with saline is necessary.

Iatrogenic pulp exposure is another common complication associated with traumatic tooth fracture or overzealous iatrogenic incisor trimming. Treatment of exposed pulp requires aseptic preparation of the site, sterile rinsing, haemostasis, drying, preparation of a small cavity and the use of an intermediate restorative material (hydroxide cement). Preoperative radiographs are necessary to assess the extent of any damage. In smaller species, sealing the surface with a drop of cyanoacrylate adhesive may be sufficient. Treated teeth need careful monitoring for evidence of inflammatory changes and infection.

Extraction of continually growing cheek teeth is possible by various methods. An intraoral or extraoral approach may be used, depending on tooth or adjacent tissue pathology. In the latter case, bone should be removed over the periapical tissues of the affected tooth. After tooth luxation, the tooth may be extracted through the surgical wound or pushed coronally and extracted intraorally. In all cases the alveolus should be flushed and debrided thoroughly to reduce the risk of inflammation.

Clinical crown adjustment

The use of a high- or low-speed dental unit with straight dental handpiece, able to reach the most mesially positioned tooth, is recommended for clinical crown adjustment. Care should be taken to avoid soft tissue and thermal damage to the pulp. Cotton swabs are helpful for cleaning the debris and saliva that accumulate in the oral cavity. The aim is to restore the normal crown height and occlusal plane.

Incisor crown height and occlusal surface adjustment can be carried out with a diamond burr in a high speed handpiece. Alternatively, in early or intermediate cases of incisor malocclusion, the author recommends that occlusal surfaces of the lower incisors are burred parallel to the anatomical occlusal plane of the upper incisors. The occlusal plane of the maxillary incisors, in this case, serves as the incline plane for the mandibular incisors. This may result in mandibular incisor crown movement towards the tongue and possible restoration of physiological occlusion.

Coronal reduction in cheek teeth should be performed when oral inspection and imaging methods show that elongated crowns are present. The coronal height is adjusted and spikes are removed using a burr on a dental handpiece. The occlusal plane is adapted depending on animal species. The degree of coronal reduction required depends on the severity of gingival hyperplasia, disease progression and the visible coronal height. If tooth growth is arrested, care should be taken when burring clinical crowns since excessive burring will prevent normal occlusion and wear for a longer period of time. Incisor and cheek teeth occlusion should be repeatedly monitored when cheek teeth coronal adjustment is performed.

Nail clippers, molar cutters and scissors should *not* be used for whole tooth trimming in any circumstance because of possible tooth fracture, tooth torsion, loss of occlusion and other pathology. Client education is essential to avoid such procedures being carried out by owners or breeders.

Caries, periodontal disease, abscesses and osteoresorptive lesions

Brachyodont teeth with caries are usually extracted (Figures 8.13 and 8.14). In larger animals, glass ionomers are used in smooth surface restoration on occlusal surfaces. Caries in elodont teeth can be removed using dental drills.

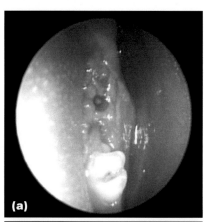

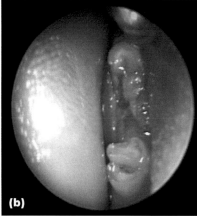

8.13 Dental caries in a rat. **(a)** The crowns of the mandibulary right M2 and M3 are missing. **(b)** The tooth most commonly affected by dental caries in myomorph rodents is the second molar (endoscopic view here shows the left mandible).

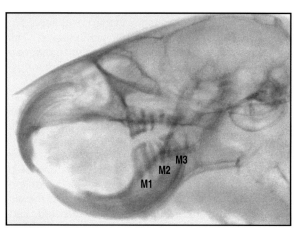

8.14 Lateral view of a hamster (inverted image). The tooth crown of mandibular M2 is missing due to dental caries.

Treatment of abscesses or osteomyelitis due to periodontal or endodontic disease should include thorough debridement, tooth extraction (if indicated), long-term antibiotic therapy and supportive care. The abscess capsule and affected bone should be dissected and removed as much as possible. The

debrided area should be marsupialized open with the skin being sutured to the underlying tissue to leave a large open wound to promote secondary healing. Local treatment consists of daily flushing and wound cleaning (Figure 8.15).

Manuka honey, povidone–iodine or potassium permanganate may be used as antiseptics and for healing support. Alternatively the wound may be packed and then closed using polymethylmethacrylate antibiotic-impregnated beads, doxycycline dental gel

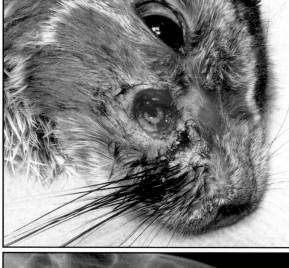

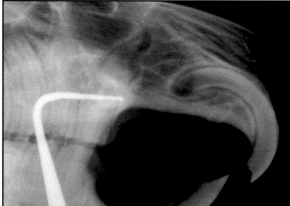

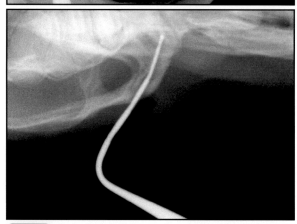

8.15 Periodontal abscessation and suspected osteoresorptive lesion in a chinchilla. Dental radiographs show probing of the abscess cavity and proving the communication with the apical parts of the right maxillary premolar and first molar.

or sponges impregnated with gentamicin. Antibiotic therapy is based on anaerobic and aerobic bacteriology results of abscess wall culture. Enrofloxacin, trimethoprim/sulphonamide, tetracyclines and/or metronidazole are the systemic drugs of choice in herbivorous rodents (see Chapter 5). In rats and mice amoxicillin clavulanate, enrofloxacin or clindamycin may be used.

Periodontal disease can be partially managed by dietary changes. Physical removal of any impacted foreign material, especially hairs and food, plaque deposits and loose teeth, is essential to permit proper healing. Periodontal pockets should be flushed with antiseptic solutions (e.g. chlorhexidine, benzydamin) and further food impaction may be minimized by local application of perioceutic products such as doxycycline gel. The latter provides physical protection for 2–4 weeks while tissues heal. Plaque may be removed by dental scaling in the early stages. In cases of severe periodontal inflammation or damage, extraction of the affected teeth should be performed.

In cases of osteoresorptive lesions, conservative therapy (monitoring), tooth extraction or coronal adjustments are the treatment options.

Pseudoneoplastic and neoplastic lesions

Possible treatment of elodontoma includes incisor extraction using an extraoral lateral or transpalatal approach. Rhinotomy with temporary stent placement is an alternative palliative treatment. In cases of neoplasia, biopsy and tumour staging is necessary for determination of prognosis and optimal treatment options.

The cheek pouches of the hamsters (especially of *Phodopus sungorus*) can become impacted with sticky food or large peanuts. Treatment consists of evacuation of impacted material and local application of antiseptic solutions under anaesthesia. Everted cheek pouch (Figure 8.16) may occur secondary to excessive grooming and cheek pouch injury. For cheek pouch replacement technique see Chapter 7.

Prevention of dental disease

Unfortunately most dental or oral cavity diseases in rodents tend to be chronic. Prevention of dental disease depends on feeding the correct diet with appropriate content for each species (see Chapter 1) and on regular veterinary consultations to ensure early diagnosis of any problems and to give the best prognosis for resolution. It is crucial to ensure good cooperation between clinician and owner and to provide client education. Dental disease is usually progressive and painful, especially in hystricomorphs, and so long-term postoperative management (including

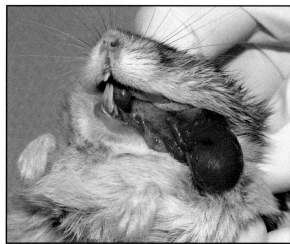

8.16 Cheek pouch eversion in a Russian dwarf hamster, due to the presence of a foreign body with cyst formation.

assisted feeding and analgesia) may be indicated. In severe cases of dental disease euthanasia should be considered in careful consultation with the owner.

References and further reading

Berkovitz BK (1972) Ontogeny of tooth replacement in the guinea pig (*Cavia cobaye*). *Archives of Oral Biology* **17**, 711–718

Capello V, Gracis M and Lennox AM (eds) (2005) *Rabbit and Rodent Dentistry Handbook.* Zoological Education Network Inc., Lake Worth, Florida

Crossley DA (2001) Dental diseases in chinchillas in the UK. *Journal of Small Animal Practice* **42**, 12–19

Crossley DA (2005) Pathophysiology of continuously growing teeth. In: *Proceedings of the 2nd Slovenian–Croatian congress on exotic pets and wild animals*, pp. 21–28, Ljubljana

Jekl V (2006) [Clinical diagnostics of intraoral pathological changes in small herbivorous mammals.] PhD Thesis, University of Veterinary and Pharmaceutical Sciences Brno, Czech Republic, 174 pp. (in Czech)

Jekl V and Knotek Z (2007) Evaluation of a laryngoscope and a rigid endoscope for the examination of the oral cavity of small mammals. *Veterinary Record* **160**, 9–13

Jekl V, Hauptman K, Gumpenberger M and Knotek Z (2007) Apical cheek teeth elongation and respiratory symptoms in degus (*Octodon degu*). *Proceedings of the 16th European Congress of Veterinary Dentistry*, pp. 12–14, Haag

Jekl V, Hauptman K and Knotek Z (2008) Quantitative and qualitative assessments of intraoral lesions in 180 small herbivorous mammals. *Veterinary Record* **162**, 442–449

Legendre LFJ (2003) Oral disorders of exotic rodents. *Veterinary Clinics of North America: Exotic Animal Practice* **6**, 601–628

Phalen DN, Antinof N and Fricke ME (2000) Obstructive respiratory disease in prairie dogs with odontomas. *Veterinary Clinics of North America: Exotic Animal Practice* **3**, 513–517

Taylor M (1999) Endoscopy as an aid to the examination and treatment of the oropharyngeal disease of small herbivorous mammals. *Seminars on Avian and Exotic Pet Medicine* **8**, 139–141

Wiggs RB and Lobprise HB (1997) Dental and oral disease in rodents and lagomorphs. In: *Veterinary Dentistry Principles and Practice*, ed. RB Wiggs and HB Lobprise, pp. 518–537, Lippincott–Raven, Philadelphia

Zuri I and Terkel J (2001) Reversed palatal perforation by upper incisors in ageing blind mole-rats (*Spalax ehrenbergi*). *Journal of Anatomy* **199**, 591–598

9

Rodents: biology, husbandry and clinical techniques in more unusual pet species

Cathy A. Johnson-Delaney

Chipmunks

Chipmunks occur in North America, Europe and Asia. The genus *Eutamias* consists of two subgenera and 24 species. The term *Eutamias* is often used as a synonym for *Tamias*, although *Walker's Mammals of the World* (Nowak, 1991) separates *Tamias* (single species *T. striatus*) from *Eutamias*. *Tamias striatus* (Figure 9.1) is the eastern American chipmunk and occurs throughout the eastern United States and southeastern Canada. It is rarely kept as a pet. Most pet chipmunks in the USA and Europe are *Eutamias sibiricus* (*Tamias sibiricus*) (Figure 9.2), the original range of which is Siberia, Mongolia, northern and central China, Korea and Hokkaido. Information in this chapter refers to this species, but is applicable to most other chipmunks of the genus *Eutamias*.

Chipmunks typically are distinguished by characteristic black-and-white stripes along the back, as well as through the eyes. The wild-type colouring is brown to grey fur with white or yellowish ventrum. They have a long bushy tail with dark guard hairs tipped with white. There are colour variations in captive-bred chipmunks, including all-cream, albino and piebald. In many of these colour variants the striping is no longer visible.

Natural habitat and biology

Eutamias sibiricus primarily inhabits forests of evergreen trees such as fir, pine and spruce as well as woodlands of deciduous trees and brush. The chipmunks reside in burrows and are active during the day. Nests may be in hollow logs and tree branches, or, in the winter, chambers tend to be burrows underground. Wild chipmunks are omnivorous, with a diet of seeds, buds, leaves and flowers. They will climb trees to obtain food. They have cheek pouches to carry food back to the nest and tend to hoard food items. They are coprophagic, allowing uptake of vitamins B and K. Biological data are summarized in Figure 9.3.

9.1 Eastern American chipmunk (*Tamias striatus*) prior to release back into the wild.

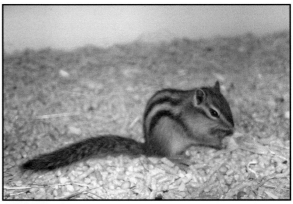

9.2 Captive pet chipmunk (*Eutamias sibiricus* (*Tamias sibiricus*)). (Courtesy of Emma Keeble.)

Lifespan in captivity	Males: up to 8 years Females: up to 12 years General: 4–6 years
Adult body weight	Depends on species: 70–142 g
Body temperature	38°C. When in torpor: a few degrees above ambient
Heart rate (beats per minute)	264–296 bpm; during torpor may drop to 3–6 bpm (Jones and Wang, 1976)

9.3 Biological data for the chipmunk (*Eutamias sibiricus*). (continues) ▶

Respiratory rate	75 breaths per minute
Food consumption	25–30 g/day per animal
Fluid consumption	75–100 ml/kg/day
Activity	Diurnal
Dentition	Incisors open-rooted: (I 1/1; C 0/0; PM 1–2/1; M 3/3) x 2 = 20–22 teeth (*Eutamias* has 2 maxillary PM, *Tamias* spp. have 1) (see also Chapter 8)
Mammary glands	4 pairs
Sexual maturity	Approximately 1 year
Sexing	Anogenital distance greater in males than females Prepuce obvious in males Testes obvious in mature males, begin seasonal enlargement in January, with breeding season commencing in March (northern hemisphere) Testes stay enlarged through to September
Oestrous cycle length	13–14 days (range: 11–21 days)
Ovulation	Spontaneous, oestrus 3 days, vocalize repeatedly Mating usually on day 2
Postpartum oestrus	No
Captive pairing	Take female to male for mating unless continuously housed as a pair Female aggressive to non-paired male when not in oestrus
Gestation	31–32 days (range 28–35 days)
Litter size	3–5 (range 1–10) Altricial (naked, blind)
Litters per year	Usually one; may have second smaller litter if wean early
Breeding season (northern hemisphere)	March–September Male testicular enlargement starts in January in the northern hemisphere, prior to onset of female oestrous cycles in March Respond to lengthening light cycle and increasing temperatures Indoor housing with constant long light days can lead to infertility
Emergence from nest	Approximately day 35 after birth
Weaning	Approximately 42 days old
Abandonment of young	Any stress, noise (television, radio, human disturbances), proximity of predators (house cats, dogs particularly) may cause the female to abandon young
Hand-rearing of orphans	Successful if >1 week old
Hand-rearing formula	Evaporated milk diluted 1:2 with water, syringe feeding every 4 hours first week, then add baby cereal, increase volume and intervals between feedings to 6–8 hours. Add probiotic Stimulate urination/defecation before and after each feeding by rubbing anogenital area with warm moist cotton wool Volumes to feed depend on overall health, stomach capacity and individual tolerances. Start at 5% of body weight and gradually increase as long as no indications of gastrointestinal upset such as gas, bloat, diarrhoea Example: 0.5 ml per 10 g body weight to start. When body weight is >100 g, feed at 7% body weight (7 ml/100 g) until weaning

9.3   (continued) Biological data for the chipmunk (*Eutamias sibiricus*).

Chipmunks do not hibernate in cold weather, but will become torpid and hoard food in their nest in preparation. In captivity, extra nest material should be supplied and food stores should not be removed. Generally pet chipmunks kept indoors at home temperatures do not exhibit the winter torpor episodes, though there is still a tendency to hoard more food in the autumn. Lifespan and health in pet chipmunks may be better if they are not allowed to follow a torpor episode pattern (Meredith, 2002).

Captive husbandry and diet
Chipmunks are not domesticated rodents and retain much of their wild behaviour in captivity. Because of this, they do not make ideal pets. They are easily stressed and may exhibit stereotypical behaviours. They also require larger enclosures than domesticated rodents of similar size. They are best kept outdoors, or at least with some outdoor access.

Housing
Chipmunks can be housed singly, in pairs, or in harem groups comprising one male and two or three females. If there is sufficient space, same-sex groups may be compatible, but usually adult males fight.

Outdoor housing should be sheltered from direct sun and prevailing weather. Indoor caging should be placed out of direct sunlight and away from human noise and disturbances. Good ventilation and air quality are essential in designing and placing housing.

Caging must be of strong metal mesh no larger than 2.5 cm spacing, with metal support structure (Figure 9.4). Minimal cage dimensions for one chipmunk are 1.2 m high by 3.5–4.5 m wide and deep, although there is no upper limit on size. Double doors with secure locking mechanisms are recommended. Outdoor habitats may be similar to walk-in aviaries in construction. Wood or heavy plastic can be used for furnishings, for nest boxes and for exercise, but wood will need frequent replacement as chipmunks gnaw incessantly. Non-toxic hardwood such as apple or other fruit trees, willow or maple branches work well for climbing and nest box construction. Polyvinyl chloride (PVC) pipes and fittings can be used for furnishings.

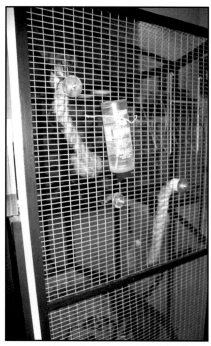

9.4 Typical chipmunk housing. (Courtesy of Emma Keeble.)

Nest boxes should have a flap door that can be closed when the chipmunk is asleep, securing the animal in the box. Nest material can be paper-based, dry hay or straw that cannot become impacted in the chipmunk's cheek pouches or entangle its toenails. The nest box should be cleaned about once a month except during the winter, when the animal should be left undisturbed.

Exercise wheels available for small pet rodents may be used. Chipmunks burrow and forage on the ground, so the base of the cage should be solid and impervious to gnawing or digging through. A deep layer (3–6 cm) of substrate such as paper pellets, shredded recycled paper substrate or hardwood chips will allow normal behaviour.

Soiled bedding should be removed frequently so that faecal material, moisture and ammonia levels do not build up in the cage. This can be done in the evening or when the chipmunk is secure in the nest box, to minimize disturbances. The cage can then be cleaned and the substrate and furnishings replaced.

Diet

The captive diet can be based on a general rodent pellet suitable for rats and mice. This can be supplemented with small amounts of vegetables, fruit, nuts and seeds. A seed-based rodent mix is inadequate as it is largely composed of sunflower seeds and peanuts, both of which are high in fat and low in calcium. Occasional treat foods can include mealworms, hard-boiled egg, cooked meat, dog food, or day-old chicks from a reputable source so that they do not have an antibiotic or antiparasitic drug level. Pregnant or lactating females require extra protein. Uneaten or hoarded fresh foods need to be removed daily to prevent mould formation. Water should be provided by sipper tube and bottle and should be changed daily.

Handling and restraint

Some hand-reared chipmunks will allow minimal handling by being cupped in the hands or held by the scruff of the neck, similar to handling of a hamster (see Chapter 2). Most are not tame and may inflict a powerful bite if handled, despite acceptance of food by hand. A lightweight net can be useful to catch the chipmunk, which can then be carefully grasped around the shoulders or scruffed. Chasing the animal should be avoided as it is very stressful. Heavy leather gloves for restraint (Figure 9.5) do not allow the dexterity and sensitivity needed to restrain the chipmunk safely. Double layers of procedure latex gloves or surgical orthopaedic gloves will afford some protection.

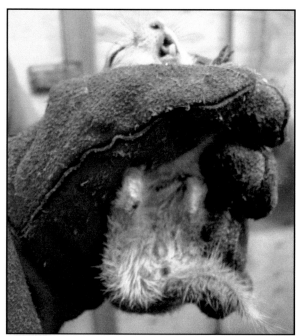

9.5 Most chipmunks resent handling. Leather gloves may be worn, but they are cumbersome and do not always allow the dexterity and sensitivity needed to restrain chipmunks safely. (Courtesy of Emma Keeble.)

The chipmunk should not be grasped by the tail as degloving injuries can occur, similar to those in gerbils and degus (see Chapter 2). For clinical examination, mild sedation with midazolam at 0.25–0.3 mg/kg i.m. is recommended. Full anaesthesia may be necessary for blood sampling or other diagnostic tests.

Diagnostic approach

Physical examination and observations

If possible, the animal should first be observed in its home cage to assess activity level, locomotion, balance, behaviours and content of the latrine area. Confinement of the awake chipmunk in a clear plastic container will allow assessment of body condition, respiratory pattern, or injury. Full examination does require sedation or full anaesthesia (see below).

Blood collection and sampling

Under anaesthesia, blood may be obtained from the jugular vein or the saphenous vein. A safe volume to withdraw depends on the body weight and condition of the chipmunk, but usually 0.1–0.2 ml can be withdrawn from most adults.

Other diagnostic sampling techniques and imaging are the same as in similarly sized rats or hamsters (see Chapters 2 and 3). Serological testing for the presence of rodent pathogens is not usually done as tests have not been validated for this species. However, many diagnostic laboratories may be able to screen wild-caught pet chipmunks for rodent-borne zoonotic infections such as lymphocytic chorio-meningitis virus, *Salmonella* spp., *Yersinia pestis* (plague), *Borrelia burgdorferi* (Lyme disease) and rabies (see also Chapters 1 and 4).

Common conditions

Diseases commonly seen in chipmunks are described in Figure 9.6. Many of the disease conditions found in other rodents, as well as their treatments, have been extrapolated to chipmunks. There are no published drug formularies for chipmunks; the author refers to dosages used in rats (see Chapter 5).

Disease	Aetiology	Clinical signs	Diagnostic tests	Treatment
Anorexia	Stress, overcrowding (subordinate animal), torpor, any systemic illness	Emaciation, poor coat condition, no faecal output Porphyrin staining around the eyes Lethargy	CBC, chemistries, radiology, ultrasonography	Correct husbandry, social situation, treat systemic illness Supportive care: fluid therapy, gavage feed, vitamin B complex for appetite stimulation
Bacterial cystitis/ urethritis	Ascending infections, concurrent urogenital infections, dehydration, calculi	Haematuria, dysuria (may vocalize), penile swelling/ protrusion, anorexia	Urinalysis, culture and sensitivity, radiology or ultrasonography to rule out concurrent uroliths	Analgesia, antibiosis, anti-inflammatories Be sure cage latrine area is kept cleaned
Bacterial enteritis	e.g. *Salmonella*. Wild rodents can act as a source; fecal accumulation in habitat	Diarrhoea, dehydration, weight loss, anorexia, stained/wet perineum, death	Faecal culture	Appropriate antibiosis, fluid therapy, supportive care Euthanasia if zoonosis (e.g. *Salmonella*)
Cage paralysis	Vitamin E deficiency, although general dietary deficiencies including calcium may contribute	Weakness, paresis, paralysis Weight loss and muscle atrophy if untreated	Review diet, elevated CPK/cholesterol Radiography to rule out fractures	Dietary supplementation with Vitamin E, other diet corrections NSAIDs and supportive care, keep in smaller habitat until strength returns
Cataracts	Unknown. Reported in older chipmunks, especially males (Meredith, 2002)	Partial/complete blindness (usually bilateral)	Ocular examination	Although surgical excision is possible, captive chipmunks appear to learn their environments and do not require treatment
Comatose, unresponsive	Torpor during winter/cold weather; end stage any disease	Low body temperature/ heart rate/respiratory rate, stays curled up, does not respond to touch	History, physical examination	Warming slowly with external heating Subcutaneous fluids if torpor
Dental disease, including incisor overgrowth, incisor fracture, cheek tooth abscess	Insufficient wear (usually diet related), trauma to mouth/teeth	Overgrown incisors, anorexia, salivation, facial soft tissue penetration, swelling May cause rhinitis May paw at mouth frequently	Oral examination, skull radiography	Bur teeth under sedation/anaesthesia (see Chapter 8) If abscess: drain, antibiosis If non-viable cheek teeth – remove Correct diet to include items for tooth wear: nuts in shell, dog biscuits, branches of hardwood
Dermatitis	Bacterial (may start with small bite wounds) Fungal (particularly if wet environment, stressed animal) May be secondary to ectoparasites	Areas of scabbing, alopecia, erythema; may be pruritic	Skin scraping, fungal/ bacterial culture	Antibiosis if bacterial Antifungal medication if fungal NSAIDs Correct stressors, husbandry (see also Chapter 5)

9.6 Common diseases of chipmunks. (continues) ▶

Disease	Aetiology	Clinical signs	Diagnostic tests	Treatment
Ectoparasites	May be indistinguishable from bacterial or fungal dermatitis without diagnostics: fleas, ticks, mange mites	Areas of alopecia, erythema with/without pruritis Parasites may be visible	Visual examination under magnification; skin scrapings, hair plucks	Appropriate topical and/or systemic preparation as used in guinea pigs for similar ectoparasites (see Chapters 5 and 10) Correct husbandry, clean out caging, furnishings, substrates. Treat environment surrounding caging if appropriate Remove ticks, submit to laboratory as may be vector for zoonoses, e.g. borreliosis
Fractures	Limbs/spine/tail Usually history of fall, fight or mishandling	Lameness, paresis, paralysis May chew affected area where there is pain	History, physical examination, radiography	Small cage confinement, analgesia, NSAIDs Amputate if severe limb fracture as splints/bandages not well tolerated; euthanasia if spinal fracture with paralysis
Hypocalcaemia	Poor diet both sexes; may follow parturition particularly if large litter, during lactation	Posterior paresis/paralysis, incoordination, tremors, collapse, semi-conscious state	Review diet/reproductive status Serum chemistry for calcium level	0.5 ml of 10% calcium gluconate s.c. (may dilute in 2–3 ml warm LRS) Calcium supplementation short term; diet correction to include calcium-rich foods
Hypothermia	Winter torpor, result of malnutrition, poor husbandry, systemic illness, shock following injury	Subnormal body temperature, slow to rouse, may stay curled up	Review diet, husbandry, history, physical examination, other diagnostic testing as appropriate	Warming slowly with external heating, subcutaneous fluids Correct underlying problems
Mammary tumours	Usually benign fibroadenomas	Mammary mass, with/without ulceration	Clinical signs, fine-needle aspiration, biopsy	Surgical removal (see Chapter 7)
Metritis/pyometra	Metritis: usually due to retained fetus. May progress to peritonitis, toxaemia Pyometra: as for other species	Vaginal discharge, abdominal enlargement, pain, anorexia and unthriftiness If lactating, may cease	Clinical signs, history, bacterial culture of discharge, abdominal ultrasonography and/or radiology	Antibiosis, supportive care, ovariohysterectomy
Neurological signs	Hypocalcaemia, waking from torpor, general malnutrition with weakness; trauma (particularly skull), toxicosis (environmental), encephalitis (bacterial)	Incoordination, paresis, paralysis, seizures, tremors, anisocoria, hypersalivation	Review history, diet, husbandry. Full workup including blood work, radiology	If trauma – assess feasibility of recovery Supportive care, NSAIDs, analgesics, antibiosis per aetiology
Pneumonia	Predisposing stressors: overcrowding, poor ventilation, damp conditions, ammonia build-up from latrine area Assumed bacterial but can contract human influenza viruses (Meredith, 2002)	Dyspnoea, tachypnoea, anorexia, unkempt coat Often fatal	Clinical signs, radiography, tracheal wash cytology and culture	Anti-anxiety relaxant such as midazolam, NSAIDs; antibiosis, bronchodilator; consider nebulization Supportive care: oxygen, heated environment, fluids, assist feeding, rest and quiet (see also Chapter 12)
Rhinitis/upper respiratory infection	May occur in association with incisor overgrowth, chronic suppurative periodontal disease; dusty or poorly ventilated environment (irritation)	Nasal discharge, upper respiratory tract stridor, epistaxis, face rubbing, conjunctivitis May see matting of forearms from grooming	Clinical signs, oral examination, ocular examination, radiography of skull, culture and sensitivity	Antibiosis, analgesia, NSAIDs; consider nebulization Supportive care: oxygen, heated environment, fluids, assist feeding, rest and quiet (see also Chapter 12) Correct dental disease if possible
Trauma (lacerations, bite wounds)	Fight wounds from cagemates (improper social combinations), predator attacks	Wounds, scabs, alopecia, pain, lameness or guarding a body area	Review social situation, husbandry, clinical signs, culture and sensitivity	Antibiosis, surgical correction if wounds severe, analgesia, NSAIDs Correct social situation and husbandry
Tumours	Masses anywhere on body, may ulcerate on surface or be self-mutilated if painful	Lumps, bumps, or (if bone tumour) lameness, pain	Clinical signs, palpation, radiology, ultrasonography, fine needle aspiration biopsy	Surgical removal if possible, analgesia, antibiosis if infected surface, supportive palliative care, euthanasia if quality of life severely compromised

9.6 (continued) Common diseases of chipmunks.

Wild-caught chipmunks may be asymptomatic hosts for a number of infectious diseases and parasites. As well those already listed, they may carry *Cryptosporidium parvum*, *Eimeria* spp., sarcoptiform mites and dermatophytes. A chipmunk brought in as a rescued animal must be considered a potential vector for zoonotic disease and precautions with handling the animal at the veterinary clinic should be considered.

General signs of illness, pain or distress in the chipmunk are similar to those seen in other rodents (see Chapter 2). Low body temperature must be interpreted with time of year and housing conditions (see above). An ill, hypothermic chipmunk needs to be warmed slowly and given warmed fluids to encourage revival from the torpid state. Fluids may be injected subcutaneously or intraperitoneally. If severe dehydration is present, intravenous or intraosseous administration of colloids and crystalloid fluids may be necessary (see also Chapter 2). Volumes for fluid and nutritional therapy are listed in Figure 9.7.

Route	Volume	Fluid type and comments
Oral (gavage, syringe feeding)	2–5 ml per feed	Oral rehydration solutions, herbivore critical care formula per body weight, human baby food cereals, vegetable stews
Subcutaneous	3–8 ml per injection site; daily requirements 75–100 ml/kg	Isotonic crystalloids
Intramuscular	Maximum volume 0.1 ml, quadriceps	Medications suitable for intramuscular injection
Intraosseous (femur, tibia)	50–70 ml/kg bolus for shock; daily requirements 75–100 ml/kg	Crystalloids, colloids
Intraperitoneal	5–10 ml maximum volume. Contraindicated if abdominal mass effect, fluid pressure pre-existing	Crystalloids, colloids
Intravenous (saphenous, jugular)	Catheter for intravenous drip. Bolus for medication injection; up to 75–100 ml/kg/day	Medications suitable for intravenous administration; crystalloids, colloids

9.7 Administration routes, fluid volumes and suggested fluids for therapy in chipmunks.

Behavioural problems

Chipmunks are extremely susceptible to stress and may remain quiescent for up to a day following a stressful event. Continued stress may result in hyperactivity and stereotypical behaviours such as circling or looping around the cage. Stressors can include catching, handling, small caging, overcrowding, insufficient nest boxes, proximity of predators (other pets, dogs, cats), electronic devices emitting electromagnetic and/or ultrasonic radiation, and transportation. Stress may exacerbate aggression from incompatible cage mates and aggression adds to the stress of the subordinate animals. Aggression may

increase in the autumn, when food-hoarding increases in preparation for hibernation (torpor) (see above).

Anaesthesia and analgesia

Inhalational anaesthetic gas, such as isoflurane or sevoflurane, can be delivered without handling the chipmunk if it is confined in a container or large canine facemask. Administration of a sedative such as midazolam at 0.25–0.3 mg/kg i.m. prior to the administration of the gas anaesthetic decreases the anxiety produced during induction, but it does require handling of the chipmunk first. Alfaxalone (Alfaxan, Vétoquinol) has been reported anecdotally in rats at a dose rate of 10–11 mg/kg i.m. or i.p. for induction/maintenance of anaesthesia; this dose rate could be extrapolated to chipmunks. Dosages of anaesthetic and analgesic agents used in rats and mice appear to be effective (see Chapter 6). The principles of pre-emptive analgesia as used in rats can be extrapolated to chipmunks. Buprenorphine at 0.1 mg/kg s.c. q6–12h has been used effectively for analgesia (Meredith, 2002). Coaxial scavenging systems designed for laboratory rodents are useful for clinical use in this and other small rodent species.

Once the chipmunk is anaesthetized in the chamber, it can be removed and anaesthesia maintained with a small facemask. It may be helpful to swab out the oral cavity and cheek areas to prevent aspiration of retained food.

Common surgical procedures

Intraoperative monitoring is as for other small rodents (see Chapter 6). Heat should be provided to maintain body temperature. As chipmunks will chew exposed sutures, all suture should be buried. Procedures for castration and ovariohysterectomy are similar to those in rats (see Chapter 7). Closed castration is preferable, to prevent abdominal herniation. Wound repair, amputations and fracture repair are problematic as the chipmunk may have already chewed the affected area; antibiotic therapy is required as well as analgesia in addition to the repair of the traumatic condition.

Duprasi

Natural habitat and biology

The duprasi or fat-tailed gerbil (*Pachyuromys duprasi*) (Figure 9.8) is infrequently found in the pet trade and has been used in a limited number of studies as a laboratory animal. It is native to the *hamadas* (patches of vegetation) of the northern Sahara Desert from western Morocco to Egypt. Its coat is yellow–grey to buffy brown, with white feet and underparts and a white spot behind each ear, and it has a bicoloured club-shaped tail. There are well developed claws on the front feet.

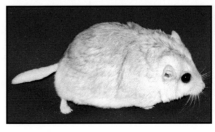

9.8 Duprasi (fat-tailed gerbil) (*Pachyuromys duprasi*). (© Jackie Roswell.)

The duprasi has open-rooted upper incisors that are slightly grooved. The dental formula is similar to that of myomorphs: (I 1/1, C 0/0, PM 0/0, M3/3) × 2 = 16. Biological data are summarized in Figure 9.9.

Lifespan	Average 3 years (4 years 5 months recorded in captivity)
Weight	60–90 g
Length	Head and body 105–135 mm, tail 45–60 mm
Sexual maturity	2.5–3.5 months
Gestation period	19–22 days
Litter size	3–6
Diet	Insectivorous
Husbandry/housing	Similar to Syrian hamster but prefers warmer ambient temperature of 24°C; provide nest box on floor of cage

9.9 Biological data for the duprasi (*Pachyuromys duprasi*).

Diet

The diet should consist of a commercial insectivore pelleted diet with additional live insects (calcium gutloaded) several times a week. A small amount of various greens, edible flowers and vegetables can be offered several times a week. Larval insects should be provided in very limited quantities and can be scattered about the cage for foraging enrichment activity. Grain- and seed-based rodent diets promote obesity in duprasi and should not be used, though the occasional seed as a treat food can be offered.

Techniques and common conditions

Handling, blood sampling, injection sites and routes of medication administration are as for domestic gerbils and hamsters (see Chapters 2 and 5). Medications and dosages used for Syrian hamsters seem to be effective and safe for duprasi, though no pharmacological trials have been documented.

The major disease problems identified in pet duprasi include obesity, malnutrition, trauma, diarrhoea and enteropathy (probably associated with bacterial pathogens) and dental malocclusion of the incisors. Differential diagnoses of diseases in the duprasi are summarized in Figure 9.10.

Prairie dog

Natural habitat and biology

The black-tailed prairie dog (*Cynomys ludovicianus*) (Figure 9.11) is native to North America. It is diurnal and does not truly hibernate. It may have dormant periods in inclement weather and tends to gain weight in the autumn as the light cycle and temperature decrease. Vocalizations include a 'bark' when excited and various chatters and growls. Prairie dogs are social animals and live in large communities or 'towns' in the wild. They are housed in large social groupings in zoos, but are frequently kept as solitary pets. They require companionship and when solitary may develop behavioural abnormalities, including self-mutilation and aggressiveness towards humans. Digging is a primary activity and they have long sharp toenails that need frequent trimming and blunting. They are not agile climbers, but many try to climb in a household environment. Biological data are summarized in Figure 9.12.

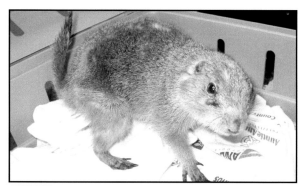

9.11 Prairie dog (*Cynomys ludovicianus*) showing typical defensive posture.

Clinical signs/disease	Aetiology	Diagnostic tests	Treatment
Diarrhoea, enteropathy	Bacterial infections Ingestion of foreign bodies	Faecal examination, culture and sensitivity, radiographs, CBC/chemistry panel	Appropriate antimicrobial therapy, NSAIDs, gastrointestinal protectants, fluid therapy, supportive care (see also Chapter 11) If foreign body impaction: enterotomy
Malocclusion	Dental trauma Tooth root infection	Skull radiographs, oral examination: conscious using an otoscope for preliminary assessment, then full examination under general anaesthesia	Burr teeth, treat underlying cause Infection: if tooth non-viable, remove; antibiosis, NSAIDs to stop osteomyelitis as with other rodents
Obesity, malnutrition	Improper diet, excess carbohydrates and fats Lack of exercise	CBC/chemistry panel, radiographs	Correct diet/husbandry Provide exercise and live insects to hunt
Trauma: wounds, fractures	Attacks from other pets Improper handling (dropped)	Radiographs; culture and sensitivity if wounds appear infected	Appropriate antimicrobials, wound care as in other rodents, NSAIDs, analgesia Fracture repair similar to birds/small mammals Correct diet/husbandry to prevent future incidents

9.10 Common diseases of the companion duprasi.

Weight	0.5–2.2 kg (males larger than females, heavier in autumn/winter)
Dentition	Open-rooted incisors, (I 1/1, C 0/0, PM 1/1, M 3/3) x 2 = 20
Body temperature	35.3–39.0°C
Torpor	Will enter torpor state if ambient temperature drops below 20.5°C for prolonged periods
Sexual maturity	2–3 years of age
Lifespan	Pets: 6–10 years
Gestation period	30–35 days
Breeding season	Spring in northern hemisphere Usually colony social situation necessary for successful captive breeding and rearing Monoestrous, seasonal, one litter per year
Litter size	2–10 (average 5)
Mammary glands	8–12
Weaning age	6 weeks
Diet in captivity	Unlimited grass hay, small amounts of various fresh greens as treats Juveniles: also pelleted guinea pig or rodent chow, and alfalfa Adults: 1–2 rodent chow blocks per week, no alfalfa hay; should not be fed peanuts, raisins, French fries, cereal, bread, dog biscuits, etc.
Housing	Large wire cages suitable for rabbits or guinea pigs Deep substrate bedding of shredded newspaper pellets or hardwood shavings for digging Provision of PVC pipes to simulate tunnels they would normally build Preferred environmental temperature range is 20.5–22°C
Unique anatomical features	Trigonal anal sacs, ducts that appear as white papillae beside the anus (Figure 9.13) Testicles descend relatively late and are more prominent during breeding season No distinct scrotal sac Hindgut fermenters: require roughage in diet.

9.12   Biological data for the prairie dog (*Cynomys ludovicianus*).

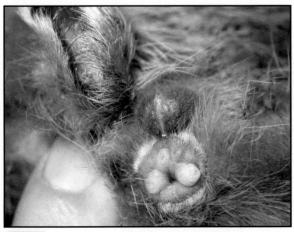

9.13   Trigonal anal sacs. These are a unique anatomical feature of prairie dogs.

Captivity regulations

Until 2003, prairie dogs in the American pet trade were harvested from the wild, though a few captive-bred animals were available. In 2003, prairie dogs housed with imported exotic rodents, principally Gambian giant rats (*Cricetomys* spp.) from Africa at pet distributors in Texas and Illinois, became infected with monkeypox (orthopoxvirus). These prairie dogs developed systemic disease with lesions in numerous organs. Initially the prairie dogs had conjunctivitis progressing to necrotizing blepharoconjunctivitis. Respiratory signs and nodular skin lesions were also found. The lesions in the prairie dog resembled monkeypox lesions in non-human primates and smallpox lesions in humans. A number of humans became infected with monkeypox.

Because of this outbreak, the US Centers for Disease Control and Prevention and the US Food and Drug Administration enacted 42 CFR 70.2, 42 CFR 71.32(b), and 21 CFR 1240.30, which placed an embargo on importation of all rodents from Africa. The regulations also prohibited the transportation or offering to transport in interstate commerce, or the sale or offering for sale, or offering for any other type of commercial or public distribution, including release into the environment, of prairie dogs and the following African rodents: tree squirrels (*Heliosciurus* spp.), rope squirrels (*Funisciurus* spp.), dormice (*Graphiurus* spp.), Gambian giant pouched rats (*Cricetomys* spp.), brush-tailed porcupines (*Atherurus* spp.) and striped mice (*Hybomys* spp.). States were also empowered to enact measures to prohibit importation, sale, distribution or display of animals that could result in transmission of infectious agents. Because of this, the number of prairie dogs seen as pets has been decreasing as the owned animals age and die. It is unlikely that these regulations will be lifted in the near future. In the United Kingdom these animals may be legally kept as pets.

Techniques

Blood collection is from the lateral or medial saphenous vein, cephalic vein, jugular vein or cranial vena cava. The last two sites require anaesthesia. Injection sites and volumes are listed in Figure 9.14.

Fluid therapy follows guidelines for guinea pigs (see Chapter 2). Unlike guinea pigs, which have the ostium anatomical structure that must be pushed through the central opening to pass a tube, prairie dogs can easily be gavage fed, using a herbivore formulation such as Critical Care or Critical Care Fine Grind (Oxbow Pet Products) or vegetable baby food. For gavaging, rather than metal feeding needles the author usually uses a red rubber French catheter size 12 or 14 softened in a cup of hot water. The tube should be premeasured and the tip lubricated with a small amount of lubricating jelly. An oral speculum with a hole in the middle to pass a catheter through can be made from a 3 ml syringe casing. It is placed in the mouth behind the incisors in the diastema space and the premeasured tube is passed into the stomach. Gavage volume can be between 5 and 10 ml/feed up to three times daily to maintain weight or until the prairie dog is eating on its own.

Route	Site	Volume
Subcutaneous	Supra/intrascapular, dorsal back	10–15 ml/site
Intramuscular	Anterior thigh	0.5 ml
Intraperitoneal	Do not administer if abdominal disease	5–10 ml
Intraosseous	Femur, tibia	1–2 ml bolus, or slow infusion if catheter placed
Intravenous	Saphenous, cephalic	3–10 ml slow bolus
Venipuncture	Cranial vena cava (under anaesthesia)	0.3–0.5 ml/kg
	Saphenous, cephalic	0.1–0.2 ml

9.14   Injection sites, venipuncture sites and volumes for therapy in prairie dogs.

Common conditions

Therapeutics that seem efficacious and non-toxic are those used for guinea pigs or chinchillas (see Chapter 5). Normal stools are similar to those of a guinea pig, which are dry and oval shaped. Urine is alkaline (pH 8–9) and clear yellow.

Wild-caught prairie dogs may carry pulmonary mites (*Pneumocoptes penrosei*) as well as potentially zoonotic infections such as *Yersinia pestis* or *Francisella tularensis*. Pulmonary mites can be diagnosed on cytology with a tracheal wash and treated with ivermectin at 200–500 µg/kg every 14 days for three treatments.

Common diseases of prairie dogs are summarized in Figure 9.15.

Obesity and dormancy

Captive prairie dogs frequently present with obesity, due to overfeeding and lack of exercise. They also may be presented in the torpid or dormant state due to the temperature in the home dropping well below 20.5°C for several days, coupled with decreasing day length. The dormant prairie dog may have elevated blood urea nitrogen levels and be slightly dehydrated and slightly hypothermic, but will rouse with warming and administration of warmed subcutaneous fluids.

Clinical signs/ disease	Aetiology	Diagnostic tests	Treatment
Dental disease: fractured teeth, malocclusion, tooth root abscesses, oral swellings/neoplasia	Fractures: falls, chewing inappropriate hard objects, trauma Abscesses may be due to improper wear, punctures from food, foreign objects Neoplasia (elodontomas): possible aetiology includes repeated mouth trauma	Oral examination under sedation or anaesthesia, skull radiographs, endoscopy of nasal cavity	Remove abscessed teeth, burr malocclusive teeth; surgical excision of neoplastic tissue; correct diet for proper tooth wear Appropriate antimicrobials, NSAIDs, analgesics for oral lesions as with guinea pigs (see Chapter 8)
Dyspnoea, with/ without sinusitis, rhinitis	*Pasteurella multocida*; pulmonary mites	Culture and sensitivity, cytology of tracheal/sinus wash; radiographs, CBC/chemistries	Appropriate antibiotics (fluoroquinolones first choice, see Chapter 5), ivermectin for mites; supportive care including nebulization, bronchodilators, NSAIDs
Neurological signs: ataxia, torticollis, stumbling, seizures	*Baylisascaris* sp. (North America) Heavy-metal toxicosis (lead, zinc) Inner ear infection Brain abscess, encephalitis	*Baylisascaris*: wild-caught or housed outdoors – exposure to skunks, raccoons; CT, MRI, or necropsy for diagnosis Heavy metals: history of chewed objects, blood lead, zinc levels, metal particulates in GI tract on radiographs CBC/chemistries, ear and oral exam	There is no treatment for *Baylisascaris* lesions For other infections: antibiotics, NSAIDs, and supportive care Heavy metal: chelation therapy (CaEDTA or D-pencillamine) Remove dangerous toys, objects
Obesity (fatty liver, lethargy)	Overfeeding and/or improper foods Initiation of winter dormancy Lack of exercise	Diet history, ambient temperature, light cycle and husbandry history. CBC/ chemistry panel, radiographs, ultrasound of liver	Correct diet (hay-based); decrease total quantity Light/temperature correction Exercise If liver disease, supportive care as appropriate To rouse from dormant condition give warmed subcutaneous fluids, provide warmth

9.15   Common diseases of prairie dogs. (continues)   ▶

Clinical signs/ disease	Aetiology	Diagnostic tests	Treatment
Open-mouthed breathing, dyspnoea, nasal/ocular discharge	Rule out oral, maxillary elodontoma or other neoplasia, nasolacrimal duct infection/blockage from tooth root abscess, sinus infection, severe respiratory tract infection	Radiographs, ophthalmic exam including nasolacrimal flush; culture and sensitivity of exudates, thorough oral examination, nasal endoscopy	Surgical excision of tumour if possible, appropriate antibiotics, NSAIDs and analgesics as needed Treatment as listed above for abscesses
Pododermatitis	Poor husbandry, dirty wet bedding Obesity, inactivity	Radiograph to assess bone/joint involvement; culture and sensitivity of edges of lesions	Treat as in guinea pigs (see Chapter 10), remove exudates, debride; appropriate antimicrobials Can try soft bandaging but likely to remove quickly and eat the bandage material Soft flooring, NSAIDs, correct sanitation/ husbandry
Self-injurious behaviour: wounding, self-amputation	Solitary animal, improper husbandry, lack of social stimulation, boredom, stereotypical behaviours Wounds may become secondarily infected, painful, pruritic	Assess husbandry Radiographs if severe, bone involved Culture and sensitivity of infected wounds	Provide companionship, social stimulation, enriched environment (larger; ability to dig; tunnels). Wound treatment as in rabbits, guinea pig Benzodiazepines may be needed to control self-injurious behaviour
Trauma, fractures, torn nails	Falls, injuries from other pets, nails caught in home furnishings, carpets	Radiographs for fractures	Trim nails Repair fractures with guidelines used for rabbits and guinea pigs (see Chapter 14)

9.15   (continued) Common diseases of prairie dogs.

Dental disease

Dental disease is common and includes fractured teeth (Figure 9.16), root abscesses, and malocclusions associated with tooth loss or overgrowth (see also Chapter 8). Maxillary teeth may abscess into the nasal cavities and sinuses, resulting in upper respiratory tract disease. Dental neoplasia (elodontoma) has been associated with chronic dental disease or mouth trauma from chewing on inappropriate objects, such as cage bars. Radiographs as well as a thorough dental examination under isoflurane anaesthesia are necessary to determine the condition of the tooth roots and bone. Prairie dogs can be intubated with a 2.0 or 2.5 mm uncuffed endotracheal tube using a blind technique or with the aid of a laryngoscope or endoscope. Removal of diseased teeth along with the creation of permanent openings in the nasal bones caudal to a tumour mass have been tried as treatment, but often the tumour cannot be effectively resected or removed. The condition is progressive. Symptomatic treatment includes NSAIDs, antibiotics, and assisted feeding.

Respiratory disease

Prairie dogs presenting with open-mouthed breathing or dyspnoea must first be screened for elodontoma blocking the nasal passages. Rhinitis can also be caused by maxillary teeth abscesses, neoplasia other than elodontoma, pulmonary mites and bacterial infections. *Pasteurella multocida* has been associated with pneumonia, rhinitis and sinusitis. A sample can be taken for bacterial culture and antibacterial sensitivity testing. The microbiology laboratory should be familiar with culturing *Pasteurella*.

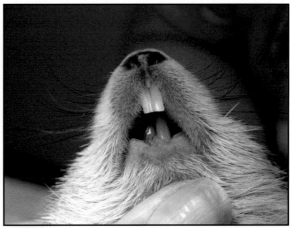

9.16   Prairie dog with fractured mandibular incisor tooth. These injuries are commonly seen in pet animals.

The author obtains material for culturing by instilling a few drops of sterile non-bacteriostatic saline into the nasal cavity as a flush, and collecting the material sneezed or dripped out. Usually this is done under mild sedation and the prairie dog is briefly held with the head down, just after the saline is instilled for collection. The animal is then placed sternally with the chest elevated and oxygen is provided using a facemask. It may continue to sneeze for a few minutes after the event. Material can be collected for cytology, staining and culture. If mites or their eggs are identified, systemic treatment with ivermectin at 0.4 mg/kg s.c. every two weeks for 2–4 treatments has been effective in the author's experience.

Treatment of bacterial respiratory disease should be based on antibiotic sensitivity and follows guidelines used for treatments in guinea pigs and rabbits for antibiotic choice. Nebulization, bronchodilators such as aminophylline at 10 mg/kg s.c. q12h, non-steroidal anti-inflammatory drugs such as meloxicam at 0.2 mg/kg orally or s.c. q24h can decrease the signs of rhinitis, sinusitis and/or pneumonia and make the prairie dog more comfortable. The author has also used ophthalmic NSAID drops placed in the eyes to reach nasal tissue and decrease inflammation, as in the rabbit. The author has effectively used flurbiprofen ophthalmic drops, 0.03% solution, at one drop for each eye twice a day to help with nasal and sinus inflammation in prairie dogs.

Neurological disease
Neurological signs including ataxia, torticollis, stumbling and seizures have been reported in pet prairie dogs. *Baylisascaris* spp. have been implicated, particularly if the pet was wild-caught or the animals are housed outdoors and exposed to skunks or raccoons. The parasite is absent from the UK. There is no treatment. Diagnosis may be aided by CT or MRI for inflammatory lesions in the brain, but the definitive diagnosis is made at necropsy. Spinal or head trauma can occur, particularly if a prairie dog falls or is dropped. Inner ear infections and brain abscesses are possible, but not reported in the literature.

Skin disease
Pododermatitis similar to that found in guinea pigs has been seen. It is usually the result of poor husbandry – dirty wet bedding combined with obesity and inactivity. Treatment may be difficult as prairie dogs do not tolerate bandages well. Soft bedding and sanitation along with systemic antibiotics and NSAIDs may be effective.

Trauma
Vertebral and long-bone fractures and fractured incisors are frequently seen due to trauma from falling in the home environment. Self-inflicted wounds, including amputation and subsequent osteomyelitis, are seen in solitary prairie dogs.

Toxicosis
Heavy-metal toxicosis may present with vague neurological or gastrointestinal signs. Both zinc and lead toxicosis have been reported, usually due to chewing on cages or other household objects. Metal densities may or may not be present in the gastrointestinal tract on radiography. Chelation is with edetate calcium disodium at 30 mg/kg s.c. q12h for 3–5 days or D-penicillamine at 30–55 mg/kg orally q12h for 1–2 weeks. Generally blood lead levels >10 μg/dl are considered diagnostic for lead toxicosis.

Surgical procedures
Ovariohysterectomy and castration are common procedures. It is preferable to perform these procedures in the first year of life as there is less body fat. Castration is easier in the spring or early summer as the testicles are descended. The testicles are lateral to the penis. A separate skin incision is made over each. The spermatic cord and vessels are best clamped and ligated using a closed technique, because of the open inguinal rings. If the testicles have not descended, a caudal coeliotomy is performed. The spermatic cords are located between the colon and bladder in a location analogous to the uterus of the female. The spermatic cord is retracted, which allows the testicle to be exteriorized. The vas deferens and vessels are then ligated and transected. Intradermal or subcuticular sutures should be used to close incisions. Postoperative analgesia is necessary, to prevent the prairie dog from chewing on and picking at the incision site.

References and further reading

Avashia SB, Petersen JM, Lindley CM *et al.* (2004) First reported prairie dog-to-human tularemia transmission, Texas, 2002. *Emerging Infectious Diseases* 10(3), 483–486

CDC, Wilson P, Grahn B *et al.* (2003) Multistate outbreak of monkeypox – Illinois, Indiana, and Wisconsin, 2003. *Morbidity and Mortality Weekly Report* 52(23), 537–540

Funk RS (2004) Medical management of prairie dogs. In: *Ferrets, Rabbits, and Rodents Clinical Medicine and Surgery, 2nd edn*, ed. KE Quesenberry and JW Carpenter, pp. 266–273. Saunders Elsevier, St Louis

Johnson-Delaney CA (1997) Special rodents: duprasi. In: *Exotic Companion Medicine Handbook for Veterinarians*, pp. 34–37. Wingers Publishing/ZEN Publications, Lake Worth, Florida

Johnson-Delaney CA (1997) Special rodents: prairie dogs. In: *Exotic Companion Medicine Handbook for Veterinarians*, pp. 18–25. Wingers Publishing/ZEN Publications, Lake Worth, Florida

Johnson-Delaney CA (2002) Other small mammals. In: *BSAVA Manual of Exotic Pets, 4th edn*, ed. A Meredith and S Redrobe, pp. 103–115. BSAVA Publications, Gloucester

Johnson-Delaney CA (2006) Common procedures in hedgehogs, prairie dogs, exotic rodents, and companion marsupials. *Veterinary Clinics of North America: Exotic Animal Practice* 9, 415–435

Jones DL and Wang LCH (1976) Metabolic and cardiovascular adaptations in the Western chipmunks, genus *Eutamias*. *Journal of Comparative Physiology B: Biochemical, Systemic, and Environmental Physiology* 105(2), 219–231

Langohr IM, Stevenson GW, Thacker HL and Regnery RL (2004) Extensive lesions of monkeypox in a prairie dog (*Cynomys* sp.). *Veterinary Pathology* 41, 702–707

Lightfoot TL (2000) Therapeutics of African pygmy hedgehogs and prairie dogs. *Veterinary Clinics of North America: Exotic Animal Practice* 3, 155–172

Mannelli A, Kitron U, Jones CJ *et al.* (1993) Role of the eastern chipmunk as a host for immature *Ixodes dammini* in northwestern Illinois. *Journal of Medical Entomology* 30(1), 87–93

Meredith A (2002) Chipmunks. In: *BSAVA Manual of Exotic Pets, 4th edn*, ed. A Meredith and S Redrobe, pp 47–51. BSAVA Publications, Gloucester

Morera N (2004) Osteosarcoma in a Siberian chipmunk. *Exotic DVM* 6(1), 11–12

Nowak RM (1991) Order Rodentia: Muridae. In: *Walker's Mammals of the World, 5th edn, Vol. II*, pp. 643–870 Johns Hopkins University Press, Baltimore

Nowak RM (1991) Order Rodentia: Sciuridae. In: *Walker's Mammals of the World, 5th edn, Vol. I*, pp. 561–642. Johns Hopkins University Press, Baltimore

Perz JF and Le Blancq SM (2001) *Cryptosporidium parvum* infection involving novel genotypes in wildlife from Lower New York State. *Applied Environmental Microbiology* 67(3), 1154–1162

Refinnetti R (1998) Homeostatic and circadian control of body temperature in the fat-tailed gerbil. *Compendium Biochemistry Physiology and Molecular Integral Physiology* 119(1), 295–300

Seville RS and Patrick MJ (2001) *Eimeria* spp. from the eastern chipmunk (*Tamias striatus*) in Pennsylvania with a description of one new species. *Journal of Parasitology* 87(1), 165–168

Slacherjt T, Ktron UD, Jones CJ *et al.* (1997) Role of the eastern chipmunk (*Tamias striatus*) in the epizootiology of Lyme borreliosis in northwestern Illinois, USA. *Journal of Wildlife Diseases* 33(1), 40–46

Vourc'h G, Marmet J, Chassagne M *et al.* (2007) *Borrelia burgdorferi* sensu lato in Siberian chipmunks (*Tamias sibiricus*) introduced in suburban forests in France. *Vector Borne Zoonotic Disease* 7(4), 637–42

Wagner RA, Garman RH and Collins BM (1999) Diagnosing odontomas in prairie dogs. *Exotic DVM* 1, 7–10

10

Rodents: dermatoses

Lesa Longley

General approach to the skin case

Clinical signs associated with dermatological disease in rodents are similar to those in other mammal species, as are aetiological categories and diagnostic investigations. It is important to acquire full husbandry details, including environmental conditions and diet. Bedding materials are often irritant, and even if not the primary cause may contribute to a worsening of clinical signs. A medical history should also be obtained. Clinical signs of in-contact animals may be significant. The history should then focus on the presenting dermatological signs (Figures 10.1 and 10.2).

Dermatoses may be associated with generalized problems. A physical examination should be performed, though it may be cursory in smaller species. The entire integument is examined, including the extremities (feet, ears and tail). At this stage, a list of differential diagnoses should be formed, allowing the veterinary surgeon to select appropriate investigative techniques (Figure 10.3).

Signalment – species, breed/strain, age, gender
Details of husbandry/diet
Health, including any skin conditions, of in-contact animals (conspecifics, other species, humans)
History of skin problem – when it began, clinical signs seen, lesion distribution, any progression
Animal's medical history and any other signs noted by owner
Physical examination – whole animal, including body weight
Detailed examination of skin (including feet, ears, tail)
Diagnostic tests (see Figure 10.2)

10.1 Investigation of skin disease in rodents.

Sample	Technique
Hair	Microscopy (trichography); fungal culture; ultraviolet (Wood's) light (detects *Microsporum* spp.)
Skin scrape	Microscopy
Material from lesion	Culture (from within intact pustule or from abscess capsule); cytology and Gram stain
Skin biopsy	Histology and special stains; electron microscopy; virus isolation
Blood	Haematology; biochemistry; serology
Trial therapy	Depends on suspected aetiology

10.2 Diagnostic tests to investigate rodent dermatoses.

Aetiology	Diagnosis	Treatment
Bacterial (often secondary)	Cytology, Gram stain, culture and sensitivity	Topical cleaning and antiseptic, systemic antibiotics
Fungal	Microscopy, culture	Antifungal agents – topical (e.g. enilconazole) or systemic (e.g. griseofulvin) and environmental decontamination
Parasitic • Ectoparasites • Endoparasites	Microscopy – hair pluck or coat brushing, superficial or deep skin scrape Perianal sellotape test	Antiparasitic agents

10.3 Differential diagnoses for rodent dermatoses. (continues) ▶

Aetiology	Diagnosis	Treatment
Viral	Histology, electron microscopy, virus isolation, serology	None
Environmental • Inappropriate (low/high) humidity • Cold • Mechanical • Poor hygiene • Inappropriate substrate • Overcrowding	Suggestive signs with identification of suboptimal environmental conditions	Correct husbandry
Behavioural • Barbering • Fighting	History, observations	Correct husbandry, improve environmental enrichment; clean wounds, treat bacterial infections (see above)
Miscellaneous • Neoplasia • Nutritional	• Histology (sometimes cytology on impression smear) or fine-needle aspirate • History, dietary evaluation	• Excise masses • Correct diet

10.3 (continued) Differential diagnoses for rodent dermatoses.

Diagnostic tests

Larger ectoparasites (e.g. ticks, fleas, lice) may be seen with the naked eye. Flea faeces may be collected using a comb or brush, and identified by the red–brown blood colour after wiping on damp cotton wool. Larger mites, such as *Cheyletiella* spp. ('walking dandruff') or *Myocoptes* spp., may be visible but require magnification for identification. Direct microscopy is useful for various samples.

Ultraviolet light may be used to detect infections of *Microsporum* species. The light is warmed beforehand and used in a darkened room. Most rodent dermatophytoses, however, are due to *Trichophyton* spp., which do not fluoresce.

Sample collection

Sample collection from rodents may necessitate sedation or anaesthesia (see Chapter 6). Analgesia should be administered if a painful procedure is performed, such as skin biopsy.

Bacterial and fungal cultures

Samples for bacterial culture are obtained from closed pustules. Hair is clipped and the skin is swabbed with 70% alcohol before opening the pustule with a sterile needle. Contamination of the culture swab from surrounding skin may produce erroneous results. If an abscess is present, a capsule sample is more likely to culture bacteria than material from the abscess centre.

Fungal culture on Sabouraud's dextrose agar takes 1–4 weeks. Hair can be sampled by plucking, or the Mackenzie brush technique (with a sterile toothbrush) can be employed.

Samples for microscopy

Tape samples: Clear adhesive tape can be used to collect surface-living mites (e.g. *Myobia* spp. and *Cheyletiella* spp.). The tape is then attached to a glass slide for microscopy at low power.

Skin scrapes: Skin scrapes are used to detect surface-living (superficial scrape) and burrowing or follicular (deep scrape) mites. The site is chosen based on the predilection site of the suspected mite, and an area with lesions but without self-trauma. The overlying hair is clipped. Wiping the skin with 5% potassium hydroxide (KOH) will dissolve keratin but also kill the mites; alternatively liquid paraffin will not kill the mites (KOH can be added later if required to clear a slide preparation). The skin is scraped in one direction using a blunted scalpel blade, and material is transferred to a microscope slide. More KOH or liquid paraffin is added to the slide and a coverslip is applied before microscopy.

Hair plucks: Hairs may be plucked from the periphery of a lesion after swabbing with 70% alcohol, cleared with 5% KOH, and examined microscopically for fungal spores and hyphae. Other abnormalities may include traumatization of the hair tip, pigment changes or follicular casts, or *Demodex* mites. The hair bulb may indicate whether anagen (growing phase) or telogen (dead) hairs are present.

Impression smears: Cytology may be useful on impression smears from exudative lesions or after scraping. Although only a superficial sample is possible, this is cheaper and less invasive than biopsy. In-house stains may be used, such as Diff-Quik® for cellular assessment, Gram stain for bacteria and lactophenol blue for fungal staining.

Skin biopsy

Full-thickness incisional or excisional skin and lesion biopsy samples can be submitted for histology and culture. The wound is closed with sutures or tissue glue. Care should be taken not to traumatize the sample during handling, and the biopsy sample should include some normal as well as abnormal skin. Samples for histology are placed on card, subcutis down, and then into 10% formalin.

Trial therapies

In some cases investigations may not be performed, perhaps due to financial considerations or health risks associated with invasive procedures, or findings are non-diagnostic. In these situations, trial therapies may be used. Commonly these include antiparasitic therapy if ectoparasites are suspected, or antibiotics in pustular disease.

Mice

Bacterial disease

Several bacteria may cause either primary or secondary dermatitis in mice. *Staphylococcus aureus* and group G *Streptococcus* may cause spontaneous ulcerative dermatitis. *Staphylococcus aureus* may result in superficial or deep infections, including disseminated abscesses in immunocompromised individuals.

Oedema and cyanosis of extremities may be associated with *Streptococcus moniliformis. Corynebacterium kutscheri* can cause furunculosis, cutaneous pyogranulomas, skin necrosis and sloughing of extremities. A severe orthokeratotic hyperkeratosis has been reported in athymic nude mice due to *Corynebacterium pseudiphtheriticum* (Ellis and Mori,

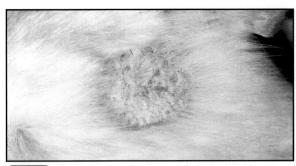

10.4 Well circumscribed area of alopecia with crusting and scale formation in a mouse. Infection with *Trichophyton mentagrophytes* was diagnosed on fungal culture in this case. (Courtesy of Anna Meredith.)

2001). *Mycobacterium chelonae* in immunocompromised mice caused granulomatous tail lesions (Mäyler and Jelinek, 2000).

Self-trauma due to acariasis or fight wounds commonly results in secondary bacterial dermatitis and abscesses, usually associated with *Staphylococcus aureus* or *Streptococcus* spp. Less often, *Pasteurella pneumotropica, Actinobacillus* spp., *Actinomyces* spp. and *Klebsiella* are cultured as opportunistic pathogens.

As the clinical signs of bacterial dermatitis are usually non-specific, cytology, histology and culture are usually necessary to identify the aetiological agent. Systemic antibiosis is ideally based on sensitivity results; many bacterial infections respond to penicillins or cephalosporins. Elimination of inciting factors and application (after clipping of hair over lesions) of topical antiseptics such as chlorhexidine 0.5–1.0% are beneficial. Topical ointments are not used, because of fastidious grooming by mice. Abscesses may be drained or surgically excised.

Fungal disease

Although dermatophytes are common in mice, they are usually asymptomatic. The most common cause of dermatophytosis is *Trichophyton mentagrophytes.* Clinical disease is usually associated with concurrent stress. Signs include hair loss and well demarcated lesions with crusts, erythema and scale (Figure 10.4). Pruritus is minimal or absent. Face, head, tail and trunk lesions are common, as are lesions on owners.

Diagnosis is by microscopic examination or fungal culture. Treatment is with oral griseofulvin or an enilconazole wash, with environmental disinfection. Husbandry issues causing stress should be addressed.

Parasitic disease

Microscopy is used to diagnose parasite infection, on hair samples, skin scrapes or biopsy. Treatment for all is ivermectin, including in-contact animals, along with cage disinfection (Figure 10.5).

Drug	Dose [species]	Comments
Antibacterial agents		
Various, topical or systemic	See Figure 5.6	Bacterial infection (primary or secondary)
Antifungal agents *(see also Figure 5.8)*		
Butenafine	Topically q24h x 10–20 days [GP]	Focal fungal lesions
Enilconazole	0.2% wash/dip 2x/week [G/M/R] 50 mg/m² topically on to groups/environment 2x/week x 20 weeks [M] (Meredith, 2006)	Dermatophytosis. Continue until two negative cultures
Fluconazole	16 mg/kg orally q24h x14 days [GP]	
Griseofulvin	25 mg/kg orally q12h x 14–60 days, or 1.5% in DMSO topically x 5–7 days [all rodents] Paediatric solution 250 mg/kg orally q10d x 3 treatments [GP] 0.75 mg (= 10 g of 7.5% powder) per kg of feed [groups of G]	Dermatophytosis. Do not use in pregnant animals (teratogenic). Side effects include diarrhoea, leucopenia and anorexia. Usually require > 21 days treatment, until two negative cultures are obtained
Itraconazole	5–10 mg/kg orally q24h [C] 20 mg/kg orally q24h [GP]	Dermatophytosis, candidiasis Usually require > 21 days treatment, until two negative cultures are obtained

10.5 Drug treatments for rodent dermatoses. C = chinchilla, D = degu, G = gerbil, GP = guinea pig, H = hamster, M = mouse, R = rat. (continues) ▶

Drug	Dose [species]	Comments
Antifungal agents continued (see also Figure 5.8)		
Ketoconazole	10–40 mg/kg orally q24h × 14 days [all rodents] 10 mg/kg orally q24h [H] 20 mg/kg orally q24h [R]	Systemic mycoses; candidiasis
Lime sulphur dip	1:40 dilution q7d × 4–6 [all rodents]	Dermatophytosis Usually require > 21 days treatment, until two negative cultures are obtained
Miconazole	Topically 1% [GP] (Burgmann, 1997)	Focal fungal lesions
	Mix 2% with sand bath (1 part miconazole with 3 parts sand), topically. Daily bath for 3 months [D]	Usually require > 21 days treatment, until two negative cultures are obtained
Mupirocin	Topically 2% q24h × 7 days [GP] (Nicholas et al., 1999)	Focal fungal lesions and pododermatitis
Terbinafine	10–30 mg/kg orally q24h × 4–6 weeks [all rodents] 40 mg/kg orally q24h or topically [GP]	
Antiparasitic agents (see also Figure 5.9)		
Amitraz	1–4 ml/l topically q7–14d × 3–6 treatments [G/H] 0.3% solution topically q7d × 4 weeks [GP] 100 ppm topically q2w × 3–6 treatments [G] 100 ppm topically q7d × 4 weeks [H]	Demodex; continue for 4 weeks after skin scrapes negative
Carbaryl powder (5%)	Topically q7d × 3–6 treatments [C/GP]	Superficial ectoparasites
Fipronil	7.5 mg/kg topically q30–60d [H/M]	Flea adulticide
Imidacloprid	< 10 mg/kg topically [C]	Flea treatment
Ivermectin	0.2–0.4 mg/kg s.c., orally, topically, q7–14d × 3 doses [M/R/H/GP/C]	Ectoparasites; use q5–7d for Demodex. Treat in-contact animals. Toxicity in some mouse strains
	1:100 dilution in 50% water & 50% propylene glycol mix topically (1–2 ml of solution per cage of mice) q10d × 3 treatments [M]	Grooming spreads drug over skin and some is ingested
	0.4 mg/kg s.c. q7–10d × 3 doses [G]	Demodex (may respond)
	0.5 mg/kg s.c. q14d [GP]	Sarcoptid mites
	8 mg/l drinking water for 4 days/week × 5 weeks [M]; 25 mg/l drinking water for 4 days/week × 5 weeks [R]	Pinworms
Selamectin	6–12 mg/kg topically, repeat in 14 days [GP] 12–24 mg/kg topically, repeat in 30 days [M/R]	Fur mites

10.5 (continued) Drug treatments for rodent dermatoses. C = chinchilla, D = degu, G = gerbil, GP = guinea pig, H = hamster, M = mouse, R = rat.

Mites

The fur mites *Myobia musculi*, *Myocoptes musculinus* and *Radfordia affinis* are commonly found, often as concurrent infections. Life cycles vary (23 days for *Myobia*, 8–14 days for *Myocoptes* and 21–23 days for *Radfordia*). Transmission is by direct contact, often from parents to offspring with lesions developing when the animal reaches maturity. Self-trauma due to pruritus results in alopecia and ulceration. The coat may appear greasy. Infection with *Myobia* may be asymptomatic in some animals, produce varying lesions, or be intensely pruritic due to an allergic response. Lesions are often around the head, neck, lateral thorax and flanks. *Myocoptes musculinus* infection produces most lesions along the back and ventrum. Treatment is usually with ivermectin by subcutaneous injection, but an ivermectin-in-water spray can be used for large colonies, or oral ivermectin administered in drinking water. An alternative is topical selamectin (see Chapter 5). Corticosteroids may reduce pruritus, but side effects may occur with long-term administration (see Chapter 16). Systemic antibiotics may be indicated if secondary bacterial infection is present. Topical preparations may be used, but they may encourage excessive grooming and further self-trauma, thus exacerbating the lesions. The use of body bandages and collars has been successful in some cases (Figure 10.6). Sedation with diazepam may also be indicated in severe cases, to prevent further self-trauma and to increase tolerance of collars or bandages. Euthanasia should be considered in severe debilitating cases.

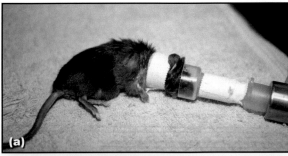
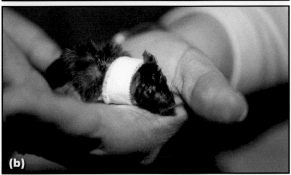

10.6 Severe skin excoriation following self-trauma due to pruritus associated with fur mite infection in a mouse. **(a)** This animal was anaesthetized and a neck bandage applied to prevent further self-trauma. **(b)** The bandage was tolerated in this case. (Courtesy of Heidi Hoefer.)

Less common mite infestations include *Psorergates simplex* (the follicle mite), *Notoedres muris* (ear mite), *Trichoecius rombousti*, *Liponyssus bacoti* and *Sarcoptes scabiei*.

Lice and fleas
The sucking louse *Polyplax serrata* is rare but can cause pruritus, dermatitis (particularly neck and back) and anaemia. This louse may be a vector for *Pasteurella tularensis*.

Fleas may be harboured by mice.

Pinworm
The pinworm *Syphacia obvelata* may produce perianal pruritus and tail-base mutilation. Clear adhesive tape applied perianally will pick up the banana-shaped eggs.

Viral disease

Mousepox
Mousepox (infectious ectromelia) has only been reported in laboratory colonies of mice. Skin lesions include a papular dermatitis, with facial and extremity swelling, necrosis and ulceration. Definitive diagnosis is by histology, electron microscopy, virus isolation, fluorescent antibody tests or serology. There is no treatment. Outcome depends on the strain of mouse, but morbidity and mortality are often high.

Other viruses
Reovirus in suckling mice causes an oily hair coat as well as systemic illness. Survivors are alopecic.

Sialodacryoadenitis virus results in periorbital pruritus, swelling and chromodacryorrhoea (see also Chapters 12 and 15).

Mammary tumours are often associated with the presence of mouse mammary tumour viruses (see Chapter 16).

Environmental disease
Correction of husbandry will prevent further environmental disease, but permanent defects may remain with the first two of the following conditions.

Ringtail
Ringtail is caused by low (<20%) environmental humidity. It occurs occasionally in mice, particularly pups. Annular constrictions on the tail result in oedema, necrosis and distal sloughing. Prevention is by ensuring sufficient humidity in enclosures. Treatment may necessitate amputation of the tail tip.

Dry gangrene
Cold temperatures and excessive grooming may produce idiopathic dry gangrene of the pinnae (and rarely distal tail).

Mechanical abrasions
Mechanical abrasions (secondary to eating through cage bars, using poorly constructed metal/water containers, or stereotypic bar chewing in individually housed mice) may result in alopecia and secondary bacterial infection.

Behavioural disease
Barbering is commonly seen in groups (particularly female groups where overcrowding or stress is present), where the dominant animal chews the facial hair and whiskers of subordinates. The behaviour may be observed or hair ends microscopically examined. Male mice that are stressed or bored are more likely to be aggressive, causing bite wounds. Treatment of both conditions is reduction of stocking density and improving environmental enrichment. Removal of the dominant animal may temporarily resolve the situation, but another usually takes over. Hair regrowth is usually within 30 days, but may take up to 90 days.

Miscellaneous skin disease

Immune-complex vasculitis
Certain laboratory strain mice may develop a pruritic secondary ulcerative dermatitis on the dorsal neck associated with immune-complex vasculitis.

Neoplasia
Spontaneous skin neoplasia is rare. Squamous cell carcinoma, papilloma and fibrosarcoma are the most prevalent. Mammary neoplasia usually carries a poor prognosis (see Chapter 16). Harderian gland tumours may occur.

Nutritional disease
Nutritional disease is rare in pet mice. Deficiencies that may lead to dermatoses include zinc, pantothenic acid, riboflavin, pyridoxine, biotin and fatty acid. Possible signs include alopecia, exfoliative dermatitis, hair depigmentation or scaling.

Alopecia

Hereditary hairlessness and keratinization defects occur rarely. Alopecia areata has been reported in one laboratory strain (Sundberg *et al.*, 1994).

Rats

Bacterial disease

Bacterial skin infections are rare, and usually secondary (to bite wounds, environmental injuries, or self-trauma from pruritus). Ulcerative dermatitis is commonly found in rats associated with *Staphylococcus aureus*, particularly in young males. Most infections produce superficial scabs and are non-pruritic; others are pruritic and can result in self-mutilation. Focal areas of alopecia or ulceration are generally over the neck and shoulders, but can be more extensive.

Other bacteria may also cause cutaneous abscesses and pyogranulomas, including *Streptococcus moniliformis*, *Pasteurella pneumotropica*, *Klebsiella pneumoniae*, *Pseudomonas aeruginosa*, *Mycobacterium lepraemurium* and *Corynebacterium kutscheri*. Sloughing of extremities may be seen with *Streptococcus moniliformis* or *C. kutscheri*.

Diagnosis and treatment are as for bacterial dermatoses in mice. Nail trimming will reduce damage from self-trauma. Underlying conditions should be identified and treated. Systemic antibiotics are often useful in treating bacterial dermatoses.

Fungal disease

Dermatophytosis is rare in rats and usually asymptomatic. Alopecia and non-pruritic scale on the dorsum and tail base may be seen, along with papules and pustules. *Trichophyton mentagrophytes* is most commonly cultured. Diagnosis and treatment are as in mice.

Parasitic disease

Mites

The rat fur mite *Radfordia ensifera* causes pruritus due to the mite allergen, leading to self-trauma. Ulcerative and crusting lesions usually affect head and shoulders. Secondary bacterial dermatitis may be associated (Figure 10.7).

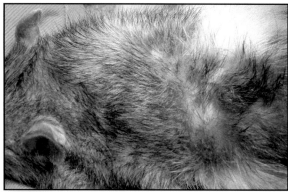

10.7 Classical lesions associated with mite hypersensitivity and secondary trauma in a rat. Ulcerative and crusting lesions usually affect head and shoulders. Secondary bacterial dermatitis may be associated. (Courtesy of Emma Keeble.)

Pruritic warty papular lesions with crusts and excoriations on the pinnae, nose and tail (and occasionally genitalia and limbs) are usually caused by the burrowing mite *Notoedres muris* (Figure 10.8). Diagnosis is usually obtained by skin biopsy, but clinical response to treatment with ivermectin is often taken as a presumptive diagnosis.

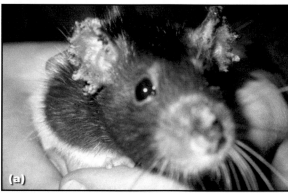
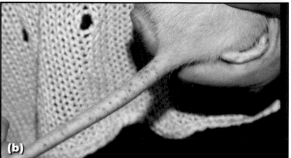
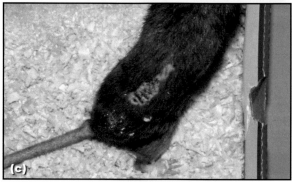
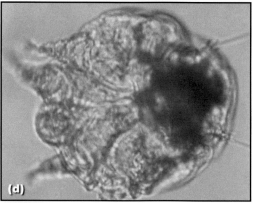

10.8 Rat infested with the burrowing mite *Notoedres muris*. Warty papular lesions typically occur on **(a)** the pinnae and nose and **(b)** the tail; and **(c)** may lead to self-trauma. **(d)** Diagnosis is based on skin biopsy and demonstration of the mite. (Courtesy of Anna Meredith.)

Other less common mites are Sarcoptidae (*Sarcoptes scabiei*, *Trixacarus diversus*, *Trixacarus caviae*, *Myobia musculi* and *Demodex* spp.) and Dermanyssidae (*Liponyssoides sanguineus* and *Liponyssus bacoti*). Deep skin scrapes or biopsy are necessary to diagnose acariasis and treatment is with ivermectin.

Lice and fleas
Lice are rare on rats. *Polyplax spinulosa* may cause clinical signs in young or debilitated animals, or those in poor husbandry conditions. This sucking louse may act as a vector for various diseases, including *Encephalitozoon cuniculi*. Treatment options include systemic ivermectin, or topical fipronil or selamectin.

Fleas may be seen on pet rats (usually from household cats and dogs). Topical preparations such as selamectin can be used to treat infestations.

Pinworm
Perianal pruritus and tail-base mutilation are seen with pinworm infection (*Syphacia obvelata*). Diagnosis and treatment are as for mice.

Viral disease

Poxvirus
Poxvirus is rare, causing erythematous papules. The lesions may crust and some will become necrotic and slough. Histology, electron microscopy and virus isolation are used to diagnose this infection.

Sialodacryoadenitis virus
Sialodacryoadenitis virus causes periorbital signs, including swelling, irritation, chromodacryorrhoea, sneezing and keratoconjunctivitis. Diagnosis is by virus isolation or antibody titres (see also Chapters 12 and 15).

Environmental disease

Ulcerative pododermatitis
Ulcerative pododermatitis causes significant morbidity in animals. Predisposing environmental factors include poor cage hygiene or wire mesh floors, particularly for obese individuals. Initially erythema and thickening are seen on the footpad, progressing to ulceration and secondary bacterial infection. Radiography may be used to assess for osteomyelitis. Husbandry should be corrected, along with the use of systemic NSAIDs and topical and systemic antibiotics. Bandages may be tolerated. Weight management is an important part of treatment in overweight animals. Surgical debridement can be useful in more severe cases. Prognosis is guarded, particularly in severe cases, where euthanasia should be considered.

Ringtail
Ringtail occurs in rats kept in low humidity (<20–40%), rarely in pet animals. Annular constrictions of the tail lead to oedema, necrosis and sloughing. Other factors may contribute, but relative humidity >50% prevents the disease.

Chromodacryorrhoea
Chromodacryorrhoea may occur in stressed animals (as in sialodacryoadenitis virus infection). Optimization of environmental conditions is important in the control of this condition (see also Chapter 15).

Behavioural disease
Barbering is rarely seen. Skin wounds with secondary bacterial infection are relatively common after fighting, especially between adult males. Bite wounds often cause abscesses.

Miscellaneous skin disease

Hyperadrenocorticism
Pituitary adenomas may produce hyperadrenocorticism (see Chapter 16). Glucocorticoid administration may cause iatrogenic Cushing's disease.

Fur yellowing and skin scaling
Aged male albino rats develop coarse yellow fur, possibly due to increased sebaceous secretions. Skin scales may be seen on the dorsum and tail. Both fur yellowing and skin scaling appear to be under androgenic control.

Neoplasia
Skin neoplasias are uncommon (see Chapter 16). Squamous cell carcinomas (often originating in the ear and spreading to the head) and papillomas are the most common. Basal and squamous cell carcinomas may invade locally, and squamous cell carcinomas may metastasize. Benign mammary fibroadenomas are commonly seen (in both sexes). The treatment of choice for all skin neoplasias is surgical excision and histopathological examination.

Tail slip
Degloving injuries to the tail ('tail slip') due to mishandling rarely occur (see Chapter 2). Treatment involves surgical amputation of the tail proximal to the lesion.

Auricular chondritis
The aetiology of auricular chondritis is not known, but may be immune-mediated, traumatic or infectious. This is not a common condition. The pinnae are swollen, nodular and erythematous, later becoming thickened and deformed. It is not usually painful. Diagnosis is by histology, showing granulomatous inflammatory foci with chondrolysis and invasion of mesenchymal cells.

Air embolism
Systemic air embolism may occur after intravenous injections, resulting in focal necrosis and ulceration.

Nutritional disease
Nutritional diseases are rare in pet rats, and are similar to those seen in the mouse.

Alopecia
Hereditary hairlessness may occur rarely. Alopecia areata has been reported in rats (McElwee and Hoffmann, 2002).

Hamsters

Bacterial disease

Trauma (such as bite wounds), rough or dirty bedding, or acariasis often predispose hamsters to secondary bacterial pyoderma and abscessation (Figure 10.9). The most common bacteria cultured are *Staphylococcus aureus*, but others include *Streptococcus* spp., *Pasteurella pneumotropica*, *Actinomyces bovis* and *Mycobacterium* spp. Treatment is as for mice. Facial abscesses (Figure 10.10) may relate to dental disease (see Chapter 8).

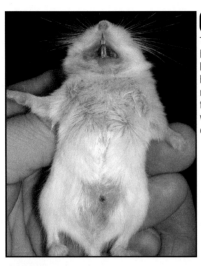

10.9
The small skin lesion on this Roborovsky hamster's ventrum responded to topical cleaning with dilute chlorhexidine.

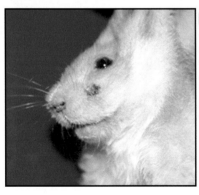

10.10
The skin lesion on this hamster's face was due to an overgrown lower incisor, which had punctured the cheek.

Experimental infection with *Treponema pallidum* subsp. *endemicum* (which causes endemic syphilis in humans) has been reported. Clinical signs include erythematous papules and ulcers. Treatment is with parenteral benzathine penicillin G or clarithromycin (Alder *et al.*, 1993).

Fungal disease

Dermatophytosis is rare, with dry circular skin lesions (or there may be no clinical signs). The most common agent is *Trichophyton mentagrophytes*. Diagnosis and treatment are as for mice.

Parasitic disease

Mites

The most common ectoparasite in hamsters is *Demodex* spp. The mite is passed from dam to suckling offspring, and is found in skin scrapes from normal animals. Animals that develop clinical signs are often immunosuppressed, have concurrent disease, malnutrition, or are aged. Skin scrapes or hair plucks are used to diagnose infection. The short fat-bodied *Demodex criceti* lives in the keratin layer and pits of the epidermal surface and is generally non-pathogenic. The cigar-shaped *D. aurati* (Figure 10.11) is found in hair follicles and causes a dry scaly alopecia, initially over the dorsum but potentially spreading. Pruritus is rare. A life cycle of 10–15 days necessitates repeat treatment with amitraz, ivermectin, or lime sulphur. Benzoyl peroxide shampoo baths may reduce mite load before treatments. Predisposing factors should be addressed.

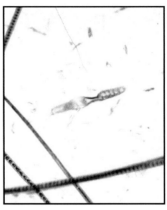

10.11
Demodex aurati from a hamster. This mite is cigar-shaped and lives in the hair follicles, causing a dry scaly alopecia. (Original magnification X40) (Courtesy of Anna Meredith.)

Other mites include the hamster ear mite *Notoedres notoedres* and the cat mange mite *N. cati*. Scabby lesions and severe pruritus are seen with the former around ears, nose, feet and perianally. *Sarcoptes scabiei*, *Trixacarus caviae* and *Liponyssus bacoti* rarely cause pruritus and dermatitis. Ivermectin, selamectin or lime sulphur is used to treat.

Fleas

Cat fleas (*Ctenocephalides felis felis*) may be found. Ticks and lice are not reported on hamsters.

Viral disease

Hamster polyomavirus

Hamster polyomavirus (HaPV) is associated with cutaneous epithelioma/ trichoepithelioma formation in Syrian hamsters. In some animals this virus produces a subclinical infection; others present with multicentric lymphoma. Once infection is endemic, lymphoma is less common and skin tumours are seen, usually around the eyes, mouth or anus. The wart-like lesions progress to cutaneous plaques and nodules, sometimes ulcerating and forming crusts. The neoplastic cells are T-lymphocytes. Biopsy is necessary for diagnosis, as skin scrapes commonly identify high numbers of *Demodex* mites.

The virus is highly contagious, spread by urine and very resistant in the environment, and it may cause high mortality in epizootics. The trichoepitheliomas are benign and do not metastasize, but large numbers may be debilitating. No individual treatment exists and disease control is by depopulation and good hygiene.

Environmental disease

Contact dermatitis
Cedar or pine shavings may cause contact dermatitis, with facial and pedal swelling and pruritus. Wood shavings may also cause a granulomatous inflammatory response, leading to degeneration of digits. These lesions regress with bedding on inert substrate such as shredded paper.

Ringtail
Ringtail, associated with low humidity, has been reported in hamsters (Besch, 1990). See also under skin diseases of mice.

Behavioural disease
Bite wounds are generally from females. Non-oestrous females are particularly aggressive towards young males, sometimes fatally wounding them. Treatment is as described for mice.

Miscellaneous skin disease
A rough or 'starey' haircoat is a non-specific sign of ageing, fighting, and other diseases.

Sebaceous scent glands
The sebaceous scent glands of Syrian hamsters may become inflamed, sometimes after rubbing against wood shavings or abrasive cage equipment. Gland impaction may also lead to self-mutilation. Treatment consists of clipping the overlying fur, cleaning the area and the use of topical antiseptics.

Neoplasia
The most common skin neoplasms are melanomas (melanotic or amelanotic) and melanocytomas, with a higher incidence in males, often on the head, back and flank gland. Diagnosis is by histology and treatment is surgical excision. Malignant melanomas may metastasize widely. Other less common skin neoplasms include carcinoma (Figure 10.12a) and pilomatrixoma (Figure 10.12b).

Epitheliotropic lymphoma (which resembles mycosis fungoides, human epidermotropic T-cell lymphoma) is the second most common skin neoplasm. Clinical signs include patchy alopecia, pruritus, exfoliative erythroderma, lethargy, anorexia and weight loss. There is no treatment and affected animals should be euthanased (see Chapter 16 for further information).

Nutritional disease
Nutritional deficiencies are rare in pet hamsters, similar to other rodents. Low dietary protein (< 16%) may result in hair loss.

Alopecia
Hyperadrenocorticism may be associated with dermatological signs, including bilaterally symmetrical alopecia, hyperpigmentation and skin thinning (see Chapter 16). Hereditary hairlessness is also reported in hamsters.

Gerbils

Bacterial disease
Acute primary dermatitis is mainly seen in young gerbils associated with *Staphylococcus aureus* infection. Morbidity and mortality may be high.

Secondary bacterial infections are common, often associated with *S. aureus*. Predisposing factors include trauma (environmental or fight wounds), acariasis and accumulated Harderian gland secretions.

The ventral abdominal sebaceous gland may become inflamed (similar appearance to early neoplastic changes) and infected, commonly with staphylococcal or streptococcal bacteria. Soft substrate such as shredded tissues should be used to reduce abrasions and aid healing. If healing does not occur the gland may be excised.

Treatment of bacterial dermatitis involves clipping of the hair and cleaning with 0.5–1% chlorhexidine and systemic antibiotics. Systemic and topical antibiotics may be indicated as well as analgesia and NSAIDs.

Fungal disease
Gerbils may very rarely have dermatophytosis with *Microsporum gypseum* or *Trichophyton mentagrophtes* infection. Both are zoonotic. Focal alopecia and hyperkeratosis are seen. See also under Mice.

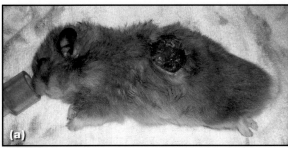

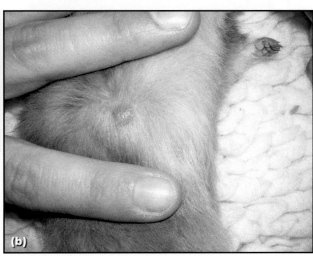

10.12 **(a)** Syrian hamster with large ulcerated skin mass. Histology confirmed a poorly differentiated carcinoma, and secondary infection with *Staphylococcus aureus* was cultured. No metastases were found and the patient did well after surgical excision with wide margins. **(b)** The same hamster presented a month later with several nodular skin lesions, which were surgically excised. Histology confirmed these to be pilomatrixomas.

Parasitic disease

Ectoparasite infections are uncommon.

Mites

Demodex meroni is species-specific, causing alopecia and scaling. Secondary bacterial infections may result in focal ulcerative dermatitis. Immunosuppression or underlying disease is often associated. Mites may be seen microscopically on hair plucks and deep skin scrapes. Amitraz is reported as the treatment of choice, though ivermectin may also be successful in the gerbil.

The fur mite *Acarus farris* may produce clinical signs (mildly pruritic alopecia with some erosions and crusts); diagnosis is by hair pluck microscopy. Environmental optimization and a single application of fipronil spray have been reported as treatment (Jacklin, 1997). Clinical signs are not reported with mouse fur mite, *Liponyssoides sanguineus*, infestation in gerbils.

Viral disease

There are no reports of viral disease resulting in dermatoses in gerbils.

Environmental disease

A rough or 'starey' coat may be seen in animals kept in excessively high humidity (> 50%), or may be a sign of ill health and stress. Pine or cedar shavings may cause matted, greasy fur.

Nasal dermatitis

The most common dermatosis (5% of gerbils) is nasal dermatitis ('sore nose' or 'facial dermatitis') (Figure 10.13). Predisposing factors are stress due to overcrowding and high humidity (> 50%) in groups of sexually mature animals, lack of grooming, and digging in abrasive substrate. Hypersecretion of porphyrin pigment from the Harderian gland accumulates at the

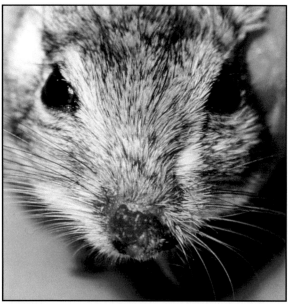

10.13 Nasal dermatitis in a gerbil. (Reproduced from *BSAVA Manual of Exotic Pets, 4th edn.*)

nares, causing irritation, self-trauma and secondary staphylococcal or streptococcal infection. Small focal areas of erythema, alopecia and crusting spread from the nares to the face, medial paws and abdomen. Extensive moist dermatitis and alopecia may result. Some individuals become anorectic and die.

Clinical signs are suggestive, with confirmation by culture and cytology from impression smears. Topical cleaning with antiseptics such as 0.5–1% chlorhexidine and systemic antibiotics are indicated, along with correction of predisposing factors. The problem usually resolves with use of soft soil or sand substrate instead of wood shavings. A sand bath may decrease Harderian gland lipids on the coat, improve fur quality and encourage grooming. Underlying stressors should be removed.

Rubbing the nose on cage wires or burrowing in bedding may result in 'bald nose' (hair loss from dorsal nose and muzzle). This may progress to nasal dermatitis. Prevention is by feeding inside the cage or housing in a glass enclosure.

Behavioural disease

Overstocking may lead to barbering, often near the head or tail base. Boredom may also result in tail chewing. Environmental enrichment such as cardboard tubes and boxes should be provided; in some cases removal of the dominant individual helps.

Fight wounds commonly lead to abscesses. For treatment, see under bacterial skin disease of gerbils. Group structure should be assessed.

Miscellaneous skin disease

Tail slip

Tail slip may occur with mishandling (see also Chapter 2). If the problem is not treated, the tail will slough or ascending infection may occur. Amputation proximal to the injury is advisable.

Neoplasia

The most common site of skin neoplasia is the ventral scent gland (particularly males), with adenomas or less commonly adenocarcinoma, or squamous or basal cell carcinomas. The lesion appears as a raised ulcerated mass and wide surgical excision is required. Local metastases to inguinal lymph nodes may occur. See also Chapter 16.

Melanomas, melanocytomas, squamous cell carcinoma of the feet and pinnae, papillomas, subcutaneous fibrosarcoma and mammary gland adenocarcinomas are also reported. Cytology/histology will diagnose the neoplasm and treatment is excision.

Aural cholesteatomas develop spontaneously in ageing Mongolian gerbils. They are non-neoplastic keratinizing epithelial masses in the middle ear, enlarging from the tympanic membrane and ear canal into the middle ear and bulla, eroding bone when contacted.

Alopecia

Cystic ovarian disease may be associated with skin signs such as symmetrical alopecia and poor coat quality. Bilateral symmetrical alopecia of flanks and lateral thighs may also be seen with skin thinning and hyperpigmentation in gerbils with hyperadrenocorticism (see also Chapters 13 and 16).

A condition where pups are born with patchy alopecia, abnormal hair pigmentation (leucotrichia) and stunted growth has an unknown aetiology (Collins, 1987). Pups are stunted and often die at weaning.

Guinea pigs

Bacterial disease

Bacterial pyoderma is common, often secondary to wounds such as bites or self-trauma, or may be predisposed by chronic skin wetting due to excessive salivation. *Staphylococcus aureus* and *S. epidermidis* are commonly isolated. Alopecia, erythema, ulcers, crusts, superficial suppuration, folliculitis and abscesses are seen. For treatment of bacterial skin disease see under Mice.

S. aureus may cause erythema and exfoliation of the epidermis by cleaving through the stratum granulosum. Lesions are seen predominantly on the ventral abdomen and medial limbs, initiated by abrasive flooring and bacterial contamination of skin wounds. Young animals may suffer high mortality.

Treponema spp., *Streptococcus* spp., *Fusobacterium* spp., *Corynebacterium* spp. and *Yersinia pseudotuberculosis* may also cause bacterial pyoderma. *Y. pseudotuberculosis* commonly affects the gastrointestinal tract, but is zoonotic and treatment is therefore not recommended. *Treponema* infection results in erythematous and then flat necrotic skin lesions. It is not possible to culture this organism; diagnosis is based on direct detection (e.g. using dark field microscopy) or using silver stains on a skin biopsy. Clinical signs and culture are used to diagnose other bacterial infections, with systemic antibiotics based on sensitivity testing. Predisposing factors or underlying causes should be corrected. Infection in guinea pigs leads to continuous immunostimulation, possibly resulting in amyloidosis and organ failure.

Streptococcus zooepidemicus is the most common cause of cervical lymphadenitis in guinea pigs, though *S. moniliformis* (potentially zoonotic) may be involved. *S. zooepidemicus* (a commensal in conjunctiva and the nasal cavity) usually gains entry to the cervical lymph nodes via small oral abrasions, bite wounds, the respiratory tract or conjunctiva. Stress increases infection susceptibility. The abscessed cervical lymph nodes present as soft, fluctuant subcutaneous ventral cervical masses. Spontaneous rupture may occur. Surgical drainage and debridement are necessary, with systemic antibiosis based on sensitivity results. Systemic infection may occur and the condition is potentially fatal in young individuals.

Fungal disease

Dermatophytosis is common, often in young animals that have incompletely developed immune systems. It is usually caused by *Trichophyton mentagrophytes*. Alopecia and scaling are usually non-pruritic and mostly affect the nose, face and ears. Kerions (moist,

raised, hairless lesions), secondary bacterial dermatitis, or delayed hypersensitivity reactions may occur. Neonates may die with severe infections.

Some animals may be asymptomatic carriers (6–14%), with clinical disease precipitated by stressors such as overcrowding, poor nutrition, high environmental temperature and humidity. Transmission, including zoonotic spread, is via direct contact or fomites. Diagnosis is by trichography and culture.

All in-contact animals should be treated and the enclosure disinfected. The environment should be disinfected, for example using a 1:10 solution of bleach and water. Fomites (including wooden hutches that cannot be treated) should be disposed of. The owner should be warned of the zoonotic potential. The affected area should be clipped. Topical miconazole, mupirocin, griseofulvin in DMSO, or butenafine may be used for focal lesions. For more generalized infections, use dips with enilconazole, miconazole or lime sulphur, or systemic griseofulvin, itraconazole, fluconazole, or terbinafine (see Chapter 5).

Cryptococcus neoformans may cause ulcerative dermatitis. *Candida albicans* and *Malassezia ovale* have induced skin lesions experimentally (Sohnle *et al.*, 1976; Rosenberg *et al.*, 1980).

Parasitic disease

Mites

Trixacarus caviae causes sarcoptic mange. The mite's life cycle is 10–14 days. Pruritus is intense, causing severe self-trauma, secondary bacterial infection and occasionally seizures. Pregnant animals may abort or resorb fetuses. Skin lesions are usually over the dorsal neck and thorax, but may progress and become generalized. Skin changes include erythema, crusts, scale and traumatic alopecia, with lichenification and hyperpigmentation developing (Figure 10.14). A leucocytosis may be seen. Asymptomatic carriers are common and clinical disease may develop when stressed (with old age, concurrent disease or hypovitaminosis C). In-contact humans may develop dermatitis.

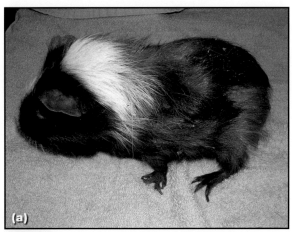

10.14 Guinea pig with acariasis: **(a)** showing hair thinning and alopecia. (continues) ▶

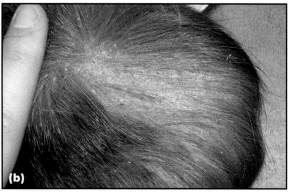

10.14 (continued) Guinea pig with acariasis:
(b) close up showing scale on skin.

Deep skin scrapes are used to diagnose infection; KOH digestion assists with visualization of mites (average 175 µm long) using microscopy. Treatment is ivermectin or 2% lime sulphur dips (see Chapter 5). In-contact guinea pigs should be treated and the enclosure disinfected. Husbandry should be optimized, including vitamin C supplementation. Analgesia (e.g. NSAIDs) may be helpful, and diazepam may be required where seizure-like activity occurs in severe cases.

Demodex caviae produces lesions typically on the head, forelegs and trunk, with alopecia, erythema, papules and crusts. Deep skin scrapes will identify mites. Treatment includes correction of underlying stressors or disease, and ivermectin or amitraz.

The guinea pig fur mite is *Chirodiscoides caviae* (Figure 10.15). It is small and non-burrowing, and usually found deep in fur over the dorsum. Clinical signs of alopecia and pruritus occur only with heavy infestation, where excessive self-grooming results in self-trauma and ulcerative dermatitis. *Sarcoptes scabiei, Myocoptes musculinus, Notoedres muris* and *Cheyletiella parasitovorax* may infest guinea pigs.

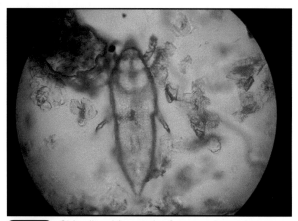

10.15 *Chirodiscoides caviae* from a guinea pig (original magnification X40).

Lice, fleas and ticks
Guinea pig lice *Gliricola porcelli* and *Gyropus ovalis* are common, feeding on hair shaft debris. Biting louse (*Trimenopon hispidum*) infection is rare. Alopecia and pruritus may be seen with heavy infestations, often in immunocompromised animals. Lice or eggs (nits) may be seen without magnification.

Fur mites and lice are transmitted by direct contact. They are identified microscopically on plucks or adhesive tape strips of hair, and can be treated with ivermectin, selamectin, 2% lime sulphur or carbaryl (see Chapter 5). Environmental disinfection should be performed to prevent reinfestation.

Fleas and ticks are rarely found on guinea pigs.

Endoparasites
The nematode *Pelodera strongyloides* is a rare cause of ventral dermatitis, diagnosed on skin scrape or biopsy. Maintenance of a clean, dry substrate is curative.

Viral disease
Poxviruses have been associated with cheilitis (see below). Experimentally, herpes simplex virus inoculated subcutaneously, intradermally or per vagina produced skin lesions (Scriba and Tatzber, 1981).

Environmental disease
Ergot poisoning may occur, with clinical signs including foot discoloration.

Ulcerative pododermatitis
Ulcerative pododermatitis is commonly seen in guinea pigs (see also Chapter 1). Predisposing factors include obesity, ageing, poor hygiene, wire flooring and hypovitaminosis C. Initially erythema, oedema and hyperkeratosis are seen. Ulceration permits secondary invasion and may affect tendons and bone (Figure 10.16). The most common isolate is *Staphylococcus aureus*, although *Corynebacterium pyogenes* may be found. Animals are reluctant to walk and vocalize frequently.

Diagnosis is by clinical signs, but radiography helps to assess for bony invasion. Besides correcting predisposing factors and supplementing vitamin C, treatment includes topical antiseptics such as silver sulfadiazine or mupirocin, systemic antibiotics

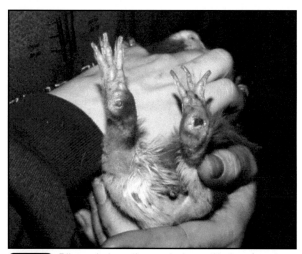

10.16 Bilateral ulcerative pododermatitis in a female guinea pig. This animal had urine excoriation of the perineum secondary to cystitis. Severe vertebral spondylosis and osteoarthritis of the stifle joints were diagnosed on radiography and were likely contributory factors in the development of the pododermatitis. (Courtesy of Emma Keeble.)

(preferably based on sensitivity results) and wound dressings. Analgesia with NSAIDs and provision of soft substrate will reduce discomfort and further progression of lesions. Surgical debridement is often ineffective. Unless recognized early, treatment is often unsuccessful, with systemic amyloidosis occurring with chronic infection.

Preputial dermatitis

Foreign materials such as bedding can become trapped in the preputial folds after mating in males (causing a foreign body reaction), or around digits or paws (causing vascular compromise). Rough cage flooring, faecal contamination or urine scalding may cause physical irritation and preputial dermatitis. Wounds should be cleaned, foreign bodies removed, and local anti-inflammatory or zinc oxide ointment applied.

Behavioural disease

Stress, overcrowding or a lack of dietary fibre may result in fur chewing, ear chewing and barbering. In group-housed animals, a dominant animal may barber subordinates, or self-barbering may occur due to boredom. Barbered hairs show broken hair shafts, associated with no skin inflammation. Incompatible animals should be separated. Environmental enrichment (addition of hay or chew toys, and multiple hides) will help to reduce this problem.

Bacteria commonly associated with abscesses following fight wounds include *Pseudomonas aeruginosa*, *Pasteurella multocida*, *Corynebacterium pyogenes*, *Staphylococcus* spp. and *Streptococcus* spp. Good drainage is not always possible, due to the thick consistency of pus; surgical excision is preferred. If complete excision is not possible, systemic antibiotics should be based on sensitivity results.

Miscellaneous skin disease

Cheilitis

Cheilitis secondary to eating abrasive and acidic food commonly has a secondary staphylococcal infection (Figure 10.17a). Poxvirus may be associated. Diagnosis is based on cytology and histopathology as well as bacterial culture and sensitivity. Treatment is debridement of ulcers, cleaning with 0.5–1.0% chlorhexidine, and systemic antibiotics for treatment of secondary bacterial infection (Figure 10.17b). Topical water-resistant muco-protectant ointments may be useful (e.g. 'Orabase', Bristol-Myers Squibb). Analgesia may be required. Lesions may be self-limiting.

Nutritional disease

Dermatoses due to nutritional deficiencies are similar to other rodents and (except for hypovitaminosis C) rare in pet guinea pigs.

Early hypovitaminosis C may result in roughened hair coat, scaling of pinnae and a mild white crusty ocular discharge. It is often an underlying factor in other guinea pig dermatoses.

The diet should be corrected as well as additional vitamin C supplementation until clinical signs resolve.

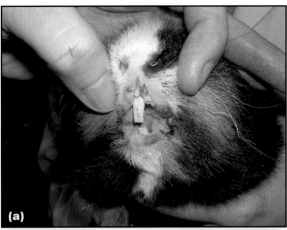
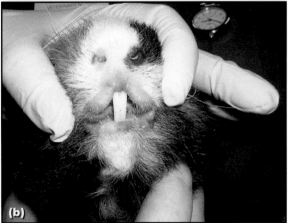

10.17 Guinea pig with cheilitis. **(a)** Note the inflammation and crusting. This animal was anorectic. **(b)** After cleaning lesions with dilute chlorhexidine. The condition responded to topical cleaning, along with systemic antibiotic and NSAID.

Alopecia

Various non-infectious causes may result in alopecia. Bilaterally symmetrical non-pruritic alopecia may be associated with cystic ovarian disease (see Chapter 13) or endocrine disease (see Chapter 16). Intensive breeding causes pregnancy-associated alopecia, via telogen defluxion associated with reduced anabolism of maternal skin. The alopecia may worsen with subsequent pregnancies. Diagnosis is based on reproductive history and exclusion of other causes of alopecia. Hair thinning may be seen in weanlings during their baby-to-adult fur transition.

Stress associated with illness is often associated with marked hair shedding. Shedding of hair by stressed or ill guinea pigs may be due to increased vitamin C requirements. Marked shedding may be seen during handling.

Guinea pigs may also have hereditary alopecia.

Scent gland impaction

Scent gland impaction may cause irritation. The anus may be occluded by sebaceous secretion circumanally in mature males, or accumulated bedding material and faeces. Secondary bacterial infections are common. The gland(s) should be washed with a mild antiseptic shampoo.

Cutaneous horns

Hyperkeratosis and cutaneous horns may develop on footpads, particularly in heavy guinea pigs or those on wire-bottomed cages. The horny growths should be clipped or filed, and a smoother substrate should be used in the cage. Overgrown claws should be trimmed.

Neoplasia

Trichofolliculoma (Figure 10.18) is the most common cutaneous neoplasm in guinea pigs. Tumours are benign, usually solitary, on the dorsum, and may discharge keratinous or haemorrhagic material from a central pore. Surgical excision is curative.

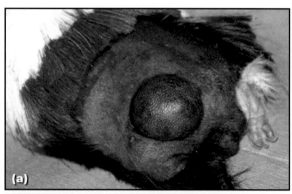

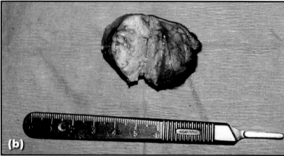

10.18 **(a)** Guinea pig with trichofolliculoma. The animal has been aseptically prepared for surgery. **(b)** Cut appearance of the trichofolliculoma following excision of the mass.

Calcification

Metastatic soft tissue calcification may produce dermal signs, with mineral deposits in soft tissue near the elbows and ribs, or in the footpads. Mineral imbalance is the suspected aetiology. There is no known treatment.

Vascular malformation

Vascular malformation in an adult female presented as an irregularly shaped violaceous plaque on the flank, which ulcerated and haemorrhaged (Osofsky *et al.*, 2004).

Chinchillas

Bacterial disease

Secondary staphylococcal infections may be associated with excess salivation due to dental disease or with dermatophytosis. The moist dermatitis is treated with topical 0.5–1.0% chlorhexidine and systemic antibiosis based on culture and sensitivity testing.

Fungal disease

Dermatophytosis is usually due to *Trichophyton mentagrophytes*, but *Microsporum gypseum* and *M. canis* may be isolated. Well circumscribed areas of alopecia, scale, crust, broken hairs and erythema are seen predominantly around the eyes, nares and mouth. Secondary bacterial infections may occur.

Transmission may be via direct contact with symptomatic or carrier animals, or indirectly via fomites. Diagnosis is by microscopy and culture of hairs. Removal of affected fur around lesions and environmental disinfection reduce transmission and zoonotic potential. Treatment is griseofulvin or topical antifungals such as enilconazole (see Chapter 5). Placing dust baths in an oven at 150°C for 20 minutes reportedly kills fungal spores.

Parasitic disease

The dense fur of chinchillas means that ectoparasites are rare. *Cheyletiella* spp. have been reported; treatment is with ivermectin if symptomatic. Fleas may cause pruritus; treatment is with products approved for use in cats and rabbits (e.g. imidacloprid).

Viral disease

No viral diseases causing dermatoses in chinchillas are reported.

Environmental disease

Matted fur may be seen in individuals without a dust bath, in a warm environment (>27°C) or in high relative humidity (>80%).

Behavioural disease

Bite wounds are common in group-housed chinchillas (females are more aggressive) and often result in abscess formation due to *Staphylococcus* and *Streptococcus* infection. Wounds may result in toe or partial ear loss. Surgical excision to remove inspissated material is recommended. Abscesses that rupture may be flushed. Systemic antibiotics are advisable.

Overcrowding, low fibre diet, boredom and other stressors may lead to fur chewing and barbering. Underlying disease such as dietary deficiencies may be associated; the barbering behaviour appears to have a heritable component. The coat has a 'moth-eaten' appearance. Husbandry optimization (with a good quality diet) reduces the problem. An underlying thyroid condition has been suggested (see Chapter 16). The dense undercoat should be removed by plucking to allow full hair regrowth, providing analgesia and sedation or light anaesthesia. Fluoxetine (5–10 mg/kg orally) has been suggested as a treatment (Meredith, 2006).

Miscellaneous skin disease

Fur-slip

'Fur-slip' may occur if animals are roughly handled, frightened or fighting (see Chapter 2). This natural defence mechanism results in a patch or patches of loosely attached fur being shed, leaving clean smooth skin. Owners should be warned of the possibility before handling. Regrowth is slow (3–5 months) and the coat may be permanently patchy.

Fur ring

Adult male chinchillas, particularly if breeding, may accumulate a ring of matted fur or smegma-like material around the penis. This fur ring can lead to paraphimosis and potentially to urinary retention. Chronic paraphimosis may result in infection and penile damage. Sedation or anaesthesia is usually required to lubricate and remove the ring. Provision of a sand bath for half an hour two to three times weekly seems to reduce the incidence of this condition. (See also Chapter 13.)

Nutritional disease

Nutritional deficiencies may result in dermatoses. Chinchillas fed a diet deficient in vitamin E, choline or methionine have impaired plant pigment metabolism, resulting in yellow–orange pigment deposition in skin and fatty tissues. Chinchillas fed a high-protein diet (>28% crude protein) may develop wavy and weak textured hair; this is known as cotton fur syndrome.

Neoplasia

Skin neoplasia has not been reported in chinchillas.

Degus

Little peer-reviewed literature has been published on dermatoses in this relatively new pet species, and information is mainly anecdotal.

Bacterial disease

Cheilitis may be seen, presenting as an inflamed oral mucocutaneous junction, often with mixed opportunistic bacterial infections. Immunosuppression may predispose. Underlying husbandry issues should be corrected. The lesions should be cleaned with 0.5–1.0% chlorhexidine solution, and systemic antibiotics are administered. See also under guinea pigs.

Abscesses may occur after bite wounds, commonly to the face, or if overgrown incisors penetrate the cheek/lip. The area should be clipped and then cleaned with 0.5–1.0% chlorhexidine. Systemic antibiotics should be administered (preferably based on culture and sensitivity results) and dental treatment as required. Surgical drainage or excision may be helpful.

Fungal disease

Dermatophytosis in degus usually presents as hairless patches on the muzzle, caudal pinnae and feet, but may be generalized. The alopecic areas can be large and are often non-pruritic (unless secondary bacterial infection is present). *Trichophyton mentagrophytes* is most commonly involved. Degu infection may trigger lupus erythematosus in humans (Boralevi *et al.*, 2003). Diagnosis is based on trichogram and culture. Affected areas should be clipped. Treatment is with topical antifungal powders such as niconazole administered in the dust bath, enilconazole washes, and/or systemic griseofulvin or ketoconazole. Treatment is continued for at least 2 weeks beyond resolution of clinical signs, and deemed successful when two sequential fungal cultures are negative. Environmental decontamination and thorough cage disinfection should be carried out.

Yeast infections may be seen, most likely secondary to other disease or associated with immunosuppression. Diagnosis is by cytology or culture. Topical antifungals such as miconazole or systemic itraconazole should be administered. Underlying risk factors should be corrected.

Parasitic disease

Mites

Infection with *Demodex* is usually associated with immunosuppression. Alopecia may be generalized, but primarily affects hindlimbs and ventrum. Diagnosis is by hair pluck microscopy and skin scrapes. Treatment includes ivermectin and correction of predisposing factors.

Pinworm

The pinworm *Helminthoxys gigantea* may cause perianal pruritus in degus (Sutton and Hugot, 1993). Diagnosis is via microscopy of a clear adhesive tape strip. Treatment is with ivermectin.

Viral disease

No viral causes of dermatoses are reported in degus.

Environmental disease

Degus without regular access to a dust bath will develop a build-up of oil on their fur.

Behavioural disease

Boredom or distress may result in fur-chewing or self-trauma. A genetic component may also be involved. The tail and/or feet are commonly affected. If stress-induced alopecia is present, signs of stereotypical behaviour may be seen or the animal may appear subdued. Environmental enrichment (larger enclosure, another degu or human companionship) should be provided and excessive stimuli, including noises and inappropriate lighting, should be removed. If the lesion has become inflamed due to self-trauma, antihistamines and an NSAID should be administered. Fluoxetine (5 mg daily orally) has also been anecdotally suggested where psychological disease is suspected.

Miscellaneous skin disease

Improper restraint using the tail, particularly if the degu is not habituated to handling, may result in struggling and a degloving injury (tail slip) exposing vertebrae. If only the brush at the tail tip is removed, the animal may bite the tip off with little haemorrhage. Amputation is recommended and will prevent haemorrhage or infection (see Chapter 7).

References and further reading

Alder J, Jarvis K, Mitten M *et al.* (1993) Clarithromycin therapy of experimental *Treponema pallidum* infections in hamsters. *Antimicrobial Agents and Chemotherapy* **37**(4), 864–867

Besch EL (1990) Environmental variables and animal needs. In: *The Experimental Animal in Biomedical Research*, ed. BE Rollin and ML Kesel, pp. 113–132. CRC Press, Boca Raton, Florida

Boralevi F, Léauté-Labrèze C, Roul S *et al.* (2003) Lupus-erythematosus-like eruption induced by trichophyton mentagrophytes infection. *Dermatology* **206**(4), 303–306

Burgmann P (1997) Dermatology of rabbits, rodents, and ferrets. In: *Dermatology for the Small Animal Practitioner,* ed. GH Nesbitt and LJ Ackerman, pp. 205–206. Veterinary Learning Systems, Trenton, NJ

Collins BR (1987) Dermatologic disorders of common small nondomestic animals. In: *Contemporary Issues in Small Animal Practice, No. 8*, pp. 235–294. Churchill Livingstone, Oxford

Ellis C and Mori M (2001) Skin diseases of rodents and small exotic mammals. *Veterinary Clinics of North America: Exotic Animal Practice* **4**(2), 493–542

Jacklin MR (1997) Dermatosis associated with *Acarus farris* in gerbils. *Journal of Small Animal Practice* **38**, 410–411

Mäyler M and Jelinek F (2000) Granulomatous inflammation in the tails of mice associated with *Mycobacterium chelonae* infection. *Laboratory Animals* **34**, 212–216

McElwee KJ and Hoffmann R (2002) Alopecia areata – animal models. *Clinical and Experimental Dermatology* **27**, 410–417

Meredith A (2006) Skin diseases and treatment of chinchillas. In: *Skin Diseases of Exotic Pets*, ed. S Paterson, pp. 195–203. Blackwell, Oxford

Nicholas RO, Berry V, Hunter PA and Kelly JA (1999) The antifungal activity of mupirocin. *Journal of Antimicrobial Chemotherapy* **43**, 579–582

Osofsky A, De Cock HEV, Tell LA *et al.* (2004) Cutaneous vascular malformation in a guinea pig (*Cavia porcellus*). *Veterinary Dermatology* **15**, 47–52

Rosenberg EW, Belew P and Bale G (1980) Effect of topical applications of heavy suspensions of killed *Malassezia ovalis* on rabbit skin. *Mycopathologia* **72**, 147–154

Scriba M and Tatzber F (1981) Pathogenesis of Herpes simplex virus infection in guinea pigs. *Infection and Immunity* **34**, 655–661

Sohnle PG, Frank MM and Kirkpatrick CH (1976) Mechanisms involved in elimination of organisms from experimental cutaneous *Candida albicans* infections in guinea pigs. *Journal of Immunology* **117**, 523–530

Sundberg JP, Cordy WR and King LE Jr (1994) Alopecia areata in aging C3H/JeJ mice. *Journal of Investigative Dermatology* **102**, 847–856

Sutton CA and Hugot JP (1993) First record of *Helminthoxys gigantea* (Quentin, Courtin & Fontecilla, 1975) (Nematoda: Oxyurida) in Argentina. *Research and Reviews in Parasitology* **53**, 141–142

11

Rodents: digestive system disorders

Michelle L. Ward

General considerations

Although interspecies differences exist in gastrointestinal anatomy, physiology and disease predisposition, dysfunction of the rodent gut is usually characterized by abnormalities in motility, secretion and/or the composition of the microbial flora. It is important to understand these general processes because, regardless of the definitive diagnosis, a critical component of therapy is supportive and aimed at restoring these functions. Moreover, many gastrointestinal disorders are multifactorial in origin and approaching the problem from first principles will facilitate diagnosis and formulation of an appropriate therapeutic plan.

Disruption to motility

Normal gastrointestinal motility is essential for digestion and absorption of nutrients. Abnormal motility of any cause will therefore result in maldigestion and malabsorption.

Gastrointestinal hypomotility (and ileus)

Hypomotility is very common and usually develops secondary to one or more environmental, behavioural and/or physiological factors (Figure 11.1). It is frequently encountered in the strictly herbivorous species as a result of inappropriate nutrition and in any species following surgery or as a sequel to systemic illness.

Insufficient dietary fibre
Anorexia
Physical and/or emotional stress
Lack of exercise
Pain
Prolonged distension of the gut (e.g. impaction/enteritis)
Excessive handling of the viscera during surgery
Acid–base imbalances
Dehydration
Electrolyte imbalances
Dysbiosis
Toxaemia

11.1 Causes of gastrointestinal hypomotility in rodents.

Gastrointestinal hypomotility leads to a reduction in appetite (which further exacerbates the problem), distension of segments of the tract, abdominal pain (primarily due to stretching of the intestinal walls) and dehydration. As the distension stimulates secretion of fluid and electrolytes into the lumen, fluid loss becomes self-perpetuating, creating a vicious cycle that can rapidly progress to cardiovascular shock.

If distension of the gut passes a critical point, a state of paralytic ileus develops, usually characterized by complete failure of peristalsis. This creates a functional obstruction. Sometimes local intestinal movements persist but are uncoordinated. Ileus is an exceptionally painful and potentially life-threatening condition. The clinical signs are summarized in Figure 11.2. Abdominal radiography is useful for diagnosis (Figure 11.3).

Trichobezoars (or 'hairballs') may form secondary to hypomotility as ingested fur in the stomach dehydrates.

Marked reduction in the amount of faeces passed
Abdominal distension
Palpably distended loops of gut
Dehydration (due to fluid sequestration in the gut and a decrease in fluid absorption)
Abdominal pain:
• Hunched posture
• Bruxism (tooth-grinding)
• Tachypnoea

NB: Rodents mask pain exceptionally well and may show limited overt signs of discomfort

---

11.2 Clinical signs of ileus in rodents.

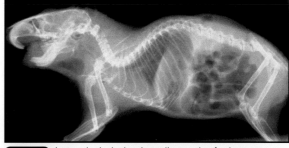

11.3 Lateral whole-body radiograph of a hamster, demonstrating generalized distension of the intestinal tract with gas, consistent with a diagnosis of ileus. In this case ileus had developed secondary to dental (and associated respiratory) disease. Note the elongation and abnormal curvature of the upper incisors, which are impinging on the upper respiratory tract.

Hypermotility

Hypermotility (often associated with diarrhoea) increases gut transit and subsequently impairs absorption. As is the case in other species, the fluid lost from the body can be appreciable.

Disruption to digestive function

The ability of the alimentary tract to digest food depends on its motor and secretory functions as well as the activity of the indigenous intestinal microflora (bacteria, yeast and protozoa). In addition, many rodents are coprophagic and any disease that impairs this behaviour will have an adverse effect on the digestive system.

Low-fibre diets, stress, infectious diseases (bacterial, viral, fungal, protozoal and parasitic), obstructions, neoplasia and toxins are amongst the aetiologies that may affect the motor and secretory functions of the gut. Hypersensitivities are a potential differential diagnosis but are not thought to be common in these species.

Factors that have the potential to adversely influence the composition of the intestinal microflora are numerous and include pathogenic organisms, administration of antibiotics, ingested toxins, increased glucocorticoid levels (e.g. secondary to stress), gastrointestinal hypomotility, dietary composition, prolonged starvation and inappetence. Such changes can be rapidly fatal.

Bacteria that are commonly isolated from the intestinal contents of rodents that have succumbed to digestive disorders include *Escherichia coli* and *Clostridium* spp. Enterotoxaemia due to release of clostridia-associated toxins is the most profound presentation. Affected rodents are depressed and anorexic with brown watery diarrhoea (containing blood or mucus) initially but rapidly become moribund and finally succumb. The prognosis is grave in most cases.

Prolonged dysfunction of the digestive system may result in specific nutrient deficiencies (e.g. hypovitaminosis C in guinea pigs).

As a general rule, infectious disease is most often encountered in young (recently weaned) animals or those housed in commercial situations (e.g. pet shops, breeding facilities, laboratories) (Figure 11.4). More often, non-infectious factors are identified as the inciting cause of enteric disease in adult pet rodents.

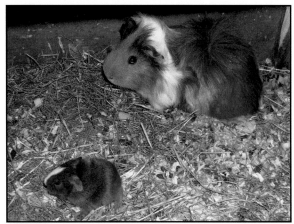

11.4 Guinea pig sow and newborn. Monitoring the appetite and faecal output of breeding and young animals is vital. These animals are more prone to infectious digestive diseases than individual pet rodents, especially if husbandry conditions are suboptimal (note the soiled bedding). In addition, even short periods of anorexia can induce hepatic lipidosis in pregnant and lactating females.

Other effects of digestive dysfunction

Gastrointestinal haemorrhage
Blood loss into the gastrointestinal tract results in anaemia. If severe enough, haemorrhage can progress to acute peripheral circulatory failure. The most likely causes of gastrointestinal haemorrhage are gastrointestinal ulceration, severe haemorrhagic enteritis, neoplasia, or heavy parasite burdens.

Hepatic lipidosis
The most common hepatic disease in pet rodents in the author's experience is hepatic lipidosis. Inappetence or anorexia of any cause may result in reduced glucose absorption from the gut (and a subsequent drop in blood glucose) which, in turn, leads to mobilization of free fatty acids. Ketoacidosis may develop and the animal becomes increasingly depressed and anorexic. Hepatic lipidosis develops rapidly and death can occur within days to weeks if the animal is not treated. Obese rodents and pregnant/lactating females are more prone to this condition.

Shock/dehydration
Severe dehydration and subsequent circulatory shock are often the cause of death in animals that succumb to gastrointestinal disease. Acute rapid distension of the stomach or intestines, regardless of cause, results in reflex effects on the heart, lungs and blood vessels. Blood pressure falls abruptly, body temperature drops below normal and there is a marked increase in heart rate. Often by the time clinical signs are apparent, the animal is unable to compensate.

General approach to rodent gastroenteropathies

Clinical presentation
Clinical signs will vary depending on the underlying problem and may be highly suggestive of a digestive upset (e.g. diarrhoea, reduced faecal output with the passage of scant dry droppings, complete cessation of faecal output, lack of coprophagy, abdominal distension) or may be entirely non-specific (e.g. lethargy, anorexia or increased appetite, weight loss, dehydration, lack of grooming and depression) (Figure 11.5). Other general signs may accompany enteropathies, including ocular porphyrin staining (e.g. in rats), hunched posture (frequently a sign of pain) and hypothermia.

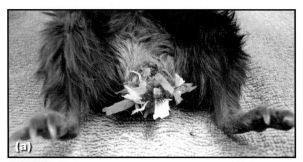

11.5 Clinical signs of digestive disease. **(a)** Specific: a guinea pig with green, mucoid diarrhoea accumulating at the anus along with some substrate material. (continues) ▶

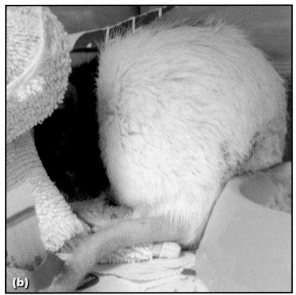

11.5 (continued) Clinical signs of digestive disease.
(b) Non-specific: a rat showing non-specific
signs of illness such as lethargy, reluctance to move,
anorexia and poor coat condition.

Signs such as hypersalivation, dysphagia, abnormalities of prehension, mastication and swallowing
and a desire but inability to eat (Figure 11.6) are commonly seen concurrently and are suggestive of an
underlying dental problem (see Chapter 8).

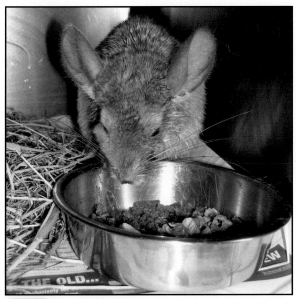

11.6 Ill rodents with poor faecal output, such as this
chinchilla, that show an interest in food but
inability to eat are often suffering from a primary dental
disorder. Note the poor coat condition and obvious weight
loss in this animal.

Vomiting and regurgitation are rarely seen in
rodents. Similarly, tenesmus is not a common presenting sign. Abdominal distension is often caused by
dilatation of the viscera (e.g. stomach or large
intestine) with gas or fluid. Ascites and advanced
pregnancy are the primary non-gastrointestinal
differential diagnoses.

Figure 11.7 summarizes the most common presenting complaints and their associated differential
diagnoses.

Clinical sign	Common differential diagnoses
Diarrhoea	Nutritional/dietary factors; environmental stressors; antibiotic-induced enterotoxaemia; bacterial enteritis; viral enteritis; candidiasis; cestodiasis; helminthiasis; protozoal enteritis; liver disease; hypovitaminosis C (guinea pigs)
Constipation/ reduced faecal output	Insufficient dietary fibre; gastrointestinal hypomotility, e.g. pain; physical or emotional stress; lack of exercise; anorexia of any cause; ileus, e.g. postoperative; acid–base imbalances; electrolyte imbalances; gastrointestinal torsion/intussusception; colorectal impaction; bacterial enteritis; helminthiasis; cestodiasis
Abdominal distension	Ileus; gastric tympany ('bloat'); ascites, e.g. associated with a hepatopathy; neoplasia; intussusception; colorectal impaction; Tyzzer's disease or other clostridial enteropathy; cryptosporidiosis
Rectal prolapse	Usually occurs secondary to diarrhoea or straining, e.g. proliferative ileitis or other cause of severe enteritis; helminthiasis
Ptyalism/ persistent facial swelling	Acquired dental disease/malocclusion and associated infections; oral trauma; oral foreign body; hypovitaminosis C (guinea pigs); cheek pouch disease (hamsters); coronavirus (rats)
Non-specific signs, e.g. depression, anorexia, poor hair coat, unthrifty appearance, hunched posture, dehydration, weight loss/poor growth	Acquired dental disease/malocclusion; ileus; hepatic lipidosis; gastric tympany; antibiotic-induced enterotoxaemia; food spoilage; unpalatable or novel diet; physical, environmental or social stressors; neoplasia; chronic liver disease; bacterial enteritis; viral enteritis; helminthiasis; cestodiasis; protozoal enteritis
Sudden death	Gastric/caecal torsion; hepatic lipidosis/ketosis; antibiotic-induced enterotoxaemia; environmental disturbances/maternal inexperience (young); bacterial enteritis; viral enteritis; helminthiasis; protozoal enteritis

11.7 Common enteric differential diagnoses of
rodents associated with digestive dysfunction
(listed according to presenting complaint). Note that many
non-digestive disorders may also cause similar clinical
signs.

History taking

A thorough history is invaluable and should include
details regarding diet, recent changes in husbandry,
the environment and the health status of in-contact
animals. Any recent medical therapy that has been
administered may be relevant, particularly antibiotics.
In young animals, the date and place of acquisition
and subsequent growth rate are important. The nature
and duration of any clinical signs that are apparent
should be noted, particularly changes in appetite or
faecal output (changes in the size, consistency and
number of pellets passed) (Figure 11.8).

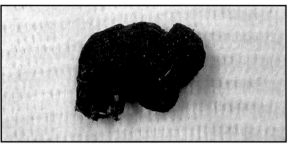

11.8 Noting the amount, size and consistency of faecal material is an important part of the history-taking procedure and clinical assessment of rodents with suspected gastroenteropathies. This dry poorly formed faecal material was being passed infrequently by a lethargic and inappetent guinea pig, suggestive of a primary or secondary enteropathy.

Physical examination

A complete physical examination should be carried out (Figure 11.9) (see also Chapter 2). The aim is to formulate a list of differential diagnoses and to assess the degree of debilitation. Common findings include:

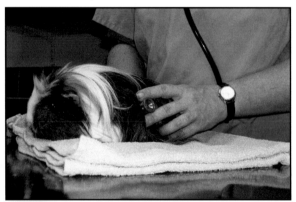

11.9 Abdominal auscultation can be a useful physical examination tool to assess the motility of the gastrointestinal tract.

- Dull, depressed demeanour
- Poor body condition
- Poor hydration status
- Perineal soiling
- Dental disease
- Abdominal distension
- Palpable abnormalities within the abdomen (e.g. distended or impacted bowel loops)
- Abnormalities on abdominal auscultation (e.g. complete lack of sounds or evidence of hypermotility).

Diagnostic tools to evaluate gastrointestinal disease

If the history and physical examination fail to provide a definitive cause for a suspected gastrointestinal disease, further diagnostic evaluation is warranted. Figure 11.10 details the most useful diagnostic tools and highlights significant findings.

Principles of treatment of gastroenteropathies

Effective treatment of gastrointestinal disease in all rodent species relies on accurate diagnosis and targeted therapeutic regimes to remove the primary cause. However, there are some aspects of treatment, largely supportive and symptomatic therapy, that are applicable to most cases.

Relieving pain

Some degree of abdominal pain is likely with most digestive disorders and alleviating this adequately is essential. Pain can be difficult to detect in many rodent species (see Chapter 6) and results in immune suppression, impaired wound healing, decreased food and water intake and therefore reduced gastrointestinal motility (which may already be reduced). Opioid and/or non-steroidal anti-inflammatory medications can be administered (see Chapter 5).

Diagnostic tool	Indications	Significant findings
Faecal wet mount	Diarrhoea	Large numbers of motile protozoa, e.g. *Giardia*
Faecal cytology/Gram stain	Diarrhoea	Bacterial (especially coliform or clostridial) or yeast overgrowth
Faecal flotation	Diarrhoea	Large numbers of coccidians, helminth eggs or cestode eggs
Perianal adhesive tape test	Diarrhoea; perianal pruritus	Detection of pinworm eggs
Aerobic and anaerobic bacterial culture and sensitivity of faeces/intestinal contents	Diarrhoea; sudden death	Pure/heavy growth of one or more pathogenic bacteria (selective media may be required, e.g. for *Salmonella*)
Oral examination under sedation/anaesthesia	Dysphagia; hypersalivation; showing interest in food despite anorexia; cheek pouch impaction (hamsters)	Malocclusion of incisors and/or cheek teeth (especially in guinea pigs, chinchillas and degus). Ulceration of the tongue or cheeks (often associated with a dental spike). Oropharyngeal infection or foreign body. Impacted/infected or ruptured cheek pouches (hamsters)
Urinalysis	Non-specific illness, e.g. dehydration, weight loss	Elevated urine specific gravity as a measure of dehydration. Altered pH e.g. acidosis. Presence of ketones, e.g. ketosis

11.10 Diagnostic tools that may be useful for evaluation of gastrointestinal dysfunction in rodents following history-taking and a complete physical examination. (continues) ▶

Diagnostic tool	Indications	Significant findings
Plain abdominal radiography	Abdominal distension; reduced or absent faecal output	Gas-filled loops of bowel that may be suggestive of ileus or an obstruction. Hepatomegaly
Positive contrast radiography (administer 5 ml/kg of a 1:1 mixture of barium sulphate mixed with water or liquidized food then radiograph hourly or as required)	To assess gut transit time in patients with hypo- or hypermotility disorders; may aid in differentiation of obstructive from non-obstructive enteropathies	Regarding gut transit time, little information is available in relation to most pet species; however, in the guinea pig some contrast is expected to have reached the colon by 4 hours post administration. Megaoesophagus (a condition that has been reported in rats and mice; Harkness and Ferguson, 1979; Randelia *et al.*, 1990). Apparent gastrointestinal obstruction. Note: coprophagy may need to be accounted for in serial radiographs as contrast material may 'reappear' in the stomach following ingestion of faeces containing barium
Fluoroscopy	Hypomotility disorders	Has the potential to assess GI motility (described in guinea pigs) (Ruelokke *et al.*, 2004)
Abdominal ultrasonography	Hepatic disease; ascites; palpable abdominal mass	Identification of focal or diffuse changes in hepatic echogenicity. Identification of soft tissue mass. Poor intestinal motility. Note: abdominal ultrasonography is frequently unhelpful in cases of ileus as gas impairs the quality of the images
Abdominocentesis (perform under general anaesthesia, ideally via ultrasound guidance, to reduce risk of visceral laceration)	Ascites	Evidence of peritonitis (inflammatory cells and/or bacteria in peritoneal fluid)
Exploratory laparotomy	Suspected gastrointestinal obstruction; cases of hypomotility that fail to respond to aggressive medical therapy after 3–5 days; palpable abdominal mass	Gastrointestinal obstruction. Intussusception. Resectable or non-resectable soft tissue mass
Liver biopsy (collect sample via exploratory laparotomy, laparoscopy or by ultrasound-guided fine-needle aspiration)	Hepatic disease	Metabolic (e.g. lipidosis), infectious, toxic, immune-mediated or parasitic changes identified on histopathology
Haematology/serum biochemistry	Non-specific illness; rarely provides a definitive diagnosis but may inform the clinician of the stability of the patient	Abnormalities related to: • PCV • Total protein • Albumin • Electrolytes • Urea • Creatinine • Hepatic enzymes
ELISA	Suspected Tyzzer's disease or viral enteritis, e.g. rat coronavirus, mouse hepatitis virus, mouse rotavirus, rat rotavirus-like agent	Positive serological test in the presence of appropriate clinical signs is suggestive of disease
PCR	Suspected Tyzzer's disease; suspected *Helicobacter* spp. infection	Positive result on faecal sample, intestinal contents or tissue samples
Cytotoxin assay	Suspected clostridial enteritis; inappropriate antibiotic administration	Identification of clostridia-associated toxin
Post-mortem examination (gross and histopathological examination of a range of tissues)	Especially useful in cases of groups of rodents suffering from gastroenteritis	Variable. For many of the infectious aetiologies this is the only reliable method of obtaining a definitive diagnosis, e.g. proliferative ileitis

11.10 (continued) Diagnostic tools that may be useful for evaluation of gastrointestinal dysfunction in rodents following history-taking and a complete physical examination.

Replacement of fluids and electrolytes

The importance of the management of fluid and electrolyte balance (Figures 11.11 and 11.12) cannot be overstated. Any alteration of gastrointestinal function will severely affect fluid balance. This, in turn, depresses gastrointestinal function further, creating a vicious cycle that must be interrupted. For more information see Chapter 2.

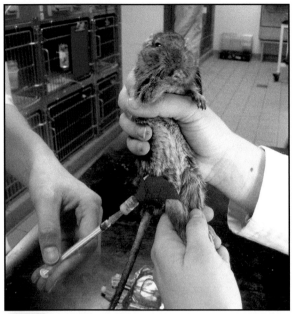

11.11 Administration of isotonic fluid to a degu via an intraosseous catheter. The patient was suffering from severe nutritional hypomotility (associated with a low-fibre diet).

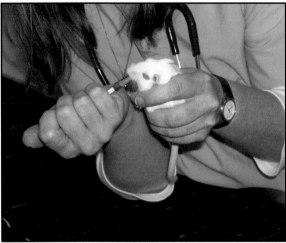

11.12 A gerbil receiving oral fluids as a supportive measure to treat mild enteritis associated with a recent change in diet.

Correcting abnormal motility

In cases with hypomotility or ileus, aggressive medical treatment can be successful and consists of fluid therapy, nutritional therapy, analgesia and stimulation of gastrointestinal motility. Metoclopramide and/or cisapride are prokinetic agents that promote normal motility (see Chapter 5 for dosage regimes). Although information relevant to pet rodents is lacking, the histamine (H2) receptor antagonist ranitidine has also been shown to have a gastric prokinetic effect in other species.

To prevent recurrence, investigation and correction of the underlying problem (e.g. high-carbohydrate low-fibre diet, dental disease, systemic illness) that predisposed to poor motility is essential. Surgical exploration is frequently unrewarding and should only be considered if diagnostic tests suggest that an obstruction is likely, or if the rodent fails to respond to appropriate and aggressive medical therapy after several days.

Unless a trichobezoar is forming an obstruction (which is very rare), it usually resolves with aggressive fluid, nutritional and prokinetic medical therapy as above.

The use of spasmolytics (e.g. butylscopolamine) to reduce motility in cases with hypermotility and diarrhoea is currently poorly understood. As such, the use of such agents is controversial and not recommended at the present time.

Temperature regulation

Hypothermia is common at initial presentation. Ensuring body temperature is maintained by providing external heat sources is important. A critical care incubator is a useful piece of equipment for hospitalizing ill rodents (see Chapter 2).

Nutritional support

Quality nutritional support is vital for any rodent that has altered gastrointestinal function, regardless of the underlying condition. In the absence of adequate caloric intake, many rodents (especially those that are overweight) will develop hepatic lipidosis within days. Additionally, rodents not practising coprophagy will rapidly become deficient in protein and vitamins. To counteract these problems, regular syringe feeding is essential for anorexic or inappetent animals (Figure 11.13). Without this form of therapy, recovery

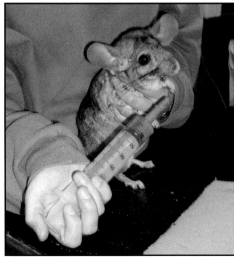

11.13 An anorexic chinchilla being fed a high-fibre commercial gruel via a catheter-tipped syringe. Feeds are given every 4–6 hours throughout the day until the animal's appetite returns to normal. The amount given is calculated on the basis of body condition, the level of debilitation and the underlying disease (if identified).

may not be possible. Most rodents tolerate this well but the process is time-consuming and requires patience. A number of companies produce high-fibre products specifically designed for the herbivorous species. Alternatively hay- or grass-based pellets may be crushed and mixed with water or puréed vegetables to produce a thick slurry. Commercial products are preferred as they are supplemented with vitamins and protein sources as well as fibre. Omnivorous species may be fed baby food. Fresh food must be available at all times (Figure 11.14). See Chapter 2 for further information.

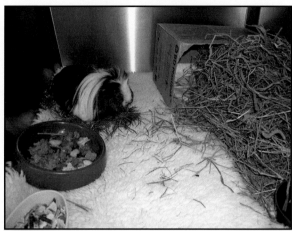

11.14 Fresh food must be offered to all rodents with gastrointestinal dysfunction, even if they are completely anorexic. This hospitalized guinea pig is being offered timothy hay, fresh grass, a variety of vegetables and small amounts of a concentrate mix with which she is familiar.

Reconstitution of the digestive flora
Nutritional support is the mainstay of restoring gut flora. Traditionally dysbiosis has been treated with the judicious use of antibiotics and supportive measures such as fluid therapy and cholestyramine, an ion-exchange resin that may reduce the effects of bacterial toxins. More recently, probiotic supplementation (e.g. *Lactobacillus*) or transfaunation (the feeding of faeces of a healthy conspecific) have been suggested as adjunctive therapeutic measures and anecdotal reports support their use.

Relieving distension
If significant distension of the gastrointestinal tract is present, attempts must be made to alleviate the problem as soon as possible. 'Bloat' is painful and has serious secondary effects on the circulation. Mild to moderate cases may be relieved with medical therapy consisting of oral simethicone (0.5–1.0 ml/kg q2–6h), fluid therapy and prokinetic medication (e.g. metoclopramide and/or cisapride). Acute, marked gastric dilatation requires immediate decompression, preferably by the passage of a stomach tube. Severe cases that cannot be resolved by other means may require decompression by percutaneous trocharization, a procedure that carries a significant risk of inducing peritonitis. Surgical correction, following initial stabilization, is required to relieve obstructive causes.

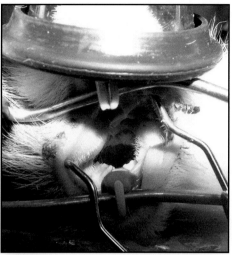

11.15 Oral examination of a guinea pig that presented with diarrhoea of 2 months' duration. Elongation of the lower premolars is evident. Such changes affect the animal's ability to chew food and can lead to a subsequent gastrointestinal disorder. Note also that one of the lower incisors is missing (previously fractured) and there is evidence of concurrent cheilitis.

Correcting dental abnormalities
Dental disease, specifically incisor and/or cheek teeth malocclusion, is one of the primary causes of gastrointestinal dysfunction in rodents (Figure 11.15). Once a patient has been stabilized, dental evaluation and correction are necessary in such cases. For further information see Chapter 8.

Common gastrointestinal diseases

The most common or significant diseases of mice, rats, hamsters, gerbils, guinea pigs, chinchillas and degus are discussed below by species. Generally, the omnivores (mice, rats, gerbils and hamsters) are prone to infectious and non-infectious diarrhoea, especially as juveniles. Dietary factors, endoparasites and opportunistic pathogens are common aetiologies. The herbivores (guinea pigs, chinchillas and degus) more frequently develop primary and secondary hypomotility disorders and disruptions to coprophagy. Low-fibre diets, stress and concurrent disease are often implicated. Figures 11.16 and 11.17 summarize the clinical and diagnostic features of selected common non-infectious and infectious conditions (see Chapter 5 for specific drug doses.)

Mice

Non-infectious diarrhoea
Diarrhoea can result from abrupt diet change, the feeding of mouldy food or engorgement on wet, fresh foods. In such cases, the mouse usually remains bright with a good appetite. The offending food item should be removed and simple balanced food (e.g. commercial rodent pellets) fed exclusively until faecal consistency improves. Fluid therapy is warranted if the patient is dehydrated and symptomatic dosing with a kaolin–pectin mixture (0.2 ml/kg orally q6–8h) may hasten clinical recovery.

Disease/agent	Species affected	Clinical signs	Diagnosis	Treatment and control	Comments
Nutritional gastroenteritis, e.g. abrupt change in diet, mouldy feed, novel food item, malnutrition	All	Diarrhoea; most animals remain bright otherwise	History; response to therapy	Remove offending food item/ correct the diet. Nutritional support (especially increasing fibre intake in the herbivores). Probiotics. Other supportive measures, e.g. fluid therapy, kaolin–pectin	
Gastric dilatation/ tympany	All	Abdominal distension; abdominal pain, e.g. tooth-grinding, dyspnoea; reluctance to move; respiratory distress	Clinical presentation; radiography	Passage of a stomach tube. Paracentesis (beware of the risk of inducing peritonitis) + treatment as for ileus	Requires immediate treatment as can be rapidly fatal. May develop secondary to anaesthesia, stress or engorgement on rich foods
Ileus	All	Reduction in faecal output – droppings absent or dry and scant; anorexia; abdominal pain, e.g. hunched posture, tooth-grinding, dyspnoea; palpably distended loops of gut; dehydration; abdominal distension	Radiography	Fluid therapy. Nutritional therapy, e.g. assisted feeding. Analgesia. Prokinetic therapy. Supplemental heat. Repeated abdominal massage. Warm, soapy enemas. Surgery if intussusception, obstruction or torsion is suspected	Identification and removal of the inciting cause is paramount
Hepatic lipidosis	All Especially obese or pregnant/ lactating females	Depression; anorexia; death within days to weeks of onset of clinical signs	History of anorexia; urinalysis (to assess for ketoacidosis); serum biochemistry; blood sample to assess acid/base balance	Assisted feeding. Fluid therapy. Multivitamin supplementation. Other supportive measures	Anecdotally medical therapy suitable for liver disease in other companion animals (e.g. lactulose, s-adenosylmethionine) may be beneficial as adjunctive therapy
Cheek pouch disease	Hamsters	Large, persistent swellings on one or both sides of the face	Examination under general anaesthesia; cytology and/or culture of cheek pouch contents	Eversion of the pouches under general anaesthesia, removal of the contents and flushing. Surgery if pouch has ruptured (see Chapter 7)	
Rectal faecal impactions	Guinea pigs (especially geriatric males)	Malodorous accumulation of soft faeces at the anus; reduced or altered faecal output	Physical examination	Regular gentle manual removal of faecal matter (usually required long term)	
Antibiotic-associated colitis (clinical signs usually occur due to *Clostridium difficile* enterotoxaemia and/or overgrowth of *Escherichia coli*)	All species, but hamsters and guinea pigs appear to be especially susceptible	Profuse diarrhoea; anorexia; poor coat quality; dehydration; hypothermia; death	History of antibiotic administration; clinical signs; post-mortem lesions (gross and microscopic); assay for *C. difficile* toxin; culture of gut contents (e.g. *E. coli*)	Usually unsuccessful. Supportive care, e.g. fluid therapy, provision of an external heat source. Transfaunation or probiotics. Antibiotics if an overgrowth of coliforms is suspected	Poor prognosis
Non-infectious intestinal dysbiosis (not associated with antibiotic administration)	All	Diarrhoea (or sometimes reduction in faecal output); abdominal pain; anorexia; weight loss; dehydration; depression; palpably enlarged mesenteric lymph nodes; acute death	Bacterial culture of faeces (to identify opportunistic pathogens); antibiotic sensitivity	Antibiotics (based on culture and sensitivity results). High fibre supplementation. Probiotics/transfaunation. Other supportive care, e.g. fluids. Nursing care. Eliminate inciting cause (if possible)	Causes include sudden dietary change, prolonged antibiotic use, stress, overcrowding and diets containing insufficient fibre and excessive fat and protein

11.16 Summary of selected non-infectious gastrointestinal disorders of rodents.

Disease/agent	Species affected	Clinical signs	Diagnosis	Treatment and control	Comments
Tyzzer's disease (*Clostridium piliforme*)	All (gerbils particularly susceptible)	Diarrhoea; dehydration; depression; lethargy; ruffled hair coat; hunched posture; unthrifty appearance; anorexia; weight loss; CNS dysfunction; death	Necropsy – liver/ intestinal histopathology; serology (ELISA); PCR	Supportive care is essential. Oxytetracycline/tetracycline may suppress clinical signs. Chloramphenicol. Decontaminate environment (use 0.5% sodium hypochlorite, peracetic acid or prolonged heat treatment). Barrier nursing or culling of affected animals. Strict quarantine. Optimizing husbandry standards	Associated with exposure to contaminated feeds or wild rodents. Poor prognosis. Predisposing factors include weaning, stress, overcrowding, concurrent disease, recent transport, immune suppression, suboptimal husbandry. Persistent infections are common; spores are difficult to eradicate
Other clostridial enteropathies, e.g. *Clostridium difficile*, *C. perfringens* type E	All	Diarrhoea (sometimes with blood or mucus); anorexia; weight loss; dehydration; lethargy; abdominal pain; death	Faecal Gram stain; faecal culture; faecal cytoxin assay	Cholestyramine 100 mg/ml in drinking water. High fibre dietary supplement. Probiotics. Antibiotics. Other supportive measures. Decontaminate environment. Toxoid vaccination has been used in chinchillas	Almost always fatal
Salmonellosis, e.g. *Salmonella enteritidis* and *S. typhimurium*	All	Diarrhoea (not always present); dehydration; depression; anorexia; weakness; gastrointestinal ulceration; weight loss; rough hair coat; gastrointestinal distension; non-GI signs, e.g. testicular enlargement, dyspnoea, conjunctivitis, abortion; sudden death (especially in guinea pigs)	Faecal culture and blood culture (use selective media)	Antibiotics and fluid therapy but treatment is not usually recommended. Thorough cleaning of environment. Prevention: thorough washing of food; good cage hygiene	Zoonotic. Exposure is via contaminated feed, animals or humans
Proliferative ileitis/ enteritis (*Lawsonia intracellularis*)	Significant disease in hamsters. Other species to a variable extent	'Wet-tail' i.e. wet perineum; foul-smelling watery diarrhoea; rough hair coat; anorexia; dehydration; abdominal pain; distended bowel loops identified on abdominal palpation	Histopathology (silver stain); electron microscopy	Supportive treatment must be aggressive. Antibiotics, e.g. enrofloxacin, trimethoprim/ sulphonamide combinations or neomycin. Bismuth subsalicylate. Quarantine. High levels of sanitation. Stress must be eliminated and any management deficiencies corrected	Poor prognosis. Primary predisposing factor is stress (e.g. weaning, poor diet, dietary change, transportation, crowding, poor hygiene). Gastrointestinal obstruction, impaction, intussusception, rectal prolapse and/or peritonitis may develop. Associated with neoplasia in rats
Enteritis due to other bacterial agents (*E. coli*, *Proteus* spp., *Yersinia* spp., *Campylobacter* spp., *Pseudomonas* spp., *Pasteurella* spp., *Listeria* spp., *Klebsiella* spp.)	All	Diarrhoea (or sometimes reduction in faecal output); abdominal pain; anorexia; weight loss; dehydration; depression; palpably enlarged mesenteric lymph nodes; acute death	Culture; antibiotic sensitivity	Antibiotics (based on culture and sensitivity results). High fibre supplementation. Probiotics/transfaunation. Other supportive care, e.g. fluids. Nursing care. Consider euthanasia if zoonotic	Some agents, e.g. *Campylobacter*, are zoonotic. Predisposing factors include sudden dietary change, prolonged antibiotic use, stress, overcrowding and diets containing insufficient fibre and excessive fat and protein

11.17 Summary of selected infectious gastrointestinal disorders of rodents. (continues) ▶

Disease/agent	Species affected	Clinical signs	Diagnosis	Treatment and control	Comments
Helicobacter spp. (many different species)	Various	Often none; weight loss; diarrhoea; rectal prolapse; death	Histopathology (silver stain); culture; PCR	None	Significance of *Helicobacter* spp. infections in rodents unclear at present. Have been associated with GI neoplasia in some species
Coronaviruses: sialodacryoadenitis virus (SDAV), Parker's rat coronavirus	Rat	Swollen cervical region; photophobia; porphyrin staining of the face; respiratory signs	Typical histopathology of salivary and other glands in the head; serology	Not usually required. Empirical therapy if ocular lesions develop	Highly infectious. Adults usually completely recover. Can exacerbate *Mycoplasma pulmonis* infection
Mouse hepatitis virus (coronavirus)	Mouse (sucklings)	Diarrhoea; weight loss; dehydration; poor growth; encephalitis with tremors and death	Serology; histopathology	Supportive therapy, e.g. fluids	Adults usually completely recover
Mouse rotavirus and rat rotavirus-like agent	Mouse and rat (sucklings)	Diarrhoea (+/− GI ulceration); adults usually asymptomatic	Serology; histopathology	Supportive therapy, e.g. fluids	May be zoonotic
Candidiasis (*Candida albicans*)	All	Diarrhoea; sudden death	Faecal examination	Antifungal drugs, e.g. amphotericin B, itraconazole, ketoconazole	Usually overgrowth is secondary to another disease
Cestodiasis (*Rodentolepis nana*, the dwarf tapeworm; *Hymenolepis diminuta*, the rat tapeworm)	All (more common in young animals)	Usually none; diarrhoea; weight loss; intestinal impaction/obstruction; unthriftiness; retarded growth; dehydration	Ova identified in faecal flotation; adult or cysticercal stages identified by necropsy/histopathology	Vector control, frequent bedding changes, treat with niclosamide, praziquantel or thiabendazole. High fibre nutritional support. Probiotics. Other supportive measures	Zoonotic threat, particularly children, so euthanasia may be considered more appropriate than treatment
Helminthiasis (e.g. *Syphacia* spp., *Aspicularis tetraptera*, *Paraspidodera uncinata*, *Dentostomella translucida*)	All	Usually none; sometimes reduced growth rate; unthriftiness; poor hair coat; diarrhoea; inappetence; anal pruritus; intestinal impaction; intussusception; rectal prolapse; cachexia; death	Pinworm ova identified on cellophane tape impressions of the anal area; faecal flotation for other helminths	Ivermectin usually effective. Piperazine. Benzimidazoles e.g. fenbendazole, tiabendazole. Levamisole. Stringent disinfection of cages and cage furniture should be carried out at the time of treatment. High fibre nutritional support, probiotics and other supportive measures if clinical signs are apparent	Not zoonotic. Control can be difficult
Coccidiosis (e.g. *Eimeria* spp.)	All (especially recently weaned animals)	Diarrhoea; death	Faecal direct smear; faecal flotation; mucosal scrapings and/or histopathology of tissues	Sulphonamides. Supportive care. Improvements in housing and husbandry	Disease usually associated with poor husbandry, overcrowding and concurrent disease
Protozoal gastroenteritis (*Giardia* spp., *Spironucleus* spp., *Trichomonas* spp., *Balantidium* spp., *Cryptosporidium* spp., *Entamoeba* spp.)	All (especially young or immuno-suppressed animals)	Usually asymptomatic; diarrhoea; failure to gain weight/weight loss; greasy coat; occasionally death	Direct faecal examination	Antiprotozoals, e.g. metronidazole – but can be difficult to eliminate completely. Benzimidazoles may be effective against *Giardia*. High fibre nutritional support. Probiotics. Other supportive measures	*Giardia* spp. and *Cryptosporidium* spp. may be zoonotic

11.17 (continued) Summary of selected infectious gastrointestinal disorders of rodents.

Bacterial enteritis

Tyzzer's disease: Tyzzer's disease is caused by *Clostridium piliforme*. Common predisposing factors are weaning, immunosuppression and suboptimal husbandry. Typical clinical signs include diarrhoea, dehydration and anorexia or occasionally sudden death. Transmission is likely through contaminated food and bedding and spores can remain viable in the environment for over a year at room temperature.

Diagnosis is not easy in the pet mouse as it requires demonstration of the characteristic clusters of intracellular bacilli in liver biopsy samples or sections of hepatic/intestinal tissue collected at post-mortem examination. Additional available aids to diagnosis include serology (ELISA) and PCR amplification of infected tissues (intestine, liver and/or myocardium). Treatment is usually unsuccessful. Prevention and control of outbreaks can be achieved by barrier housing, good husbandry practices and strict quarantine.

Other bacterial gastroenteropathies: These include:

- Other clostridial enteropathies (e.g. *C. perfringens* or *C. difficile*)
- Salmonellosis (rare, but significant due to its zoonotic potential)
- *Escherichia coli* (only pathogenic in immunodeficient mice)
- *Lawsonia intracellularis* (associated with proliferative enteritis, typhlitis or colitis)
- *Corynebacterium kutscheri* septicaemia of stressed or immunosuppressed mice (causes disseminated abscesses in many organs, including the liver)
- *Helicobacter* spp., which occupy the caecum and colon of the mouse with variable presence in the liver and can cause typhlocolitis and hepatitis
- Colonic hyperplasia disease (transmissible murine colonic hyperplasia) caused by *Citrobacter freundii.*

Viral enteritis/hepatitis
Many viruses have been associated with enteritis and hepatitis in the mouse. Most have been identified in laboratory settings and their prevalence in the pet mouse population is unknown. Examples include mouse hepatitis virus (coronavirus), epizootic diarrhoea of infant mice (rotavirus), lymphocytic choriomeningitis virus, reovirus, murine norovirus 1 (calicivirus), mouse cytomegalovirus and mousepox (ectromelia virus). Treatment of suspected viral enteropathies is largely supportive.

Endoparasites

Pinworms (oxyurids): Pinworms (*Syphacia obvelata, Aspicularis tetraptera*) are ubiquitous and usually non-pathogenic but heavy infestations can present with rectal prolapse secondary to straining, poor hair coat, mucoid enteritis, anal pruritus, intestinal impaction and intussusception. Diagnosis is achieved by microscopic examination of tape applied to the perianal skin (*Syphacia*) and by faecal smear or flotation (*Aspicularis*). Ivermectin, piperazine citrate and the benzamidazoles (e.g. fenbendazole) are effective at resolving clinical disease though complete elimination of these parasites is difficult (see Chapter 5 for dose rates). Stringent disinfection of cages and cage furniture should be carried out at the time of treatment.

Cestodiasis: *Rodentolepis* (previously *Hymenolepis*) *nana*, the dwarf tapeworm, and *Hymenolepis diminuta*, the rat tapeworm, may infect mice. Both species are potentially zoonotic but *H. diminuta* requires an intermediate host and so is less of a public health concern. Clinical disease is rare, though diarrhoea and retarded growth can be seen with heavy infestations. Diagnosis can be made by faecal flotation or by identification of adult cestodes at necropsy. Treatment with praziquantel may be effective. The benefits of therapy may have to be weighed against the zoonotic hazard the host poses.

Spironucleus (Hexamita) muris *and* ***Giardia muris:*** These protozoal organisms are found in the small intestine and caecum. They can cause enteritis and diarrhoea in young mice and occasionally death. Older animals are generally asymptomatic. Treatment with metronidazole or oxytetracycline can be effective at resolving clinical signs but does not completely eliminate the organism (see Chapter 5 for dose rates). The benzimidazoles are also effective against *Giardia* spp.

Cryptosporidiosis: In mice, *Cryptosporidium parvum* colonizes the upper small intestine and *C. muris* is found within the stomach. Both are mildly pathogenic and may lead to malnutrition, especially in young animals with concurrent illness. Diagnosis is possible by faecal examination but usually histopathology of tissues sampled at necropsy is required. Treatment of suspected cases is largely supportive.

Gastric yeast: *Candida albicans* is present in the mouse gastrointestinal tract as a commensal organism. Disruption of gut function or prolonged use of antibiotics may permit overgrowth.

Rats

Non-infectious digestive disorders

Diarrhoea of dietary origin: This can result from the overfeeding of treat items or a sudden change in dietary composition. Most rats will remain bright with a good appetite despite showing altered faecal consistency. For treatment, see under non-infectious diarrhoea of mice above.

Megaoesophagus: This has been reported in the rat (Harkness and Ferguson, 1979). Clinical signs include accumulation of food around the mouth and dyspnoea. Contrast radiography will confirm the diagnosis but the prognosis is poor.

Bacterial digestive diseases

Tyzzer's disease: Tyzzer's disease (*Clostridium piliforme*) is most prevalent in weanlings. For clinical signs, diagnosis and treatment see under Mice.

Other bacterial enteropathies: Other bacteria that have been associated with enteropathies in rats include *Campylobacter* spp. (isolated from young rats with mild diarrhoea) and *Lawsonia intracellularis* (observed in the epithelium of rat intestinal adenocarcinomas). Rats are capable of becoming infected with *Salmonella enteritidis* and *S. typhimurium*. Clinically affected animals typically present with distension of the ileum and caecum and may develop gastrointestinal ulceration. Subclinical carriers also exist. Due to the zoonotic nature of salmonellosis, consideration should be given to euthanasia of animals diagnosed with this disease.

Viral digestive diseases

Infectious diarrhoea of infant rats (IDIR): IDIR is a rotavirus-like disease that principally affects suckling rats (less than 2 weeks of age) (Vonderfecht *et al.*, 1984). Diarrhoea (with or without ulceration) is typical and growth rates are poor. Treatment is largely supportive but the disease is potentially zoonotic so euthanasia may need to be considered.

Coronaviruses: Sialodacryoadenitis virus and Parker's rat coronavirus are common amongst pet rats and highly infectious. They may cause transient inflammation and swelling of the cervical salivary and lacrimal glands as well as respiratory disease (see also Chapters 12 and 15). Mortality is low and many infected rats remain asymptomatic. No treatment is required unless ocular lesions are severe. The signs usually resolve but residual (histopathological) lesions may persist within the affected glands.

Endoparasites

Pinworms: The pinworms of the rat include *Syphacia muris*, *Syphacia obvelata* and *Aspicularis tetraptera*. Pinworms do not cause clinical disease in this species, but infected young rats may exhibit a reduced growth rate. For diagnosis, treatment and control see under Mice.

Cestodes: The rat is the definitive host of both *Rodentolepis* (previously *Hymenolepis*) *nana* and *Hymenolepis diminuta*. Disease only occurs if burdens are heavy. Individual tapeworms can grow up to 150 mm in length. *R. nana* has a direct life cycle and is a concern given the potential for interspecies and zoonotic spread. For diagnosis and treatment see under Mice. Euthanasia may be considered more appropriate than treatment, given the zoonotic status of this parasite.

Protozoa: *Giardia muris* and *Spironucleus muris* are pathogenic flagellates of the small intestine. Disease tends to be restricted to young or immunosuppressed animals. For treatment see above under Mice.

Coccidia: *Eimeria* spp. are generally non-pathogenic in rats. Disease only tends to occur when husbandry standards are poor. Treatment is with sulphonamides.

Hepatitis

Hepatitis may be caused by systemic bacterial infections with organisms such as *Corynebacterium kutscheri*. Diagnosis is usually made via histopathology and bacterial culture of liver samples (e.g. biopsy). Treatment includes general supportive measures (e.g. fluid therapy, nutritional support) and appropriate antibiotics (ideally based on culture and sensitivity).

Hamsters

The most common syndrome seen in hamsters is described by the confusing term 'wet-tail'. Although some people use 'wet-tail' to refer to proliferative ileitis specifically, most often it is used as a lay term for diarrhoea or enteropathy, regardless of aetiology (Figure 11.18). As such it can occur at any age and may be due to a variety of factors, including pathogenic and opportunistic bacteria, parasitic infections and/or stress.

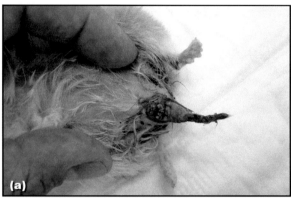
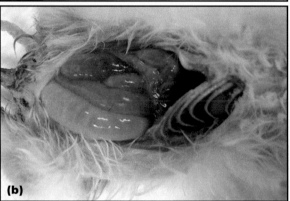

11.18 **(a)** Severe excoriation of the anogenital area secondary to diarrhoea (frequently termed 'wet tail') in an 8-week-old Syrian hamster. **(b)** Post-mortem examination revealed markedly distended intestinal loops. A diagnosis of proliferative ileitis (transmissible ileal hyperplasia) secondary to infection with *Lawsonia intracellularis* was made on histopathological examination. (Courtesy of Emma Keeble.)

Non-infectious diseases

Cheek pouch disease: This usually presents as large persistent swellings on one or both sides of the face. Most cases are caused by impaction of food material. Under general anaesthesia the pouches can be everted and flushed. Infection, abscessation and rupture may also occur. Infections are diagnosed via cytology and culture of cheek pouch swabs. Rupture requires surgical correction. See also Chapters 7 and 8.

Antibiotic-associated enterocolitits: Many antimicrobial agents are highly toxic to hamsters, even at very low doses. For this reason, empirical antibiotic therapy for any condition must be carefully considered. Enterocolitis has been reported following administration of lincomycin, clindamycin, ampicillin, vancomycin, erythromycin, cephalosporins, gentamicin, bacitracin and penicillin. Treatment with these drugs may lead to an overgrowth of coliforms and *Clostridium difficile*. *C. difficile* has an associated toxin which promotes haemorrhagic ileocolitis. Clinical signs include anorexia, poor coat quality, dehydration and profuse diarrhoea. The prognosis is very poor and most hamsters die within 4–10 days. Therapy should start immediately by discontinuing the causative antibiotic and providing a *Lactobacillus* probiotic supplement and supportive care (see Chapter 2). Antibiotics that are generally effective against Gram-negative organisms may be given with caution if an overgrowth of coliforms is suspected. Long-term use of vancomycin has been advocated by some authors. Bovine antibodies against toxigenic *C. difficile* given orally have been shown to protect hamsters against experimental antibiotic-associated enterotoxaemia (Lyerly *et al.*, 1991). Chapter 5 discusses antibiotic therapy in more detail.

Neoplasia: The incidence of alimentary neoplasia is low. Most reported tumours are benign (e.g. gastric squamous papillomas and intestinal adenomas). Small intestinal lymphosarcoma has also been reported (Manci *et al.*, 1984).

Polycystic disease: This benign congenital condition can be an incidental finding in this species. Cysts can be present on many organs, most commonly the liver. The disease is often asymptomatic but clinical signs such as abdominal distension or unexplained 'weight gain' may be seen (E. Keeble, personal communication). See Chapter 13 for further details.

Amyloidosis: Although more commonly associated with renal disease, amyloidosis may affect the liver and spleen. Clinical signs include anorexia, oedema, ascites and decreased serum albumin. Treatment is largely supportive and reducing dietary protein is recommended.

Bacterial diseases

Proliferative ileitis: Also known as transmissible ileal hyperplasia, this is a very common and often fatal condition in the hamster caused by infection with *Lawsonia intracellularis*. It usually affects young animals (2–8 weeks old) and spreads via the faecal–oral route. The major predisposing factor is stress (weaning, poor diet, dietary change, transportation, crowding, poor hygiene). The clinical signs include a wet perineum, foul-smelling watery diarrhoea, unkempt hair coat, anorexia, dehydration, discomfort on abdominal palpation and distended intestinal loops (see Figure 11.18b). Gastrointestinal obstruction, impaction, intussusception, rectal prolapse and/or peritonitis may be present. The prognosis is poor and diagnosis relies on a silver stain of tissues (harvested during post-mortem examination) submitted for histopathology. Treatment, if attempted, must be aggressive. Antibiotics can be effective if given early in the course of disease. Enrofloxacin, trimethoprim/sulphonamide combinations or tetracycline are

recommended. Metronidazole, neomycin or chloramphenicol are alternatives (see Chapter 5 for dose rates). Supportive therapy is essential and bismuth salts (2–5 mg/kg orally q6–8h) may provide useful adjunctive therapy. Quarantine of affected individuals and high levels of sanitation are required for control of the disease in group situations. Stress must be eliminated and any management deficiencies corrected.

Tyzzer's disease: Tyzzer's disease is caused by *Clostridium piliforme*, which multiplies exclusively within hepatic, intestinal epithelial or myocardial cells. Weanlings are most often affected and factors such as poor sanitation, intestinal parasitism and the feeding of an inappropriate diet may precipitate a clinical outbreak. Clinical signs include sudden-onset pale yellow watery diarrhoea, depression, dehydration, lethargy and death. Typhlitis and hepatitis are the typical pathologies associated with infection. Treatment with tetracycline can be attempted but the mortality rate can be high regardless.

Other bacteria: Salmonellosis (e.g. *Salmonella typhimurium*) is uncommon in hamsters and, when present, does not usually cause enteritis. Instead general illness may be seen associated with septicaemia, multifocal necrosis of the liver and hepatosplenomegaly. Zoonotic transmission has occurred and, given that an asymptomatic carrier state can develop following treatment, euthanasia is recommended. Similarly, many hamsters carry the potentially zoonotic bacterium *Campylobacter jejuni* asymptomatically. Treatment with oral erythromycin has been described for clinically affected animals with diarrhoea (Hrapkiewicz and Medina, 2007) but euthanasia may be considered in individual cases.

Parasitic diseases

Pinworms: Hamsters may be infected with pinworms of the genus *Syphacia*. The worms are of low pathogenicity but do have the potential to spread to other rodent species. For diagnosis, treatment and control see under Mice.

Cestodes: Several species of tapeworm may infect hamsters. Most infections are asymptomatic but heavy burdens may result in diarrhoea. Of note is *Rodentolepis* (previously *Hymenolepis*) *nana*, the dwarf tapeworm, which has a direct life cycle and can cause disease in other rodents and in humans. For diagnosis, treatment and control see under Mice.

Protozoa: Although rarely the primary cause of disease, *Giardia* spp. and *Spironucleus* spp. may contribute to gastrointestinal disease.

Gerbils

Non-infectious diseases

Antibiotic-associated enterocolitis: Typhlocolitis/colitis with mortality due to *Clostridium difficile-*

associated enterotoxaemia has occurred following oral amoxicillin and metronidazole therapy.

Gastric dilatation: Gaseous distension of the stomach may occur secondary to intestinal ileus/anorexia and feeding inappropriate or stale diets. The clinical signs include abdominal tympany, tooth-grinding and dyspnoea. Cardiovascular compromise can rapidly develop. Immediate treatment is essential by passage of a wide-bore stomach tube or direct aspiration with a needle and syringe. Fluid therapy and analgesia are vital supportive measures.

Ileus: Ileus is a relatively common sequela to anaesthesia, malocclusion or periods of anorexia. Droppings are absent or dry and scant. Increased gas is present in the small intestine on radiography. Treatment as for other species is with fluids, nutritional support, prokinetics and probiotics (see above under general considerations).

Amyloidosis: This is a disease of older gerbils. The liver, spleen and lymph nodes are common sites of amyloid deposition (see also Chapter 13). The disease often accompanies chronic renal disease. Clinical signs, when present, include dehydration, weight loss, anorexia and death. There is currently no known effective treatment for suspected cases and definitive diagnosis relies on histopathology of affected organs (most commonly sampled during post-mortem examination).

Neoplasia: Intestinal adenocarcinoma has been reported (Vincent and Ash, 1978).

Bacterial disease

Tyzzer's disease: Caused by *Clostridium piliforme*, this is the most common infectious disease of gerbils. It is most frequently seen at weaning age but can also affect adults. Mongolian gerbils appear to be extremely susceptible. Predisposing factors include stress, poor sanitation, overcrowding, concurrent disease and recent transport. Diarrhoea may be present or absent. Acute infection is characterized by lethargy and death within 48 hours. Chronic infection may present as depression, anorexia, weight loss, ruffled hair coat, hunched posture, watery diarrhoea, head tilt, ataxia and death. Transmission is by the faecal–oral route (e.g. via infected bedding). Initial enteric infection spreads rapidly to the liver, heart and central nervous system. Ante-mortem diagnosis is difficult. Typically post-mortem observation of intracytoplasmic bacilli on histopathology of affected organs is diagnostic. Serological screening (ELISA) is available and may aid diagnosis. Treatment is rarely successful but oxytetracycline or tetracycline for 30 days has been shown to reduce mortality in groups. Chloramphenicol is an alternative antibiotic and supportive care is essential. In colony situations, isolation and/or culling of affected animals may be necessary as a carrier state may develop after treatment. Cages, feeding and watering equipment should be sterilized. The disease can be prevented by improving husbandry and hygiene standards and reducing stress levels. Interspecies transmission is an important consideration.

Salmonellosis **(S. typhimurium, S. enteritidis)*:*** Adult gerbils are fairly resistant to salmonellosis but disease can occur in the young (3–10 weeks of age). Clinical signs include dehydration, depression, emaciation, rough hair coat, weight loss, abdominal distension and/or moderate to severe diarrhoea. Sudden death may occur in some cases. Focal hepatitis, splenic necrosis, suppurative orchitis, interstitial pneumonia and purulent to pyogranulomatous leptomeningitis have also been reported (Percy and Barthold, 2007). Infected cockroaches have been implicated as a source. Concurrent parasite burdens can exacerbate disease. Asymptomatic carriers may result after recovery and euthanasia may be considered appropriate, as zoonotic and interspecies transmission are possible. Diagnosis is made by isolation of the causative organism using appropriate bacterial media. *Salmonella* may be recovered post mortem from sites such as the small intestine, liver, spleen and blood.

Citrobacter rodentium: Infection with this organism has been reported from a laboratory animal facility in Spain (De La Puente-Redondo *et al.*, 1999). Clinical signs included haemorrhagic diarrhoea, rough hair coat and wasting. The mortality rate was high.

Escherichia coli: *E. coli* may cause enteritis. Diagnosis is by faecal culture and treatment is with antibiotics based on sensitivity screening.

Helicobacter: Naturally occurring *Helicobacter* infections (e.g. *H. hepaticus, H. bilis*) can occur. The incidence and significance in gerbils is yet to be determined.

Parasitic diseases

Pinworms: Gerbils can become infected with several species of oxyurids, including *Syphacia* spp. and *Aspicularis tetraptera* from mice and rats. Gerbils are the primary natural host of *Dentostomella translucida*, which resides in the proximal small intestine and large intestine. As a general rule, pinworms rarely cause clinical disease in gerbils. However, rectal prolapses have been reported associated with heavy burdens (Keeble, 2002). For diagnosis, treatment and control see under Mice.

Tapeworms: Species such as *Hymenolepis diminuta* and *Taenia crassicollis* are usually subclinical in gerbils. Severe infections with the dwarf tapeworm *Rodentolepis* (previously *Hymenolepis*) *nana* may result in debilitation, dehydration and mucoid diarrhoea. For diagnosis and treatment see under Mice.

Protozoa: Coccidiosis (*Eimeria* spp.), *Trichomonas*, *Entamoeba muris* and *Giardia* spp. may occasionally cause clinical disease. Diagnosis is by faecal examination.

Guinea pigs

Non-infectious diseases

Ileus: Gastrointestinal ileus is very common in guinea pigs. Clinical signs include anorexia and reduced faecal output. Treatment is supportive and should consist of removal of the inciting cause, assisted feeding, analgesia, fluids, supplemental heat, gentle abdominal massage and prokinetic therapy.

Gastric dilatation, caecal torsion and typhlitis: Guinea pigs are susceptible to acute abdomens characterized by sudden onset gaseous distension ('bloat'), pain, anorexia and profound weakness. Death will ensue rapidly due to respiratory impairment and possibly vascular shock. Radiographically, large sections of stomach or caecum are found to be distended by gas and sometimes fluid (Figure 11.19). The aetiology may not always be identifiable but considerations include impactions from hairballs, dietary indiscretion, bacterial gastroenteritis, anaesthesia and gut adhesions from prior abdominal surgeries. Gastric dilatation may also occur as an advanced stage of gastrointestinal hypomotility. In these cases inappropriate diets (low fibre, high carbohydrate) are implicated. Treatment consists of decompression by stomach tube or trocharization with a fine needle. Anti-gas formulations (e.g. simethicone 0.2 ml/kg orally; repeat dose 3–4 hours after initial dose if required) may be helpful but the prognosis is guarded unless treatment is started promptly. Failure to improve with decompression and early medical therapy warrants surgical intervention, but the outcome of surgical cases is generally poor.

Caecal torsion and acute idiopathic typhlitis occur sporadically in this species. Animals are often found dead with no recent history of illness.

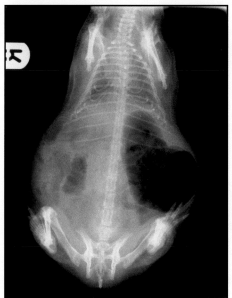

11.19 Dorsoventral radiograph of a guinea pig with acute gastric tympany. The stomach is markedly distended with gas. Acute abdominal distension developed in this animal 3 days after anaesthesia and surgery (cystotomy to remove a urolith). Aggressive medical therapy led to complete resolution of the gastric distension.

Antibiotic toxicity: Guinea pigs are exquisitely sensitive to many antibiotics. In susceptible individuals (up to 50% of guinea pigs), treatment with antibiotics, especially those with a Gram-positive spectrum, may destroy the normal bacterial intestinal flora (predominantly streptococci and lactobacilli) and permit an overgrowth of Gram-negative organisms and clostridia. Some guinea pigs, on the other hand, tolerate the same antibiotics reasonably well. Penicillins, cephalosporins, lincomycin, clindamycin, erythromycin, bacitracin, spiromycin, streptomycin and tetracyclines have been implicated. Oral administration carries the highest risk, but some parenteral and topical formulations have also been reported to cause problems. Enterotoxaemia (associated with secretory diarrhoea and haemorrhagic typhlitis) due to elaboration of the toxin associated with *Clostridium difficile* and/or an overgrowth of *Escherichia coli* is an all too common fatal consequence. In addition to diarrhoea, clinical signs include anorexia, dehydration and hypothermia and are apparent 1–5 days after antibiotic administration. Diagnosis is usually based on the history, clinical signs and post-mortem lesions. Bacteriology and an assay for *C. difficile* toxin can confirm suspicions. Treatment is usually unsuccessful and the disease is frequently fatal. Treatment involves supportive measures (fluid therapy, probiotics or transfaunation). Chloramphenicol may suppress further clostridial overgrowth. Control of this syndrome relies on the careful and discriminate use of broad-spectrum antibiotics in the guinea pig (see Chapter 5). Probiotics administered at the time of antibiotic treatment are reported anecdotally to reduce the risk of toxicity.

Non-antibiotic-related dysbiosis: In addition to antibiotics, many other factors (e.g. diet change, stress, appropriate but prolonged antibiotic therapy) may alter the enteric microflora and can initiate dysbiosis and subsequent enterotoxaemia. Diarrhoea may or may not be present. Enterotoxaemia may present as anorexia, rapid weight loss, dehydration, depression or acute death. Diagnosis is based upon history and the isolation of an offending organism or toxin. Treatment is difficult and largely supportive (e.g. fluid therapy and transfaunation).

Hypovitaminosis C (scurvy): Guinea pigs with hypovitaminosis C will infrequently present with diarrhoea. Usually there will be concurrent clinical signs such as a swollen joints or a reluctance to move. This disease is discussed in more detail in Chapter 14.

Rectal faecal impactions: Aged guinea pigs (particularly males) commonly develop faecal impactions consisting of soft faeces within the anus (Figure 11.20). A loss of muscle tone and an inability to practice coprophagy are thought to contribute. Clinical signs usually relate to abnormal faecal output and a malodorous accumulation of faecal matter in the anus. Regular gentle manual extraction of the faeces is required (sometimes on a long-term basis).

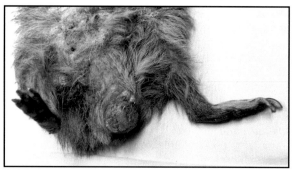

11.20 Geriatric guinea pigs, especially males, are prone to develop impactions of faecal matter in the rectum. This is thought to be due to a loss of muscle tone and cessation of coprophagy.

Fatty infiltration of the pancreas: This is frequently identified incidentally on post-mortem examination of elderly animals and is thought to be a normal part of the ageing process.

Fatty infiltration of the liver: This is most commonly seen in obese animals suffering from the metabolic/nutritional form of pregnancy toxaemia (see Chapter 13). Multifocal periportal necrosis of the liver can occur with the circulatory form of pregnancy toxaemia. Treatment relies on fluid therapy and nutritional and hepatic support.

Liver contusions: Liver contusions with subsequent haemorrhage into the peritoneal cavity may occur secondary to trauma (e.g. mishandling, being trodden on). Such injuries are usually fatal.

Metastatic mineralization: Incidental mineralization of various organs, including the stomach and colon, has been reported. Treatment is not recommended and the cause is presently unclear.

Neoplasms: Intestinal neoplasia appears to be rare, though bile duct tumours have been reported.

Bacterial enteritis

Tyzzer's disease: Spontaneous cases of Tyzzer's disease (caused by *Clostridium piliforme*) have been reported in guinea pigs. The highest risk animals are those that are immunocompromised, stressed and young. Clinical signs include an unthrifty appearance, lethargy, watery diarrhoea and sudden death. Definitive diagnosis is made by histopathological evaluation of intestine or liver samples, collected post mortem. Treatment is usually unrewarding. Prevention is by good husbandry practices and stress reduction, especially at the time of weaning.

Salmonellosis: In guinea pigs this is an uncommon but usually highly lethal (> 50% mortality) disease. The most common isolates are *Salmonella typhimurium* and *S. enteritidis*. The source is usually infected water or food. Key predisposing factors include stress, pregnancy, malnutrition and age (very young and very old animals are at the highest risk). Clinical signs include anorexia, depression, weight loss, light-coloured soft faeces or diarrhoea, scruffy hair coat,

weakness, conjunctivitis, abortion and dyspnoea. Chronic cases may show progressive weight loss and poor general condition. Hepatomegaly and spleno-megaly (sometimes with focal lesions) frequently develop along with septicaemia. Definitive diagnosis is made on the basis of culture of the faeces, blood or spleen using media selective for *Salmonella*. Treatment is not usually recommended, because of the potential for an inapparent carrier state to develop and the risk of zoonotic and interspecies spread. If attempted, anti-biotics (based on sensitivity testing) and fluids are the mainstay of therapy. The environment should be thoroughly disinfected. Prevention is achieved by good cage hygiene and thorough washing of fresh food.

Lawsonia *infection (adenomatous intestinal hyperplasia):* Segmental epithelial hyperplasia of the duodenum attributed to *Lawsonia intracellularis* has been observed in guinea pigs receiving steroid therapy. Clinical signs included diarrhoea, weight loss and death. The intracellular organisms were identified by electron microscopy.

Other causes of bacterial diarrhoea: Bacterial enteritis may also be caused by *Yersinia pseudotuberculosis*, *Clostridium perfringens*, *Escherichia coli*, *Pseudomonas aeruginosa*, *Listeria monocytogenes*, non-antibiotic-induced *Clostridium difficile* infection and *Citrobacter freundii*. These are generally acquired by faecal contamination of food. Stress and dietary changes are thought to be predisposing factors. For most bacterial infections, treatment is with appropriate antibiotics (ideally on the basis of culture and sensitivity) and supportive care. *Y. pseudotuberculosis* is a zoonotic condition and therefore treatment for this infection is not advised; affected animals should be euthanased.

Viral disease

A wasting syndrome, caused by a coronavirus or related virus, has been reported in weanling guinea pigs characterized by diarrhoea, anorexia, rapid weight loss and acute death with low levels of morbidity and mortality (Jaax *et al.*, 1990). It causes an acute to subacute necrotizing enteritis involving primarily the distal ileum.

Parasitic diseases

Candidiasis: *Candida albicans* is part of the normal enteric flora of the guinea pig. Antibiotic therapy may result in an overgrowth. Diagnosis is by faecal examination or cytology of oral lesions. Recommended treatment options include itraconazole (5 mg/kg orally q24h) or ketoconazole (10–40 mg/kg orally q24) for 2 weeks. Lesions in the oral cavity can be treated topically with nystatin.

Nematodes: Infections with gastrointestinal helminths in guinea pigs are predominantly due to the nematode *Paraspidodera uncinata*, a member of the Oxyuridae family. The nematode develops and resides in the colon and caecum and typical oxyurid eggs can be found by faecal flotation. The life cycle is direct. Clinical signs are predominantly mild or absent; however, heavy infections may cause cachexia, enteritis, unthriftiness and a rough coat. Sanitation is an important control measure. Treatment of patent infections is effective using fenbendazole, levamisole, piperazine or thiabendazole.

Cestodes: Cestode infections are caused by *Rodentolepis* (previously *Hymenolepis*) *nana* (the dwarf tapeworm) or *Hymenolepis diminuta*. The source of infections with *H. diminuta* (which requires an intermediate host) is either a flea infestation in a multi-pet household or outdoor housing with access to insects such as beetles or cockroaches. Zoonotic transmission is a concern with *R. nana*. Praziquantel is the treatment of choice.

Protozoans: *Cryptosporidium wrairi* is a major cause of small intestinal disease in guinea pigs, especially juveniles, weanlings and immunosuppressed animals. Transmission is by ingestion of oocysts in contaminated water, food and fomites. Clinical signs include failure to gain weight, weight loss, greasy coat, diarrhoea and death. Morbidity and mortality rates vary from negligible to up to 50%. Immunocompetent guinea pigs recover within 4 weeks and become resistant to reinfection. At necropsy the small and large intestines usually contain watery ingesta. Examination of fresh faeces or mucosal scrapings with phase contrast microscopy is the most reliable method of diagnosis. Electron microscopy will also identify organisms. There is no effective treatment but sulphonamides may suppress outbreaks. Environmental oocysts can be killed with 5% ammonia or by freezing (< 0°C) or extreme heat (> 65°C). Cryptosporidiosis is potentially zoonotic, a consideration when deciding whether treatment of a particular animal is warranted.

Eimeria caviae is the intestinal coccidian of guinea pigs. It is usually non-pathogenic but occasionally causes colitis, watery diarrhoea and death, especially in recently weaned animals. Predisposing factors include overcrowding, poor husbandry and concurrent disease. Good sanitation will disrupt the life cycle of the parasite. Diagnosis is by faecal flotation, mucosal scrapings and/or histopathology of tissues. Treatment is with sulphonamides and is usually effective if combined with improvements in housing and husbandry.

Balantidium caviae and *Giardia duodenalis* are relatively non-pathogenic but may be identified on faecal examination.

Chinchillas

Non-infectious diseases

Non-infectious hypomotility and enteritis: Non-infectious causes of digestive disease are more common in the pet chinchilla than infectious aetiologies, in the author's experience. Poor nutrition is the most frequent cause. Hypomotility disorders are a common presentation, frequently associated with anorexia and acquired dental disease. Colic and faecal impactions may subsequently develop.

Diarrhoea may develop due to inappropriate feeding (mouldy hay, overfeeding of fresh, rich or carbohydrate-laden foods), stress and abrupt dietary change. Non-infectious diarrhoea is often acute in onset and the chinchilla usually remains bright.

Choke and bloat: Oesophageal choke may present as drooling, retching, anorexia and dyspnoea. The offending item is often a treat (e.g. raisin, nut), bedding material or, in postparturient females, the placenta. Bloat or gastric tympany can result after overeating rich foods, sudden diet alterations and as a sequel to gastroenteritis. Clinical signs include abdominal distension, reluctance to move and dyspnoea. Ideally a stomach tube should be passed to relieve the gas. In an emergency a needle or trochar may be passed transabdominally but there is a significant risk of contamination of the peritoneal cavity with gastric contents. Analgesia, fluid therapy and nutritional support are vital adjunctive measures.

Trichobezoars: Gastric trichobezoars may form secondary to behavioural fur-chewing. Clinical signs are non-specific and include anorexia and lethargy. Diagnosis may be achieved by plain or positive contrast radiography. Medical treatment with fluids, high-fibre syringe feeds and gastric motility stimulants is recommended.

Antibiotic toxicity: Gram-positive spectrum antibiotics such as lincomycin, clindamycin, erythromycin and ampicillin are best avoided where possible as they suppress normal chinchilla gut flora. The implications of such changes and the associated clinical signs are similar to those seen in guinea pigs (see above). For further information see Chapter 5.

Constipation/intestinal stasis: Constipation and/or intestinal stasis is more common than diarrhoea and may present as straining and the passage of thin, short, hard faecal pellets. Insufficient dietary fibre is the primary cause and dietary correction is essential to prevent recurrence. Treat items such as raisins and grains must be removed from the diet. Laxatives marketed for cats can be used if there is no response to dietary and other supportive therapy. If fibre intake is reduced as a result of dental pathology, the underlying problem must be addressed to achieve resolution of clinical signs (see Chapter 8). Non-dietary causes include obesity, lack of exercise, intestinal obstruction and intestinal compression secondary to pregnancy.

Intestinal torsion and impaction: Chronic constipation or gastroenteritis can lead to intestinal torsion, impaction or intussusception. Radiographically, severely distended gas-filled loops of bowel are apparent. Animals may sit hunched or stretch out due to abdominal pain. Impactions and trichobezoars can usually be treated medically (with fluids, gut stimulants and warm soapy enemas) but intussusception, torsion and obstructions require surgery.

Rectal prolapse: Rectal prolapse may occur secondary to severe constipation or diarrhoea, stress or parturition. The prolapse can be replaced and retained with a purse-string suture. Gently soaking oedematous tissue in concentrated sugar solution may aid in reducing swelling. The primary problem must be corrected. Prolapses may be related to a colorectal intussusception and in some cases a volvulus of the small intestine. The prognosis in these cases is very poor.

Liver disease: Hepatic lipidosis is a common sequel to prolonged anorexia. Liver failure associated with metronidazole therapy has been reported anecdotally.

Chinchillas with liver disease generally present with non-specific signs of illness, such as anorexia, lethargy and weight loss. Diagnostic aids include serum biochemistry, abdominal imaging (radiography and/or ultrasonography) and liver biopsy (collected via ultrasound guidance, laparoscopy or exploratory laparotomy). Treatment includes fluid therapy, nutritional support and multivitamin supplementation. Anecdotally, medical therapy suitable for the treatment of liver disease in other companion animals (e.g. lactulose, s-adenosylmethionine) appears to be beneficial when combined with general supportive measures.

Bacterial enteritis

Infectious diarrhoea: This is most common in breeding females and young chinchillas, especially those kept under suboptimal husbandry conditions. Many bacteria have been implicated, including *Pseudomonas* spp., *Pasteurella* spp., *Proteus* spp., *Salmonella* spp., *Klebsiella pneumoniae* and *Escherichia coli*. The clinical signs include listlessness, dehydration, soft or liquid faeces or a complete absence of faeces. Bacterial enteritis may progress, if severe, to septicaemia. Predisposing factors are sudden dietary change, inappropriate or prolonged antibiotic use, stress, overcrowding and diets containing insufficient fibre and excessive fat and protein. Treatment is with appropriate antibiotics, aggressive fluid therapy and quality nursing care.

Enterotoxaemia: This is caused by *Clostridium perfringens* types A and D. Young chinchillas (2–4 months) are most susceptible. The clinical signs include diarrhoea, abdominal pain and sudden death. Immunization with toxoid in the laboratory setting has prevented disease (Hrapkiewicz and Medina, 2007).

Listeriosis: Although fur-ranched chinchillas appear to be highly susceptible to infection with *Listeria monocytogenes*, it is uncommon in pet chinchillas. Predisposing factors include feeding silage or beet pulp. Listeriosis is a caecal disease with blood-borne dissemination. The main target organ is the liver, where the bacteria multiply within hepatocytes. Neurological signs may accompany the enteric signs (e.g. anorexia, malaise, diarrhoea, depression). Peracute cases die within 48–72 hours of the onset of clinical signs. See also Chapter 14.

Pseudotuberculosis: Acute or chronic disease with *Yersinia enterocolitica* and *Y. pseudotuberculosis* can occur in chinchillas. The acute form is characterized by septicaemia. Chronically affected animals are anorexic and depressed. Weight loss, intermittent diarrhoea, palpably enlarged mesenteric lymph nodes and sudden death may be seen. Systemic spread results in granulomatous lesions in various organs. A 'chinchilla strain' of *Y. enterocolitica* persists enzootically among chinchilla stock worldwide. Tetracycline therapy can be attempted but treatment is usually unrewarding and may be considered inappropriate, given that yersiniosis is zoonotic.

Intestinal parasitism

Parasitism is generally uncommon in pet chinchillas. Coccidia, cestodes and nematodes are rare. Healthy chinchillas harbour large numbers of *Giardia* in their intestines. Poor husbandry and stress can lead to overgrowth and predispose animals to opportunistic infections. Diarrhoea is the primary clinical sign, accompanied by inappetence and poor coat condition, and severe cases can be fatal. Chinchillas may serve as intermediate hosts for the cestodes *Taenia serialis*, *T. pisiformis*, *Echinococcus granulosus* and *Rodentolepis* (previously *Hymenolepis*) *nana*.

Degus

Less is known about the gastrointestinal diseases of degus than other rodent species. As a general rule, they share many disease predispositions with the guinea pig and chinchilla. Non-infectious diarrhoea (due to dietary indiscretion), hypomotility, gastric dilatation and hepatic lipidosis are common problems. Treatment is as for other species. Degus appear to have a high pain threshold and as such will often only show clinical signs very late in the course of a particular disease, compared with other species. As such, supportive care often has to be more aggressive and recovery may be prolonged.

Hepatocellular carcinoma and splenic haemangioma have also been reported in degus (Donnelly, 2004b).

References and further reading

De La Puente-Redondo VA, Gutierrez-Martin CB, Perez-Martinez C *et al.* (1999) Epidemic infection caused by *Citrobacter rodentium* in a gerbil colony. *Veterinary Record* **145**(14), 400–403

Donnelly TM (2004a) Disease problems of chinchillas. In: *Ferrets, Rabbits and Rodents – Clinical Medicine and Surgery, 2nd edn*, ed. KE Quesenberry and JW Carpenter, pp. 255–265. WB Saunders, St Louis

Donnelly TM (2004b) Disease problems of small rodents. In: *Ferrets, Rabbits and Rodents – Clinical Medicine and Surgery, 2nd edn*, ed. KE Quesenberry and JW Carpenter, pp. 299–315. WB Saunders, St Louis

Fallon MT (1996) Rats and mice. In: *Handbook of Rodent and Rabbit Medicine*, ed. K Laber-Laird, *et al.* pp. 1–38. Elsevier, Oxford

Flecknell P (2002) Guinea pigs. In: *BSAVA Manual of Exotic Pets, 4th edn*, ed. A Meredith and S Redrobe, pp. 52–64. BSAVA Publications, Gloucester

Goodman G (2002) Hamsters. In: *BSAVA Manual of Exotic Pets, 4th edn*, ed. A Meredith and S Redrobe, pp. 26–33. BSAVA Publications, Gloucester

Harkness JE and Ferguson FG (1979) Idiopathic megaesophagus in a rat (*Rattus norvegicus*). *Laboratory Animal Science* **29**(4), 495–498

Harkness JE and Wagner JE (1995) *The Biology and Medicine of Rabbits and Rodents, 4th edn*. Williams and Wilkins, Baltimore

Hoefer HL and Crossley DA (2002) Chinchillas. In: *BSAVA Manual of Exotic Pets, 4th edn*, ed. A Meredith and S Redrobe, pp. 65–77. BSAVA Publications, Gloucester

Hrapkiewicz K and Medina L (2007) *Clinical Laboratory Animal Medicine: An Introduction, 3rd edn*. Blackwell Publishing, Ames, Iowa

Huerkamp MJ, Murray KA and Orosz SE (1996) Guinea pigs. In: *Handbook of Rodent and Rabbit Medicine*, ed. K Laber-Laird *et al.*, pp. 91–149. Elsevier, Oxford

Jaax GP, Jaax NK, Petrali JP *et al.* (1990) Coronavirus-like virions associated with a wasting syndrome in guinea pigs. *Laboratory Animal*

Science **40**(4), 375–378

Keeble E (2002) Gerbils. In: *BSAVA Manual of Exotic Pets, 4th edn*, ed. A Meredith and S Redrobe, pp. 34–46. BSAVA Publications, Gloucester

Laber-Laird K (1996) Gerbils. In: *Handbook of Rodent and Rabbit Medicine*, ed. K Laber-Laird, *et al*., pp. 39–58. Elsevier, Oxford

Lipman NS and Foltz C (1996) Hamsters. In: *Handbook of Rodent and Rabbit Medicine*, ed. K Laber-Laird, *et al*., pp. 59–89. Elsevier, Oxford

Lyerly DM, Bostwick EF, Binion SB and Wilkins DT (1991) Passive immunization of hamsters against disease caused by *Clostridium difficile* by use of bovine immunoglobulin G concentrate. *Infection and Immunity* **67**(2), 527–538

Manci EA, Heath LS, Leinbach SS and Coggin Jr JH (1984) Lymphoma-associated ulcerative bowel disease in the hamster (*Mesocricetus auratus*) induced by an unusual agent. *American Journal of Pathology* **116**(1), 1–8

O'Rourke DP (2004) Disease problems of guinea pigs. In: *Ferrets, Rabbits and Rodents – Clinical Medicine and Surgery, 2nd edn*, ed. KE Quesenberry and JW Carpenter, pp. 245–254. WB Saunders, St Louis

Orr HE (2002) Rats and mice. In: *BSAVA Manual of Exotic Pets, 4th edn*, ed. A Meredith and S Redrobe, pp. 13–25. BSAVA Publications, Gloucester

Percy DH and Barthold SW (2007) *Pathology of Laboratory Rodents and Rabbits, 3rd edn*. Blackwell Publishing, Ames, Iowa

Randelia HP, Panicker KN and Lalitha VS (1990) Megaesophagus in the mouse: histochemical and ultrastructural studies. *Laboratory Animals* **24**, 78–86

Richardson VCG (2000) *Diseases of Domestic Guinea Pigs, 2nd edn*. Blackwell Publishing, Oxford

Richardson VCG (2003) *Diseases of Small Domestic Rodents, 2nd edn*. Blackwell Publishing, Oxford

Ruelokke ML, Arnbjerg J and Martensen MR (2004) Assessing gastrointestinal motility in guinea pigs using contrast radiography. *Exotic DVM* **6**(1), 31–36

Strake JG, Davis LA, LaRegina M and Boschert KR (1996) Chinchillas. In: *Handbook of Rodent and Rabbit Medicine*, ed. K Laber-Laird *et al*., pp. 151–182. Elsevier, Oxford

Swanson SJ, Snider C, Braden CR *et al.* (2007) Multidrug-resistant *Salmonella enterica* serotype Typhimurium associated with pet rodents. *New England Journal of Medicine* **356**(1), 21–28

Vincent AL and Ash LR (1978) Further observations on spontaneous neoplasms in the Mongolian gerbil, *Meriones unguiculatus*. *Laboratory Animal Science* **28**(3), 297–300

Vonderfecht SL, Huber AC, Eiden J *et al.* (1984) Infectious diarrhoea of infant rats produced by a rotavirus-like agent. *Journal of Virology* **52**(1), 94–98

12

Rodents: respiratory and cardiovascular system disorders

Gidona Goodman

Introduction

Veterinary knowledge of rodent respiratory disease was initially based on laboratory animal medicine. As these pets have increased in popularity, and owners are more inclined to present them to the veterinary surgeon, diagnostic techniques and treatment options have improved. Respiratory disease is one of the most common problems encountered in pet mice and rats, mainly caused by *Mycoplasma pulmonis*. In guinea pigs *Bordetella bronchiseptica* is the most common respiratory pathogen. Respiratory disease is less common in hamsters and chinchillas and rare in gerbils and degus.

Animal husbandry, environmental conditions and immune status all play a part in pathogenesis. Inadequate husbandry such as overcrowding, poor ventilation and high humidity may contribute to respiratory disease.

Laboratory rodents are used in cardiovascular research but in practice cardiovascular disease is rarely seen except in chinchillas, hamsters and gerbils. It is described at the end of this chapter.

General approach to respiratory cases

Clinical signs and examination

Clinical signs in respiratory disease may be vague, with animals typically presenting with poor coat condition, lethargy, reduced appetite or anorexia and porphyrin staining around the nose and eyes (Figure 12.1). Excessive porphyrin staining could be a result of general illness with decreased grooming, or there may be obstruction of the lacrimal ducts due to rhinitis.

Animals may present with ocular or nasal discharge, sneezing or dyspnoea and an abdominal breathing pattern. Head tilt as a result of otitis may occur due to invasion of the middle ear via the Eustachian tube. One or a combination of the above signs may be present.

If the animal is overtly dyspnoeic, handling for clinical examination can exacerbate the signs. Oxygen therapy (placement in an oxygen chamber) should be started prior to clinical examination. Respiratory sounds such as snuffling and wheezing may be audible without auscultation. A characteristic 'clicking' respiratory noise can be detected in some individuals. Animals can be auscultated in the container in which they are presented, or, to reduce stress, rats can sit

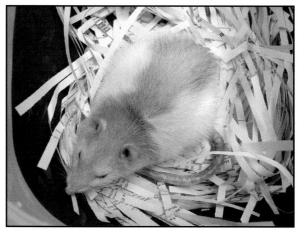

12.1 Rat with non-specific clinical signs associated with respiratory disease – weight loss, poor coat condition and porphyrin staining around the nose and eyes. (Courtesy of Emma Keeble.)

on the client's arm rather than being restrained for auscultation. Auscultation of the lung fields can be unrewarding if lung tissue is consolidated.

Diagnosis

A presumptive diagnosis of respiratory disease is often based on clinical signs, signalment and response to therapy. Common presenting clinical signs and associated causes are shown in Figure 12.2. A definitive diagnosis, in cases of infectious respiratory disease, should be based on bacterial culture and include antibiotic sensitivity.

In an animal presented with rhinitis a bilateral deep nasal swab should be taken (Figure 12.3) rather than exudate alone, since the latter results in only secondary pathogens or bacteria being isolated. A conjuctival scraping obtained using a bacteriology swab can be examined if the rhinitis is accompanied by conjunctivitis, for example with *Chlamydophila*. The conjunctival smear stained with Giemsa may then reveal intracytoplasmic inclusions.

When pneumonia is suspected tracheal lavage can be performed in rats as small as 300 g. The technique for tracheal lavage in rodents is similar to that for other mammals. The patient is anaesthetized, either by gaseous anaesthetics or by injectable agents, and sterile saline at 2 ml/kg is introduced into the trachea via an intravenous catheter plastic sheath without the stylet in place. The sample is then aspirated (see also Chapter 2).

Sign	Rat	Mouse	Guinea pig	Chinchilla
Abortion			*Bordetella bronchiseptica*; *Streptococcus pneumoniae*	
Conjunctivitis	*Pasteurella pneumotropica*; coronavirus	*Pasteurella pneumotropica*	*Chlamydophila caviae*	
Death	*Streptococcus pneumoniae*	Sendai virus	*Bordetella bronchiseptica*; adenovirus	
Dyspnoea	*Mycoplasma pulmonis*; *Corynebacterium kutscheri*; CAR bacillus	Sendai virus	*Bordetella bronchiseptica*; adenovirus	
Head tilt (otitis)	*Pasteurella pneumotropica*; *Mycoplasma pulmonis*; *Streptococcus pneumoniae*	*Pasteurella pneumotropica*; *Mycoplasma pulmonis*	*Streptococcus pneumoniae*	
Pericardial effusion	*Streptococcus pneumoniae*		*Streptococcus pneumoniae*	
Pneumonia	*Streptococcus pneumoniae*; *Mycoplasma pulmonis*; CAR bacillus	*Mycoplasma pulmonis*	*Streptococcus pneumoniae*; *Bordetella bronchiseptica*	*Pasteurella*; *Streptococcus*; *Bordetella*
Reproductive tract infection	*Mycoplasma pulmonis*; *Pasteurella pneumotropica*	*Pasteurella pneumotropica*	*Bordetella bronchiseptica*; *Chlamydophila caviae*	
Rhinitis	*Streptococcus*; *Mycoplasma pulmonis*; *Klebsiella pneumoniae*; CAR bacillus	*Mycoplasma pulmonis*	*Streptococcus pneumoniae*; *Bordetella bronchiseptica*; *Chlamydophila caviae*; adenovirus; *Klebsiella* spp.; *Staphylococcus* spp.	*Pasteurella*; *Streptococcus*; *Bordetella*; *Pseudomonas aeruginosa*

12.2 Common presenting signs of respiratory disease in rodents and associated infectious agents.

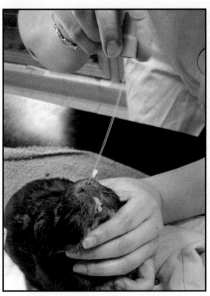

12.3 A deep nasal swab is recommended for culture and sensitivity testing. Heavy sedation or general anaesthesia, with application of topical local anaesthetic, is required. (Courtesy of Emma Keeble.)

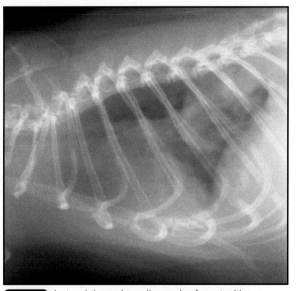

12.4 Lateral thoracic radiograph of a rat with pneumonia and lung consolidation.

It is important to select the correct microbial transport medium and sample storage technique. Some bacteria, e.g. *Mycoplasma*, can be difficult to isolate. *M. pulmonis* is best isolated using an appropriate selective transport medium. Samples should be kept refrigerated and ideally reach the laboratory within 24–48 hours, as the bacterium is fastidious in its growth. However, cultures may fail to detect 25–30% of infected rats (Percy and Barthold, 2001).

Radiography of the thorax (ventrodorsal, left and right lateral views) and skull will help in determining the extent and prognosis of disease. This includes changes in the lungs (Figure 12.4), nasal passages and tympanic bullae (see also Chapter 3).

Although not routinely used in pet rodents, serological tests exist for various common pathogens as a screening tool in laboratory rodents. These include: *Mycoplasma pulmonis*, *Corynebacterium kutscheri*, Sendai virus, adenovirus, coronavirus, cilia-associated respiratory (CAR) bacillus infection, pneumonia virus of mice and *Streptococcus pneumoniae*. Serological tests for *Mycoplasma* (e.g. ELISA) can fail to detect subclinical infections and may remain seronegative for up to 4 months post exposure and cross-react with other rodent mycoplasmas such as *M. arthritidis*. High concentrations of specific antibodies are associated with severe disease and a large number of organisms in the respiratory tract, rather than elimination of the organisms and resolution of lesions (Schoeb *et al.*, 1996). For serology a minimum of 50 μl of serum is needed; a positive result indicates exposure to disease.

Companies that provide serological screening services in the UK include Harlan UK Ltd, Charles River and Surrey Diagnostics. The University of Missouri Research Animal Diagnostic and Investigative Laboratory (RADIL) provides serological screens in the USA.

Treatment

From the outset, clients should be made aware that in many cases therapy does not eliminate the disease but only alleviates the clinical signs.

As some of these cases are presented with reduced appetite, anorexia and lethargy, fluid and nutritional support should be provided in conjunction with medical therapy (see Chapter 2).

Animals not requiring an oxygen-enriched environment should be housed on dust-free bedding, such as newspaper, in a well ventilated cage in the hospital or at home. Animals with severe dyspnoea should be placed in an oxygen chamber. An incubator or even a plastic rodent carrier can serve as a chamber. Humidified oxygen can be supplied via a T-piece and the chamber sealed with transparent plastic to enable easy monitoring of the patient (Figure 12.5). Provision of additional heat is recommended, either via a purpose-built incubator or with heat mats or hot-water bottles.

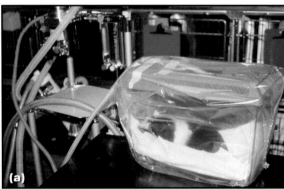

(a)

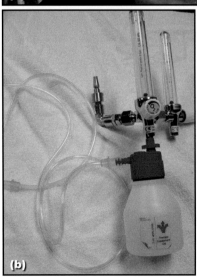

(b)

12.5

(a) Dyspnoeic guinea pig in an oxygen chamber for supportive care. **(b)** Humidified oxygen therapy unit. (Courtesy of Emma Keeble.)

Nebulization

Aerosol therapy is used in conjunction with systemic therapy for administration of antimicrobials, mucolytics, bronchodilators or mucokinetics.

Although nebulization is frequently used for small mammals, drug efficacy in respiratory syndromes in these species is not known. Alternatively clients can place the animal in a bathroom filled with steam. The nebulizer should deliver small particles, as the optimal particle size for the trachea is 2–10 μm and for the peripheral airway 0.5–5 μm. Animals are nebulized in their carrier, covered cage or hospital incubator (Figure 12.6). Nebulization is recommended for 30–45 minutes two to three times daily with 5 ml of fluid at a time. A list of nebulizing agents can be found in Figure 12.7.

Mucolytics such as bromhexine (0.3 mg per animal on food) can also be given orally as well as bronchodilators such as clenbuterol and terbutaline. There are no published dose rates for rodents and the author has used them empirically at dose rates for

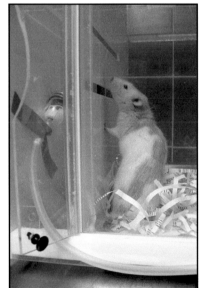

12.6

Nebulization is well tolerated even by small rodents. Animals may be nebulized in their carrier, covered cage or hospital incubator. (Courtesy of Emma Keeble.)

Drug	Dosage
Mucokinetics	
Saline	
F10	1:250 dilution
Mucolytic	
Acetylcysteine	50 mg as a 2% solution (dilute with saline)
Antimicrobials	
Gentamicin	5 mg/ml saline [a]
Enrofloxacin	10 mg/ml saline [a]
Tylosin	10 mg/ml saline [a]
Bronchodilator	
Aminophylline	3 mg/ml [a]

12.7 Agents used for aerosol therapy in rodents. [a] Based on avian dose rates (Carpenter, 2005)

dogs and cats. Often the choice of product is based on the availability of paediatric solutions, which are easier to administer. It is important to inform the client of the off-label use of these products and obtain informed signed consent in the UK.

Antimicrobial therapy

If infectious respiratory disease is suspected, antimicrobial therapy (ideally based on culture and sensitivity) is started. Figure 12.8 lists common infectious agents according to species affected and appropriate antimicrobial therapy. The author does not regularly use corticosteroids as part of the treatment regime, due to concerns with potential immunosuppression. In cases of severe pneumonia, corticosteroids may be given at anti-inflammatory dose rates (e.g. dexamethasone at 0.5 mg/kg s.c., i.m.). NSAIDs, such as meloxicam (0.3–0.6 mg/kg orally or s.c. q24h), can be given if the animal appears to be in discomfort (see Chapter 6).

Infectious agents	Drug	Dose rate and frequency	Notes and references
Mice and rats			
Mycoplasma pulmonis	Chloramphenicol	30–50 mg/kg orally, s.c., i.m. q8–12h	
	Doxycyline	5 mg/kg orally q12h for 7–21 days	Not for young or pregnant animals
	Enrofloxacin	5–10 mg/kg orally, s.c., i.m. q12h; 50–200 mg/l drinking water for 7 days	Limit s.c. or i.m. injections as this may cause local irritation
	Trimethoprim/sulfamethoxazole	30 mg/kg q12h orally, s.c., i.m.	
	Tylosin	10 mg/kg s.c. 10 mg/kg orally q24h; 500 mg/l drinking water	Carter *et al.* (1987) NB: prepare daily
	Macrolide antibiotics used include erythromycin (20 mg/kg orally q12h), azithromycin and clarithromycin (all have paediatric syrups available in the UK)		Human mycoplasmal infections have been shown to develop resistance to macrolide antibiotics (Carter *et al.*, 1987)
Streptococcus pneumoniae	Penicillin	22,000 IU/kg s.c., i.m. q24h	
CAR bacillus	Sulfamerazine	500 mg/l in the drinking water	Useful to prevent disease
	Ampicillin	500 mg/l drinking water for 4 weeks	Reduces development of respiratory tract changes but failed to prevent or eliminate disease (Matsushita and Suzuli, 1995)
Corynebacterium kutscheri	Tetracycline	10–20 mg/kg orally q8–12h	
	Chloramphenicol	30–50 mg/kg orally, s.c., i.m. q8–12h	
Pasteurella pneumotropica	Enrofloxacin	In drinking water at 25.5 mg/kg; 85 mg/kg for 14 days	Goelz *et al.* (1996); Ueno *et al.* (2002); Matsumiya and Lavoie (2003)
Pneumocystis carinii	Trimethoprim/sulphonamide ('Borgal 24%'; Intervet)	6.25 ml added to 10 litres of drinking water (150 mg/ml)	
Hamsters			
Pasteurella Streptococcus	Chloramphenicol	30–50 mg/kg orally, s.c., i.m. q8–12h	
	Enrofloxacin	5–10 mg/kg orally, s.c., i.m. q12h	Limit s.c. or i.m. injections as these may cause local irritation
	Trimethoprim/sulfamethoxazole	30 mg/kg orally, s.c., i.m. q12h	
Guinea pigs			
Bordetella bronchiseptica	Chloramphenicol	50 mg/kg orally q12h	
	Enrofloxacin	5–10 mg/kg orally, s.c., i.m. q12h	Limit s.c. or i.m. injections as these may cause local irritation
	Trimethoprim/sulfamethoxazole	30 mg/kg orally q12h	
Chlamydophila caviae	Topical tetracycline eye ointment or systemic enrofloxacin	q6–12h 5–10 mg/kg orally, s.c., i.m. q12h	Limit s.c. or i.m. injections as these may cause local irritation

12.8 Antimicrobial agents used in rodent respiratory disease.

Common respiratory diseases

Infectious diseases

Infectious respiratory disease is common in rats and guinea pigs but rare in gerbils and degus. Bacterial respiratory infections are reported to be the second most common type of infection in hamsters. However, hamsters seem to be more resistant to infectious respiratory disease than other rodents and only a few cases are seen in the clinical situation, in the author's experience.

Some of the causal bacteria are opportunist pathogens, such as *Bordetella* in rats. Other infections, such as mycoplasmosis, are acquired and animals remain infected for life. Inadequate housing conditions (e.g. overcrowding and poor ventilation) and dietary deficiencies, such as hypovitaminosis C in guinea pigs, can all predispose to respiratory disease.

Bacterial disease

Bordetella bronchiseptica: *B. bronchiseptica* is a significant respiratory pathogen of guinea pigs. In rats it is an opportunistic pathogen concurrent with other respiratory pathogens. It has also been reported in hamsters and gerbils. In chinchillas, it has been reported as a single pathogen or in combination with *Streptococcus* and *Pasteurella*. Species such as rats, dogs and rabbits can harbour *B. bronchiseptica* in the upper respiratory tract and be a source of infection. The organism is transmitted by direct contact, aerosol and fomites, with possible interspecies transmission. The incubation period is 3–7 days.

B. bronchiseptica is a Gram-negative aerobic rod or coccobacillus with an affinity for ciliated respiratory epithelium. Guinea pigs can develop immunity and eliminate the disease but a small percentage may remain carriers (Percy and Barthold, 2001). Young guinea pigs and animals kept in suboptimal conditions are more susceptible to disease, especially in the winter.

In guinea pigs, *B. bronchiseptica* causes pneumonia with consolidation of lung lobes. Pleuritis and purulent exudates in the tympanic bullae may also be present.

The nasal passages and trachea frequently contain mucopurulent or catarrhal exudates. Haematogenous spread to distant organs can occur (Huerkamp *et al.*, 1996). It can be fatal for pregnant animals and they may deliver stillborn pups or abort. Metritis with vaginal discharge and pyosalpinx is also seen.

Guinea pigs may present with ocular and nasal discharge (Figure 12.9), abnormal respiratory sounds and dyspnoea. These animals may become anorexic and lethargic and in these cases prognosis is guarded. In-contact animals may be carriers and should be monitored for clinical signs of the disease.

Treatment should be based on bacterial culture and sensitivity testing on a deep nasal swab. Some of the more common antibiotics used are listed in Figure 12.8.

A study into the efficacy of various commercial vaccines in protecting guinea pigs against *B. bronchiseptica* concluded that these vaccines did not give

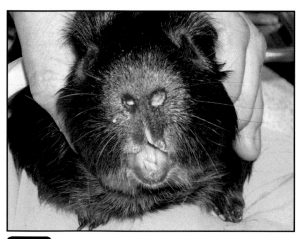

12.9 Unilateral nasal discharge in a guinea pig.

complete protection but decreased the incidence and severity of pulmonary lesions (Matherne *et al.*, 1987). The vaccines used included commercial porcine *B. bronchiseptica* vaccines, human diphtheria–pertussis–tetanus vaccine and an autogenous bacterin (0.2 ml i.m.). Several other sources quote the use of the canine or porcine vaccine for bordetellosis. They also administered 0.2 ml intramuscularly, with a booster given 2–3 weeks later followed by an annual booster. The vaccines should not contain aluminium hydroxide as this can cause a hypersensitivity reaction.

CAR (cilia-associated respiratory) bacillus infection: CAR bacillus is a Gram-negative filamentous rod that adheres to ciliated epithelial respiratory cells. Its pathogenic potential as a potentiator of *M. pulmonis* respiratory disease has been demonstrated most clearly in rats (Fallon, 1996). Disease has been reported in conventionally kept laboratory rats as well as wild rats. Clinical signs are identical to those in rats with severe *M. pulmonis* infection and often there is indeed concurrent mycoplasma infection. Presumptive diagnosis is based on commercial serological tests.

Chlamydophila caviae: *C. caviae* is common in guinea pig colonies, infecting guinea pigs 2–8 weeks of age. Animals are often asymptomatic and the disease is self-limiting. Clinical signs include bilateral conjunctivitis and less frequently rhinitis, genital tract infection and abortion. The mode of transmission in guinea pigs is unknown, but inhalation and direct sexual contact are the most likely routes (Huerkamp *et al.*, 1996) with an incubation period of 2–4 days. Diagnosis is based on conjunctival scrapings. Intracytoplasmic inclusions can be demonstrated on the conjunctival scrapings using immunofluorescent antibodies or Giemsa stain.

Treatment options include topical tetracycline eye ointment or systemic enrofloxacin.

Corynebacterium kutscheri: *C. kutscheri* is a Gram-positive bacterium. Mice, rats and hamsters are natural hosts. It is thought to be transmitted via the faecal–oral route, direct contact and aerosol. The organism is frequently harboured as an inapparent infection, but chronic carrier status with shedding is a problem. Clinical disease is associated with immunosuppression, concurrent infection and poor husbandry.

In rats, clinical signs are related to pulmonary lesions with dyspnoea, weight loss, anorexia and hunched posture. In mice there is more generalized disease due to necropurulent lesions in multiple organs, with polyarthritis and visceral lesions in kidney and liver. An ELISA test is available for detection of seropositive animals. Treatment options are listed in Figure 12.8.

Murine respiratory mycoplasmosis (MRM): *Mycoplasma pulmonis* infection is ubiquitous in pet rodents. It is the most common cause of respiratory disease in rats and less common in mice. It has been isolated from Syrian hamsters and guinea pigs, but without clinical disease, and also reported in gerbils. To the author's knowledge it has not been reported in chinchillas.

Transmission is by aerosol, *in utero* or at birth. The infection is persistent for life, even though infected rats may have relatively high antibody titres.

M. pulmonis colonizes the respiratory epithelium, nasal passages and middle ear (Figure 12.10). The infection can progress to bronchopulmonary disease and is enhanced by various environmental and host-related factors. These include excessive ammonia levels (above 25 ppm), concurrent infection such as CAR bacillus, rat coronavirus, sialodacryoadenitis virus (SDAV) or Sendai virus, and vitamin A and E deficiencies. The age, strain and immunity of the rat as well as the virulence of the mycoplasma strain also play a part in the progression of the infection. Clinical presentation can range from subclinical infection to severe dyspnoea and debilitating weight loss. Endometritis has also been observed in the author's experience (see also Chapter 13).

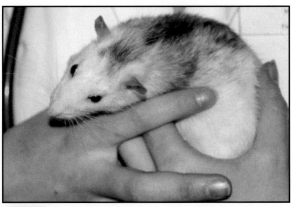

12.10 Rat with head tilt due to *Mycoplasma pulmonis* infection. (Courtesy of Emma Keeble.)

In mice, *M. pulmonis* causes chronic pneumonia, suppurative rhinitis and occasional otitis media. Mice tend to develop pulmonary abscesses.

A presumptive diagnosis is often based on clinical signs, although radiography and tracheal lavage may be useful (see above). Differential diagnoses or concurrent bacterial infections include *Pasteurella pneumotropica*, *Bordetella bronchiseptica*, *Corynebacterium kutscheri*, CAR bacillus and *Klebsiella pneumoniae*.

On gross pathology lesions may not be obvious and often correlate poorly with clinical signs. Although the lungs may externally appear normal in the majority of infected rats and mice, the clinical signs and microscopic changes may suggest infection (Schoeb *et al.*, 1996). The lung may have a cobblestone appearance with bronchial inflammation and atelectasis. Abscesses and purulent exudates may be present in lung (Figure 12.11), ear, and reproductive tract with possible regional lymph node enlargement.

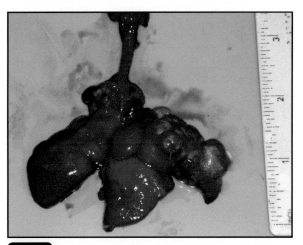

12.11 Lung from a rat with *Mycoplasma* infection.

Treatment rarely resolves the clinical signs. Infected animals tend to respond to treatment initially, but relapses with increasingly more severe clinical signs are likely to lead to a guarded long-term prognosis. Antibiotics used to treat mycoplasma infections are listed in Figure 12.8. Environmental factors such as overcrowding, poor ventilation and environmental dust contamination contribute to the severity of clinical signs. Animals should be housed on dust-free bedding, such as newspaper, rather than wood shavings. Glass vivaria are not recommended, due to poor ventilation; instead a well ventilated cage and room are ideal.

Figure 12.12 gives a detailed treatment plan for *M. pulmonis* infection in rats. In-contact animals are potential carriers and should be monitored for clinical signs. Apart from laboratory rats, there is no recognized source of pet rats officially free from *M. pulmonis* in the UK.

Pasteurella pneumotropica: *P. pneumotropica* is a Gram-negative bacterium with mice, rats, hamsters and guinea pigs as natural hosts. It is also reported in gerbils. It is a potential opportunistic commensal bacterium in mice and rats, complicating mycoplasma and Sendai virus infections. Outbreaks of disease are mainly seen in immunocompromised animals. Clinical symptoms include conjunctivitis, otitis, subcutaneous abscesses and reproductive tract infections. For diagnosis and treatment see above.

Diagnostics
Bacteriology (culture and sensitivity testing)
Radiography (for prognosis)
Serology

Mild infection (few clinical signs)
7–10 day course of antibiotics
Use newspaper and shredded paper as bedding
Ensure adequate ventilation and hygiene

Moderate infection
10–14 day course of antibiotics
Use newspaper and shredded paper as bedding
Ensure adequate ventilation and hygiene
Place in room with steam
Mucolytic/ bronchial secretolytic
Bronchodilators
Aerosol therapy

Severe infection
Treatment as for moderate infection, plus:
Supportive care, fluid therapy
Oxygen therapy
Hospitalization

12.12 Management of *Mycoplasma pulmonis* infection in rats. It is important to monitor closely for recurrence of clinical signs. Some cases may require chronic therapy. Euthanasia may be indicated in severe non-responsive or chronic cases.

Streptococcus pneumoniae: *S. pneumoniae* is a Gram-positive bacterium often seen in pairs under the microscope. It is a respiratory pathogen for rats and guinea pigs, but only subclinical infections have been described in mice (Fallon, 1996). *Streptococcus* is also reported in hamsters, gerbils and chinchillas. Pneumococci can be commensals in the mouse and rat respiratory system as well as the middle ear.

Young and pregnant guinea pigs are more susceptible to infection with *S. pneumoniae*. Although a respiratory pathogen in guinea pigs, pregnant guinea pigs may abort (see also Chapter 13). Young rats tend to be more severely affected than older rats, with sudden death occurring. Clinical signs include suppurative rhinitis, otitis media and interna leading to head tilt and circling, pneumonia and pleural and pericardial effusion. For diagnosis and treatment see above.

Transmission is by aerosol and direct contact. It is not known whether rodent infections are acquired from humans, hence it should be considered a potential anthropozoonosis (Percy and Barthold, 2001).

Streptococcus zooepidemicus: *S. zooepidemicus* more commonly causes suppurative lymphadenitis of the cervical lymph nodes in guinea pigs. In young animals, a more acute form causes cardiovascular or respiratory disease. Treatment with antibiotics has generally not been successful.

Viral disease

Adenovirus: Adenovirus is a host-specific DNA virus affecting guinea pigs. This disease is mainly reported in laboratory animals and transferred via horizontal transmission with an incubation period of 5–10 days.

Adenovirus infection is subclinical in healthy adult guinea pigs, but fatalities can reach 100% in young and elderly animals. Clinical signs such as dyspnoea, nasal discharge and lethargy are rarely seen prior to death. Hence diagnosis tends to be at post-mortem examination or via serology. Treatment consists of supportive care and is usually unsuccessful. In laboratory settings, animals will be obtained from adenovirus-free colonies or screened serologically while in quarantine.

Coronaviruses of rats: Sialodacryoadenitis virus (SDAV) and Parker's rat coronavirus (RCV) are both strains of rat coronavirus. SDAV causes sialoadenitis and dacryoadenitis. Coronavirus is very contagious and is transmitted by direct contact and aerosol.

Endemic (enzootic) infections within a colony cause only mild signs, with conjunctivitis in sucklings. In an outbreak (epizootic), cervical swelling surrounding the submandibular salivary glands, corneal lesions, conjunctivitis, keratitis and porphyrin staining are seen. Diagnosis is based on clinical signs and serology. Antibiotic therapy is given to combat secondary bacterial infection. Animals will recover, as they usually remain active and feeding. Serological screening is used to ensure SDAV-free rat colonies in laboratory settings.

Sendai virus: Sendai virus is an RNA virus from the paramyxovirus family (parainfluenza 1). Mice, rats and hamsters are natural hosts. The virus is very contagious and is transmitted via direct contact or aerosol. In adult mice the disease may present with mild respiratory distress. In acute outbreaks, neonatal and weanling fatalities may be seen. Adults generally recover within 2 months. Concurrent mycoplasmal infection will exacerbate clinical signs. Clinical disease is rarely observed in rats and hamsters, and gerbils can be carriers of Sendai virus.

A related virus in mice, pneumonia virus of mice (PVM), is an opportunistic pathogen in immunologically compromised mice.

Parasitic disease

Pneumocystis carinii: *P. carinii* is an atypical protozoal respiratory pathogen in immunodeficient laboratory rodents. Pet mice and rats may harbour *P. carinii* asymptomatically. Detection of carriers via PCR on tracheal lavage is difficult and transmission is via direct contact.

Choke in chinchillas

In chinchillas the entrance of the trachea (glottis) can become occluded with food or a foreign body, causing irritation and leading to oedema. Initially the animal appears startled, coughs and attempts to dislodge the foreign body. The animal's condition tends to deteriorate rapidly, followed by suffocation and death.

Neoplasia

Primary pulmonary neoplasia is rare in pet rodents. A primary bronchoalveolar carcinoma with renal and hepatic metastases has been diagnosed on post-mortem examination in a mature male degu (Anderson *et al.*, 1990). The majority of reports of primary lung tumours originate from laboratory rodent publications and are usually species, age and strain related. For example, primary pulmonary tumours are common in ageing BALB, GR and A strains of mice (Percy and Barthold, 2001). The majority of pulmonary tumours reported in guinea pigs are benign papillary adenomas, whereas primary malignant tumours of the lung are rare (Percy and Barthold, 2001).

Pulmonary metastatic neoplasia originating from a mammary gland neoplasia in a chinchilla and a hepatocellular carcinoma in a degu have been diagnosed on post-mortem examination. In mice, metastatic tumours are seen originating from mammary gland and liver tumours.

Radiographic evidence of pulmonary neoplasia may be present in advanced cases but usually neoplasia is diagnosed on post-mortem examination.

Cardiovascular disease

Cardiac disease in chinchillas

Heart murmurs in chinchillas are often picked up incidentally during clinical examination without associated clinical signs. Further investigation is warranted if a chinchilla is presented with episodes of syncope, or what is described by the owner as a seizure or epileptic fit, and a heart murmur is detected. Blood samples are taken to rule out other underlying causes of seizures or fits, such as lead poisoning or bacterial infections (e.g. *Listeria monocytogenes*). Echocardiography, ultrasonography and radiography should also be performed. There has been only one published report on cardiac disease in chinchillas (Hoefer and Crossley, 2002).

Tricuspid valve regurgitation and hypertrophic cardiomyopathy (HCM) have been diagnosed on echocardiography by the Exotic Animal Service, University of Edinburgh, UK. Repeat ultrasound scans are recommended at intervals of 3–6 months. In some cases the grade of the heart murmur progresses and symptomatic treatment (diuretics) has been prescribed if warranted.

Cardiomyopathy and valvular disease have been seen on post-mortem examination of chinchillas presenting with heart failure and acute dyspnoea. Pleural effusion, pulmonary oedema and cardiomegaly have been seen radiographically (Hoefer and Crossley, 2002).

Cardiovascular disease in hamsters

The left atrium is the most common location of cardiac thrombosis in hamsters. Cardiomyopathy, vascular disease, coagulopathy and amyloidosis have been suggested as contributors to thrombus formation. Clinical signs include hyperpnoea, tachycardia, cyanosis and cold extremities and should raise suspicion in ageing hamsters. Reported empirical treatments (detailed in Figure 12.13) include digoxin, diuretics, angiotensin-converting enzyme inhibitors,

Drug	Dose rate and frequency
Digoxin	0.05–0.1 mg/kg orally q12–24h
Furosemide	2–10 mg/kg orally, s.c. q12h
Verapamil	0.25–0.5 mg s.c. q12h for 4 weeks

12.13 Agents used for cardiovascular disease in hamsters.

anticoagulants and verapamil (0.25–0.5 mg s.c. q12h for 4 weeks) (Kuo *et al.*, 1984).

Cardiovascular disease in gerbils

Arteriosclerosis and focal myocardial degeneration have been reported in ageing gerbils (Vincent *et al.*, 1979). On standard diets, about 10% of the animals became obese and some showed decreased glucose tolerance, elevated serum immunoreactive insulin and diabetic changes in the pancreas and other organs. Some animals exhibited hyperactivity of the adrenal cortex associated with hyperglycaemia, hyperlipidaemia and degenerative vascular disease.

References and further reading

Anderson WI, Steinberg H and King JM (1990) Bronchioalveolar carcinoma with renal and hepatic metastases in a degu (*Octodon degus*). *Journal of Wildlife Disease* **26**(1), 129–130

Carpenter JW (2005) Rodents. In: *Exotic Animal Formulary, 3rd edn*, ed. JW Carpenter, pp. 377–408. Elsevier-Saunders, St Louis

Carter KK, Hietala S, Brooks DL and Baggot JD (1987) Tylosin concentration in rat serum and lung tissue after administration in drinking water. *Laboratory Animal Science* **37**(4), 468–470

Fallon MT (1996) Rats and mice. In: *Handbook of Rodent and Rabbit Medicine*, ed. K Laber-Laird *et al.*, pp. 1–38. Pergamon, Oxford

Goelz MF, Thigpen JE, Mahler J *et al.* (1996) Efficacy of various therapeutic regimens in eliminating *Pasteurella pneumotropica* from the mouse. *Laboratory Animal Science* **46**(3), 280–285

Hoefer HL and Crossley DA (2002) Chinchillas. In: *BSAVA Manual of Exotic Pets, 4th edn*, ed. A Meredith and S Redrobe, pp. 65–75. BSAVA Publications, Gloucester

Huerkamp MJ, Murray KA and Orosz SE (1996) Guinea pigs. In: *Handbook of Rodent and Rabbit Medicine*, ed. K Laber-Laird *et al.*, pp. 91–150. Pergamon, Oxford

Kuo TH, Ho KL and Wiener J (1984) The role of alkaline protease in the development of cardiac lesions in myopathic hamsters: Effect of verapamil treatment. *Biomedical Medicine* **32**(2), 207–215

Matherne CM, Steffen EK and Wagner JE (1987) Efficacy of commercial vaccines for protecting guinea pigs against *Bordetella bronchiseptica* pneumonia. *Laboratory Animal Science* **37**(2), 191–194

Matsumiya LC and Lavoie C (2003) An outbreak of *Pasteurella pneumotropica* in genetically modified mice: treatment and elimination. *American Association for Laboratory Animal Science: Contemporary Topics* **42**(2), 26–28

Matsushita S and Suzuli E (1995) Prevention and treatment of Cilia-Associated Respiratory Bacillus in mice by use of antibiotics. *Laboratory Animal Science* **45**(5), 503–507

Percy DH and Barthold SW (2001) *Pathology of Laboratory Rodents and Rabbits, 2nd edn*. Iowa State University Press, Ames

Porter WP, Bitar YS, Strandberg JD and Charache PC (1985) Absence of therapeutic blood concentrations of tetracycline in rats after administration in drinking water. *Laboratory Animal Science* **35**(1), 71–75

Schoeb TR, Davis JK and Lindsey JR (1996) Murine respiratory mycoplasmosis, rat and mouse. In: *Monographs on Pathology of Laboratory Animals: Respiratory System, 2nd edn*, ed. TC Jones *et al.*, pp. 117–128. Springer, Berlin

Ueno Y, Shimizu R, Nozu R *et al.* (2002) Elimination of *Pasteurella pneumotropica* from a contaminated mouse colony by oral administration of enrofloxacin. *Experimental Animals* **51**(4), 401–405

Vincent AL, Rodrick GA and Sodeman WA Jr (1979) The pathology of the Mongolian gerbil (*Meriones unguiculates*): a review. *Laboratory Animal Science* **29**(5), 645–651

13

Rodents: urogenital and reproductive system disorders

Heidi Hoefer and La'Toya Latney

Urogenital tract disease

Clinical signs

Clinical signs of urinary tract disease may include the following: loss of appetite, anorexia, polydipsia, polyuria, pyuria, anuria, isosthenuria, haematuria, stranguria, dysuria, cachexia and dehydration.

Indications of pain include a hunched posture or sensitivity to manipulation of the back or dorsum.

Diagnosis

Diagnosing renal disease in all rodents generally follows the same considerations used in small animal medicine. This includes a thorough physical examination, evaluation of blood chemistry (e.g. BUN, creatinine, calcium, phosphorus, albumin, total protein), determination of azotaemia, urinalysis, urinary sediments, cytology, culture, and diagnostic imaging viewed in conjunction with clinical signs.

Treatment

A generalized treatment protocol, depending on the stage of renal function, should include diuresis, a reduced protein diet, phosphate binders (calcium glubionate or calcium carbonate), vitamin and iron supplementation to support bone marrow red blood cell regeneration, avoidance of potentially nephrotoxic medications (e.g. aminoglycosides, non-steroidal anti-inflammatories), appropriate antibiotic therapy where indicated, gastrointestinal support (antacid and H2 blockers: famotidine 0.50 mg/kg orally q24h; sucralfate 1 ml/kg orally q8h) and agents to increase appetite (diazepam: 0.2–0.3 mg/kg orally, s.c. q12h;

vitamin B complex 5–10 mg/kg s.c., i.m.; steroids for pain and appetite stimulation: prednisolone 0.5–1 mg/kg orally q12–24h). Antibiotic drugs that the authors would use in the first instance, pending bacterial culture results, include trimethoprim/sulphonamide at 30 mg/kg orally q12h and, if indicated, enrofloxacin at 10 mg/kg orally q12h. If required, iron dextran may also be given intramuscularly at 1 unit/100 g body weight as a one-off dose.

Figure 13.1 gives normal urinalysis values for rodents. For normal blood chemistry parameters, see Chapter 4.

Reproductive disease

Reproductive disease can be diagnostically challenging. However, imaging and a thorough physical examination often supply clues towards diagnosing commonly seen diseases. Given the range of reproductive disorders and variance in clinical signs between species, each set of clinical signs and treatment protocols will be discussed under individual sections.

Mice

There are some unique observations noted with regard to normal renal and reproductive physiology when evaluating mice. Proteinuria is normal in adult mice and is most pronounced in sexually mature male mice (Percy and Barthold, 1993). Male mice also have ejaculatory plugs, which is a normal finding.

Species	Urine volume (ml/24 h)	pH	Specific gravity	Protein (g/l)	Novel characteristics
Mouse	0.5–2.5	7.3–8.5	1.034–1.058	< 0.10	Naturally proteinuric
Rat	13–23	7–7.4	1.022–1.050	< 0.30	Naturally proteinuric
Hamster	5.1–8.4	Basic	1.050–1.060	N/A	
Gerbil	2–4 drops	N/A	N/A	N/A	Natural acetone, bilirubin, glucose and protein
Guinea pig	N/A	8–9.0	N/A	N/A	Calcium carbonate crystalluria
Chinchilla	N/A	N/A	N/A	N/A	
Degu	N/A	N/A	N/A	N/A	

13.1 Normal urinalysis parameters for rodents.

Urinary diseases

Hydronephrosis
A thorough palpation coupled with diagnostic imaging (radiography and/or ultrasonography) can aid in the diagnosis. Hydronephrosis occurs unilaterally and bilaterally and is commonly seen on necropsy. It is seen more frequently in male mice, likely secondary to proteinaceous plugs or obstructive urinary or urethral calculi. Signs of urine scalding and dermatitis can be observed in cases of partial obstructions. Analysis of the animal's biochemical profile and urinalysis will help to discern renal function and prognosis.

Interstitial nephritis
As in other species, there are several pathogens that can cause tubulointerstitial disease. Common murine bacterial and viral aetiologies include *Pseudomonas aeruginosa*, *Proteus mirabilis*, *Staphylococcus aureus* and lymphocytic choriomeningitis virus (LCMV). Clinical signs include a hunched posture, pain on back manipulation, dehydration, loss of appetite, weight loss and lethargy. Urinalysis and serum biochemistry evaluation are invaluable in staging advanced renal damage. Urine culture and sensitivity testing is recommended. Pre-emptive antimicrobial therapeutics and diuresis should be attempted as supportive care. It is important to note that LCMV is a zoonotic concern. If the virus is suspected at any point, the owner and hospital staff should handle cases with great care. Definitive diagnosis is confirmed by ELISA and PCR analysis of tissue samples (see Chapter 14).

Amyloidosis
Spontaneously occurring and senescence associated, even in wild mouse strains, amyloidosis is a uniquely prevalent uropathy that should always be considered when a murine patient presents with signs of urinary disease. This can also be a secondary manifestation of systemic disease or stress.

Amyloid is a beta-pleated protein created as a native biological product, though it is not catabolized. Deposition can occur in the renal glomeruli, renal interstitium, myocardium, aorta, adrenal cortex, thyroid gland and other tissues. It is known to cause renal papillary necrosis (Percy and Barthold, 2003). This progressive disease process irreversibly damages the nephrons, resulting in decreased glomerular filtration and life-threatening chronic renal failure. Diagnosis is confirmed by histology on post-mortem examination, but patients should be managed as one would manage small animal chronic renal failure.

Chronic glomerulonephritis and glomerulopathy
This is seen in older polydipsic mice and is more prevalent in certain strains. Antigen–antibody complexes damage the basement membrane of the glomeruli. This occurs as an autoimmune disease in some strains, while other causes include persistent bacterial and retroviral infections. Signs of renal insufficiency, blood chemistry abnormalities and proteinuria are present. Care of these patients should follow supportive therapy treatment protocols as used in managing chronic renal failure in other species.

Suppurative pyelonephritis/nephritis
The causes previously listed for interstitial nephritis also commonly cause suppurative pyelonephritis. It is important to note that *Proteus mirabilis* and *Pseudomonas aeruginosa* have been reported to incite sporadic disease in mice (Casey, 1981). *Streptococcus agalactiae* has also been reported as a cause of pyelonephritis and subsequent septicaemia (Fisher, 2006). *Corynebacterium kutscheri* is a prevalent cause of pathological liquefactive necrotic lesions. The initial source of the infection can originate from two routes: ureteral ascension or haematogenous infection. Abscessation results from a haematogenous nidus at the level of the glomeruli, whereas the renal pelvis is primarily assaulted from ureteral ascension. Both routes of infection can destroy renal architecture. Although many cases are confirmed at necropsy, it would be valuable to perform urine cytology, pending a urine culture, and begin pre-emptive antibiotic therapy in addition to concurrent supportive therapy for renal disease.

Leptospirosis
Leptospira has several pathogenic serovars but *L. ballum* is most commonly found in clinically normal mice. These mice can shed organisms in their urine throughout their lives as a result of naturally acquired infection. Given that leptospirosis is a serious zoonotic concern, it is always essential to note the importance of this pathogen to owners, as it can cause signs of a flu-like illness in people. A serological diagnosis can be made on microscopic agglutination test, PCR or ELISA. Exposure to wild mice is the likely source of infection in pet animals. If diagnosed, euthanasia is indicated due to the zoonotic risk.

Obstructive uropathies
The most common causes of obstructive uropathies include preputial gland infections and bulbourethral gland infections. Preputial gland infections in both males and females can occur from a number of bacterial causes, including *Staphylococcus aureus* and *Pasteurella pneumotropica* (Percy and Barthold, 1993). *P. pneumotropica* is the major cause of bulbourethral gland infections in males (Donnelly, 1997). Male mice often present with mutilation of the penis as a result of the bulbourethral infection. Treatment includes isolation of the affected mouse, cleaning and debridement of the affected area, and treatment with antibiotics. Ejaculatory plugs are commonly found in males and are most frequently diagnosed by clinicians at necropsy. This is not an abnormal finding and should not be mistaken for an obstructive cause of urinary disease. (See also Chapter 7.)

Other uropathies
Chloroform fumes have been found to cause renal tubular necrosis, especially in male mice (Percy and Barthold, 1993).

Diabetic nephropathy has been documented in db/db strains of laboratory mice and presents with an albuminuria; it is used as a model to study human diabetic nephropathy (Fisher, 2006).

Although not commonly diagnosed, *Klossiella muris* sporocysts can be seen on urine cytology of wild mice. This renal protozoan usually causes a non-pathogenic and asymptomatic disease in wild mice. Control of this disease involves strict hygiene and administration of coccidiostats (Fisher, 2006).

Reproductive diseases

Mucometra and cystic endometrial hyperplasia
Mucometra is commonly seen when large groups of pregnant mice do not whelp. Pyometra and neoplasia should be ruled out as differentials. Cytology of the vaginal discharge can aid in diagnosis.

Aged female mice commonly present with cystic endometrial hyperplasia. Secondary bacterial infections should be ruled out as well. Antibiotic therapy should be implemented if secondary bacterial infections are suspected. Ovariohysterectomy is indicated for pyometra and cystic endometrial hyperplasia.

Mammary adenocarcinoma
Mice are known to develop mammary adenocarcinomas spontaneously. Owing to a variety of factors, including exposure to murine retroviruses, carcinogens, hormones and stress, mammary tumours are commonly diagnosed on palpation. Firm nodular masses can be felt along the mammary chains. Mammary tissue can be found on the length of ventrum, spanning the inguinal area, axillary region and extending dorsally over the scapulae.

Mammary adenocarcinomas are locally invasive and can metastasize to the lung. Attempted treatment involves surgical excision (see Chapter 7), but recurrence is very common and is associated with a poor prognosis.

Fibroadenomas and hyperplastic nodules involving the mammary glands are possible, but less common. For further information see Chapter 16.

Rats

It is important to note that renal tubular production of alpha globulins results in normal proteinuria in male rats. This form of proteinuria can be distinguished from the loss of serum proteins in the urine, in cases of chronic progressive nephropathy, by performing a urine protein electrophoresis. Females have cyclic uterine eosinophilic infiltrates and this is a normal finding (Percy and Barthold, 1993).

Rats have an extensive network of mammary tissue that spans from the elbow to the inguinal region. The six mammary glands include cervical, thoracic, abdominal, mammary papillae, inguinal and preputial (O'Malley, 2005).

Urinary diseases

Chronic progressive nephropathy
Also known as 'old rat nephropathy', this well documented phenomenon is the most commonly diagnosed nephropathy in rats. Associated with ageing (over 12 months of age), signs include weight loss, significant proteinuria (>10 mg/dl; Johnson-Delaney,

1998), isosthenuria and elevated plasma creatinine consistent with renal insufficiency. Traditionally, predisposing factors have been identified, including age, high-protein diets, gender (higher incidence in males), strain (Sprague Dawleys are over-represented) and hormonal influence. Prolactin has also been suspected in the development of the disease (Fisher, 2006). Secondary renal hyperparathyroidism should also be considered. Radiographic evidence may include mineral deposits seen in the kidney, gastric mucosa, lungs or tunica media of arteries. Evaluation of urine cytology and sediments can help to diagnose this disease. Proteinaceous casts may be shed in urine. Radiography and ultrasonography can be helpful in discerning the extent of renal damage and prognosis. Treatment includes a low-protein diet and supportive care.

Hydronephrosis
This condition is a hereditary trait in Brown Norways, Gunn and Sprague Dawley strains. Commonly found incidentally on necropsy, only severe bilateral hydronephrosis causes clinical disease. Although uncommon, urolithiasis can be associated with hydronephrosis. Ultrasonography can be used to elucidate renal pelvis dilatation. Differential diagnoses should include pyelonephritis, renal papillary necrosis and polycystic disease.

Nephrocalcinosis
This disease is found in pet rats and incidentally in laboratory rats. It is linked to dietary factors (low magnesium and high calcium to phosphorus ratios). Females have a higher incidence, as oestrogens have a role in inciting disease development. Disease induction has been achieved in castrated males and spayed females on oestrogen therapy; it is therefore suggested that ovariectomy can prevent disease development (Johnson-Delaney, 1998). Diagnosis can be made on ultrasonography and radiography, with calcium phosphate deposition in the renal interstitium and corticomedullary junction (Fisher, 2006). Treatment includes lower dietary calcium intake and adequate magnesium intake, low-protein diet and supportive care for renal disease.

Suppurative pyelonephritis/nephritis
Suppurative pyelonephritis and nephritis is seen in older male rats, with *Pseudomonas*, *Escherichia coli*, *Proteus mirabilis* and *Klebsiella* commonly isolated. Extended antibiotic therapy (4–6 weeks) and supportive care are warranted if diagnosed on urine culture.

Parasites
Pet rats have been diagnosed with renal parasitism. *Klossiella hydromyos* is a renal coccidian and sporocysts are diagnosed on urine cytology. Rarely clinically apparent, it is controlled by improved sanitation and coccidiostats in the drinking water (Johnson-Delaney, 1998).

Bladder threadworms (*Trichomoides crassicauda*) are commonly found in rats 8–12 weeks old and operculated eggs can be seen on urine cytology. Signs are usually subclinical but can include ill thrift, dysuria and urinary calculi. On occasion the worms can ascend to the kidney and incite a chronic pyelitis and urolith formation. Ivermectin and sanitation are used for control.

Other uropathies

Rare uropathies include leptospirosis, urinary calculi, urinary plugs, renal papillary hyperplasia, polycystic renal disease and neoplasia. Documented neoplastic conditions include renal cortical epithelial carcinoma, adenoma, adenocarcinoma, renal pelvic epithelial papilloma, transitional cell carcinoma (Dontas and Khaldi, 2006) and squamous cell carcinoma. Metastatic tumours to the kidney include lipoma, liposarcoma, fibrosarcoma, haemangiosarcoma and leiomyosarcoma (Fisher, 2006).

Reproductive diseases

Mycoplasmal endometritis and pyometra

Mycoplasma pulmonis is a ubiquitous life-threatening infection of rats, and is the most common cause of lower respiratory disease. The organism has an affinity for the epithelial cells of the respiratory tract, middle ear and endometrium. Intrauterine transmission can occur, but postnatal infection via aerosol is more likely in pups exposed to infected dams. Leucocytes and cellular debris are present in endometrial glands in cases of chronic endometritis (Percy and Barthold, 1993). In addition to respiratory distress, infertility is a common clinical sign. Treatment modalities have been limited to controlling clinical signs. The authors have had success with enrofloxacin (10 mg/kg orally q12h for 14 days) and doxycycline (75 mg/kg s.c. depot q7d), meloxicam (1 mg/kg orally q24h for 3–5 days), oxygen therapy, and nebulization with albuterol (add 0.5 ml albuterol sulfate to 4 ml saline, nebulize q8–24h) in managing chronic cases. See Chapter 12 for further details.

Neoplasia

Mammary tumours are commonly diagnosed in male and female rats, with an 80–95% incidence of fibroadenomas (Percy and Barthold, 1993). These benign masses can be found along the ventrum and are commonly found around the axillary region (Figure 13.2). They can become quite large and highly mobile and are not locally invasive. To improve ambulation and prevent ulceration due to their sheer size, surgical excision is recommended. Surgery is straightforward and carries a favourable prognosis, but recurrence is very common.

Studies have shown that prolonged administration of growth hormone increases the incidence of fibroadenoma formation, and increased oestrogen administration increases the incidence of adenocarcinomas (Orr, 2002). Ovariectomy has been shown to reduce the incidence of fibroadenomas *and* pituitary tumour development (Hotchkiss, 1995) (see also Chapter 7). Fibroadenomas are found commonly with pituitary tumours (90% incidence). Although less common (<10%), adenocarcinomas carry a graver prognosis. Other less commonly documented neoplastic conditions include interstitial cell tumours (Percy and Barthold, 1993). See Chapter 16 for further information.

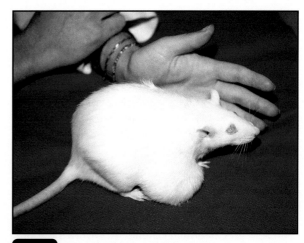

13.2 Rat with mammary tumour.

Hamsters

Hamster urine is naturally very thick and creamy and should not be mistaken for pyuria. Female hamsters have a characteristic vaginal discharge. During their 4-day oestrous cycle, a creamy white stringy discharge with a distinctive odour exudes from the vaginal orifice. This is normal and should not be mistaken for pus, as pyometra is relatively rare in hamsters.

Urinary diseases

Arteriolar nephrosclerosis and amyloidosis

These two diseases have a high incidence in geriatric female hamsters. Many studies in Syrian hamsters have tried to elucidate further both pathological mechanisms; amyloidosis has been documented as a common spontaneous lesion in geriatric hamsters (Kamino *et al.*, 2001). Arteriolar nephrosclerosis has been likened to 'old rat nephropathy' syndrome in comparison with disease incidence and pathology (Fisher, 2006). It is believed that excess dietary protein, chronic viral infections and intrarenal hypertension are all contributing causes. Amyloidosis is often concurrently seen with arteriolar nephrosclerosis. Both degenerative glomerular diseases present with 'nephrotic syndrome' clinical signs, which include anorexia, oedema, ascites, proteinuria, hypercholesterolaemia, hypoalbuminaemia and hyperglobulinaemia (Goodman, 2002). Polyuria, polydipsia and haematuria can also be seen. Both terminal diseases are managed with chronic renal failure therapeutics.

Polycystic disease

This is primarily an incidental finding on necropsy, whereby cysts are most commonly found within the liver and epididymis in older male hamsters. They have been documented as also involving the renal pelvis. The aetiology is unknown, but it is thought to be congenital in nature. The patient usually presents with an enlarged abdomen and a quick clinical diagnosis can be made on digital palpation and ultrasonography. Treatment involves palliative draining of the cysts, though recurrence is likely in 2–4 weeks (Capello, 2002).

Hamster polyomavirus
This virus is the cause of transmissible lymphoma in hamsters. Multicentric lymphoma commonly involves the kidney, and viral transmission occurs through environmental contamination with infected urine. Documented cases have been reported in a pet Syrian hamster as young as 8 weeks old (Simmons *et al.*, 2001). For further information see Chapters 10 and 16.

Zoonoses

Leptospirosis: Leptospira ballum can infect hamsters from contaminated mice. This zoonotic disease should always be considered if a hamster presents with jaundice and haemoglobinuria. A severe nephritis, haemolytic anaemia and hepatitis ensue within 4–6 days. Treatment can be attempted, but hamsters are extremely susceptible and infection results in high mortality.

Lymphocytic choriomeningitis: This arenavirus causes a chronic fatal wasting disease in young hamsters. Wild mice are the natural host; disease transmission occurs through organisms shed in saliva and urine. Congenital infection can also occur. Confirmed cases should be euthanased to minimize the serious zoonotic potential to human handlers.

Other uropathies
Less common documented uropathies include diabetic nephropathy and urolithiasis.

Diabetic nephropathy: It is important to note that hamsters are being used as new laboratory animal models for type 2 diabetic nephropathy studies. In one study, golden hamsters have been shown to metabolize diets high in saturated fat in a similar way to humans, predisposing them to diabetic nephropathies (Popov *et al.*, 2003). Concurrent findings revealed elevated creatinine concentrations, renal azotaemia and nodular glomerulosclerosis and nephropathy. This emphasizes the importance of keeping pet hamsters on a formulated rodent diet.

Urolithiasis: Although not commonly diagnosed, there have been documented cases of urolithiasis. The aetiology is unknown but a solely dry food diet may be a predisposing factor (Capello, 2002). Crystalluria with a basic urine pH is seen. Radiography can help with a diagnosis. Surgical management is discussed in Chapter 7.

Reproductive diseases

Cannibalism of young
Hamsters are well known for this behavioural disposition, which occurs most frequently in groups of stressed primiparous females. Chinese hamsters are more prone to this behaviour. It is important to instruct owners to provide the mothers with plenty of food, water and nesting material. Handling the young and their nest should be reduced for 1–2 weeks. Continued stress could result in litter desertion and cannibalism.

Endometritis/pyometra
This has been clinically observed in hamsters, but it is rare. Mistaking a normal oestrous vaginal discharge leads to misdiagnosis. Cytology of the discharge and ultrasonography should elucidate whether there is a true pyometra. Ovariohysterectomy is the treatment of choice.

Vaginal haemorrhage is an abnormal finding. There have been documented cases of uterine endometrial adenocarcinoma (Goodman, 2002) (see Chapters 7 and 16).

Other reproductive diseases
Less commonly documented reproductive diseases include mastitis and spontaneous haemorrhagic necrosis of the CNS of fetal hamsters.

Mastitis: Mastitis has been well documented in hamsters and has several causes, the most common being beta-haemolytic *Streptococcus*, *Pasteurella pneumotropica*, *Escherichia coli*, *Staphylococcus aureus* and *Pseudomonas aeruginosa* (Percy and Barthold, 1993). Cutaneous and cervical abscesses may result. Broad-spectrum antibiotics should be administered pending bacterial culture and sensitivity testing.

Spontaneous haemorrhagic necrosis of the CNS: This disease of fetal hamsters can become very relevant if the dam is not provided with an adequate amount of dietary vitamin E. Pups are usually stillborn or weak at birth and are cannibalized by the dam.

Gerbils

Gerbil kidneys are extremely well adapted for concentrating urine. When performing urinalysis, it should be remembered that their urine is usually alkaline and normally contains small amounts of protein, glucose, bilirubin and acetone (see Figure 13.1).

Urinary diseases
Chronic uropathies
Renal pathology associated with amyloidosis, bacterial nephritis, glomerulonephritis, hydronephrosis and nephrocalcinosis are discussed collectively here because they are all viewed as significant causes of chronic uropathies in gerbils. One retrospective study reported that of 141 gerbils examined post mortem, the following disease incidence was revealed: 16% chronic interstitial nephritis, 18% chronic tubular necrosis, 14% chronic glomerulonephropathy, 9% glomerular and interstitial amyloidosis, and 6% glomerulonephrosis; pyelonephritis, hydronephrosis, and nephrocalcinosis were also noted (Bingel, 1995). In the same study an incidence of 5% renal haemangiomas and 1.5% haemangiosarcomas was noted.

Clinical signs of chronic renal disease are similar to those discussed above for other rodents: anorexia, polydipsia, polyuria, weight loss, anorexia and signs of cystitis. Blood chemistry reveals elevated creatinine and BUN; urinalysis and urine culture can help to identify the inciting cause of renal failure. Therapeutic protocols are as detailed for managing chronic renal failure at the beginning of this chapter.

Reproductive diseases

Ovarian cystic disease

This condition is remarkably common in older females. Cysts can affect one or both ovaries and do reduce reproductive performance (Keeble, 2002). Ultrasonography and radiography can provide a quick diagnosis. Many clinicians percutaneously aspirate cysts, but recurrence is very common – at times within the same week. Ovariohysterectomy is the treatment of choice (Lewis, 2003).

Neoplasia

The following neoplastic conditions have been documented in gerbils: granulosa and thecal cell tumours, uterine leiomyoma, mammary gland adenocarcinoma, uterine adenocarcinoma, testicular teratomas, and seminomas (see Chapter 16).

Guinea pigs

Guinea pig urine is characteristically thick, cloudy white in colour and alkaline, and contains calcium carbonate and ammonium phosphate crystals. Female guinea pigs have a bicornuate uterus and vaginal membranes that seal the vaginal orifice except during copulation or parturition (O'Malley, 2005). The vaginal membrane has rarely been seen clinically by the authors. The urethral opening is separate from the vagina, which is particularly important in identifying the specific origin of abnormal discharges. Boars have a very thin os penis and perineal sac glands that often become impacted with caseous secretions, faeces, hair and other debris (O'Malley, 2005).

Urinary diseases

Urolithiasis

This is most commonly seen in middle-aged to older cavies (> 2.5 years old). Females are thought to be predisposed because their urethral orifice is close to the anus, allowing for faecal bacteria (*Escherichia coli*) and subsequent ascending infections to cause cystitis. Calculi can form in the kidneys, ureters, bladder or urethra. Ongoing calculi studies at the University of California, Davis have shown most calculi to be composed of calcium carbonate (Michelle Hawkins, personal communication, 2007). Calcium phosphate, calcium oxalate and magnesium phosphate (struvite) can also be found. While the exact aetiology is unknown, the major speculated causes include high calcium and oxalate diets and bacterial infections, including *Streptococcus pyogenes*, *Proteus mirabilis* and *E. coli*.

Clinical signs can be vague and are governed by the size and location of the stone. They include haematuria, stranguria, dysuria, anuria, pollakiuria, inappetence, hunched posture (abdominal pain), vocalization when attempting to urinate, and a fluffed haircoat appearance. Some guinea pigs in pain present for anorexia and lethargy without urinary signs due to pain, especially with ureteral stones.

Uroliths are diagnosed on radiographs. Proper positioning for radiographs is essential, because distal ureteral stones are common and can resemble a cystic location radiographically (Figure 13.3). Ultrasonography can help further elucidate the presence of hydronephrosis and hydroureter, identify whether there are stones within the renal pelvis and assess renal architecture. Urinalysis and culture should also be performed as standard in these cases.

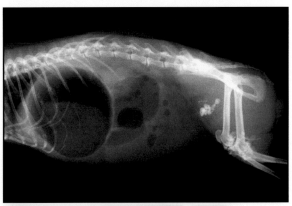
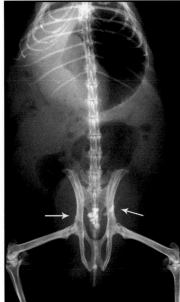

13.3
Radiographs of a sedated male 4-year-old guinea pig with uroliths. Note that in the lateral view, the calculi appear to be in a cystic location, but the ventrodorsal view reveals that the stones are actually in both ureters (arrows), as well as the bladder, the distal urethra, and the right kidney. The guinea pig also has extensive gastrointestinal gas, indicating gut stasis, and calcifications of both stifles (arthritis).

Medical treatment has been unrewarding. Initial treatment should include antibiotic therapy, pain management and diet modification. Dissolution therapy has been used in animals with acidic urine to inhibit calcium stone crystallization in the urine, using potassium citrate at 150 mg/kg divided q12h. Citrate reduces urinary saturation of calcium salts by binding calcium, reducing ion activity and alkalinizing the urine (Hoefer, 2004). Although guinea pigs have alkaline urine, some clinicians believe that potassium citrate therapy may help and in the authors' experience this treatment aids in inhibiting stone formation following surgical stone removal.

Dietary modifications are aimed at reducing high calcium and oxalate content in the urine. Alfalfa-based pellets and hay should be avoided. Foods high in oxalates, such as kale, spinach, parsley, celery and strawberries, should be given sparingly. Vitamin C also has high oxalate content, but the daily nutritional requirement (25–100 mg/kg/day) administered to guinea pigs is unlikely to cause hyperoxaluria (Hoefer, 2004). The authors have observed that feeding Timothy hay and a Timothy hay-based pelleted diet, which is lower in calcium and higher in fibre, not only reduces the likelihood of urolith formation but also improves dental health.

Surgical management via cystotomy is routine. Presurgical chemistry profiles should be performed to assess kidney function. Ureteral stones should be milked down into the bladder for removal, and a 5F red rubber catheter can be placed antegrade from the bladder into the urethra to prevent small urinary stones from migrating into the urethra during the cystotomy (Hoefer, 2004) (see also Chapter 7). Prognosis is guarded, given the high rate of recurrence.

Cystitis and urinary tract infections

Cystitis, commonly noted in older sows, is likely to be caused by an ascending infection from faecal bacterial contamination of the urethra. Common isolates include *E. coli* and *Streptococcus*. *Chlamydophila caviae* has been a reported cause of asymptomatic, transient cystitis in male guinea pigs (Rank *et al.*, 1981). It is important to take radiographs to discern whether uroliths are also present. Haematuria, pyuria, malodorous urine, dysuria and stranguria are all clinical signs. Vocalization during urination and hunched postures indicate pain. Buprenorphine (0.02 mg/kg s.c., i.m. q8h) can be administered to provide analgesia. A chemistry profile and urinalysis should be performed to classify a renal or postrenal azotaemia. The authors have found gentle warm sterile saline bladder flushes using a 3.5F red rubber catheter to be therapeutic in cases of severe pyuria. Trimethroprim/ sulphonamide antibiotics should be administered pending urine culture results.

Chronic interstitial nephritis

This can be noted with several other active disease processes, including the aforementioned chronic urolithiasis (obstructive urolithiasis, hydronephrosis, hydroureter). Diabetes mellitus and hyperglycaemia have also been reported to cause a chronic interstitial nephritis. Chronic pododermatitis caused by staphylococci has been shown to cause consequent renal amyloidosis (Schaeffer *et al.*, 1997). *Encephalitozoon cuniculi* has been reported to cause subacute interstitial nephritis in gnotobiotically reared guinea pigs, but the prevalence of this parasite is unknown in pet guinea pigs (Boot *et al.*, 1998). Diagnosis is made by chemistry profiles, urinalysis, ultrasonography and cystograms. Medical management is based on treatment of the underlying cause of nephritis, but should include supplemental fluid therapy and antibiotic therapy.

Renal disease associated with pregnancy toxaemia

Seen in obese sows 2 weeks prior to parturition, signs of pregnancy toxaemia are abrupt and include lethargy, fluffed coat appearance, possible dyspnoea, anorexia, severe depression and recumbency.

Hypoglycaemia, metabolic acidosis, ketonuria, proteinuria and acidic urine (pH 5–6) are consistent clinical findings. The proteinuria occurs as a result of proximal tubule necrosis and subcapsular renal haemorrhaging (Fisher, 2006). Immediate medical therapy should include intravenous administration of dextrose-supplemented fluids and oral glucose therapy. More detail on pregnancy toxaemia is given below.

Metastatic calcification

This occurs in guinea pigs over 1 year of age. Many are asymptomatic, but clinical signs may include muscle stiffness and unthriftiness (see also Chapter 14). Soft tissue mineralizations can be seen on radiographs. Diets that are rich in calcium and phosphorus but low in magnesium are thought to be the cause of the mineralized lesions. Mineralization can occur in soft tissues around the ribs and elbows, but can also include the lung, trachea, heart, aorta, liver, kidney and stomach (Percy and Barthold, 1993). Diagnosis is made from radiographs; ultrasonography, a chemistry profile and urinalysis should also be performed to evaluate kidney and circulatory function. Diet modification and supportive care are indicated in managing cases where kidney, respiratory or circulatory function is compromised.

Other uropathies

Other less commonly clinically encountered uropathies include klossiellosis, cytomegalovirus infection, renal cysts, transitional cell carcinoma, segmental nephron nephrosis, lymphocytic choriomeningitis virus infection, and renal failure after oxalate ingestion.

Klossiella cobayae, a renal coccidian, is uncommon; clinical signs are often absent, and diagnosis is made on renal histopathology. Its mode of transmission is through infective urine, and medical treatment includes improved sanitation and trimethroprim/ sulphonamide antibiotic therapy.

Cytomegalovirus inclusion bodies are usually an incidental finding at necropsy, as guinea pigs are inapparent hosts for this naturally occurring herpesvirus (Fisher, 2006).

Renal cysts and nephronephrosis are also an incidental necropsy finding. Segmental nephrosclerosis is thought to have several aetiologies, including autoimmune disease, high-protein diet, infectious diseases and vascular disease (Schaeffer and Donnelly, 1997).

Lymphocytic choriomeningitis virus is rarely found in guinea pigs but can cause hindlimb paralysis and meningitis. No treatment is currently available.

There is a documented report of renal failure following the ingestion of peace lily leaf (oxalate ingestion) with similar idiopathic clinical signs to those seen in the feline syndrome (Holowaychuk, 2006).

Reproductive diseases

Ovarian cystic disease

This is the most common reproductive disease of guinea pigs in both authors' experience. Cystic retes ovarii occur in middle-aged to older sows (Schaeffer and Donnelly, 1997). Bilateral symmetrical truncal alopecia is the most common clinical sign, but vaginal bleeding from cystic endometrial hyperplasia can be seen. It is frequently associated with a decline in reproductive performance in sows older than 15 months. One study revealed that there is no correlation between reproductive history and prevalence of cysts, but that there is a correlation between cyst size and age, and between cyst prevalence and age (Nielsen *et al.*, 2003). Mucometra, endometritis, and fibroleiomyomas have been associated with cystic retes ovarii (Percy and Barthold, 1993).

Diagnosis can be made from a thorough abdominal palpation and is confirmed on ultrasonography. The cysts can become very large, up to 2 cm in diameter, are often bilateral, and can be singular or multi-lobulated. Percutaneous fine-needle aspiration of the cysts reveals a clear serous fluid. In the authors' experience therapy including percutaneous drainage of the cysts (Figure 13.4), and hormone therapy with leuprolide acetate injections (100 µg/kg s.c.) given once every 3 weeks, provides temporary improvement. Other clinicians have successfully used gonadotrophin-releasing hormone (GnRH) therapy administered at 25 µg per guinea pig every 2 weeks for two injections (Mayer, 2005). Other hormone therapies include intramuscular injections of human chorionic gonadotrophin (hCG) at 1000 USP, repeated in 7–10 days, but they have been associated with allergic reactions and reduced effectiveness (Mayer, 2005). Ovariohysterectomy is the treatment of choice (see Chapter 7).

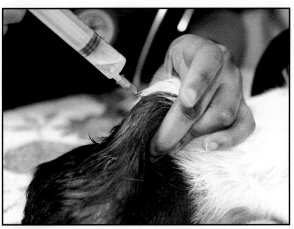

13.4 Percutaneous fine-needle aspiration of an ovarian cyst in a sedated guinea pig. An aseptic technique is required. The cystic ovary is immobilized against the lateral abdominal wall using one hand whilst the other aspirates the contents using a needle and syringe.

Dystocia

This condition presents in breeding sows more than 6 months of age. It results from the physiological consequence of complete pelvic symphysis fusion at an early age (6–8 months). Other causes include obesity, primiparity, uterine inertia, and small litters resulting in large fetuses (Nakamura, 2002). Hypovitaminosis C has also been implicated as a cause of dystocia (Bishop, 2002). Clinical signs of dystocia include straining, contractions, vocalization and biting at the flanks, anxiousness, depression and occasional bloody or green discharge. Radiographs are warranted to determine fetal size and position. If pelvic symphysis dilatation is less than 20–25 mm, immediate Caesarean section is indicated (O'Rourke, 2004). If the pelvis is dilated, oxytocin at 0.2–0.3 IU/kg i.m. can be administered. If there is no response after 15–20 minutes, Caesarean section should be considered (see Chapter 7) and the prognosis is guarded at best.

Pregnancy toxaemia

This is common 2 weeks prior to parturtion and occurs when the energy requirements needed to sustain the fetuses and lactation exceed energy intake (Bishop, 2002). The sow then catabolizes fat in an effort to sustain herself, resulting in metabolic acidosis, ketosis and an abrupt decline requiring immediate medical intervention. Predisposing factors include obesity, change in diet, environment, lack of exercise, large fetal loads, heat stress and primiparity (Nakamura, 2002). Clinical signs include lethargy, fluffed coat appearance, possible dyspnoea, anorexia, severe depression, incoordination and recumbency. Diagnostic observations include ketonuria, proteinuria, hypoglycaemia, hyperlipidaemia, hyperkalaemia and aciduria. Treatment includes immediate intravenous fluid therapy supplemented with dextrose, calcium gluconate, oral glucose and magnesium sulphate (advocated as an arteriolar dilator). Corticosteroids are indicated if the downed sow presents in shock.

Another recognized form of pregnancy toxaemia involves the heavy gravid uterus compressing blood vessels and nerves, leading to vascular and neurological dysfunction. Hypertension will be seen with compression of the renal vessels. Blood pressure measurements will help to differentiate the conditions. If hypertension is present, immediate Caesarean section is warranted. In cases of pregnancy ketosis, hypotension can be managed with corticosteroids and intravenous fluid therapy with crystalloids and colloids. If ischaemia occurs, the animal can suffer fatal disseminated intravascular coagulation (Bishop, 2002). Prevention includes an energy-rich diet in late pregnancy and discouraging obesity.

Vaginitis and pyometra

A condition that can be seen in breeding and non-breeding sows, this usually occurs when the vaginal area becomes impacted with wood chips, sawdust and other particulate substrates. Diagnosis can be made on vaginal examination; and concurrent pyometra can be diagnosed on palpation, radiography and ultrasonography. The most commonly isolated organisms are *Bordetella bronchiseptica* and haemolytic *Streptococcus*, but other pathogens include *Escherichia coli*, *Arcanobacterium pyogenes* and *Salmonella*. *Toxoplasma gondii* has also been documented to cause infertility and abortion (Bishop, 2002). Treatment involves immediate broad-spectrum antibiotic therapy pending culture and gentle dilute chlorhexidine lavage of the vaginal vestibule. Surgery is the treatment of choice (see Chapter 7).

Mastitis

Soiled housing, abrasive bedding, trauma by young, early weaning, or dead offspring can predispose a sow to an infectious cause of mastitis. *Pasteurella*, *Klebsiella*, *E. coli*, *Staphylococcus*, *Streptococcus* and *Pseudomonas* are all implicated as infectious isolates. Treatment includes antibiotic therapy, administration of analgesics such as meloxicam or buprenorphine, warm compresses, and fostering and weaning the young. Necrotic mammary tissue warrants surgical resection (see Chapter 7). Systemic infections can become quickly fatal to the sow and the young.

Neoplasia

Reported neoplastic conditions include mammary adenocarcinoma and fibroadenomas, granulosa cell tumour (Burns *et al.*, 2001), teratomas, uterine fibroma and leiomyomas (Percy, 1993). (See also Chapter 16.)

Other reproductive disorders

Pregnancy alopecia is a less common reproductive disorder and may result from hypovitaminosis C (Nakamura, 2002). Pseudopregnancy is rare and results in lactations lasting for 15–17 days. Stress can inhibit milk production, causing agalactia. Fetal resorption can result from poor nutrition and severe mite infestation. *Bordetella bronchiseptica* infections can result in abortion (Percy and Barthold, 1993).

Boars naturally form copulatory plugs. Orchiditis and epididymitis can result from sexual transmission from a sow, fight wounds from another boar or through haematogenous spread (Bishop, 2002). Antibiotic therapy is warranted pending cultures; *Streptococcus* and *Bordetella* are commonly isolated.

Other documented reproductive disorders include uterine torsion (rare), superfetation, haemorrhagic syndrome and penile papillomas. Superfetation is very rare and results from carrying fetuses from two separate matings from two different oestrous cycles; the litters are born 35 days apart. Haemorrhagic syndrome is a fatal diathesis condition resulting from vitamin K deficiency (Nakamura, 2002). Gravid uterine compression of the liver has also been implicated in liver dysfunction and subsequent compromise (Bishop, 2002). Prognosis is poor and treatment includes vitamin K supplementation and supportive care.

Chinchillas

Chinchillas present with urogenital disorders less commonly than other rodents. It is important to note that female chinchillas have normal waxy vaginal plugs that are expelled after successful mating (Hoefer and Crossley, 2002) (Figure 13.5).

Urinary diseases

Fur rings

Fur rings are commonly encountered in male chinchillas as excessive hair around the penis. Gentle digital expulsion of the penis from the prepuce and careful physical examination allows for a quick diagnosis (Figure 13.6). Hair can be removed with

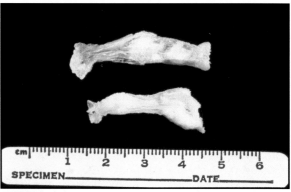

13.5 Normal waxy vaginal plugs. These are expelled from female chinchillas after successful mating. (Reproduced from *BSAVA Manual of Exotic Pets, 4th edn.*)

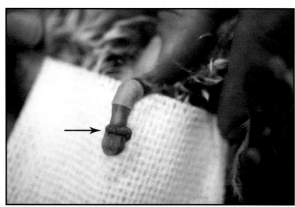

13.6 Fur ring in a male chinchilla. (Reproduced from *BSAVA Manual of Exotic Pets, 4th edn.*)

forceps. Strangulating rings can lead to paraphimosis and ureteral obstruction, which is quite painful. Sterile lubrication can be applied to aid in the removal of such rings. (See also Chapter 10.)

Chronic renal failure and urolithiasis

Both diseases are relatively uncommon. In the authors' experience, clinical signs are similar to those encountered in other rodents with chronic renal disease: anorexia, weight loss, inappetence, stranguria, dysuria, anuria, pollakiuria, hunched posture (pain) and lethargy. Diagnosis includes urinalysis and radiography. Treatment includes medical management of chronic renal failure.

Reproductive diseases

Dystocia

Dystocia can be occasionally diagnosed in chinchillas, whereby uterine inertia, malpositioned fetuses, oversized fetuses and uterine torsion are all possible causes (Hoefer and Crossley, 2002). Radiography can aid in the determination of fetal position. Chinchillas in labour exceeding 4 hours require surgical intervention. Caesarean section (see Chapter 7) is well tolerated in chinchillas. Other less commonly reported reproductive disorders include pyometra, stump pyometra (Kottwitz, 2006) and, very rarely, uterine leiomyosarcoma (Donnelly, 1997).

Degus

Although degus have been well studied in laboratory research, information is very limited for pets. Degus rarely present with urogenital disorders, but some are being observed more frequently in practice.

Urinary diseases

Diabetic nephropathy

Diabetic nephropathy is well described in laboratory degus (see Chapter 16). Degus develop spontaneous diabetes mellitus and islet amyloidosis (Murphy *et al.*, 1980). A characteristic clinical sign is cataract formation (Figure 13.7). Predisposing factors include an improper diet, such as fruits and pelleted diets high in sugar. Diagnosis can be made by serum chemistry profile, ultrasonography and demonstration of glucosuria on urinalysis. Renal architecture can be observed on ultrasonography. Treatment includes dietary modification (high-protein, low-fibre, low-fat, no-sugar rat diet; vegetables instead of fruit) and supportive care. Sorbinil, an aldose reductase inhibitor, has been used in treating and preventing diabetic nephropathy and cataract formation, but it is currently not available in the United States or in the UK (Datules, 1989). Diabetic degus have higher aldose reductase activity. This enzyme is involved in an alternative glucose reduction biochemical pathway, seen in diabetic degus who suffer from impaired glucose tolerance. Sorbinil inhibits aldose reductase, thereby preventing development of secondary diabetic complications, such as diabetic nephropathy and cataract formation.

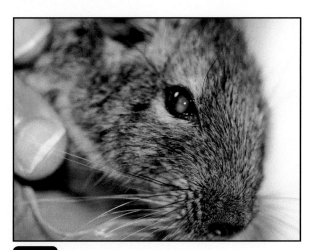

13.7 Mature cataract in a male degu.

Renal neoplasia

Renal neoplasia is very rare, but there is one documented case of renal transitional cell carcinoma (Lester *et al.*, 2005).

Reproductive disease

Dystocia (Figure 13.8) has been documented. Malpositioned fetuses can be the cause. Pregnancy toxaemia is very rarely seen in practice but presents as described above for the guinea pig.

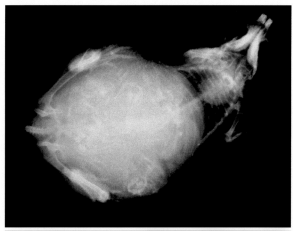

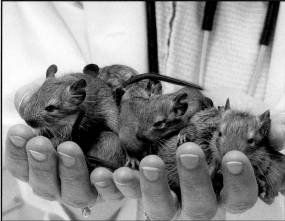

13.8 Dorsoventral radiograph of a degu with dystocia: eight pups can be seen. Seven of the pups survived following Caesarean section. (Courtesy of Dan Johnson.)

References and further reading

Bingel SA (1995) Pathological findings in an aging Mongolian gerbil (*Meriones unguiculatus*) colony. *Laboratory Animal Science* **45**(5), 597–600

Bishop CR (2002) Reproductive medicine of rabbits and rodents: guinea pigs. *Veterinary Clinics of North America: Exotic Animal Practice* **5**(3), 519–535

Boot R, van Knapen F, Kruijt BC *et al.* (1988) Serological evidence for *Encephalitozoon cuniculi* infection (nosemiasis) in gnotobiotic guinea pigs. *Laboratory Animal* **22**, 337–342

Burns RP, Paul-Murphy J and Sicard GK (2001) Granulosa cell tumor in a guinea pig. *Journal of the American Veterinary Medical Association* **218**(5), 726–728

Capello V (2002) Pet hamster medicine and surgery, part III: infectious, parasitic and metabolic diseases. *Exotic DVM* **3**(6), 27–32

Casey HW and Irving GW (1981) Bacterial, mycoplasmal, mycotic, and immune-mediated diseases of the urogenital system. In: *The Mouse in Biomedical Research. Vol. II. Diseases*, ed. HL Foster *et al.*, pp. 43–53. Academic Press, New York

Datiles MB and Fukui H (1989) Cataract prevention in diabetic *Octodon degus* with Pfizer's sorbinil. *Current Eye Research* **8**, 233–237

Donnelly TM (1997) Disease problems of small rodents. ed., In: *Ferrets, Rabbits and Rodents: Clinical Medicine and Surgery*, ed. EV Hillyer and KQ Quesenberry, pp. 312–315. WB Saunders, Philadelphia

Donnelly TM and Brown CJ (2004) Guinea pig and chinchilla care and husbandry. *Veterinary Clinics of North America: Exotic Animal Practice* **7**(2), 351–373

Dontas IA and Khaldi L (2006) Urolithiasis and transitional cell carcinoma of the bladder in a Wistar Rat. *Journal of the American Association of Laboratory Animal Science* **45**(4), 64–67

Fisher PG (2006) Exotic mammal renal disease: causes and clinical presentation. *Veterinary Clinics of North America: Exotic Animal Practice* **9**(1), 52–62

Goodman G (2002) Hamsters. In: *BSAVA Manual of Exotic Pets, 4th edn*, ed. A Meredith and S Redrobe, pp. 26–33. BSAVA Publications, Gloucester

Hawkins M (2007) *Owbox Pet Products 2005 Guinea Pig Urinary Calculus Study.* (Publication pending; personal communication)

Hoefer HL (2004) Guinea pig urolithiasis. *Exotic DVM* **4**(2), 23–25

Hoefer HL and Crossley DA (2002) Chinchillas. In: *BSAVA Manual of Exotic Pets, 4th edn*, ed. A Meredith and S Redrobe, pp. 65–75. BSAVA Publications, Gloucester

Holowaychuk MK (2006) Renal failure in a guinea pig (*Cavia porcellus*) following ingestion of oxalate containing plants. *Canadian Veterinary Journal* **47**(8), 787–789

Hotchkiss CE (1995) Effect of surgical removal of subcutaneous tumors on survival of rats. *Journal of the American Veterinary Medicine Association* **206**, 1575–1579

Johnson-Delaney CA (1997) Special rodents: degus. In: *Exotic Companion Medicine Handbook for Veterinarians*, pp. 27–32. Wingers Publishing/ZEN Publishing, Lake Worth, Florida

Johnson-Delaney CA (1998) Disease of the urinary system of rats and mice. *Exotic Pet Practice* **3**(9), 65–68

Johnson-Delaney CA (2002) What veterinarians need to know about degus. *Exotic DVM* **4**(4), 39–42

Johnson-Delaney CA (2006) Common procedures in hedgehogs, prairie dogs, exotic rodents, and companion marsupials. *Veterinary Clinics of North America: Exotic Animal Practice* **9**(2), 415–435

Kamino K, Tillemann T, Boschmann E and Mohr U (2001) Age-related incidence of spontaneous non-neoplastic lesions in a colony of Han:AURA hamsters. *Experimental Toxicological Pathology* **53**(2-3), 157–164

Kashuba C, Hsu C, Krogstad A and Franklin C (2005) Small mammal virology. *Veterinary Clinics of North America: Exotic Animal Practice* **8**(1), 107–122

Keeble E (2002) Gerbils. In: *BSAVA Manual of Exotic Pets, 4th edn*, ed. A Meredith and S Redrobe, pp. 34–46. BSAVA Publications, Gloucester

Kottwitz J (2006) Stump pyometra in a chinchilla. *Exotic DVM* **8**(5), 24–28

Lester PA, Rush HG and Sigler RE (2005) Renal transitional cell carcinoma and choristoma in a degu (*Octodon degus*). *Contemporary Topics in Laboratory Animal Science* **44**(3), 41–44

Lewis W (2003) Cystic ovaries in gerbils. *Exotic DVM* **5**(1), 12–13

Martinho F (2006) Dystocia caused by ectopic pregnancy in a guinea pig (*Cavia porcellus*). *Veterinary Clinics of North America: Exotic Animal Practice* **9**(3), 713–716

Mayer J (2003) The use of GnRH therapy to treat cystic ovaries in a guinea pig. *Exotic DVM* **5**(5), 36

Murphy JC, Crowell TP, Hewes KM *et al.* (1980) Spontaneous lesions in the degu. In: *The Comparative Pathology of Zoo Animals*, ed. RJ Montali and G Migaki, pp. 437–444. Smithsonian Institution Press, Washington DC

Nakamura C (2002) Reproduction and reproductive disorders in guinea pigs. *Exotic DVM* **2**(2), 11–16

Nielsen TD, Holt S, Ruelokke ML and McEvoy FJ (2003) Ovarian cysts in guinea pigs: influence of age and reproductive status on prevalence and size. *Journal of Small Animal Practice* **44**(6), 257–260

O'Malley B (2005) *Clinical Anatomy and Physiology of Exotic Species*. Elsevier Saunders, Philadelphia

O'Rourke DP (2004) Disease problems of guinea pigs. In: *Ferrets, Rabbits and Rodents: Clinical Medicine and Surgery, 2nd edn*, ed. K Quesenberry and J. Carpenter, pp. 245–254. WB Saunders, St Louis

Orr HE (2002) Rats and Mice. In: *BSAVA Manual of Exotic Pets, 4th edn*, ed. A Meredith and S Redrobe, pp. 13–25. BSAVA Publications, Gloucester

Percy DH and Barthold SW (1993) *Pathology of Laboratory Rodents and Rabbits*. Iowa State University Press, Ames, Iowa

Popov D, Simionescu M and Shepherd PR (2003) Saturated-fat diet induces moderate diabetes and severe glomerulosclerosis in hamsters. *Diabetologia.* **46**(10),1408–1418

Rank RG, White HJ, Soloff BL and Barron AL (1981) Cystitis associated with chlamydial infection of the genital tract in male guinea pigs. *The American Venereal Disease Association* **700**, 203–210

Schaeffer DO and Donnelly TM (1997) Disease problems of guinea pigs and chinchillas. In: *Ferrets, Rabbits and Rodents: Clinical Medicine and Surgery*, ed. EV Hillyer and KQ Quesenberry, pp. 261–270. WB Saunders, Philadelphia

Simmons JH, Riley LK, Franklin CL and Besch-Williford (2001) Hamster polyomavirus infection in a pet Syrian hamster (*Mesocricetus auratus*). *Veterinary Pathology* **38**(4), 441–446

14

Rodents: neurological and musculoskeletal disorders

Simon Hollamby

Introduction

Neurological and musculoskeletal disorders in rodents are characterized by clinical case reports from exotic pet practice in addition to aetiologies more commonly documented under laboratory conditions. This makes it difficult to determine the actual incidence of many neurological and musculoskeletal disorders that may present in practice and whether this has changed over time.

The causes of neurological and musculoskeletal disorders can be traumatic, infectious, neoplastic, nutritional, metabolic, toxic, degenerative, idiopathic, iatrogenic, genetic or congenital, or a combination of these. Neurological and musculoskeletal diseases can be species specific or affect multiple species, be geographically restricted or generalized, and be part of a multisystemic disorder or have pathology isolated exclusively to these organ systems. Disease can very frequently have a husbandry component.

History, physical examination and diagnostic procedures

Given the diversity of aetiologies it is useful to have a working knowledge of the biology, dietary, reproductive and social systems of the rodent species commonly presented. The history should concentrate on four questions:

- What is the origin of the pet rodent?
- What type of environment does it currently live in and how long has it been there?
- With whom does it share this environment?
- How is it sustained within this environment?

A general clinical examination should be performed as described in Chapter 2. Initial assessment of the neurological and musculoskeletal system should be performed without restraint. Examination of the neurological system should extrapolate as much as possible and where applicable from well described feline and canine examination techniques. Assessment of cranial nerve function has been described in rabbits but not rodents (Keeble, 2006). An ophthalmological examination should always be attempted, as described in Chapter 15. Mentation, posture (placing reactions), pain response (withdrawal reflex) and sensation should be assessed with the caveat that not all species will respond, and different individuals may not respond in a similar way. Many species that are preyed upon will either freeze or struggle in response to restraint, making examination challenging. A further limitation to neurological examination in many rodent species is their diminutive size.

Diagnostic procedures as described in this manual are often necessary to obtain a specific diagnosis or to differentiate the primary aetiology from the secondary complaint (e.g. traumatic fractures may be an indication of metabolic bone disease).

Selected neurological and musculoskeletal conditions

Figures 14.1 to 14.5 summarize differential diagnoses for neurological and musculoskeletal disease in mice, rats, hamsters, gerbils, guinea pigs and chinchillas. The sections below follow the same order of clinical presentations as in these figures. Figure 14.6 suggests diseases that might be seen in other rodent species.

Clinical presentation	Differential diagnoses
Head tilt, torticollis, circling, ataxia	*Clostridium piliforme* (Tyzzer's disease), otitis media and interna (secondary to *Pseudomonas aeruginosa*/ *Mycoplasma pulmonis*, *Pasteurella pneumotropica*, *Streptococcus pneumoniae* (R) subclinical infection (M), pituitary adenoma
Muscular weakness, reluctance to move	Heat stress, mousepox (M), diabetes mellitus
Lameness, abnormal gait	*Streptobacillus moniliformis* (M), osteoarthrosis (M), *Mycoplasma arthritidis* (R, rare), skeletal trauma
Paresis, paralysis	Lymphocytic choriomeningitis virus (LCMV), spinal trauma, mouse poliovirus infection (Theiler's meningoencephalitis virus), murine encephalomyelitis virus, spontaneous degeneration of the spinal cord and peripheral nerves (radiculoneuropathy) (R)

14.1 Summary of differential diagnoses of mouse (M) and rat (R) neurological and musculoskeletal disease.

Clinical presentation	Differential diagnoses
Head tilt, torticollis, circling, ataxia	Neoplastic disease of the nervous system (glioblastoma, astrocytoma), *Clostridium piliforme* (Tyzzer's disease)
Muscular weakness, reluctance to move	Vitamin E deficiency, amyloidosis, exercise restriction
Lameness, abnormal gait	Traumatic fractures, pododermatitis, osteoarthritis of the femorotibial joint
Paresis, paralysis	Traumatic spinal injuries, lymphocytic choriomeningitis virus (LCMV)

14.2 Summary of differential diagnoses of hamster neurological and musculoskeletal disease.

Clinical presentation	Differential diagnoses
Head tilt, torticollis, circling, ataxia	Aural cholesteatomas, *Clostridium piliforme* (Tyzzer's disease), otitis media and interna, aural papilloma/polyp
Convulsions, seizures	Epilepsy, lead toxicity
Lameness, abnormal gait	Traumatic fractures
Paresis, paralysis	Streptomycin toxicity, traumatic spinal injuries

14.3 Summary of differential diagnoses of gerbil neurological and musculoskeletal disease.

Clinical presentation	Differential diagnoses
Head tilt, torticollis, circling	Otitis interna and media, severe reactions to *Trixicarus caviae* infections, streptoccocal lymphadenitis, ototoxicity, *Baylisascaris* infection, gentamicin toxicity
Convulsions, seizures	Heat stress, pregnancy toxaemia, trauma, hypocalcaemia, systemic bacterial infections, *Clostridium piliforme* (Tyzzer's disease), toxoplasmosis, lymphocytic choriomeningitis virus (LCMV)
Muscular weakness, reluctance to move	Vitamin E deficiency, hypervitaminosis D, osteoarthritis, heat stress, malnutrition, vitamin C deficiency
Lameness, abnormal gait	Ulcerative pododermatitis, hypervitaminosis D, metastatic calcification, abnormal leg position in neonates due to dystocia, overgrown nails, osteosarcomas, vitamin C deficiency, *Histoplasma capsulatum*
Paresis, paralysis	Trauma, osteoarthritis (infectious and spontaneous), histoplasmosis, iatrogenic (intramuscular drug administration), vitamin D deficiency,
Abnormal behaviour	Rabies (very rare)

14.4 Summary of differential diagnoses of guinea pig neurological and musculoskeletal disease.

Clinical presentation	Differential diagnoses
Head tilt, torticollis, circling, ataxia	Listeriosis, thiamine deficiency, otitis media and interna, *Baylisascaris* infection, aflatoxicosis
Convulsions, seizures	Heat stress, lead toxicosis, epilepsy, toxoplasmosis, *Frenkelia*, herpesvirus 1 infections (human herpesvirus), calcium:phosphorus imbalances (muscle spasms), lymphocytic choriomeningitis virus (LCMV)
Lameness, abnormal gait	Fractures (tibia common)
Paresis, paralysis	Traumatic spinal injuries
Abnormal behaviour	Rabies

14.5 Summary of differential diagnoses of chinchilla neurological and musculoskeletal disease.

Species	Condition
Degu	Epilepsy
Prairie dog	*Baylisascaris* infection, rabies, pododermatitis, tularaemia (rare), traumatic fractures, toxoplasmosis
Squirrel	West Nile virus, *Baylisascaris* infection, toxoplasmosis
Chipmunk	West Nile virus, traumatic fractures

14.6 Selected neurological and musculoskeletal diseases in other rodent species.

Disorders associated with head tilt, torticollis, ataxia, circling and rolling

Otitis media

In the guinea pig, otitis media is usually subclinical as few cases progress to the inner ear. *Bordetella bronchiseptica*, *Streptococcus zooepidemicus* and *S. pneumoniae* are commonly isolated. Clinical signs include head tilt, ataxia, circling and torticollis (see also Chapter 12). Middle ear infections are often associated with pneumonia, or may occur by extension of nasopharyngeal bacterial flora. Surgical correction (bulla osteotomy) has not been described in guinea pigs, and conservative therapy via antibiotic/anti-inflammatory administration is not curative (Huerkamp *et al.*, 1996). Damage to the CNS may cause similar signs.

Otitis media is frequently seen in young chinchillas (Figure 14.7) and, rarely, will spread to the internal ear or cause a meningoencephalitis (Strake *et al.*, 1996). It can be initiated by trauma or respiratory infections. Inflammation of the tympanic membrane and narrowing of the ear canal can trap debris and allow bacterial proliferation. Surgery to reopen the canal, together with prolonged courses of topical and/or systemic antibiotics, based on culture and sensitivity, may lead to resolution. Radiographs are necessary to rule out involvement of the chinchilla's very large tympanic bullae. Bulla osteotomies may be performed in chinchillas to allow flushing and drainage.

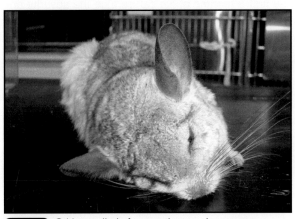

14.7 Otitis media is frequently seen in young chinchillas and may present with a head tilt as in this case. (Courtesy of Emma Keeble.)

Listeria monocytogenes

Listeria monocytogenes has caused sporadic disease as well as outbreaks in chinchillas raised for the fur trade. It has less commonly been seen in laboratory and pet chinchillas. Chinchillas may present with abortion, enteritis and encephalitis, but more often acute death is the only clinical sign, with diagnosis being made post mortem. Treatment once clinical signs have developed is usually unrewarding (Wilkerson *et al.*, 1997).

Mycoplasma pulmonis and *Streptococcus pneumoniae*

Mycoplasma pulmonis can cause an otitis media or interna in rats, and less commonly mice, and is often seen as an extension of a respiratory infection (see

Chapter 12). The main signs observed are a head tilt and ataxia. If antibiotic culture and sensitivity are not possible, enrofloxacin at 10 mg/kg alone, or combined with doxycycline at 5 mg/kg orally q12h (Carpenter, 2005), may be used but the prognosis is often poor. Some affected animals may be able to adapt to a head tilt with time and their food and water intake should be monitored carefully.

Similar signs may be seen with *Streptococcus pneumoniae* infections in rats.

Aural papillomas, polyps and cholesteatomas

Aged gerbils can develop head tilts due to aural papillomas, polyps and cholesteatomas. Due to their vertically orientated ear canals allowing good drainage, bacterial middle/inner ear infections are less common causes of head tilt in this species. Aural cholesteatomas occur spontaneously in older gerbils. More than 50% of gerbils over 2 years of age have cholesteatomas. They comprise masses of keratinized epithelium that form on the outer surface of the tympanic membrane and external auditory canal. The tympanic membrane is displaced inwards, causing increased pressure leading to middle ear inflammation and bone necrosis. No treatment has been described.

Baylisascaris spp.

Infection with the nematode parasite *Baylisascaris* spp. has been reported in a number of rodent species (chinchillas, woodchucks, grey squirrels) where the parasite's natural host species occur (raccoon, skunk). Transmission is via ingestion of infected raccoon faeces, with affected animals displaying a range of neurological signs including head tilt, ataxia, recumbency, paralysis and death. Diagnosis is by history, clinical signs and histopathological demonstration of ascarid larvae in the cerebrum, midbrain and medulla. Larvae may not always be seen in neural tissue and so multiple sections should be examined. Migrating larval granulomas may be seen in other organs and may support a diagnosis. Eosinophilic pleocytosis of the cerebrospinal fluid has been noted in acute infections in humans. Larval isolation and identification is definitive. Treatment with albendazole may slow progression of signs, especially with early intervention or infections with low numbers of migrating larvae, but anthelmintic treatment will not be effective in reversing neural larval migrans. No specific dose rates for rodents are known, but two ruffed lemurs with probable infection showed gradual improvement (though not complete resolution of signs) on 5 mg/kg orally q8h for 14 days, repeated in 4 months (Kazacos, 2001). Treatment with steroids did not appear to improve treatment efficacy significantly in experimentally infected mice.

Protozoan parasites

Toxoplasma gondii and *Frenkelia* spp. are two protozoan parasites that are reported to infect chinchillas. *Frenkelia microti* is a sarcocystis-like coccidium that has birds of prey as definitive hosts and a range of small mammals as intermediate hosts. There are only two reports of *Frenkelia* infection in chinchillas. One case was an incidental finding post mortem, while the second case was concomitantly infected with *T. gondii* (Dubey *et al.*, 2000). The clinical significance of *Frenkelia* infection in chinchillas is unknown. Lobulated macroscopic tissue cysts in the cerebrum of wild rodent species appear to be incidental findings. Clinical signs with toxoplasmosis include weight loss, anorexia, depression, incoordination, lethargy, rolling, loss of balance, cyanosis and dyspnoea. Diagnosis is by serology or PAS/Giemsa staining of histological sections. Treatment of active infections can be attempted with trimethoprim/sulphonamide at 30 mg/kg orally q12h or sulfadimethoxine at 30 mg/kg orally q24h as required, but this will not remove encysted bradyzoites.

Pituitary hyperplasia and adenomas

These are very common in older rats, particularly non-breeding females. Usually a chronic deterioration is seen, with inappetence, weight loss, muscle atrophy, chromodacryorrhoea and neurological signs associated with vestibular nerve dysfunction (head tilt, ataxia, circling; Figure 14.8). Increased hormonal secretions stimulate mammary gland hyperplasia and neoplasia (e.g. prolactin) and possible hyperadrenocorticism (e.g. ACTH). Although the prognosis is poor, it has been reported that dietary restriction (80% of *ad libitum* feeding) and reduction of protein intake may reduce the incidence of pituitary neoplasia (Keeble, 2001).

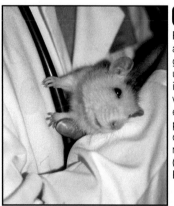

14.8

Rat with head tilt. This animal's condition gradually deteriorated until it became inappetent with marked weight loss. It was euthanased and a pituitary adenoma was diagnosed on post-mortem examination. (Courtesy of Emma Keeble.)

As these tumours may be oestrogen dependent, early ovariohysterectomy has been suggested as a possible way of decreasing the incidence of pituitary adenoma. It has been speculated that the anti-oestrogen drug toremifene at 12 mg/kg orally q24h may be a useful prophylactic agent in female rats to prevent formation of pituitary and mammary tumours (Keeble, 2001). Supportive care is indicated, but the long-term prognosis in these cases is poor and affected animals commonly deteriorate.

West Nile virus

This virus has been reported as infecting black-tailed prairie dogs (*Cynomys ludovicianus*), grey squirrels (*Scuirus carolinensis*), fox squirrels (*S. niger*) (Kuipel *et al.*, 2003) and eastern chipmunks (*Tamias striatus*) in the United States. Hamsters experimentally infected with WNV showed lethargy and decreased food consumption and grooming activity 6–7 days post inoculation. By 7–10 days most hamsters were showing neurological signs, including hindlimb paralysis, tremors, difficulty in walking, circling and loss of balance, and most affected hamsters died between days 7 and 14. Residual neurological signs remained in the survivors (Xiao *et al.*, 2001). Diagnosis in eastern fox squirrels was through histopathology, immunohistochemical staining of selected tissues (heart, brain, liver, lung, kidneys), reverse transcriptase PCR and viral RNA extraction. Lymphoplasmacytic inflammation was seen in the brain, heart, kidney and liver. Inflammatory lesions seen in squirrels, especially in the myocardium, were severe (Kuipel *et al.*, 2003).

Disorders associated with convulsions/seizures

Epilepsy

Selectively bred lines of gerbils develop an inherited form of spontaneous epilepsy (Figure 14.9), usually beginning around 2 months of age and often increasing in incidence and severity until 6 months old. Seizures are caused by a deficiency of glutamine synthetase, the enzyme that catabolizes glutamate, an excitatory neurotransmitter. Stressors such as handling or introduction to a novel environment can precipitate seizures. The incidence in gerbils is between 20% and 40% and signs can range from mild hypnosis to myoclonic convulsions with severe seizures lasting up to approximately 5 minutes. Frequent handling in the first 3 months of life can reduce the severity and incidence of seizures. There is no permanent damage and treatment is rarely required (Scotti *et al.*, 1998). Cases of spontaneous epilepsy have also been seen in chinchillas and degus.

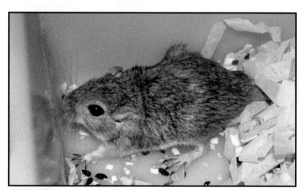

14.9 Epileptiform seizure in a young gerbil. Spontaneous epilepsy is common in selectively bred lines of gerbils and is inherited. Frequent handling in the first 3 months of life can reduce the severity and incidence of seizures. (Courtesy of Emma Keeble.)

Heat stress

Any small rodent may be vulnerable to heat stress but chinchillas, due to their dense fur coat, and guinea pigs can be particularly susceptible. Prostration, excess salivation, shallow rapid respiration and death can occur in guinea pigs exposed to ambient temperatures above 28°C but effects may be seen even as low as 21°C, especially in obese, stressed or pregnant individuals. Treatment is by immediate immersion in a cold-water bath. Subcutaneous or intraperitoneal administration of 25 ml of isotonic fluids kept at room temperature may also be beneficial. Although not attempted by this author in guinea pigs, cold-water enemas have proved effective in treating hyperthermia in a range of larger mammalian species. Normal daily water intake for guinea pigs is estimated to be 100 ml/kg.

The prognosis for treating heat stress in guinea pigs is usually poor. Care should always be taken when transporting guinea pigs in cars during hot weather. Guinea pigs housed outdoors should always have access to shade and should never be kept in glass buildings, such as greenhouses.

Mites
Severe infestations with the mite *Trixacarus caviae*, which can be intensely pruritic, may cause fitting in guinea pigs (see also Chapter 10).

Human herpes simplex 1 virus
Human HSV 1 caused seizures, disorientation, recumbency and lethargy secondary to an ocular infection in a 1-year-old chinchilla. The infection was diagnosed post mortem where a non-suppurative meningitis and polioencephalitis with ulcerative keratitis, uveitis, optic neuritis and a purulent rhinitis with presence of intranuclear inclusion bodies characterized the disease. The source of the infection could not be traced in this case, but the authors (Wohlsein *et al.*, 2002) suggested that the most likely route would be close contact with a human who had a herpetic lesion. They also cautioned that infected chinchillas represent a potential zoonotic risk of infections for humans.

Lead poisoning
Lead poisoning has the potential to occur in any rodent species as an acute or chronic disease, depending on exposure. A report on a chinchilla described acute convulsions and blindness (Hoefer, 1995) while a second report described seizures with both cases having blood lead concentrations in excess of 300 µg/dl. Both cases were responsive to chelation therapy with edetate calcium disodium at 30 mg/kg s.c. q12h for 5 days (Morgan *et al.*, 1991).

In addition to chelation therapy, it is important to remove the source of the lead and treat clinical signs, as required. Most small rodent species can be sedated to treat seizures with diazepam at 3–5 mg/kg i.m. or midazolam at 1–2 mg/kg i.m. Gerbils may be particularly vulnerable to lead poisoning due to the urine concentrating ability of their kidneys and their gnawing behaviour.

Lymphocytic choriomeningitis virus
LCMV is an arenavirus that is endemic in wild house mice (*Mus musculus*) worldwide. Infection rates of wild mice vary geographically, with some reports describing rates from 3% to 40% (Childs *et al.*, 1992). Hamsters, and less commonly gerbils, guinea pigs and chinchillas, can also become infected and spread is usually thought to be through contact with wild rodents. Transmission can be through direct contact or via aerosol, urine, saliva or *in utero*. Infections are usually asymptomatic, with some individuals clearing the infection (usually immunocompetent adults) while others persistently shed the virus. Neonatal hamsters

may be acutely affected with blepharitis, facial oedema and chronic seizures. Young hamsters can develop a chronic wasting disease associated with an immune-mediated glomerulonephritis. Signs include weight loss, depression, photophobia and seizures. Diagnosis is by pathology or serological tests (ELISA and immunofluorescent antibody staining).

LCMV can be a significant zoonosis, with serological studies in urban US locales reporting an almost 5% human infection rate (Childs *et al.*, 1991). The virus can be transmitted to humans through exposure to rodent urine, faeces, saliva or blood. In immunocompetent individuals, infection produces mild self-limiting flu-like symptoms or is asymptomatic. Aseptic meningitis can occur but is rarely fatal. In humans that are immunocompromised, LCMV can cause serious systemic infections with vasculitis and lymphocytic infiltrates occurring in multiple organs. LCMV during pregnancy can cause spontaneous abortion or severe birth defects and is likely greatly underreported as a congenital causative factor for these pregnancy outcomes. Two fatal clusters of LCMV infection in organ transplant recipients have been reported (Amman *et al.*, 2007). In one case the organ donor had been exposed to a hamster infected with LCMV.

Serological testing of pet rodents is available in the United States but the US Center for Disease Control does not recommend testing pet rodents as they suggest the results can be inaccurate and misleading (Center for Disease Control, 2005). Measures that practitioners can take to limit the zoonotic risk posed by pet rodents include encouragement of sentinel surveillance at pet stores, encouraging clients to take steps to exclude wild rodents and practice hygienic pet handling and husbandry techniques, and advising against immunocompromised and pregnant persons owning pet rodents.

Rabies
Although rodents are not natural reservoirs of the rabies virus, 621 cases were recorded in rodents or lagomorphs out of 87,700 animal cases reported in the United States between 1992 and 2002 (Eidson *et al.*, 2005). Where sylvatic strains occur, practitioners should always consider rabies infection in rodents with neurological signs and housing conditions that would allow exposure.

Disorders associated with reluctance to move, lethargy, lameness, paresis or paralysis

Osteoarthritis and ulcerative pododermatitis
Swelling and ulceration of the footpads is common in guinea pigs and often associated with bacterial infection, the aetiological agent most often being *Staphylococcus aureus*. Osteoarthritis has been documented to occur spontaneously in guinea pigs but can also be associated with pododermatitis. Ensuring a non-abrasive substrate and adequate room for exercise along with preventing obesity will all help to reduce the chance of pododermatitis developing. A detailed description of the condition can be found in Chapter 10. Vitamin C deficiency in guinea pigs may also

present as lethargy and reluctance to move. Pododermatitis is fairly common in captive prairie dogs (Boschert, 2005) and obese rats, while osteoarthritis is commonly seen in aged mice and rats.

Fractures

Fractures in small rodents occur as a result of falls, being dropped, or accidental crushing (Figure 14.10). Entrapment of small rodent limbs in spoked exercise wheels can also be a cause of fractures. Size, high activity levels and the tendency of some rodent species (e.g. rats) to chew at bandages, splints and other external stabilization devices can limit repair options and complicate healing. Non-complicated fractures normally heal rapidly in small rodents, with callus formation in as little as 7–10 days. The principles of splinting are the same as for dogs and cats. Stable closed fractures in smaller species (e.g. rats, mice) may heal satisfactorily without further stabilization. If fracture repair without further stabilization (secondary union) is attempted, all climbing devices and obstacles should be removed from the patient's environment and there should be no direct contact with cage mates. Amputation may be indicated for comminuted fractures, with pet rodents such as rats generally coping well with the loss of a limb.

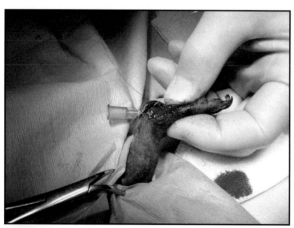

14.10 Calcaneal fracture in a guinea pig. This was successfully stabilized using a hypodermic needle as an intramedullary pin in combination with a monofilament orthopaedic wire tension band. Fractures are common in rodents and often occur secondary to trauma following mishandling. (Courtesy of Emma Keeble.)

Fractures of the tibia occur commonly in chinchillas as a result of their long thin hind limbs being inappropriately grasped for restraint. As in rabbits, surgical repair of fractures is complicated in chinchillas by bones being thin and fragile. External fixators combined with bandages have been recommended for fracture repair in chinchillas (Donnelly, 2004). It is useful to assess via radiography whether pathological bone disease has contributed to a traumatic fracture.

Radiculoneuropathy

Posterior paresis associated with a spontaneous radiculoneuropathy characterized by progressive spinal nerve root degeneration by a primary segmental demyelination has been documented in ageing laboratory rats over 18 months old (Gilmore, 2005).

Streptomycin toxicity

Acute streptomycin toxicity has been reported in gerbils treated with the neomycin–streptomycin group of antibiotics (see also Chapter 5). Gerbils treated with a single 50 mg injection of a penicillin/dihydro-streptomycin/procaine combination developed depression, flaccid paralysis and death within minutes of administration (Wightman et al., 1980).

Aminoglycoside antibiotics

Aminoglycoside antibiotics are ototoxic and nephrotoxic and their effects have been well studied in guinea pigs as models for human hearing research (see also Chapter 5). Aminoglycosides can also cause an ascending flaccid paralysis with respiratory arrest, coma and death, due to neuromuscular blockade of skeletal muscles (Harkness and Wagner, 1995). A study by Conlee et al. (1989) showed albino guinea pigs to be more susceptible to ototoxicity than pigmented animals. Aminoglycosides should always be administered with fluids, especially in older animals. A general dose rate for gentamicin in guinea pigs, chinchillas, rats, mice and hamsters is 2–4 mg/kg s.c. q8–24h. However, some studies suggest that the least nephrotoxic dosing schedule for aminoglycosides is once-daily dosing, such as with gentamicin at 6 mg/kg s.c. q24h in guinea pigs (Campbell et al., 1996).

Disorders associated with nutritional deficiencies and excesses

Vitamin C deficiency

Guinea pigs cannot endogenously synthesize vitamin C (L-ascorbic acid) as they lack the gene that controls production of L-gulonolactone oxidase thus preventing the conversion of L-gulonolactone to ascorbic acid. Clinical signs include anorexia, lethargy, unkempt coat, hypersalivation, lameness or a 'stiff gait' (Figure 14.11), vocalization when handled due to pain, swellings at the costochondral junctions and enlarged limb joints. Diarrhoea, oculonasal discharge, fractures and bacterial infections secondary to immunosuppression may also be seen. Clinical signs are usually more severe in young growing animals, whereas adults with marginal deficiencies and animals in early-stage disease may only present with anorexia and lethargy.

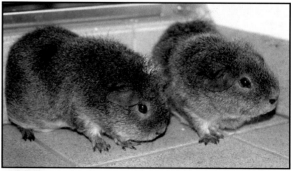

14.11 Rex guinea pigs with vitamin C deficiency. These animals presented with stiffness of all four limbs and a shuffling gait. A diagnosis was made based on clinical signs and history. The animals responded well to vitamin C supplementation. (Courtesy of Emma Keeble.)

Radiology may reveal enlargement of the epiphyseal region of long bones and the costochondral junctions. Due to the effects of deficiency on blood vessel integrity, post-mortem examination may reveal haemorrhage into joints (especially the stifle), skeletal muscle, the gingivae, intestine and subcutaneous tissues. The diversity of clinical signs seen is attributable to ascorbic acid's critical role in the formation of the structural protein, type IV collagen.

Treatment involves administration of vitamin C at 50 mg/kg daily. This is best given subcutaneously until clinical improvement is noted (usually approximately 7 days); thereafter it can be given orally. It may be best to avoid intramuscular injections, given that abnormal collagen synthesis precipitates skeletal muscle haemorrhage and myofilament fragmentation. Vitamin C is water soluble and so toxicity due to overdose is highly unlikely. Resolution of clinical signs may take 7 days. Guinea pigs presented with chronic disease, no matter what the aetiology may be, should be supplemented with vitamin C as tissue levels are maintained for approximately 4 days only.

Guinea pigs require vitamin C at 10 mg/kg daily for maintenance and 30 mg/kg daily during pregnancy. The easiest way to achieve this is by adding vitamin C tablets to the drinking water at 200–400 mg/l. Water should be changed daily, due to the instability of vitamin C. While adequate vitamin C is now present in most commercial guinea pig foods (not rabbit food) the labile nature of this vitamin means that inadequate or prolonged storage can decrease levels to below maintenance. Commercial foods, stored in a cool and dry area, should be used within 90 days of the production date.

Vitamin D and osteoporosis

Osteoporosis in guinea pigs has been associated with excess dietary vitamin D, usually due to oversupplementation with cod liver oil in animals receiving adequate hay and sunlight. Clinical signs include reluctance to move and hindlimb paresis. Similar signs may be seen in inactive obese cage-confined individuals; this condition is often termed cage paralysis.

Vitamin E and muscular dystrophy

Guinea pigs can develop muscular dystrophy caused by diets deficient in vitamin E (often due to inappropriate storage under hot moist conditions). Vitamin E deficiency is characterized by joint stiffness, lameness, lethargy and weakness due to muscle necrosis. There will be elevated levels of serum CPK. At post-mortem examination, skeletal muscles appear pallid with proliferation of sarcolemmal nuclei. Treatment of clinical cases is with daily dosing of vitamin E at 5–10 mg/kg orally until signs resolve.

Metastatic calcification

Metastatic calcification can cause muscle and joint stiffness, as well as weight loss, renal failure and more commonly acute death. It is most often seen in aged guinea pigs and is thought to be due to diets high in calcium and phosphorus and low in magnesium and potassium. It is most often diagnosed as an incidental post-mortem finding. Calcium deposits may be seen in the lungs, aorta, heart, kidneys, liver, skeletal muscle and commonly in the soft tissue around the elbows and ribs. Mineralization is irreversible once present, but nutritional disease in the guinea pig can be prevented by provision of an adequate diet. The diet should contain 0.3–0.4% magnesium, 0.4–1.4% potassium, 0.9–1.1% calcium and 0.6–0.7% phosphorus. The correct ratio of Ca:P is 1.5:1.0. The diet should contain 50 mg/kg of vitamin E and no more than 1600 IU of vitamin D/kg.

Pregnancy toxaemia and hypocalcaemia

Pregnancy toxaemia and hypocalcaemia are not uncommon in guinea pigs. Pregnancy toxaemia is most commonly seen in obese primiparous sows 7–14 days prior to or 1 week after parturition. However, since the predisposing factors also include obesity, fasting, diet change and environmental stressors, boars and virgin sows are also susceptible. Uterine blood vessel ischaemia associated with visceral displacement due to large litter size can also precipitate this condition. Acute death occurs commonly, but affected animals can become progressively anorectic, stop drinking and become prostrate with muscle fasciculations, incoordination and death occurring within 5 days of onset of signs. See Chapter 13 for more detail.

Hypocalcaemia associated with pregnancy and lactation has an onset and clinical signs similar to those seen with pregnancy toxaemia, but it is more commonly seen in obese multiparous sows.

References and further reading

Amman BR, Pavlin, Albarino CG *et al.* (2007) Pet rodents and fatal lymphocytic choriomeningitis in transplant patients. *Emerging Infectious Diseases* [serial on the Internet]. 13. Cited 16 July 2007. Available from http://www.cdc.gov/EID/content/13/5/719.htm

Boschert KR (2005) Rodents. In: *The Merck Veterinary Manual, 9th edn,* ed. CM Kahn. Merck and Co, Whitehouse Station, New Jersey

Campbell BG, Bartholow S and Rosin E (1996) Bacterial killing by use of once daily gentamicin dosage in guinea pigs with *Escherichia coli* infection. *American Journal of Veterinary Research* **57**(11), 1627–1630

Carpenter J (2005) *Exotic Animal Formulary, 3rd edn.* Elsevier, St Louis

Center for Disease Control (2005) *Interim Guidance for Minimizing Risk for Human Lymphocytic Choriomeningitis Virus Infection Associated with Rodents,* July 29, 2005 / 54(Dispatch); 1-3 cited 22 February 2008. Available from http://www.cdc.gov/mmwr/preview/mmwrhtml/mm54d729a1.htm

Childs JE, Glass GE, Ksiazek *et al.* (1991) Human–rodent contact and infection with lymphocytic choriomeningitis and Seoul viruses in an inner city population. *American Journal of Tropical Medicine and Hygiene* **44**, 117–121

Childs JE, Glass GE, Korch GW *et al.* (1992) Lymphocytic choriomeningitis virus infection and house mouse (*Mus musculus*) distribution in urban Baltimore. *American Journal of Tropical Medicine and Hygiene* **47**, 27–34

Conlee JW, Gill SS, McCandless PT *et al.* (1989) Differential susceptibility to aminoglycoside ototoxicity between albino and pigmented guinea pigs. *Hearing Research* **41**, 43–52

Donnelly TM (2004) Disease problems of chinchillas. In: *Ferrets, Rabbits and Rodents Clinical Medicine and Surgery, 2nd edn,* ed. KE Quesenberry and JW Carpenter, pp. 255–265. WB Saunders, St Louis

Dubey JP, Clark TR and Yanis D (2000) *Frenkelia microti* infection in a chinchilla (*Chinchilla laniger*) in the United States. *Journal of Parasitology* **86**, 1149–1150

Eidson M, Matthews SD, Willsey AL *et al.* (2005) Rabies virus infection in a guinea pig and seven pet rabbits. *Journal of the American Veterinary Medical Association* **227**, 932–935

Gilmore SA (2005) Spinal nerve root degeneration in aging laboratory rats: a light microscopic study. *The Anatomical Record* **174**(2), 251–257

Harkness JE and Wagner JE (1995) *The Biology and Medicine of Rabbits and Rodents, 4th edn*. Williams and Wilkins, Media, Pennsylvania

Hoefer HL (1995) Chinchillas. In: *Proceedings of the North American Veterinary Conference*. Orlando, Florida, pp. 672–673

Hrapkiewicz K, Medina L and Holmes DD (1998) *Clinical Laboratory Animal Medicine – An Introduction, 2nd edn*. Iowa State University Press, Ames, Iowa

Huerkamp MJ, Murray, KA and Orosz, SE (1996) Guinea pigs. In: *Handbook of Rodent and Rabbit Medicine, 2nd edn*, ed. K Laber-Laird, MM Swindle and P Flecknell, pp. 91–150. Elsevier Science, Oxford

Kazacos KR (2001) *Baylisascaris procyonis* and related species. In: *Parasitic Diseases of Wild Mammals, 2nd edn*, ed. WM Samuel, MJ Pybus and AA Kocan. Iowa State University Press, Ames, Iowa

Keeble E (2001) Endocrine diseases in small mammals. *In Practice* **23**, 570–585

Keeble E (2006) Nervous and musculoskeletal disorders. In: *BSAVA Manual of Rabbit Medicine and Surgery, 2nd edn*, ed. A Meredith and P Flecknell, pp. 103–116. BSAVA Publications, Gloucester

Kiupel M, Simmons HA, Fitzgerald SD *et al.* (2003) West Nile virus infection in eastern fox squirrels (*Sciurus niger*). *Veterinary Pathology* **40**, 703–707

Meingassner JG and Burtscher H (1977) Double infection of the brain with *Frenkelia* species and *Toxoplasma gondii* in *Chinchilla laniger*. [In German] *Veterinary Pathology* **14**, 146–153

Meredith A and Redrobe G (ed.) (2002) *BSAVA Manual of Exotic Pets, 4th edn*. BSAVA Publications, Gloucester

Morgan RV, Pearce LK, Moore FM *et al.* (1991) Demographic data and treatment of small companion animals with lead poisoning: 347 cases (1977–1986). *Journal of the American Veterinary Medical Association* **199**, 98–102

Najecki D and Tate B (1999). Husbandry and management of the degu. *Laboratory Animal Magazine* **28**, 54–62

National Research Council (1991) *Infectious Diseases of Mice and Rats*. National Academy Press, Washington DC

O'Rourke D (2004) Disease problems of guinea pigs. In: *Ferrets, Rabbits and Rodents Clinical Medicine and Surgery, 2nd edn*, ed. KE Quesenberry and JW Carpenter, pp. 245–254. WB Saunders, St Louis

Percy DH and Barthold SW (1993) *Pathology of Laboratory Rodents and Rabbits*. Iowa State University Press, Ames, Iowa

Richardson VCG (1997) *Diseases of Small Domestic Rodents*. Blackwell Science, Oxford

Richardson VCG (2000) *Diseases of Domestic Guinea Pigs, 2nd edn*. Blackwell Science, Oxford

Scotti AL, Bollag O, Nitsch C *et al.* (1998) Seizure patterns in Mongolian gerbils subjected to a prolonged weekly test schedule: evidence for kindling-like phenomenon in the adult population. *Epilepsia* **39**, 567–576

Strake JG, Davis LA, LaRegina M *et al.* (1996) Chinchillas. In: *Handbook of Rodent and Rabbit Medicine*, ed. K Laber-Laird, MM Swindle and P Flecknell, pp. 151–181. Elsevier Science, Oxford

Wightman SR, Mann PC and Wagner JE (1980) Dihydrostreptomycin toxicity in the Mongolian gerbil, *Meriones unguiculatus*. *Laboratory Animal Science* **30**(1), 71–75

Wilkerson MJ, Melendy A and Stauber E (1997) An outbreak of listeriosis in a breeding colony of chinchillas. *Journal of Veterinary Diagnostic Investigation* **9**, 320–323

Wohlsein P, Thiele A, Fehr M *et al.* (2002) Spontaneous human herpes virus type 1 infection in a chinchilla (*Chinchilla lanigera f. dom.*). *Acta neuropathologica* **104**, 674–678

Xiao SY, Guzman G, Zhang H, Travassos da Rosa APA and Tesh RB (2001) West Nile Virus infection in the golden hamster (*Mesocricetus auratus*): a model for West Nile Encephalitis. *Emerging Infectious Diseases* **7**(4), 714–721

15

Rodents: ophthalmology

Fabiano Montiani-Ferreira

Basic ocular anatomical features of rodents

The anatomy and physiology of the eyeball (bulbus oculi) is fairly uniform among most rodent species, but they do show some interesting structural differences regarding the bony orbital anatomy.

Bony orbital anatomy

Three elements constitute the zygomatic arch in rodents: (i) the zygomatic bone; (ii) the zygomatic process of the maxillary bone; and (iii) the zygomatic process of the temporal bone. The presence of a prominent and well developed zygomatic process of the maxillary bone is what differentiates the zygomatic arch of rodents from that of dogs and cats.

The shape of the zygomatic arch varies considerably among rodent species. In chinchillas and guinea pigs it is flat and wide rostrally, making the infraorbital region of these two species look very robust. In smaller rodents, like gerbils, hamsters, mice and rats, the zygomatic arch is elongated and proportionally thinner and delicate. The orbital shape tends to be ovoid in rats, mice and hamsters and circular in chinchillas and guinea pigs. In its general outline, the zygomatic arch may be convex, as it is in rats, mice, chinchillas and guinea pigs, or concave, as in gerbils and hamsters (Figure 15.1).

Eyeball and eyelids

Following the same common pattern of most mammals, nocturnal species of rodent (in comparison with diurnal species) have larger eyes (Figure 15.2a), which is manifest partly as especially broad corneal surfaces, to maximize the amount of light received by the retina. Most rodents have eyes that were evolutionarily adapted for night vision.

Mice and rats have three lacrimal structures: the intraorbital gland; the extraorbital gland; and the Harderian gland. The intraorbital gland is located deep in the retrobulbar space. The extraorbital gland is located near the base of the masseter muscle and commonly has been misinterpreted as a neoplasm because of its unusual location. The Harderian gland is U-shaped and located posterior to the globe in the orbit.

The majority of rodent species are born with the eyelids closed, opening on the 12th to 14th day of life. Chinchillas and pacas (*Cuniculus paca*) have rudimentary third eyelids. Another common feature for most rodents is the presence of a large (proportionally to its small globe) spherical lens that occupies a considerable part of the eye. Most rodents have circular pupils, but chinchillas curiously have vertical elliptical pupils that contract to small vertical slits (Figure 15.2b).

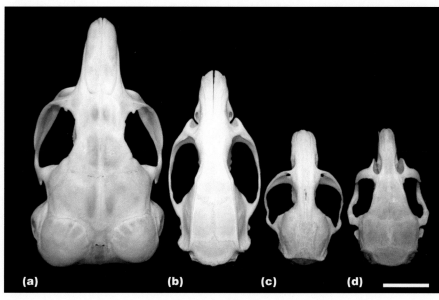

15.1 Dorsal view of skulls of four different rodent species (without the mandible): **(a)** chinchilla; **(b)** albino Wistar rat; **(c)** golden hamster; **(d)** gerbil. Note the convex shape of the zygomatic arch in (a) and (b), and its concavity in (c) and (d), as well as its thin aspect in (b) and (c); the proportionally larger interorbital breadth in (a) and (d), and the round shaped orbit in (a). Bar: 10 mm. (Courtesy of Marcello Machado.)

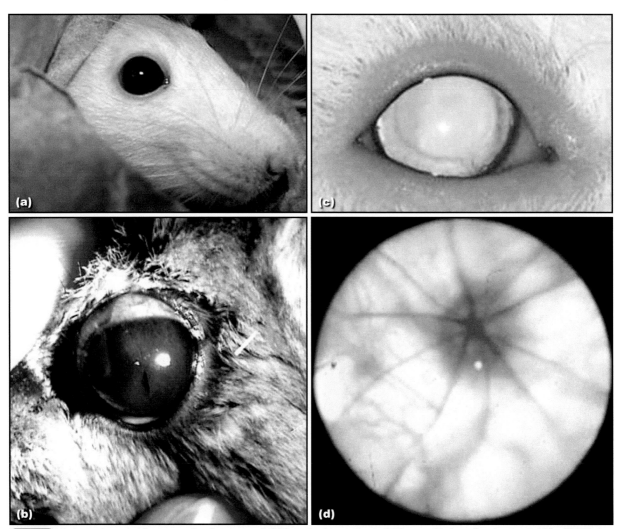

15.2 Selected normal features of rodent eyes. **(a)** Note the large eyes of this rat with heavily pigmented iris. **(b)** Note the slit pupil of the chinchilla eye. **(c)** Albino guinea pig: note the semi-transparent appearance of the iris. It is even hard to tell the pupillary margins. The overall red appearance of the eye is due to the lack of pigment and predominant reddish fundic reflection. **(d)** Note the reddish appearance of the fundus of this albino rat. Additionally, note the holangiotic retina with arterioles and venules that radiate from the optic disc like spokes on a bicycle wheel.

The uveal tissues of albino rodents, like other parts of their bodies, have no pigment. This gives a bright red semi-transparent appearance when illuminated by ophthalmic instruments (Figure 15.2c). The same principle applies to the fundus of albino rodents (Figure 15.2d). Some rodents possess a tapetum lucidum.

Mice and rats have a rod-dominated holangiotic retina with arterioles and venules that radiate from the optic disc like spokes on a bicycle wheel (Figure 15.2d). Guinea pigs have paurangiotic and chinchillas have anangiotic, atapetal retinas. The optic nerve head of mice and rats often appears small (Figure 15.2d), cupped, or possibly colobomatous, because optic nerve fibres do not become myelinated until after leaving the eye through the poorly developed lamina cribosa.

Rats have an orbital plexus formed by deep orbital veins. In contrast, mice have a large dilated channel, a venous sinus.

Physical restraint and ophthalmic examination

A protocol for ophthalmic examination is shown in Figure 15.3. Physical restraint is an important issue when performing an ophthalmic examination in pet rodents (see Chapter 2 for restraint techniques). If smaller rodents are restrained by the scruff of the neck, transitory exophthalmos is likely to occur, particularly in hamsters (see Figure 15.4a). Sedation may rarely be required for ophthalmological examination, such as the collection of conjunctival cytological samples.

The first step of the examination should always be to observe the animal from arm's length (about 66 cm) looking for general symmetry of the head and eyes, the blink rate and the presence of discharges. At this point, the eyelid–globe position should be assessed for entropion, ectropion, third eyelid protrusion, strabismus and exophthalmos/enophthalmos.

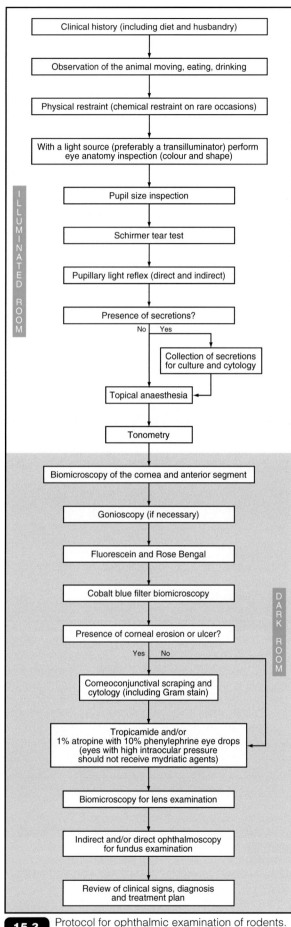

Clinical history (including diet and husbandry)

↓

Observation of the animal moving, eating, drinking

↓

Physical restraint (chemical restraint on rare occasions)

↓

With a light source (preferably a transilluminator) perform eye anatomy inspection (colour and shape)

↓

Pupil size inspection

↓

Schirmer tear test

↓

Pupillary light reflex (direct and indirect)

↓

Presence of secretions?
No — Yes

Collection of secretions for culture and cytology

↓

Topical anaesthesia

↓

Tonometry

↓

Biomicroscopy of the cornea and anterior segment

↓

Gonioscopy (if necessary)

↓

Fluorescein and Rose Bengal

↓

Cobalt blue filter biomicroscopy

↓

Presence of corneal erosion or ulcer?
Yes — No

Corneoconjunctival scraping and cytology (including Gram stain)

↓

Tropicamide and/or 1% atropine with 10% phenylephrine eye drops (eyes with high intraocular pressure should not receive mydriatic agents)

↓

Biomicroscopy for lens examination

↓

Indirect and/or direct ophthalmoscopy for fundus examination

↓

Review of clinical signs, diagnosis and treatment plan

ILLUMINATED ROOM

DARK ROOM

15.3 Protocol for ophthalmic examination of rodents. (Modified from Montiani-Ferreira, 2001.)

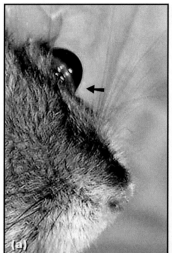

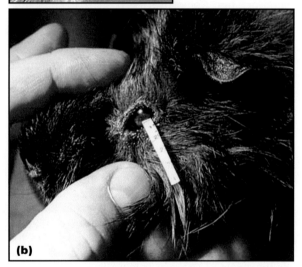

15.4 Ophthalmic examination in rodent species. **(a)** This hamster was restrained by the scruff of the neck and transitory exophthalmos occurred (arrow). **(b)** Use of the conventional 6 mm-wide Schirmer tear test (STT) strip in a guinea pig. Normal production can be low in this species (about 1–2 mm). (Courtesy of Giuseppe Visigalli.)

The head and eyes should be observed from different directions; for example, also from above the head to check for exophthalmos/enophthalmos.

Mydriasis

Mydriatics have variable effects in rodents. Those with pigmented irides (see Figure 15.2a) are more resistant to the pharmacological effect of mydriatics, possibly because the drug binds to melanin in the iris, reducing availability to the synaptic terminal. Repeated application of 1% atropine with 10% phenylephrine every 5 minutes three to four times usually achieves mydriasis (Kern, 1989).

The large size of the lens in most rodent eyes results in distortion of the fundus image during ophthalmoscopy, causing the retina to seem to float in the vitreous cavity. Because of its small size, the mouse fundus is difficult to examine but it can be done using +30 to +40 dioptre indirect ophthalmoscopy lenses. Alternatively, a rapid convenient way to examine the mouse fundus can be performed using an ordinary stereoscopic dissecting microscope. This method provides more information than ophthalmoscopic examination because of the higher magnification of the microscope and the three-dimensional information it provides. The following steps can be accomplished in a few minutes (Pinto and Enroth-Cugell, 2000):

1. In a mouse under general anaesthesia, the pupil is dilated and the head positioned to allow the line of sight of the eye to be colinear with the optical axis of the microscope.
2. The cornea is covered with a droplet of solution with approximately the same index of refraction as the cornea (0.98% NaCl with 2% methylcellulose, 400 centipoise).
3. A piece of thin glass, such as a microscope cover glass, is placed over the solution at an angle that directs glare away from the microscope.

Tonometry

The Schiøtz tonometer cannot be used in most rodents because of its large footplate. However, the portable Tono-Pen™ XL applanation tonometer is ideal for use in most rodents, especially those with corneal diameters over 9 mm. Sometimes it is possible to obtain reliable readings even in corneal diameters as small as 5 mm. In the author's experience, tonometry using the Tono-Pen™ is uncomplicated in rats, guinea pigs and chinchillas whereas obtaining good readings in mice and hamsters with this instrument is quite challenging and results are, perhaps, a bit imprecise. Another option for performing tonometry in small rodents is the handheld rebound tonometer called TonoLab.

Lacrimal production

Measurement of lacrimal production is also possible in chinchillas and guinea pigs using the conventional 6 mm-wide Schirmer tear test (STT) strips (see Figure 15.4b). Normal parameters for STT for chinchillas are quite similar to those of other small animals, at 20.00 ± 7.8 mm/minute (Montiani-Ferreira, 2001). On the other hand, in guinea pigs, in the author's experience the results for STTs are quite low with a great variance (around 2.5 ± 2.0 mm/minute).

For practical purposes, the traditional Schirmer test filter paper strip can be cut in half lengthwise to 3 mm for smaller species. This procedure makes STT possible in small rodents with small conjunctival sacs, such as gerbils, mice and hamsters. Furthermore, the procedure results in a longer length of wetted strip length, improving the margin of error of the test. However, normal values using this technique have not been established.

Examination for associated conditions

In addition to the large number of primary conditions the eye may develop, it may also show changes secondary to systemic abnormalities. A thorough examination of the eye may prove to be a valuable step in investigating systemic disease. For instance, eye discharge can be associated with respiratory diseases, and enophthalmic (shrunken) eyes can be associated with dehydration.

As mentioned previously, most rodents possess proportionally large and prominent eyeballs. Because of that, traumatic injuries to other parts of the body may cause secondary ophthalmic lesions. Thus, when traumatic injuries are observed, the clinician should closely examine the eyes.

Eye diseases can also be seen secondary to dental disease of the maxillary teeth in many rodents, particularly guinea pigs and chinchillas. Thus, a thorough dental examination can prove invaluable for veterinary ophthalmologists examining a rodent patient.

Ophthalmological diseases

Microphthalmos and anophthalmos

Several experimental models of microphthalmos exist in the rat. In addition to these, spontaneous microphthalmos can occur as an incidental finding in standard non-microphthalmic strains.

Anophthalmos has been reported in the rat, as in many other species, but generally only in specifically anophthalmic strains rather than occurring as an incidental finding in otherwise normal rats, as does microphthalmos (Williams, 2002).

Disorders of the eyelids and periocular infections

Periocular and/or retrobulbar abscesses may be caused by tooth-root infections. These can be associated with blepharitis, conjunctivitis and epiphora, hemifacial swelling and asymmetry, exophthalmos, proptosis, exposure keratitis (Figure 15.5) and generalized sepsis (see also Chapter 8).

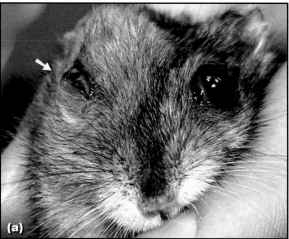

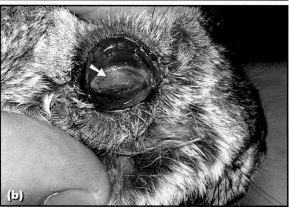

15.5 Representative cases of ophthalmic conditions caused by tooth-root infections. **(a)** Periocular abscess with blepharitis and hemifacial swelling causing marked facial asymmetry (arrowed) due to a cheek tooth-root infection in the right eye of this hamster. **(b)** Exposure keratitis (arrowed), chemosis and exophthalmos due to a retrobulbar abscess in a chinchilla, secondary to a tooth-root infection (an apical abscess).

Blepharitis can be a component of infectious conjunctivitis in hamsters and gerbils (see below for a more detailed discussion).

Periocular dermatitis is common in gerbils. Dermatitis in the periocular region combined with involvement of the tarsal glands (tarsal adenitis) may aggravate the severity of the disease considerably. Blepharitis has also been reported secondary to dermatophyte infections in young guinea pigs (Gaarder and Kern, 2001).

Treatment may vary but usually includes abscess drainage or surgical debridement and curettage combined with a broad-spectrum systemic antibiotic or antifungal therapy.

In some cases, as a result of the healing process, scar tissue formation can lead to secondary eyelid conformational problems (entropion or ectropion). Primary entropion has also been reported in some rodents, particularly guinea pigs, and a simple surgical technique (Hotz–Celsus procedure) can correct the defect.

Epiphora and chromodacryorrhoea in rats and mice

Epiphora can be associated with obstruction of the nasolacrimal duct as a result of dental root infection, malocclusion, overgrowth of the incisors or neoplasia. Corrective dentistry may treat this problem and prevent it from recurring (see also Chapter 8).

The most common abnormality associated with the lacrimal structure of mice and rats is dacryoadenitis, or inflammation of the Harderian gland. Rats and mice sometimes produce profuse amounts of porphyrin in their Harderian gland secretions. The porphyrin-filled tears overflow and dry on and around the eyelids, forming a dark red crust, which can be mistaken for dried blood; this condition is called chromodacryorrhoea. The red–brown staining can involve the periorbital fur and the fur of the front paws, since rats and mice groom their eyes with their front paws. Nutritional deficiencies, physiological stresses, mycoplasmosis and sialodacryoadenitis are important causes of chromodacryorrhoea. Dacryoadenitis in rats and rarely mice can be associated with the sialodacryoadenitis virus (SDAV), which is a coronavirus that is closely related antigenically to mouse hepatitis virus and Parker's rat coronavirus. SDAV is a common pathogen in rats and disease can occur as an enzootic infection in breeding colonies or as epizootics in susceptible populations (see also Chapter 12).

Histological abnormalities of the affected gland include diffuse oedema, necrosis and widespread inflammation with the presence of a mixed population of inflammatory cells (McGee and Maronpot, 1979). Treatment is supportive and directed at preventing secondary bacterial disease, as no specific therapy exists. Thus, red periocular staining in laboratory animals or pet rats should be a warning sign of potentially severe systemic disease or stress. Because it can resemble dried blood, patients may be presented for what their owners describe as 'bleeding from the eyes'. A useful way to tell blood from porphyrin is the fact that dried porphyrin glows pink under ultraviolet light, whereas blood does not.

Conjunctivitis and other conjunctival diseases

Conjunctivitis is commonly seen in rodents, especially hamsters, and the resulting exudate may commonly result in the eyelids sticking together (Figure 15.6). Keratoconjunctivitis sicca (KCS) is sporadically diagnosed in several species of rodent and should be considered in the differential list of diagnoses for ocular discharge (Figure 15.7).

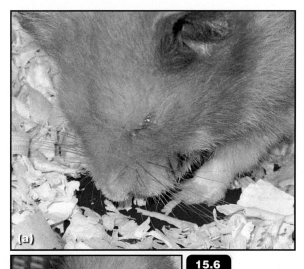

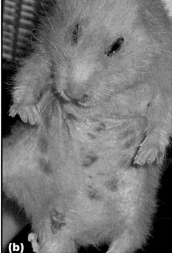

15.6 Representative cases of conjunctivitis in rodents. **(a)** Note that the resulting exudate made the eyelids of the left eye stick together. In this case, the conjunctivitis was associated with severe respiratory disease. **(b)** This bilateral blepharoconjunctivitis case was associated with a skin infection caused by *Staphylococcus* spp. (Courtesy of Carlos Alexandre Pessoa.)

Cause	Examples
Conformational lid abnormalities	Entropion, ectropion, trichiasis (Texel animals are at risk), lid tumours
Systemic, often immunosuppressive conditions	Respiratory disease
Spread of infection from elsewhere	Skin, ears, lips and teeth
Tear film abnormalities	Keratoconjunctivitis sicca (dry eye)
Irritants	Chemicals, fumes, dust

15.7 Secondary causes of conjunctivitis in rodents.

Important items to bear in mind while examining the eye with discharge and inflamed conjunctiva are:

- Careful history taking and examination may reveal the predisposing factors
- A Schirmer tear test (STT) is indicated whenever the conjunctiva is inflamed
- Blepharitis commonly accompanies chronic cases of conjunctivitis
- Eyelid and orbital conformational abnormalities frequently result in secondary conjunctivitis
- Palpebral neoplasms may cause conjunctival hyperaemia when in contact with the conjunctiva
- Abnormal hair and eyelashes (trichiasis, ectopic cilia) can also predispose the conjunctiva and corneal surface to inflammation. It is important that this is checked in Texel guinea pigs, in which the coat is composed of short bristly hairs.

Bacterial conjunctivitis

Bacteria, especially Gram-positive species, can frequently be cultured in low numbers from the normal conjunctival sac of most mammals. It is important to remember this fact when evaluating bacterial cultures from the conjunctiva. Bacterial conjunctivitis is more commonly the result of a predisposing factor that allows an overgrowth of invading bacteria, or even bacteria that are not part of the normal conjunctival flora. Many bacteria and viruses are associated with conjunctivitis in rodents, including *Streptococcus pneumoniae*, *Pasteurella pneumotropica*, *Salmonella* spp., *Streptococcus* spp., *Mycoplasma pulmonis*, *Pseudomonas aeruginosa*, *Streptobacillus moniliformis*, Sendai virus, mousepox and lymphocytic choriomeningitis virus, among others. In guinea pigs, cases of conjunctivitis have been reported as being associated with *Chlamydophila caviae* and *Listeria monocytogenes* infections. In rats, as in mice, mycoplasmosis is one of the most common causes of conjunctivitis not associated with intraocular lesions.

Conjunctival scrapings for cytology and swabs for culture are indicated if the conjunctivitis is severe or is chronic or recurrent. Typical intracytoplasmic inclusion bodies may be seen on conjunctival cytological examination of guinea pigs suspected to suffer from a *Chlamydophila caviae* infection. The inflammatory cell picture is not always helpful in pointing to aetiology.

Treatment for bacterial conjunctivitis: As a general rule any underlying abnormality or predisposing factor for conjunctivitis should always be treated along with the ocular signs. A broad-spectrum antibiotic such as triple antibiotic ophthalmic solution (neomycin–bacitracin–polymyxin) or trimethoprim–polymyxin eye drops should be instilled every 6 hours.

Topical corticosteroids may be useful as long as any infection is treated appropriately and there is no corneal ulceration. Topical ocular steroid therapy can retard corneal healing and can thus cause perforation of the globe if there is thinning of the cornea or sclera. Several potential side effects due to long-term use of topical steroids have been reported in several species, such as an increase in intraocular pressure (steroid-induced ocular hypertension), cataract formation, and enhanced ocular susceptibility to and severity of fungal and viral infections. Additionally, there is a risk of developing systemic signs such as polydipsia, polyphagia, polyuria and other iatrogenic hyperadrenocorticism signs. In the author's opinion, however, when topical steroids are used in the short term and with caution, they are safe and very efficient drugs that save many eyes.

If the response to treatment is poor, the diagnosis should be re-evaluated. As already mentioned, conjunctivitis and discharge may be associated with upper airway infection in rodents; therefore, systemic antibiotics are commonly prescribed as well.

Non-infectious causes of conjunctivitis

Conjunctivitis in guinea pigs has also been reported secondary to vitamin C deficiency (scurvy) (see also Chapter 14). Other non-infectious primary causes of conjunctival discharge in rodents include ocular irritation from soiled bedding, stress, multiple vitamin deficiencies, water deprivation and lack of grooming.

Bedding material and ammonia vapours from urine-soaked bedding can contain substances that are particularly irritating for the cornea and conjunctiva and may contribute to or cause conjunctivitis and ocular discharge. Red cedar shavings contain aromatic hydrocarbons and should not be used as bedding material. The use of this type of bedding can cause severe conjunctivitis, with chemosis and ocular discharge. Hay may also be problematic for guinea pigs, because small pieces of hay in the diet or used as bedding material may become lodged in the conjunctiva and cause corneal ulceration. Treatment for non-infectious causes of conjunctivitis includes removal of the primary agent and application of topical steroids, provided that there is no corneal ulcer.

Conjunctival nodules

Differential diagnoses for conjunctival irritation with nodules are lymphosarcoma and a syndrome known as pea eye. The pea eye syndrome (Figure 15.8) is unique to guinea pigs and appears as a nodule that protrudes from the inferior conjunctival sac, unilaterally or bilaterally. The nodule is habitually composed of glandular tissue consistent with lacrimal or zygomatic

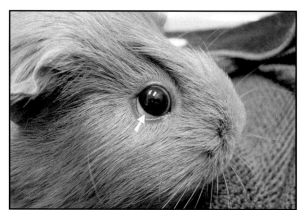

15.8 Guinea pig with 'pea eye syndrome'. Note the nodule that protrudes from the inferior conjunctival sac (arrowed). (Courtesy of Daniel H Johnson.)

glands. Generally there is a history of weight gain prior to the consultation. No treatment is usually necessary, though the nodules may cause minor ectropion and exposure conjunctivitis. If the latter two ophthalmic signs are severe enough, surgical removal of the nodule may be necessary.

Corneal diseases

Corneal dermoids
Corneal dermoids have been reported in a number of guinea pigs. Dermoids are most commonly found on the cornea; however, corneoscleral and sceral dermoids have also been reported. This congenital disease manifests as a mass consisting of skin and its dermal appendages (including hair) localized at the corneal surface (Figure 15.9). A corneal dermoid is considered a choristoma (normal tissue in an abnormal location). Surgical excision to reduce irritation and improve vision of the affected eye is the ideal treatment. The surgical excision creates a corneal epithelial defect. Thus, antibiotic eye drops are prescribed post-surgically for 10 days. Although rare in rodents and small laboratory animals, dermoids should be considered in the differential diagnoses of conjunctival and corneal abnormalities.

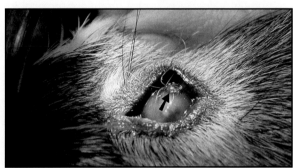

15.9 This guinea pig was diagnosed with a corneal dermoid. In this case a patch of normal skin tissue is abnormally located in the cornea (arrowed). Surgical excision is the treatment for the condition. (Courtesy of Daniel H Johnson.)

Corneal dystrophy
Corneal dystrophy (or degeneration) is a common abnormality of the rodent cornea. It usually appears as small dense white punctate opacities. The environment seems to influence the occurrence of these corneal opacities. It has been proposed that bacteria in faecal material convert urinary urea to ammonia, which then contacts the cornea and causes necrosis of the corneal epithelium. This change eventually results in scarring and mineralization of the stroma with dysplasia of the overlying epithelium. When the environment is improved the lesions also seem to improve. Prognosis for retaining vision is good, but leucomas (whitish corneal scars) are a common consequence.

Corneal lymphosarcoma
Lymphosarcoma is rare in guinea pigs but has been reported to infiltrate the cornea (Steinberg, 2000). Diagnosis is based on the cytology of biopsy samples of conjunctival tissue. Ocular lymphosarcoma is usually an incidental finding, as part of the systemic illness. Ocular prognosis depends on the systemic remission of the neoplasia.

Corneal ulcers
Most rodent species are prone to corneal ulcers. The majority of such ulcers are discrete (Figure 15.10a) and do not cause visible corneal craters or pit-like defects like those typically diagnosed in dogs or cats. In a number of cases, corneal ulcers become infected by microorganisms (more commonly bacteria), progress to an ulcerative keratitis with stromal invasion and start to be clinically more evident (Figure 15.10b). Thus, corneal ulcers and ulcerative keratitis in rodents may be separated into three groups of lesions: (i) epithelial defects not severely infected; (ii) stromal ulcers; and (iii) stromal keratitis that closely resembles stromal abscesses.

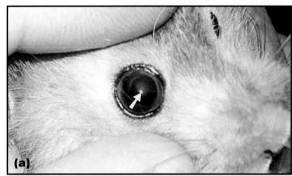

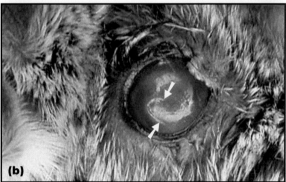

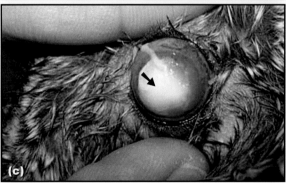

15.10 Corneal ulcers and stromal abscesses in rodents. **(a)** There is a very discrete superficial corneal epithelial defect in this hamster. The epithelial defect created a corneal opacity (arrowed). **(b)** A deeper ulcer with more evident margins (arrowed) and mild stromal bacterial invasion. The ulcer was stained with fluorescein dye. **(c)** Note the conjunctivitis, thick mucopurulent discharge and severe white purulent stromal plaque (arrowed) in this chinchilla suffering from a stromal abscess. (continues) ▶

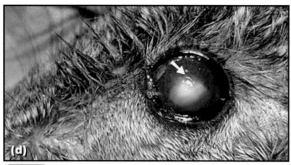

15.10 (continued) Corneal ulcers and stromal abscesses in rodents. **(d)** Note the intense stromal keratitis and vascularization (arrowed) partially obscuring the stromal abscess in this gerbil.

Epithelial defects: An uncomplicated superficial corneal epithelial defect is manifested frequently as a discrete ulcer (see Figure 15.10a), usually traumatic in origin, and is easily diagnosed with fluorescein staining. Initial treatment is generally a broad-spectrum antibiotic (e.g. a triple antibiotic such as a combination of neomycin and polymyxin B with gramicidin or bacitracin). Typically, superficial ulcers will re-epithelialize (heal) within 3–5 days. Chinchillas with ear infections and exposure keratitis due to suppression of the blink reflex usually start with superficial epithelial defects but can progress to stromal keratitis if not treated early.

Stromal ulcers: In the author's experience, conventional stromal ulcers are the least common form of presentation, but they do occur occasionally. When facing such a condition the clinician should try to identify and treat the cause (e.g. trauma or eyelid abnormalities). These ulcers may vary in deepness, but even the superficial ones are potentially serious and should be watched carefully for progression to a corneal abscess or a melting or deep ulcer. There is often a variable amount of corneal oedema and vascularization and accompanying anterior uveitis (miotic pupil, flare or even hypopyon), which adds to the discomfort and is clinically evident as anorexia. For these ulcers culture, sensitivity and cytology are indicated.

Antibiotics are selected on the basis of cytology (Gram staining of bacteria present; Figure 15.11) and modified if necessary once culture results are available. Selection of antibiotic will also depend on

Observation	Choice of antibiotic
No organisms observed	Triple antibiotic eye drops
Gram-positive cocci	Triple antibiotic eye drops and cephazolin drops (i.v. solution 50 mg/ml used topically as eye drops)
Gram-positive rods	Triple antibiotic eye drops
Gram-negative cocci	Ciprofloxacin, ofloxacin, gentamicin or tobramycin eye drops
Gram-negative rods	Ciprofloxacin, ofloxacin or tobramycin eye drops

15.11 Guide to antibiotic selection on the basis of cytology and Gram staining.

the severity and progression of the ulcer. If the ulcer is infected, antibiotics should be given frequently (e.g. initially every 2 hours).

Additionally, 1% atropine may be needed to dilate the pupil in order to relieve painful spasm of the ciliary muscle and miosis as well as to prevent synechia formation, but it should not be used more than four times a day, 5 minutes before or after the antibiotic eye drop instillation. Consideration should be given to hospitalization to treat and monitor corneal healing, or, if that is not possible, daily rechecks are recommended until the defect shows signs of healing. Lighting can be subdued during the treatment as this could help to alleviate ocular pain.

The author has no experience with the use of autologous serum in rodents. The principle of its use applies to any species and so it may be of use in rodents as part of a deep stromal ulcer treatment protocol. Blood should be drawn from the patient (or from another animal of the same species) and spun down; serum should be drawn off and stored in the refrigerator in a dropper bottle or serum tube for up to 14 days. Serum is non-toxic and should be used topically as many times a day as possible, with a 5-minute interval before or after instillation of any other topical drug.

Another valuable part of a treatment protocol for deep melting ulcers that perhaps might be extrapolated from canine and feline ophthalmology is the use of acetylcysteine (5–10%) and 0.17% sodium ethylenediamine tetra-acetic acid (EDTA). Acetylcysteine and/or EDTA can be instilled hourly, in addition to the other indicated drugs, for anti-melting effect until stromal liquefaction ceases. It may be necessary to use serum, EDTA and acetylcysteine simultaneously in severe cases.

It is important to remember that topical corticosteroids should never be used for the treatment of corneal ulcers. If stromal ulcers deepen or get larger in diameter, surgical management should be considered.

Stromal keratitis (stromal abscess): Stromal keratitis or abscesses are quite common in rodents. In these lesions, epithelial migration proceeds over a traumatic corneal injury, which then seals infectious agents (bacterial, fungal or both) in the underlying stroma (see Figure 15.10c,d). In the author's experience, chinchillas in particular are often presented with this condition. Patients have conjunctivitis and a thick mucopurulent discharge (see Figure 15.10c). Under slit lamp biomicroscopic examination of the cornea, a white plaque can be observed, corresponding to purulent stromal infiltrate, which is sometimes surrounded by an intense stromal keratitis and vascularization (see Figure 15.10d). Corneal vascularization may partly obscure the abscess (see Figure 15.10d). Uveitis may be present as well. Treatment involves intensive topical and occasional systemic antibiotics (and, if indicated, antifungals), iridocycloplegics, and topical and systemic anti-inflammatory drugs. In some cases surgical drainage of the abscess is necessary. Surgery also provides material for culture and cytology to obtain an aetiological diagnosis. These stromal abscesses are often septic, but on occasion they are sterile. In most septic cases *Staphylococcus* spp. or *Pasteurella* spp. are isolated from the infection site.

Diseases of the lens

Lens luxation

Abnormalities of the lens are frequently detected during the ophthalmic examination. Abnormalities of the zonular fibres that normally hold the lens in position may occur, resulting in luxation of the lens from its normal position into the anterior chamber (Figure 15.12) or into the vitreous chamber. Lens luxation may cause glaucoma; and glaucoma may cause lens luxation. Thus it is important to determine which disease came first. A primary luxated lens can obliterate the pupillary space. This might cause disruption or blockage of the flow of the aqueous humour through the pupil.

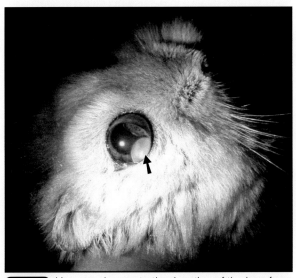

15.12 Hamster demonstrating luxation of the lens from its normal position into the anterior chamber (arrowed). (Courtesy of Giuseppe Visigalli.)

When lens luxation occurs secondarily to glaucoma, it usually occurs late in the disease once the elevated pressure within the eye has caused the zonular ligaments to tear. In such cases, attention must be given to resolving the pain associated with glaucoma.

Treatment of lens luxation *per se* usually involves surgical excision of the lens (intracapsular facectomy). This intraocular surgical procedure is invasive and requires constant rechecks in order to diagnose and treat postoperative inflammation or bacterial infection as well as its consequences.

Cataracts

The opacification of the lens, lens capsule or both is called a cataract. Cataracts (Figure 15.13) are quite common in pet rodents. They develop when the normal biochemical mechanisms of lens metabolism have been damaged, resulting in altered hydration status and subsequent osmotic effects. Numerous causes for cataracts have been identified. The most common aetiologies are discussed below.

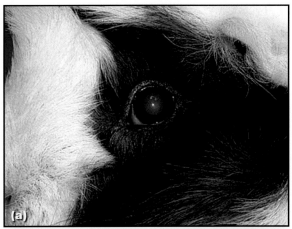

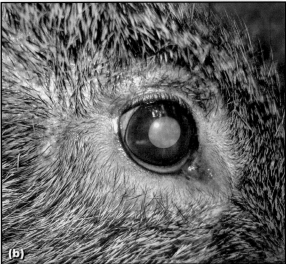

15.13 Cataracts in rodents. **(a)** Mature cataracts in a guinea pig. (Courtesy of Marc H Kramer.) **(b)** Mature cataracts in an agouti with diabetes mellitus.

Heritability/genetics: This is one of the most common causes of cataracts. Cortical cataracts of suspected genetic origin have been reported in strains of Abyssinian and English short-haired guinea pigs (Kern, 1989; Lawton, 2002).

Metabolic: Diabetes mellitus is the most common cause of metabolic cataract in several rodent species (Figure 15.13b) and is related to abnormal metabolism of glucose by the lens. These cataracts are always bilateral and form rapidly. In diabetic cataracts, hyperglycaemia overwhelms normal metabolic pathways in the lens. The consequent disruption of lens fibre membranes leads to protein precipitation and cataract formation.

Anaesthesia-related: Cataractous change can be observed in mice during anaesthesia. It depends on the type of anaesthetic agent used; for example, it has been associated with the ketamine/xylazine combination, but it has also been observed with the use of isoflurane. The pathophysiology of the condition is not fully known, but hypotheses include suppression of the blink reflex, drying of the corneal surface and degree of mydriasis during the procedure; all of these seem to lead to transcorneal water loss and alteration of aqueous humour and lens composition and osmolarity (Beaumont, 2002), leading to cataract formation. These opacities are usually transient and resolve soon after recovery from anaesthesia in most cases.

Intraocular disease: Cataracts have also been associated with intraocular diseases in rodents such as uveitis, glaucoma, lens luxation and retinal disease.

Nutritional: L-Tryptophan deficiency can cause cataracts in guinea pigs and rats, whereas L-tryptophan overdose seems to cause cataracts in rodents as well as humans. Nutritional cataracts due to excessive dietary levels of galactose, sucrose and xylose have been reported in laboratory rats (Gaarder and Kern, 2001).

Other possible causes: Cataracts can be associated with ocular malformations such as microphthalmos. Perforating injury to the cornea and lens frequently induces cataract formation, but rarely does blunt trauma cause cataracts to form.

Other causes include electric shock, radiation and toxins (including the release of posterior segment metabolic by-products in rats with retinal dystrophy) or degeneration and iatrogenic causes, such as long-term use of steroids.

Treatment of cataracts: The only treatment for cataracts is surgical removal. Cataract surgery is almost always an elective procedure. As such, other major health problems and ophthalmic abnormalities should be addressed before cataract surgery is considered. A complete ophthalmic examination should always be performed. Often electroretinography will be performed to check retinal function and modern ocular ultrasound systems can be used to detect any evidence of retinal detachment, which would preclude the surgical correction of cataracts. Selection of appropriate candidate eyes or animals for lens extraction is an important consideration for a successful outcome. Various ocular diseases that would complicate or obviate the need for cataract surgery include keratitis, KCS, uveitis, glaucoma, lens subluxation and retinal diseases, especially progressive retinal atrophy (PRA) or retinal detachment.

Phacoemulsification is certainly the most efficient technique currently available for cataract surgery for most animals and human beings. The equipment has a high purchase price, but most veterinary ophthalmologists already have or work with a phacoemulsification unit. The technique uses ultrasonic energy to fragment the opaque lens, which is then aspirated. This can be performed through a 3 mm incision, which is quite a large incision for most rodent eyes. Other complicating factors for phacoemulsification surgery in rodents, besides the small size of the globe of most species, are the large size of the lens, comparatively large corneal incision (3 mm) and the high price of the surgery. Even though all of these disadvantages exist, phacoemulsification has been performed in larger rodents such as chinchillas, guinea pigs and agoutis. For mice and rats, needle aspiration of cataractous lenses may be attempted in carefully selected cases.

Uveal disease

Two studies have been reported of young mice with a coloboma that is usually located in the ventral quadrant of the iris, resulting in a small ventrally displaced pupil (Rubin and Daly, 1982; Beaumont, 2002). A coloboma is a notch-like defect originating from a congenital abnormality due to a failure of some portion of fetal tissue to close. It may involve the choroid, retina, optic nerve, ciliary body or iris.

Synechiae and uveitis in mice are not commonly observed, though uveitis is occasionally seen in aged mice. Spontaneous intraocular neoplasms are considered relatively rare in these species. Melanoma has been reported as one of the most common ocular neoplasms in rats (Magnusson *et al.*, 1978).

Blood in the anterior segment should not necessarily be taken to indicate uveal inflammation as it is often associated with persistent embryonic vasculature around the lens and iris. Similarly, blood in the vitreous body is often related to persistent hyaloid vessels.

Glaucoma

Glaucoma has been reported in rats. Chronic glaucoma cases develop buphthalmos in rodent species, just as in dogs and cats. Glaucoma in rodents has been associated with persistent pupillary membranes that result in pupil-block glaucoma, or peripheral anterior synechiae causing angle-closure glaucoma.

Mean intraocular pressure in Lewis rats measured by applanation tonometry has been reported as 13.9 ± 4.2 mmHg (Williams, 2002). In an investigation using chinchillas, the mean intraocular pressure was 20.0 ± 7.8 mmHg (Montiani-Ferreira, 2001).

Retinal disease

Reported causes of retinal diseases leading to blindness in rats and mice include primary genetic defects or secondary diseases, as a result of another condition such as uveitis caused by SDAV or excessive light exposure.

Excessive light exposure is a common and important cause of degenerative retinal disease in rodents under research-type settings. It is probably not a common condition in pet rodents, but the possibility should be always considered when facing degenerative retinal disease in rodents. Predisposing factors are photoperiodicity, illumination intensity and temperature. Even low intensities of light over a long period of time can produce changes in the retina (Semple-Rowland and Dawson, 1987).

Mice and rats have been found to show a variety of inherited retinal problems, including various retinal degenerations. Many strains of mouse with retinal disease exist and are used as biological models for the study of human retinal disease.

A recent report documents a spontaneous rod-function disorder, as observed by electroretinography, in a group of consanguineous guinea pigs (Racine *et al.*, 2003).

Rats and mice are probably the most widely used animal model in the retinal electrophysiology literature. Recently the guinea pig also has been suggested as a superior model for comparative electrophysiological investigations (Racine *et al.*, 2005).

Orbital disease and exophthalmos

Retrobulbar diseases causing exophthalmos (protrusion or prominence of the eye) are occasionally seen in pet rodents. Common clinical signs of retrobulbar disease are progressive exophthalmos and the inability to retropulse the eye. Possible causes of orbital disease include trauma, foreign body, fungal or parasitic infections, sinus infection, inflammation of the zygomatic salivary gland (often associated with a mucocele), orbital tumours, and encephalic tumours with orbital extension (Figure 15.14).

Exophthalmos in rodents may be commonly related to dental disease, as previously mentioned. A tooth-root abscess may result in maxillary sinusitis and orbital disease (see Figure 15.5b). Careful examination of the teeth is indicated in any rodent with exophthalmos.

Neoplasms of the Harderian gland can also cause exophthalmos and are fairly common in mice. Severe exophthalmos with consecutive exposure keratitis

has been reported as a consequence of an osseous choristoma of the ciliary body in a guinea pig (Schmidt *et al.*, 2007).

Some diagnostic procedures that may be helpful in evaluating orbital disease in rodents include: (i) skull radiographs, dental radiographs and orbital ultrasonography; and (ii) clinical pathology (CBC, serum chemistry profile, cytology of fine-needle aspirates, culture and sensitivity). When available, a computed tomography scan is especially helpful in diagnosing intracranial, orbital and retrobulbar disease.

It is worth mentioning that buphthalmos is a common clinical sign of chronic glaucoma but is not a common clinical sign of retrobulbar disease. Proptosis, which is a forward displacement of the globe that traps the eyelid margins behind the equator of the globe, is usually a consequence of trauma and should also be differentiated from buphthalmos and exophthalmos (Figure 15.15).

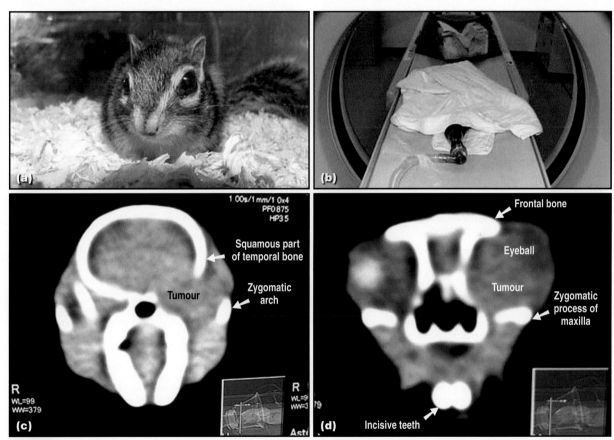

15.14 **(a)** Chinese chipmunk (*Tamias sibiricus*), 5-year-old male, presenting with exophthalmos in the left eye. **(b)** The patient was anaesthetized and a CT scan analysis of its head was performed. **(c)** A tumour at the base of its brain also invading the orbit was diagnosed. **(d)** In this CT scan section it is possible to appreciate the forward dislocation of the left eyeball (exophthalmos). (Courtesy of Yasutsugu Miwa.)

Exophthalmos	Buphthalmos	Proptosis
Normal sized globe protrudes from the orbit	Ocular radii (corneal and scleral) increased, making the whole globe enlarged	Globe protrudes from the orbit
Examined from above: globe is positioned rostrally	Examined from above: enlarged globe is not displaced at the equatorial region	Examined from above: globe is positioned rostrally

15.15 Clinical signs and medical manoeuvres that may help to differentiate between exophthalmos, buphthalmos and proptosis in rodents. (continues) ▶

Exophthalmos	Buphthalmos	Proptosis
Resists retropulsion	Retropulses normally	Resists retropulsion but degree of resistance depends on the retrobulbar tissue oedema and/or damage and the integrity of the bony orbit
Normal globe and corneal diameter	Increased globe and corneal diameter	Usually normal globe and corneal diameter
Often visual	Usually blind	May be visual or blind
Eyelid margins visible	Eyelid margins visible	Eyelid margins not visible
Common aetiology: retrobulbar disease	Common aetiology: glaucoma (primary or secondary)	Common aetiology: trauma

15.15   (continued) Clinical signs and medical manoeuvres that may help to differentiate between exophthalmos, buphthalmos and proptosis in rodents.

Acknowledgements

The author would like to acknowledge Dr Marcello Machado, UnC, Canoinhas, SC, Brazil and FMVZ/USP, SP, Brazil as a co-author for the section on basic ocular anatomical features of rodents in this chapter and also wishes to thank Dr Gillian Shaw (The Johns Hopkins University, Baltimore, Maryland) for her help in the preparation of this chapter. A special thanks to Pedro Primo Bombonato and Marina Moreira from the Veterinary Anatomy Museum, FMVZ/USP, Brazil.

References and further reading

Alessandrini G (1907) Dermoid centrale della cornea in una cavia cobaya schreb. *Il Progresso Ophthalmologico* **3**, 88–89

Balazs T and Rubin L (1971) A note on the lens in aging Sprague-Dawley rats. *Laboratory Animal Science* **21**, 267–263

Beaumont SL (2002) Ocular disorders of pet mice and rats. *Veterinary Clinics of North America: Exotic Animal Practice* **5**(2), 311–324

Bellhorn RW (1973) Ophthalmological disorders of exotic and laboratory animals. *Veterinary Clinics of North America* **3**, 345–356

Bisaria KK and Narayan D (1973) The lamina cribrosa in some mammals (a histological study). *Indian Journal of Ophthalmology* **21**, 178–181

Brunschwig A (1928) A dermoid of the cornea in a guinea pig. *American Journal of Pathology* **4**, 371–374

Burnie D and Wilson DE (2001) *Animal.* Dorling Kindersley, London

Chan R (1932) A corneo-scleral dermoid in a guinea pig. *American Journal of Ophthalmology* **15**, 525–526

Elbroch M (2006) *Animal Skulls: a Guide to North American Species.* Stackpole Books, Mechanicsburg, Pennsylvania

Gaarder JE and Kern TJ (2001) Ocular disease in rabbits, rodents, reptiles and other small exotic animals. In: *Fundamentals of Veterinary Ophthalmology, 3rd edn*, ed. D Slatter, pp. 593–599. WB Saunders, Philadelphia

Gupta BN (1972) Scleral dermoid in a guinea pig. *Laboratory Animal Science* **22**, 919–921

Hanna PE, Percy DH, Paturzo F and Bhatt PN (1984) Sialodacryoadenitis in the rat: effects of immunosuppression on the course of the disease. *American Journal of Veterinary Research* **45**, 2077–2083

Hubert MF, Gillet JP and Durand-Cavagna G (1994) Spontaneous retinal changes in Sprague Dawley rats. *Laboratory Animal Science* **44**, 561–567

Kern TJ (1989) Ocular disorders of rabbits, rodents and ferrets. In: *Current Veterinary Therapy X*, ed. RW Kirk and JD Bonagura, pp. 125–129. WB Saunders, Philadelphia

Kirschner SE (1997) Ophthalmologic disease in small mammals. In: *Ferrets, Rabbits and Rodents. Clinical Medicine and Surgery*, ed. EV Hiller and KE Quesenberry, pp. 339–345. WB Saunders, Philadelphia

Lawton MPC (2002) Exotic species. In: *BSAVA Manual of Small Animal Ophthalmology, 2nd edn*, ed. S Petersen Jones and S Crispin, pp. 285–295. BSAVA Publications, Gloucester

Magnusson G, Majeed S and Offer JM (1978) Intraocular melanoma in the rat. *Laboratory Animals* **12**, 249–252

McGee MA and Maronpot RR (1979) Harderian gland dacryoadenitis in rats resulting from orbital bleeding. *Laboratory Animal Science* **29**, 639–641

Montiani-Ferreira F (2001) Ophthalmology. In: *Biology, Medicine and Surgery of South American Wild Animals*, ed. MF Fowler and Z Cubas, pp. 437–456. Iowa State University Press, Ames, Iowa

Montiani-Ferreira F, Petersen-Jones S, Cassotis N *et al.* (2003) Early postnatal development of central corneal thickness in dogs. *Veterinary Ophthalmology* **6**, 19–22

Mouse Models for Ocular Disease. http://www.jax.org/

Munger RJ (2002) Veterinary ophthalmology in laboratory animal studies. *Veterinary Ophthalmology* **5**, 167–175

Ollivier FJ, Samuelson DA, Brooks DE *et al.* (2004) Comparative morphology of the tapetum lucidum (among selected species). *Veterinary Ophthalmology* **7**, 11–22

Otto G, Lipman NS and Murphy JC (1991) Corneal dermoid in a hairless guinea pig. *Laboratory Animal Science* **41**, 171–172

Pinto LH and Enroth-Cugell C (2000) Tests of the mouse visual system. *Mammalian Genome* **11**, 531–536

Popesko P, Rajtová V and Horák J (2003) *A Color Atlas of Anatomy of Small Laboratory Animals.* WB Saunders, Philadelphia

Racine J, Behn D, Simard E and Lachapelle P (2003) Spontaneous occurrence of potentially night blinding disorder in guinea pigs. *Documenta Ophthalmologica* **107**, 59–69

Racine J, Joly S, Rufiange M *et al.* (2005) The photopic ERG of the albino guinea pig (*Cavia porcellus*): a model of the human photopic ERG. *Documenta Ophthalmologica* **110**, 67–77

Rubin LF and Daly IW (1982) Ectopic pupil in mice. *Laboratory Animal Science* **32**, 64–65

Schmidt W, Hertslet S, Hetzel U *et al.* (2007) High resolution imaging in a case of osseous choristoma of the ciliary body of a guinea pig. Abstracts: European College of Veterinary Ophthalmologists, European Society of Veterinary Ophthalmology, International Society of Veterinary Ophthalmology, and the Italian Association of Veterinary Ophthalmology, Genoa, Italy, May 30–June 3, 2007. *Veterinary Ophthalmology* **10**(5), 323–335

Seely JC (1987) The Harderian gland. *Laboratory Animal Science* **16**, 33–39

Semple-Rowland SL and Dawson WW (1987) Cyclic light intensity threshold for retinal damage in albino rats raised under 6 lx. *Experimental Eye Research* **44**, 643–661

Steinberg H (2000) Disseminated T-cell lymphoma in a guinea pig with bilateral ocular involvement. *Journal of Veterinary Diagnostic Investigation* **12**, 459–462

Taradach C and Greaves P (1984) Spontaneous eye lesions in laboratory animals: incidence in relation to age. *Critical Reviews in Toxicology* **12**, 121–147

van der Woerdt A (2003) Ophthalmologic diseases in small pet mammals. In: *Ferrets, Rabbits and Rodents Clinical Medicine and Surgery, 2nd edn*, ed. KE Quesenberry and JW Carpenter, pp. 421–428. WB Saunders, Philadelphia

Williams DL (2002) Ocular disease in rats: a review. *Veterinary Ophthalmology* **5**, 183–191

Young C, Festing MFW and Barnett KC (1974) Buphthalmos (congenital glaucoma) in the rat. *Laboratory Animal* **8**, 21–31

16

Rodents: neoplastic and endocrine disease

Hannah Orr

Introduction

A variety of endocrine and neoplastic conditions are commonly observed in rodents in clinical practice. Only some of these diseases are reported in the literature and the successful diagnosis and treatment of such diseases is even more rarely described. There are many reasons for this, but the problems are principally: the small size of most of these species; the difficulty in obtaining adequate or repeated samples; interpreting test outcomes when rodent responses to an established cat or dog test can be highly variable; and the paucity of information on reference ranges. This chapter will list the main endocrine and neoplastic diseases likely to be encountered, give a guide to aetiology, clinical signs and the differential diagnoses and, where possible, describe treatment or management regimes. An overview of the diseases discussed for each species is given in table form at the end of each section. Figure 16.1 gives blood glucose ranges in rodent species.

Mice

An overview of neoplastic and endocrine diseases in mice is given in Figure 16.2.

Neoplastic disease

There are many strains of mice, which vary in genetic background and husbandry conditions. Therefore there is a wide range of neoplastic conditions that may be observed. Common tumours are mammary neoplasia (described below), pulmonary tumours (including alveogenic and bronchogenic carcinomas and alveolar cell adenomas), lymphomas, hepatic carcinomas, testicular interstitial cell tumours and ovarian tumours.

Mammary neoplasia

In mice these are most likely to be malignant carcinoma/adenocarcinoma. Endogenous mouse mammary tumour viruses (MMTVs) have been observed to influence the onset and incidence in laboratory mice, as do mouse strain, environmental stressors (e.g. intensive breeding or overcrowding) and the presence of certain hormones and chemical carcinogens.

They present as enlarging masses under the skin of the flanks or ventral body (Figure 16.3), and because of the extent of mammary tissue in mice they

Species	Blood glucose (mmol/l)	Blood glucose upper limit* (mmol/l)
Mouse	3.3–12.7[a]	13.89[c]
Rat	4.7–7.3[a]	12.05[c]
Hamster	3.6–7.0[a]	11.11[#c]
Gerbil	2.8–7.5[a]	–
Guinea pig	3.3–6.9[a]	6.94[c]
Chinchilla	3.3–6.1[a]	6.67[c]
Degu	4.12–4.56[b]	6.7[d]

16.1 Blood glucose ranges in rodent species. * Upper limit for blood glucose concentration after fasting period; # Syrian; (Sources: [a] Keeble, 2001; [b] Opazo, 2004; [c] Oglesbee, 1996; [d] Datiles and Fukui, 1989)

	Differential diagnoses	Clinical signs	Notes	Treatment
Tumours				
Mammary neoplasia	Abscesses, seroma, galactocele, cyst	Fleshy infiltrative mass on ventrum, axilla, scapula or flank	Cytology on FNA, or histology post surgical removal	Supportive care until euthanasia or surgical removal but prognosis guarded
Endocrine disease				
Diabetes mellitus	Cystitis, renal disease	Polyuria, polydipsia; persistent glycosuria; blood glucose severely elevated	Rarely seen – experimental or genetically modified animals or those on certain high-fat diets	None described in clinical setting

16.2 Neoplastic and endocrine diseases of mice.

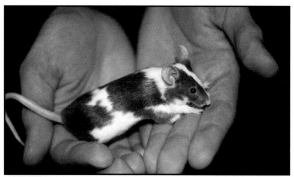

16.3 Female mouse with a mammary tumour in the right axilla. (Courtesy of Emma Keeble.)

may appear from the neck down to the inguinal region. They can be differentiated from abscesses or other tumour types by fine-needle aspiration cytology or post surgery by dissection and/or histological examination of the mass. Although they can be treated by surgical excision, this can be difficult as they are soft, fleshy, vascular and invasive. It can be challenging not to cause significant tissue damage and haemorrhage (see also Chapter 7). Prognosis should be guarded since mice are expert at hiding signs of illness and metastatic spread is common. Figure 16.4 outlines management where excision is not undertaken.

Endocrine disease

Diabetes mellitus
This condition is only reported with any frequency in certain strains of laboratory mice and it tends to be in genetically altered animals or those being fed high fat (obesogenic) diets. For general information on supportive care and treatment/management see Hamsters.

Rats

An overview of neoplastic and endocrine diseases in rats is given in Figure 16.5.

Neoplastic disease
The most common neoplastic lesion in rats is mammary gland neoplasia (see Figure 13.2). Other tumour types are said to occur in specific strains, but it is hard to make generalizations for domestic rats. These are pituitary, adrenal and thyroid gland neoplasms, lipoma, mononuclear cell leukaemia, testicular and uterine neoplasia, adnexal gland tumours (e.g. of Zymbal's gland, located at the base of the external ear (Figure 16.6), preputial gland (males), and clitoral gland (females)) and various epithelial cutaneous neoplasms (Toft, 1992; Haseman *et al.*, 2003).

Surgical management:

- If the mass is sympathetic to removal (i.e. it is fairly superficial and movable), surgery is likely to increase the quality of life and the lifespan
- Tumours can grow rapidly. Unless fine-needle aspiration/cytology results can be processed in-house, inadvisable delays may occur while waiting for results to return before commencing removal of the mass

Conservative management:

- If the owner does not opt for removal, the key issue is quality of life prior to euthanasia
- Superficial tumours can be measured with callipers to give an objective guide to speed of growth
- Care should be taken if using body weight to monitor health and welfare since masses in small rodents can contribute a significant proportion of their body weight
- The owner should be advised that at some stage the mass may begin to inhibit movement and may ulcerate if it drags on the cage floor
- The animal should be handled and checked daily
- Daily food intake should be measured

16.4 Management of mammary masses in mice and rats.

	Differential diagnoses	Clinical signs	Notes	Prevention, treatment and prognosis
Tumours				
Mammary tumours	Abscess/es, seroma, galactocele, cyst	Solitary or multiple masses in region of mammary chain	Aged animals (over 18 months, females – more common) Diagnosis: cytology on FNA, or histology post surgical removal	Prevention: early dietary restriction to 70% of ad lib intake. Early neutering may reduce the incidence Treatment: surgical removal.
Zymbal's gland tumour	Abscess, otitis	Large (frequently ulcerated) mass within, or just below, external ear canal	Gland: sebaceous, surrounds external ear canal Tumour: invasive, not metastatic	Surgical removal of lobulated invasive gland complex Prognosis poor
Testicular tumour	Abscess, orchitis, testicular torsion	Testis greatly enlarged. Involves one or both testes; if unilateral, other testis atrophied	Incidence varies between strains, and increases with age. Usually interstitial cell adenomas. Benign	Surgical removal recommended
Lymphoma	Pituitary adenoma, diabetes mellitus	Anaemia, weight loss, icterus, depression and the characteristic blood leucocyte counts	Blood leucocyte counts of up to 400,000/ml³, splenomegaly and possible hepatomegaly	Prognosis poor

16.5 Neoplastic and endocrine diseases of rats. (continues) ▶

	Differential diagnoses	Clinical signs	Notes	Prevention, treatment and prognosis
Endocrine disease				
Pituitary adenomas	Diabetes mellitus, otitis interna, chronic progressive nephropathy, radiculoneuropathy, pseudopregnancy, *Encephalitozoon cuniculi*, murine, encephalomyelitis virus	May present concurrently with mammary tumour. Neurological signs: depression, unresponsiveness, anorexia (pituitary cachexia), weight loss, muscle atrophy, vestibular nerve dysfunction causing ataxia, head tilt, circling and seizures, polyuria, polydipsia	Common. Incidence increases with age, higher in females. Neurological signs due to compression atrophy of surrounding brain areas. Check brain at PM examination for definitive diagnosis	Prevention: low-protein diet, dietary restriction. Early neutering may reduce the incidence Treatment: supportive care. Prognosis poor
Diabetes mellitus	Pituitary adenoma, chronic progressive nephropathy	Polyuria, polydipsia. Persistent glucosuria. Blood glucose severely elevated	Rarely seen spontaneous disease. Experimental models exist	Insulin ('Caninsulin' – Intervet), s.c. q12h, start at 1–2 IU and titrate dose

16.5 (continued) Neoplastic and endocrine diseases of rats.

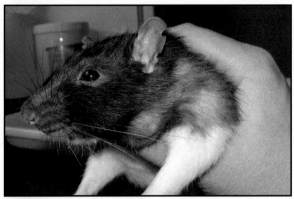

16.6 Rat with a mass at the ear base. This was diagnosed as a Zymbal's gland tumour.

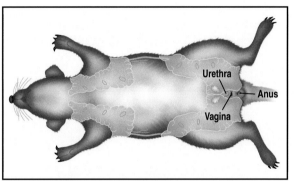

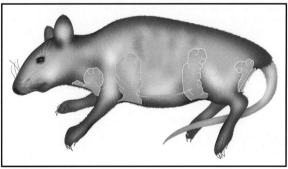

16.7 Anatomical extent of mammary tissue in a female rat.

Mammary neoplasia

Unlike mice, mammary fibroadenomas are the commonest tumour in female rats (80–90% incidence), the majority of the rest being carcinomas. They occur most often in aged females, are slow growing and do not metastasize. They may also occur in male rats. These can be solitary or multiple along the mammary chain. Anatomically, the mammary gland tissue extends on either side of the ventral midline from axillary to inguinal regions (Figure 16.7). Thus tumours may arise in the submandibular region, scapular region, on the flanks or at the tail base.

These tumours can grow very large (10 cm in diameter) and may impair mobility or ability to eat if not closely monitored. Large tumours are prone to cutaneous ulceration and secondary infection. In such cases the cytological appearance can become confused as the neoplastic component becomes obscured by inflammatory cells (Garner, 2007). One laboratory study, restricting food intake to 80% of *ad libitum* feeding, reduced the incidence of mammary tumours in female rats fivefold (Tucker, 1979). Tamoxifen, an antioestrogen used in the treatment of human breast cancer, has been shown to induce hepatic cancer in rats and is therefore not recommended (Keeble, 2001). Another study showed that serum prolactin levels in females with mammary tumours were 25 times that

of 6-month-old virgin females (Percy and Barthold, 1993). There have been attempts to draw a link between mammary tumours and the occurrence of prolactin-producing pituitary adenomas (they often occur in the same animal, suggesting they are related) but no conclusive correlations have been found. In a rat, a good prognosis may be given if the lesions are successfully removed (see Chapter 7). For treatment and management see Figure 16.4.

Pituitary gland neoplasia

This is one of the more commonly encountered tumours of the endocrine system seen in older male and female rats (laboratory animal strains such as the Sprague Dawley and Wistar are particularly affected). The majority are interpreted on histopathology to be chromophobe adenomas. A higher incidence is reported in females, particularly non-breeding females, and factors such as genetics and diet may play a significant role in their development. In one study, dietary restriction gave rise to a significantly lower incidence of the disease in both males and females (Tucker, 1979).

Mortality is usually due to increased intracranial pressure and compression atrophy of surrounding brain areas, leading to a gradual deterioration in health and signs such as head tilt, depression and hydrocephalus. For clinical signs, see Figure 16.5. Supportive care may prolong the lifespan of affected animals, but the prognosis is poor and euthanasia is indicated once severe clinical signs develop. The tumours are usually benign; on post-mortem examination they are often grossly apparent (up to 1 cm diameter) and reddish brown with a haemorrhagic appearance.

Endocrine disease

Diabetes mellitus
Rats are used as models of experimentally induced diabetes, which is rare as a spontaneous condition, occurring only in certain strains of rat. It may also occur iatrogenically secondary to corticosteroid administration (E Keeble, personal communication). These animals can become immunosuppressed and susceptible to secondary bacterial or ectoparasite infection. Diagnosis is based on glucosuria and very elevated blood glucose levels (see Figure 16.1 for normal values).

Diabetes can be controlled using twice daily subcutaneous injections of insulin; Caninsulin (Intervet) is a medium-duration product. An anecdotal dose rate of 1–2 IU/kg has been recommended. Urine glucose should be checked twice daily and the insulin dose titrated according to the results. Keeble (2001) reported that a final stabilization was achieved with 10 IU insulin/kg given twice daily by subcutaneous injection. Supportive care is discussed in Figure 16.8.

Hamsters

An overview of neoplastic and endocrine diseases in hamsters is given in Figure 16.9.

Attention to husbandry will reduce welfare problems. The following supportive care often improves survival time and quality of life:

- When appropriate, try to house affected rodents in pairs, but monitor the affected animal's food intake
- Control food intake, feed a high-fibre diet and avoid sugary or fatty foods (e.g. carrots or sunflower seeds)
- Depending on the severity of any polyuria:
  - House with deep absorbent bedding and change bedding each day
  - Provide a raised sleeping area with extra bedding for warmth
  - Use plastic or cardboard tunnels suspended from the cage top to keep them dry; this gives animals that can climb continued access to refuges ('bolt-holes')
- Provide a warm wet pellet mash in a bowl, or syringe-feed mash, rather than offering dry food. This assists in maintaining hydration (do not wait for signs of dehydration – provide this from the start)
- If possible, train the owner to administer subcutaneous fluids (every 2–3 days in severe cases with clinical signs of dehydration)
- Record the animal's weight weekly

Suggest that further consultations are required:

- If stabilized and disease returns (e.g. polydipsia/polyuria recurs or glycosuria is detected on urinalysis)
- When dehydration or pain are suspected
- If body weight *loss* is approaching 15% of what would be viewed as a healthy normal weight for that animal

---

16.8 Supportive care for diabetes mellitus.

	Differential diagnoses	Clinical signs	Notes	Treatment
Tumours				
Lymphoma	As for transmissible lymphoma below	Solitary or multiple tumours affecting skin, lymph nodes, spleen, liver and other organs	Occurs in aged animals	Poor prognosis. Orcutt (2005) mentions anecdotal reports of chemotherapy based on protocols in other species
Epitheliotropic (cutaneous) lymphoma	Ectoparasites, dermatophytosis, hyperadrenocorticism	Lethargy, weight loss, patchy alopecia, scales and crusts	Resembles mycosis fungoides in humans; exclude other causes and diagnoses by histopathology of skin biopsy, or FNA cytology	Poor prognosis, disease progresses rapidly
Transmissible lymphoma: hamster polyomavirus infection	Transmissible ileal hyperplasia (causes palpable enlargement of terminal ileum), spontaneous lymphoid tumours, skin problems e.g. *Demodex* folliculitis	Two disease pictures: lymphoma outbreak in naïve colony, or low level of cutaneous tumours and subclinical infection in established infection	In a colony epizootic outbreaks are unmistakable	Once infection is established in a colony it cannot be eradicated without culling the colony

16.9 Neoplastic and endocrine diseases of hamsters. (continues) ▶

	Differential diagnoses	Clinical signs	Notes	Treatment
Tumours continued				
Adrenal cortical tumours		See Cushing's syndrome below	Most often adenoma or adenocarcinoma	
Normal flank/ ventral scent glands	Neoplasia	Normal anatomical gland; flank glands in Syrian hamster, ventral in Djungarian/dwarf hamster	Can easily be mistaken by owners for tumour	Reassurance of the owner
Endocrine disease				
Hyperadreno-corticism/ Cushing's syndrome	Ectoparasites, dermatophytes, hypothyroidism, epitheliotropic lymphoma	Bilateral symmetrical flank / thigh alopecia, hyperpigmentation, skin thinning, hepatomegaly polydipsia, polyuria polyphagia, behavioural changes	High plasma cortisol/ corticosterone; note that these also rise with stress such as handling or transport. Increased SAP	One report of effective treatment with metyrapone, 8 mg orally daily for 1 month (Bauck *et al.*, 1984)
Diabetes mellitus	Tyzzer's disease	Chinese hamster in poor body condition, hyperglycaemia, polyuria, polydipsia, glycosuria, ketonuria, hyperphagia	Inherited condition; autosomal recessive in some lines, polygenic in others	Prevention: onset delayed by restricting food or fat intake Treatment: s.c. injection of NPH insulin, start at a low dose and titrate to effect by monitoring urine glucose level

16.9 (continued) Neoplastic and endocrine diseases of hamsters.

Neoplastic disease

Male hamsters have large pendulous testes and darkly pigmented sebaceous flank (Syrian/Golden) or ventral (Djungarian/dwarf) glands. Clients may mistake these for neoplastic disease (see Chapter 1 for normal anatomy).

Syrian hamsters

Reported commonly occurring benign neoplasms include intestinal polyps (adenoma), stomach papill-oma, adrenal adenoma and splenic haemangioma. Of the malignant neoplasms, lymphoma is common (see later) and intestinal adenocarcinoma and adrenal carcinoma also occur. For further information on tumours of the adrenal gland see Hyperadrenocorticism.

Dwarf hamsters

This species is reported to have a high incidence of spontaneously occurring neoplasia, particularly of the skin (Figure 16.10), oral cavity and mammary glands (Cooper *et al.*, 1991; Lawrie and Megahy, 1991).

Chinese hamsters

Uterine tumours (adenocarcinoma) presenting at post-mortem examination as firm white masses involving the cervical area and with the ability to metastasize are reported to occur commonly (Strandberg, 1987). The presenting clinical sign of uterine tumours is generally vaginal haemorrhage (see also Chapter 13). The author could find no information in the literature on prognosis and treatment of this condition in Chinese hamsters.

Lymphoma

Lymphoma is the most common neoplastic disease to affect hamsters. There are various forms, one of which arises secondarily to infection with hamster polyoma-virus and is described below. In aged Syrian hamsters

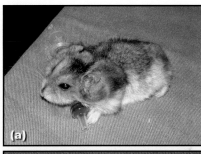
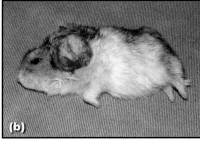

16.10
(a) Russian dwarf hamster with a cutaneous mass. A diagnosis was not obtained in this case and the animal was euthanased.
(b) Gross appearance of the incised mass at post-mortem examination.

lymphomas arise that are not associated with ham-ster polyomavirus. These are multicentric, often involving multiple lymph nodes, spleen, liver and other body organs. Cutaneous epitheliotropic lymphoma resembling mycosis fungoides in humans has been observed in aged adult hamsters (Harvey *et al.*, 1992) (Figure 16.11). Clinical signs include lethargy, weight loss, patchy alopecia and exfoliative erythroderma (scale and crusts). Diagnosis is by exclusion of other causes (e.g. ectoparasites) by skin scrape, fine-nee-dle aspiration cytology and histology of skin biopsy. Prognosis is poor, owing to the progressive nature of the dermatosis and associated deterioration in body condition. Lesions are often painful and secondary bacterial infection and demodicosis are common.

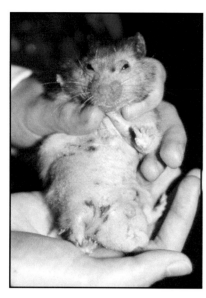

16.11 Syrian hamster with lesions secondary to cutaneous epitheliotropic lymphoma (mycosis fungoides). (Courtesy of Anna Meredith.)

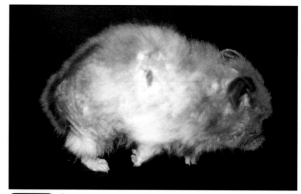

16.12 Syrian hamster with suspected hyperadrenocorticism (Cushing's syndrome) and secondary infection with *Demodex* mites. (Courtesy of Gidona Goodman.)

Transmissible lymphoma – hamster polyoma virus (HaPV) infection: There are two lymphoma disease pictures seen following infection with HaPV. In groups of animals where infection is established it exists subclinically. Young animals are seemingly protected and in older animals that become infected occasional cases are seen of a cutaneous form that causes keratinizing skin tumours of the hair follicle (epitheliomas), mostly on the face or feet. Animals that present with the problem may have solitary or multiple lesions. In naïve breeding groups, when the virus is first introduced it results in epizootics of lymphomas amongst young hamsters, with a prevalence of 80% within 4–30 weeks of exposure (a diagnostic sign, as lymphoma is normally seen at a very low incidence and in older animals). The lymphomas present as multiple tumours affecting skin, lymph nodes, spleen, liver and other body organs. Affected animals are often in poor body condition, with palpable abdominal masses. Virus transmission is via the urine. Barthold (1991) present a thorough review of HaPV biology. Once infection is established in a colony it cannot be eradicated without culling the colony. For further information see Percy and Barthold (1993) and Figure 16.9.

Endocrine disease

Hyperadrenocorticism (Cushing's syndrome)
This condition is most common in older male animals, adrenocortical adenoma being one of the most common benign neoplasms in the Syrian hamster (Figure 16.12). For clinical signs, see Figure 16.9.

Diagnosis of hyperadrenocorticism is generally presumed on the basis of history and clinical signs. Definitive diagnosis should include elevated blood cortisol (normal range 13.8–27.6 nmol/l) and/or alkaline phosphatase (normal range 8–18 IU/l, raised >40 IU/l). As hamsters secrete both corticosterone and cortisol, it has been suggested that both should be measured to assess adrenocortical function accurately. The practicalities of obtaining blood to run these tests may prove problematic (see Chapter 2). Note that cortisol and corticosterone levels rise through stress due to handling and restraint (Ottenweller *et al.*, 1985) and during pregnancy (Brink-Johnsen *et al.*, 1981). Treatment has been described with metyrapone (8 mg orally daily) or surgical removal of the affected gland via flank laparotomy (though this would not be curative in pituitary-dependent disease).

Descriptions of clinical cases are scant in the literature; the only histopathological report involved three related Teddy Bear hamsters. They presented with alopecia and hyperpigmentation of the skin, but no polyuria/polydipsia. Post-mortem and histopathological examination demonstrated that one animal had an adrenocortical adenocarcinoma and another a pituitary chromophobe adenoma. The third case was not definitively diagnosed by post-mortem examination, because the animal responded to treatment (metyrapone, for 1 month) and after 12 weeks the animal's hair had regrown (Bauck *et al.*, 1984). A blood sample taken prior to treatment demonstrated high plasma cortisol. Another reported case was diagnosed on the basis of alopecia, hyperpigmentation, thin skin and elevated serum alkaline phosphatase secondary to hepatomegaly (Adamcak *et al.*, 1998). There is one report in the literature of urine cortisol/creatinine ratio being used as a screening test for a suspected case of Cushing's syndrome (Martinho, 2006). A 24-hour sample was collected in the home cage with all the bedding removed to reduce the effect of stress on cortisol excretion. The ratio in that case was significantly increased compared with the laboratory's reference range, but no reference range is established for hamsters.

Diabetes mellitus
Genetically linked spontaneous diabetes mellitus is reported in some lines of Chinese hamster. Its transmission was first observed as a recessive factor in hamsters in 1957 during inbreeding of a laboratory colony (Meier and Yerganian, 1959). The disease arises through degranulation of the beta cells and a primary deficiency in insulin synthesis. Clinical signs can be apparent from 18 days of age and are usually evident by 90 days. Animals exhibit weight loss, glucose intolerance, mild to severe hyperglycaemia, glycosuria, ketonuria, polydipsia/polyuria (50–70 ml urine/day in animals weighing 25 g) and hyperphagia.

Non-fasting glucose levels rise above 16.65 mmol/l in diabetics. As with other species, blood glucose levels are sensitive to handling and collection techniques. Also, insulin metabolism and blood glucose levels may vary in hamsters due to aestivation and hibernation cycles. Urine specific gravity is reported to rise from normal values of 1.018 to >1.029 in glycosuric animals (Meier and Yerganian, 1961). Caloric restriction *per se* or reduction of dietary fat (replacing animal fat with vegetable fat) can delay onset of hyperglycaemia and hyperinsulinaemia in pre-diabetics. Diabetic hamsters show a reduction in urinary glucose output when fed low fat diets (40 g fat/kg of feed *ad libitum*). Treatment with hypoglycaemic drugs has been reported in breeding females to maintain inbred lines (Meier and Yerganian, 1961). This was with neutral protamine (NPH) insulin; doses ranging from 2 to 40 IU were reported and some animals required increasing doses over a period of weeks. Treatment should be instigated with a low dose; urine glucose should be checked twice daily and the insulin dose titrated according to the results to establish a regime. For supportive care, see Figure 16.8.

Gerbils

An overview of neoplastic and endocrine diseases in gerbils is given in Figure 16.13.

Neoplastic disease

Most reviews of rodent neoplasia report a high incidence of spontaneous tumours in gerbils. Female reproductive tract neoplasms are most frequent, with ovarian tumours making up the largest proportion, followed by uterine tumours. Neoplasia of the reproductive tract may present as a vulval discharge due to secondary bacterial infection. A differential diagnosis is pyometra. Next most common are those involving the integument, with the ventral scent gland having the largest proportion of problems (see below). Adrenal gland adenomas and adenocarcinomas are reported in gerbils (see below for hyperadrenocorticism). One study reported that 37% of *Helicobacter*-infected gerbils developed gastric adenocarcinoma in 62 weeks (Watanabe *et al.*, 1998).

Ventral scent gland

Gerbils have a large ventral abdominal scent gland that is androgen dependent, thus the gland is larger in males. It is used for territorial marking and scent identification of pups. Owners may mistake the normal gland for a tumour, though in old animals it may become neoplastic (Figure 16.14) and/or infected. Infection causes erythema and ulceration and can be similar in appearance to neoplasia. If neoplasia is suspected (e.g. a raised ulcerated gland does not respond to topical or systemic antibiotic treatment in an older animal), a wide excisional biopsy is recommended. Histology should be performed to obtain a diagnosis and prognosis. Adenomas and squamous and basal cell carcinomas have all been reported. Castration has been advocated at the time of excision due to the androgen link with this gland. Local spread to inguinal lymph nodes has been reported in advanced cases (Keeble, 2002). (See also Chapter 10.)

	Differential diagnoses	Clinical signs	Notes	Treatment
Tumours				
Integumentary, including ventral gland lesions	Normal prominent scent gland; inflammation and infection of the scent gland; abscesses of the skin	Ulceration, erythema and proliferation of scent gland	Sebaceous gland adenomas and carcinomas. Squamous cell carcinomas, melanomas, and subcutaneous fibrosarcomas most common	Based on stage of disease and whether surgical removal possible
Adrenal cortical adenomas and carcinomas/ Cushing's syndrome	As described above for hamsters	As described above for hamsters	Adrenal gland is normally large, adrenal to body weight ratio one of largest of known species	As described above for hamsters
Ovarian tumours	Cystic ovaries; pyometra; pregnancy; retained fetus; uterine neoplasia	Abdominal distension; vulval discharge	Granulosa cell, leiomyomas and thecal cell most commonly reported	Based on stage of disease and whether surgical removal possible
Endocrine disease				
Cystic ovaries	Tumour; pregnancy/ retained fetus; ascites; respiratory disease	Infertility, decreased litter size; abdominal distension; respiratory difficulties in severe cases	Unilateral/bilateral, approx 20% aged females affected. Cyst size increases with age	Removal of affected ovary/ies Percutaneous drainage is not curative
Diabetes mellitus	Primary cystitis	PU/PD; secondary cystitis	Occurs as a sequel to obesity	Weight reduction may alleviate signs, but care must be taken to avoid hepatic lipidosis

16.13 Neoplastic and endocrine diseases of gerbils.

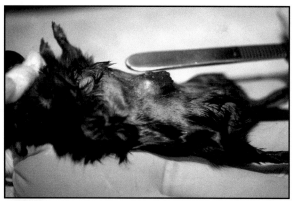

16.14 Gerbil with ventral scent gland neoplasia. (Courtesy of Heidi Hoefer.)

Endocrine disease

Cystic ovaries

Cystic ovaries occur commonly in gerbils, with the incidence reported as between 20% and 50% of aged female gerbils. Cysts can be up to 5 cm in diameter and can be uni- or bilateral. Clinical signs include palpable masses, or abdominal distension and respiratory difficulties in severe cases. Breeding can continue in the presence of cysts, but litter sizes are reduced and severely affected females do become infertile. Percutaneous drainage has been performed, but removal of the affected ovary or ovariohysterectomy is recommended.

Diabetes mellitus

Diabetes mellitus may occur secondary to obesity, since this leads to hyperglycaemia and glucose intolerance. Blood insulin levels increase and pancreatic changes occur. Clinical signs include polyuria/polydipsia and secondary cystitis. Diagnosis can be based on urinalysis (glycosuria) and raised blood glucose levels. Weight reduction may resolve the signs but sudden dietary changes should be avoided as rapid weight loss may induce hepatic lipidosis. Sunflower seeds are a common cause of obesity in gerbils. Total daily food intake should not exceed 4–10 g.

Hyperadrenocorticism

Cushing's syndrome rarely occurs in this species, though it has been reported in ageing animals. Clinical signs, diagnosis and treatment are as described above for hamsters.

Guinea pigs

An overview of neoplastic and endocrine diseases in guinea pigs is given in Figure 16.15.

	Differential diagnoses	Clinical signs	Notes	Treatment
Tumours				
Cavian leukaemia	Cervical lymphadenitis ('lumps')	Lymphadenopathy, splenomegaly, hepatomegaly, anaemia, signs of liver/kidney failure if organs infiltrated	Animals can be aleukaemic with lymphoma, but leukaemic animals typically have a WBC count over 25,000/mm³	After onset of signs the clinical course is rapid, 2–5 weeks
Pulmonary neoplasia	On radiography: metastatic neoplasia, abscesses, foreign bodies, granulomas	Most frequently detected incidentally on thoracic radiographs	Account for 35% of spontaneous tumours, question as to whether truly neoplastic disease	Rarely cause clinical disease
Trichoepithelioma	Abscess; cervical lymphadenitis	Subcutaneous mass (may be large), aspiration of sebum on FNA	Can become secondarily infected	Excision recommended. Wound closure techniques may be required if mass is large
Ovarian neoplasia	Bladder tumour; ovarian cyst	Haematuria; may be palpable (up to 7 cm in diameter) If haemorrhagic then weakness, depression, collapse	Account for 25% of spontaneous tumours Rarely metastasize	If collapsed due to haemorrhage then supportive care to stabilize Surgical removal – ovariohysterectomy
Mammary neoplasia	Abscess/es; mastitis	Mass in region of mammary gland	Uncommon; rarely these metastasize to lungs	Surgical excision, thoracic radiograph may be prudent
Endocrine disease				
Cystic ovaries	Barbering, ectoparasites, dermatophytosis, alopecia of pregnancy, fetal masses, cystic/enlarged kidneys or ovarian neoplasia on abdominal palpation	Bilateral symmetrical alopecia – flanks and rump, enlarged external genitalia, abdominal distension, infertility	May be bilateral multiple, thin walled up to 7 cm diameter Can be diagnosed on palpation, radiography or by ultrasound examination	Temporary remission with HCG administration; percutaneous drainage is reported, surgical treatment by ovariohysterectomy is recommended

16.15 Neoplastic and endocrine diseases of guinea pigs. (continues) ▶

	Differential diagnoses	Clinical signs	Notes	Treatment
Endocrine disease continued				
Diabetes mellitus	Cystitis, chronic renal failure, urolithiasis, stress, ketosis, anorexia, hepatic lipidosis, inherited cataracts, cataracts secondary to metastatic calcification	Glycosuria with secondary cystitis, hyperglycaemia, cataracts, breeding problems, anorexia, polyuria, polydipsia, haematuria	Glycosuria and hyperglycaemia can result from handling or transport stress, see text for diagnostic tests (e.g. GTT)	Dietary therapy often controls the clinical signs, insulin rarely required. Spontaneous remission is reported. Oral hypoglycaemic drugs (e.g. glipizide) may also be useful
Endocrine alopecia	Dermatophytosis, ectoparasites, barbering, vitamin deficiencies, ovarian cysts	Bilateral flank alopecia in late pregnancy or with repeated breeding (non-pruritic)	'Alopecia of pregnancy'	Rest from breeding and this will resolve following parturition and an improvement in condition
Hyperadrenocorticism (Cushing's disease)	Cystic ovarian disease, vitamin C deficiency, alopecia of pregnancy, barbering	Bilateral symmetrical non-pruritic alopecia, weight loss, polydipsia, anorexia, bilateral exophthalmos	Diagnosis based on adrenal gland ultrasonography, salivary cortisol levels and ACTH response test	Trilostane 2–6 mg/kg orally q24h; side effects observed at higher doses; monitor basal salivary cortisol levels

16.15 (continued) Neoplastic and endocrine diseases of guinea pigs.

Neoplastic disease
Spontaneous tumours in guinea pigs are rare but certain breeds have a genetic susceptibility to spontaneous neoplasia.

Cavian leukaemia
This is a B-cell leukaemia, which may be associated with an endogenous retrovirus of the lymphopoietic system, though Harkness *et al.* (2002) stated that the tumour is more likely transplantable than transmissible. Animals present most often as young adults (typically over 2 years old) with multiple enlarged lymph nodes (e.g. cervical, axillary, inguinal) (Figure 16.16). Organs such as the spleen and liver are also enlarged and this may be detected on abdominal palpation. Often a leukaemic disease (WBC counts typically >25,000/mm³ and can exceed 180,000/mm³) occurs; however, animals with aleukaemic lymphoma may present. Many animals maintain good body condition and are bright and alert until late in the disease course, when they may have rough hair coats, dull eyes, lethargy, anaemia and icterus. Lymph node fine-needle aspiration and cytology may aid diagnosis. Definitive diagnosis is by clinical signs allied with demonstration of neoplasia by lymph node or liver biopsy. Prognosis is poor; the disease tends to have a course of 2–5 weeks. Single treatments of cyclophosphamide have been reported to be curative, but relapses within 10–30 days also occurred (Huerkamp *et al.*, 1996).

Pulmonary neoplasia
Bronchogenic tumours are not uncommon incidental findings in older guinea pigs and are most frequently benign papillary adenomas. They can be multicentric and involve multiple lobules and, if seen on radiographs, may be mistaken for metastatic cancer, abscesses or granulomas. At post-mortem examination they appear as solitary circumscribed small white nodules in the lung periphery. It has been called into question whether these changes are truly neoplastic or are reactive changes associated with infectious agents or foreign bodies.

Cutaneous and subcutaneous neoplasia
Skin and subcutaneous tumours are the second most commonly reported neoplasia of guinea pigs. The majority are benign trichoepithelioma, which are usually cystic (Figure 16.17). They can arise anywhere on the body, but usually occur on the dorsum and may contain sebum, hair and keratin debris. Aspiration of

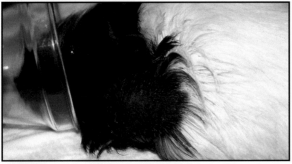

16.16 Guinea pig with enlarged submandibular lymph node. This animal had generalized lymphadenopathy. Lymph node biopsy confirmed the diagnosis of lymphoma. The animal was euthanased four weeks later when it became lethargic and anorexic. (Courtesy of Emma Keeble.)

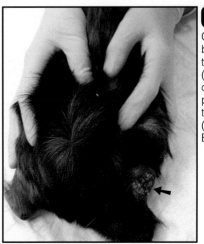

16.17
Guinea pig with benign trichoepithelioma (arrowed). These occur commonly, particularly along the dorsum. (Courtesy of Emma Keeble.)

sebum from a subcutaneous mass suggests a benign cystic neoplasm. These cysts can grow to a large size and become secondarily infected. They may go on to ulcerate and discharge. Complete excision with removal of the capsule is recommended. Although guinea pigs do have plenty of loose skin dorsally, wound closure techniques such as undermining or skin flaps may be required if the excised mass is very large.

Reproductive tract neoplasia

Ovarian tumours are most commonly unilateral teratomas and are seen in females over 3 years of age. They can result in a greatly enlarged ovary (>7 cm) and may be detected on palpation. Although they seldom metastasize, they can implant on the surfaces of the abdominal viscera. Clinical signs can include weakness, depression and collapse if there is intra-abdominal haemorrhage from the tumour. Ovariohysterectomy is the treatment of choice. Uterine tumours tend to be benign and are most often fibromas and leiomyomas. Infection and pyometra can arise secondarily to any uterine neoplasia. Mammary tumours can occur in males and females, the most common benign tumours being adenomas and fibroadenomas, with the most prevalent malignant tumours being adenocarcinomas. Recorded sites of metastasis include regional lymph nodes, lungs, pleura and abdominal viscera. Treatment is by excision with 5–10 mm margins and removal of local lymph nodes if possible. A thoracic radiograph may be prudent before removing mammary masses.

Endocrine disease

Endocrine alopecia ('alopecia of pregnancy')

Bilateral non-pruritic flank alopecia frequently occurs in sows in advanced pregnancy and early lactation, particularly in animals that have been bred repeatedly and are in poor condition. Nutritional and genetic factors may be involved. In pregnant animals the hair loss may be associated with reduced anabolism of maternal skin during fetal growth and the high metabolic demands of pregnancy. Diagnosis is based on reproductive history and ruling out other causes (see Figure 16.15). The hair loss usually occurs over the flanks and rump and will diminish and resolve if further breeding is delayed and the animal's condition (i.e. health and husbandry) is improved. If repeated breeding with mating at postpartum oestrus occurs, this condition is likely to progress.

Hyperadrenocorticism (Cushing's disease)

This condition has recently been described in a 4-year-old female guinea pig, associated with bilateral symmetrical alopecia, polydipsia, weight loss and bilateral exophthalmos (Zeugswetter *et al.*, 2007). Diagnosis was based on: abdominal ultrasonography that demonstrated enlarged adrenal glands; measurement of basal salivary cortisol values; and adrenocorticotropic hormone (ACTH) response testing. The latter two tests have been validated in guinea pigs and in this case showed hypercortisolism and hyperreactivity of the adrenals in the affected guinea pig when compared with control animals. Treatment with 2–6 mg trilostane orally once daily was successful. Careful monitoring of basal salivary cortisol concentrations was essential to ensure adequate therapy and reduce potential side effects at higher dose rates (inappetence and weight loss).

Cystic ovaries

This is a fairly common disease in female guinea pigs of 1½–5 years of age. An incidence of 76% has been reported at post-mortem examination (Keller *et al.*, 1987). Animals present with non-pruritic alopecia (usually bilateral and symmetrical; Figure 16.18), abdominal distension, enlargement of the external genitalia and failure to breed. Masses may be palpated on abdominal examination and confirmation of diagnosis can be made by radiography or ultrasonography, which aids in differentiation of cysts from ovarian tumours. Cysts can be as large as 7 cm in diameter and may be unilateral or bilateral and singular or multilobular. A temporary response may be seen with the administration of human chorionic gonadotrophin; recommended dose regimes vary but include 100 IU i.m. once weekly for three doses, or once a fortnight for two doses. Percutaneous drainage is reported but is not curative. Surgical treatment by ovariohysterectomy is the treatment of choice. (See also Chapter 13.)

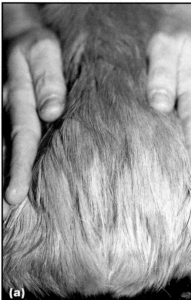
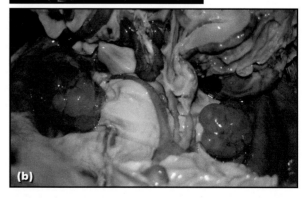

16.18 **(a)** Bilateral symmetrical alopecia in a female guinea pig. Cystic ovaries were palpable on examination and confirmed with ultrasonographic examination. **(b)** Post-mortem dissection of a female guinea pig with bilateral cystic ovarian disease. (Courtesy of Emma Keeble.)

Diabetes mellitus

Spontaneous disease is reported in the guinea pig with a variety of suggested aetiologies. Clinical signs tend to occur in animals over 6 months old and include polyuria/polydipsia, glucosuria (100–2500 mg/100 ml), hyperglycaemia with secondary cystitis, chronic weight loss and cataracts in more advanced cases. Various breeding problems are reported in colony situations. Diagnosis is based on clinical signs and results of glucose tolerance testing (GTT). For GTT the animal has blood glucose levels measured following an 18-hour fast. An oral glucose challenge is then given at 1.75 g/kg body weight. Glucose values after dosing will be at least double the fasting baseline in diabetics and only 1–1.5 times the baseline value in normal animals. Caution must be exercised in interpreting mild glycosuria and blood glucose elevation since they can rise transiently and return to normal without post-mortem changes consistent with diabetes. Additionally, ascorbic acid may interfere with laboratory determinations for glycosuria (Lang *et al.*, 1976). As with other species, blood glucose levels are sensitive to handling and collection techniques. Treatment should be with a high-fibre diet; most animals do not require insulin treatment and spontaneous remission does seem to occur (evidenced by lack of glycosuria). Insulin therapy is reported with NPH insulin started at 1 IU every 12 hours and titrated to effect. Vannevel (1998) reported that an owner was able to monitor urine glucose by training the animal to urinate in response to being offered a food reward. The successful use of oral hypoglycaemic drugs such as glipizide has been reported anecdotally for type II non-insulin-dependent diabetes mellitus.

Chinchillas

An overview of neoplastic and endocrine diseases in chinchillas is given in Figure 16.19.

	Differential diagnoses	Clinical signs	Notes	Treatment
Tumours				
Rare isolated reports			See general discussion	
Endocrine disease				
Diabetes mellitus	Renal disease, cystitis, stress, ketosis, anorexia, hepatic lipidosis	Polyuria, polydipsia, anorexia/reduced appetite, weight loss, (early) cataracts, depression	Persistent glycosuria, ketonuria and elevated blood glucose levels aid diagnosis	Increased dietary fibre, insulin therapy, though no successful treatment is documented
Fur chewing			Not truly an endocrine problem – see discussion in text	

16.19   Neoplastic and endocrine diseases of chinchillas.

Neoplastic disease

Spontaneous tumours in chinchillas (Figure 16.20) are rarely reported. This could be due to a truly low incidence of neoplasia or because, until relatively

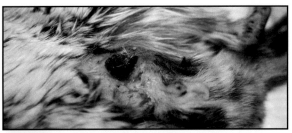

16.20   Ulcerated mammary tumour in a female chinchilla. This was confirmed as an adenocarcinoma on excisional biopsy. (Courtesy of Gidona Goodman.)

recently, chinchillas were bred mainly for fur production. Earlier information on diseases focuses on problems that impacted on commercial fur production.

Endocrine disease

Fur chewing

This problem is recognised to have a multitude of influences (see also Chapter 10). It has been hypothesized that it is linked with hyperplasia and thyroid over-activity; this has not been shown to be the case, however, and it is more likely that thyroid and adrenal hormone secretion are altered as a normal response to the hair loss.

Diabetes mellitus

Only one case of diabetes mellitus treatment is reported in the literature (Marlow, 1995) even though this is the most commonly observed endocrine disease in chinchillas. For clinical signs see Figure 16.19. Diagnosis is based on glycosuria, ± ketonuria and elevated blood glucose levels (>20 mmol/l). In Marlow's report a 5-year-old overweight female chinchilla presented with polyuria, polydipsia and cataracts. Urine dipstick demonstrated a heavy glycosuria with ketonuria. Blood glucose was >22 mmol/l. Treatment was instigated with daily intramuscular injections of insulin (Caninsulin, Intervet) at 2 IU, gradually increasing the dose. Initially a good response to treatment was observed, but it proved impossible to stabilize the condition and the animal was euthanased. Histopathological examination of the pancreatic islets revealed prominent vacuolation consistent with a diagnosis of diabetes mellitus.

Degus

An overview of neoplastic and endocrine diseases in degus is given in Figure 16.21.

Neoplastic disease

According to a study by Murphy *et al.* (1980) the incidence of neoplasms in degus appears to be low. The study describes pathological changes in 189 degus in a laboratory colony, ranging in age up to 60 months. Of the 189 animals examined, seven had neoplastic disease (3.7%). With the exception of one degu (2 years old with a lipoma) all the other neoplasms were in aged animals. Three of the tumours were malignant (two hepatic carcinomas and a sarcoma in a cervical lymph node) and four benign (two hepatomas, a lipoma and a haemangioma of the spleen).

	Differential diagnoses	Clinical signs	Notes	Treatment
Tumours				
Low incidence			See general discussion	
Endocrine disease				
Diabetes mellitus	See differential diagnoses for guinea pig	Raised blood glucose, glycosuria and cataracts	GTT (glucose tolerance test) is used in laboratory animals to diagnose spontaneous onset diabetes	Dietary control prevents or delays onset

16.21 Neoplastic and endocrine diseases of degus.

Endocrine disease

Diabetes mellitus

This is the most frequently reported disease of degus (Murphy *et al.*, 1980). It develops spontaneously in laboratory-housed animals and can be controlled by diet. Wild degus are herbivores, feeding on leaves, bark, and seeds of shrubs and forbs, and they practise coprophagy. Lee (2004) reported that degus should not be fed root vegetables or fruit due to the high sugar and carbohydrate content, which may lead to hyperinsulinaemia and consequent cataract development and kidney failure. Najecki and Tate (1999) reported that degus develop spontaneous diabetes, which is thought to result from feeding high-sugar diets. A low-sugar diet consisting of guinea pig chow with no added sugar is recommended. This appeared to reduce the incidence of cataracts in the degu colony. Diabetic animals have altered glucose tolerance test (GTT) results, high blood glucose, glycosuria and may develop cataracts. A diabetic degu (induced diabetes model) may develop cataracts within 4 weeks (Datiles and Fukui, 1989). The author could find no reference describing the method for GTT or treatment of diabetes with insulin therapy in degus.

References and further reading

Adamcak A, Kaufman A and Quesenberry K (1998) What's your diagnosis: generalized alopecia in a Syrian hamster. *Laboratory Animal* **27**(6), 19–20

Barthold SW (1991) Hemolymphatic tumours. In: *The Pathology of Tumours in Laboratory Animals, III. Tumours of the Hamster*, ed. V Turusov and U Mohr. IARC Scientific Publications, Lyon, France

Bauck (Brouwer) L, Orr JP and Lawrence H (1984) Hyperadrenocorticism in three Teddy Bear hamsters. *Canadian Veterinary Journal* **25**(6), 247–250

Brink-Johnsen T, Brink-Johnsen K and Kilham L (1981) Gestational changes in hamster adrenocortical function. *Journal of Steroid Biochemistry* **14**, 835–839

Cooper JE, Knowler C and Pearson AJ (1991) Tumours in Russian hamsters (*Phodopus sungorus*). *Veterinary Record* **128**, 335–336

Datiles MB and Fukui H (1989) Cataract prevention in diabetic *Octodon degus* with Pfizer's sorbinol. *Current Eye Research* **8**(3), 233–237

Garner MM (2007) Cytological diagnosis of diseases of rabbits, guinea pigs and rodents. *Veterinary Clinics of North America: Exotic Animal Practice* **10**, 25–49

Goodman G (2002) Hamsters. In: *BSAVA Manual of Exotic Pets, 4th edn*, ed. A Meredith and S Redrobe, pp. 26–33. BSAVA Publications, Gloucester

Greenacre CB (2004) Spontaneous tumours of small mammals. *Veterinary Clinics of North America: Exotic Animal Practice* **7**, 627–651

Harkness JE, Murray KA and Wagner JE (2002) Biology and diseases of guinea pigs. In: *Laboratory Animal Medicine, 2nd edn*, ed. JG Fox *et al.*, pp. 203–246, Academic Press, Orlando

Harvey RG, Whitbred TJ, Ferrer L and Cooper JE (1992) Epidermotropic cutaneous T-cell lymphoma (mycosis fungoides) in Syrian hamsters (*Mesocricetus auratus*). A report of six cases and the demonstration of T-cell specificity. *Veterinary Dermatology* **3**(1), 13–19

Haseman JK, Ney E, Nyska A and Rao GN (2003) Effect of diet and animal care/housing protocols on body weight, survival, tumour incidences and nephropathy severity of F344 rats in chronic studies. *Toxicological Pathology* **31**, 674–681

Hejna M and Myers P (2006) 'Octodon degus' (on-line), Animal Diversity Web. Accessed July 25, 2007 at http://animaldiversity.ummz.umich.edu/site/accounts/information/Octodon_degus.html

Hillyer EV, Quesenberry KE and Donnelly TM (1997). Guinea pigs and chinchillas. In: *Ferrets, Rabbits and Rodents Clinical Medicine and Surgery*, ed. EV Hillyer and KE Quesenberry, pp. 244–281. WB Saunders, Philidelphia

Huerkamp MJ, Murray KA and Orosz SE (1996) Guinea pigs. In: *Handbook of Rodent and Rabbit Medicine*, ed. K Laber-Laird *et al.*, pp. 91–149. Pergamon Press, Oxford

Keeble E (2001) Endocrine diseases in small mammals. *In Practice* **23**, 570–585

Keeble E (2002) Gerbils. In: *BSAVA Manual of Exotic pets, 4th edn*, ed. A Meredith and S Redrobe, pp. 34–46. BSAVA Publications, Gloucester

Keller LS, Griffith JW and Lang CM (1987) Reproductive failure associated with cystic rete ovarii in guinea pigs. *Veterinary Pathology* **24**, 335–339

Laber-Laird K, Swindle M and Flecknell PA (eds) (1996) *Handbook of Rodent and Rabbit Medicine*. Pergamon, Elsevier Science, Oxford

Lang CM, Munger BL and Hershey MD (1976) Diabetes mellitus in the guinea pig. *Diabetes* **25**(5), 434–443

Lawrie AM and Megahy IW (1991) Tumours in Russian hamsters. Letter to the *Veterinary Record* **128**(17), 411–412

Lee TM (2004) *Octodon degus*: a diurnal, social, and long-lived rodent. *ILAR Journal* **45**(1), 14–24

Marlow C (1995) Diabetes mellitus in a chinchilla. *Veterinary Record* **136**(23), 595–596

Martinho F (2006) Suspected case of hyperadrenocorticism in a Golden Hamster (*Mesocricetus auratus*). *Veterinary Clinics: Exotic Animal Practice* **9**, 717–721

Meier H and Yerganian GA (1959) Spontaneous hereditary diabetes mellitus in Chinese hamster (Cricetulus-Griseus). 1. Pathological findings. *Proceedings of the Society for Experimental Biology and Medicine* **100**(4), 810–815

Meier H and Yerganian G (1961) Spontaneous hereditary diabetes mellitus in the Chinese Hamster (Cricetulus Griseus). *Diabetes* **10**(1), 19–21

Murphy JC, Crowell TP, Hewes KM *et al.* (1980) Spontaneous lesions in the degu (Rodentia Hystricomorpha: *Octodon Degus*). In: *The Comparative Pathology of Zoo Animals*, ed. RJ Montali and G Migaki, pp. 437–444. Smithsonian Institution Press, Washington DC

Najecki DL and Tate BA (1999) Husbandry and management of the degu (*Octodon degus*). *Laboratory Animal* **28**(3), 54–57

Oglesbee B L (1996) Enfermedades de las aves y de los anumales exoticos de compania. In: *Manual Clinico De Pequenas Especies*, ed. SJ Birchard and RG Sherding, pp. 1481–1687. McGraw Hill Interamericana, Mexico.

Opazo JC (2004) Blood glucose concentration in caviomorph rodents. *Comparative Biochemistry and Physiology – Part A: Molecular and Integrative Physiology* **137**(1), 57–64

Orcutt C J (2005) Common hamster diseases and treatment. In: *The North American Veterinary Conference – 2005 proceedings*, pp. 1358–1360

Ottenweller JE, Tapp WN, Burke JN and Natelson BH (1985) Plasma cortisol and corticosterone concentrations in the golden hamster (*Mesocricetus auratus*). *Life Science* **37**, 1551–1558

Percy DH and Barthold SW (1993) *Pathology of Laboratory Rodents and Rabbits*. Iowa State University Press, Ames, Iowa

Strandberg JD (1987) Neoplastic diseases. In: *Laboratory Hamsters*, ed. GL Van Hoosier, Jr, and CW McPherson, pp. 157–168. Academic Press, New York

Toft JD (1992) Commonly observed spontaneous neoplasms in rabbits, rats, guinea-pigs, hamsters and gerbils. *Seminars in Avian and Exotic Pet Medicine* **1**(2), 80–92

Tucker MJ (1979) The effect of long-term food restriction on tumours in rodents. *International Journal of Cancer* **23**, 803–807

Vannevel J (1998) Diabetes mellitus in a 3-year-old, intact, female guinea pig. *Canadian Veterinary Journal* **39**, 503

Wagner JE and Farrar PL (1987) Husbandry and medicine of small rodents. *Veterinary Clinics of North America: Small Animal Practice* **17**(5), 1061–1087

Watanabe T, Tada N, Nagai H, Sasaki S and Nakao M (1998) *Helicobacter pylori* infection induces gastric cancer in Mongolian gerbils. *Gastroenterology* **115**, 642–648

Zeugswetter F, Fenske M, Hassan J and Kunzel F (2007) Cushing's syndrome in a guinea pig. *Veterinary Record* **160**, 878–880

17

Ferrets: biology and husbandry

John Chitty

Introduction

The ferret is a small carnivore of the Family Mustelidae, which also contains stoats, weasels, otters and badgers. The domestic ferret *Mustela putorius furo* (so-named from the Latin *putor*, stench, and *furonem*, thief) is a domesticated version of the European polecat, *M. putorius putorius*. (It should be noted that the black-footed ferret, *Mustela nigripes*, is not a colour variety of the domestic ferret but a wild species native to North America.)

There is evidence for the domestication of the ferret from approximately 1800 BC – approximately the same time as the cat became domesticated. There are references in both Greek and Roman literature to tame ferrets being used for hunting. This is their major role and ferrets are still used for hunting in many countries, though notably not in the United States or Japan, where they are kept almost exclusively as pets.

Ferrets are usually used for bolting rabbits: the ferret is slipped into a burrow and its presence flushes the rabbits out. The hunter will be waiting with gun or hawk, or the escape runs may be covered with nets so that rabbits are flushed into these and then killed by the hunter. Classically ferrets were muzzled to prevent them from killing their own prey and remaining underground to consume it, but this is rarely done now. Apart from hunting rabbits for sport or to eat, ferrets are also used for pest control of rabbits and rodents. In addition, their natural inclination to enter a run has been exploited to gain access to otherwise inaccessible areas; for example, they might be used to carry a cable through a pipe.

In spite of being efficient hunters, ferrets have engaging, playful and friendly personalities and are easily handled. They are also attractive and very active, which means that they are now kept for a much wider variety of reasons:

- **Showing** – ferrets are attractive animals and come in a wide variety of colours (see later). As well as appearance, ferrets are judged on health and character.
- **Racing** – ferrets are very inquisitive and love entering any tube that resembles a rabbit burrow. Races are used in many zoos and country shows as fund-raising entertainments and ferret clubs regularly hold race meetings. In a race, food is placed several feet from one end of a tube (typically long lengths of drain pipe with several bends). There are often wire-covered 'windows' cut in the pipe to enable viewing during the race. The winner is the first ferret to exit the pipe completely.
- **Fur** – now a minimal use, but previously ferrets have been farmed for their fur ('fitch').
- **Laboratory research** – ferrets are widely used in laboratories. While this has resulted in much data that may help the veterinary surgeon treating ferrets, especially with respect to welfare and husbandry, it must be remembered that the ferrets used in laboratories often belong to specific lines. This means that some aspects of their medical management may differ from the pet or working ferret. Laboratory use will not be covered in this chapter.
- **Pets** – ferrets are becoming increasingly popular as domestic pets and may be obtained from pet shops as well as directly from breeders. While their character does make them suitable as pets, they must be well handled from an early age, especially if children are present in the house – even friendly ferrets sometimes will give a 'curiosity nip' and this can be very damaging to a child. Ferrets do mix with dogs and cats but must be introduced when young and should never be left alone with a dog or cat. They are not suitable to mix with pet rabbits or other small mammals.

Biology

The European polecat is a small mustelid carnivore found throughout temperate northern Europe. Across Europe its numbers are declining, though in the UK it is now recovering in terms of both numbers and distribution following heavy persecution by gamekeepers in the 19th century. The name polecat comes from the French *poule-chat* (chicken cat) and in Old English it was known as the foulmart, distinguishing it from the related 'sweetmart' (pine marten) that lacks a defensive scent.

The gait of the polecat (and of the ferret) is ambling when walking, with the head held low, and becomes more sinuous as they run, with much arching of the back. They are active hunters, using hearing and smell as the main senses in locating prey when exploring burrows and cavities. They are basically nocturnal, though nursing females may hunt in daylight.

Wild polecats tend to nest in underground burrows – usually rabbit burrows. They have a home territory that may contain several sleeping burrows as well as above-ground couches (resting places). In some cases they have been known to nest in farm buildings, preying on rodents.

They are not fussy in terms of prey taken: rodents, rabbits, hares, hedgehogs, small birds, eggs, amphibians, reptiles and a wide range of invertebrates are all consumed.

Polecats are generally solitary, with young leaving the mother and dispersing in their first autumn. However, while territorial, they are known to tolerate other polecats in their territory as long as food is plentiful.

Wild polecats can interbreed easily with their domestic descendant, the ferret. Domestic ferrets may become lost while hunting and can adapt to living in the wild, which means that there may be hybridization between polecat and feral ferret. Rehabilitators and veterinary surgeons working with wildlife casualties therefore have a duty to identify polecats correctly before re-releasing them. This is not always straightforward. While ferrets (even so-called polecat-ferrets, i.e. domesticants whose facial markings broadly resemble those of the wild polecat) tend to be paler than the wild counterpart, the darker domestic varieties are very similar. The Vincent Wildlife Trust (see end of chapter for address) publishes an excellent illustrated leaflet on this subject.

Biological data for the domestic ferret are given in Figure 17.1. It should be noted that there may normally be a variation in body weight between seasons, with both male (hob) and female (jill) ferrets laying down fat stores over winter. In some cases this may result in a 20% change in body weight. It is important that owners become familiar with their pet ferret's normal variations and that veterinary surgeons working with ferrets understand that weight loss in spring may be normal. In males there is some crossover, as they will 'bulk up' with increasing testosterone in spring, becoming much more muscular and losing body fat.

Body weight[a]	Male (hob): 1–2 kg Female (jill): 500–900 g
Lifespan	5–15 years, but rare to see ferrets older than 10 years
Body temperature	37.8–40°C
Resting heart rate	200–400 bpm
Resting respiratory rate	33–36/minute

17.1 Biological data for ferrets. [a] Note: there will normally be seasonal variation (e.g. laying down fat stores over winter) of as much as 20%.

Anatomy and physiology

Ferrets are long thin carnivores with short legs, adapted for hunting in tunnels and cavities (Figure 17.2). Many of their features are similar to those of the dog or cat. Figure 17.3 illustrates the internal anatomy. The following provides a brief summary of

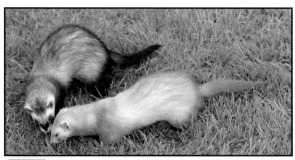

17.2 Note the long thin body shape.

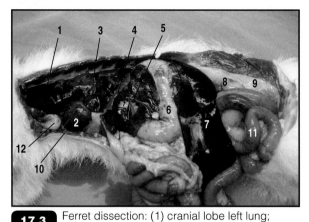

17.3 Ferret dissection: (1) cranial lobe left lung; (2) heart; (3) caudal lobe left lung; (4) diaphragm; (5) liver; (6) stomach (note large size of full stomach); (7) spleen (this is an old ferret, euthanased with barbiturate – both factors contribute to a very large spleen); (8) left kidney; (9) sublumbar fat; (10) sixth rib cut; (11) small intestine; (12) fat deposits in site of thymus gland.

the more important features, i.e. those where the ferret differs greatly from other species and those that have medical or surgical relevance.

Skeleton

Skull

The skull is approximately twice as long as it is wide, but the facial region is quite short. The dorsal surface is flattened and there are large surfaces for attachments of the large temporal muscles.

The jaws are short and the transverse articular fossa (into which the articular condyle of the mandible fits) possesses a postarticular process that prevents dislocation when the jaws are opened widely. The lower jaw fits inside the upper, allowing for a shearing action when chewing.

The teeth are adapted to a carnivorous diet with little need for mastication (Figure 17.4). The dental formula (permanent teeth) is: I 3/3, C 1/1, P 3/3, M 1/2. The last upper premolar and the first lower molar are the enlarged shearing carnassial teeth. The canines are long and pointed and the tips of the upper canines may slightly protrude when the mouth is closed. The upper incisors are longer than the lower (Figure 17.5). Deciduous teeth (I 4/3, C 1/1, M 3/3) erupt from 3 to 4 weeks of age. These are replaced by the permanent teeth between 50 and 74 days of age, starting with canines and lower first molar and ending with the fourth premolar and second molar of the mandible.

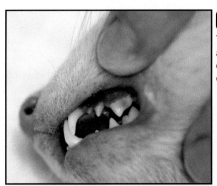

17.4 The teeth are adapted to a carnivorous diet.

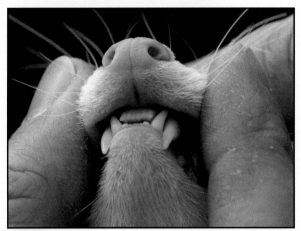

17.5 The upper incisors are longer than the lower and normally are rostral to the lower when the mouth is closed.

Vertebral column

The vertebral formula is: C7, T15, L5–7, S3 (fused), Cd18. The vertebrae are comparatively large for the size of animal and the entire column is extremely flexible. The lumbar vertebrae have very large transverse processes allowing for attachment of the trunk muscles. The cranial and caudal articular processes interdigitate to allow extensive dorsoventral flexion with limited lateral movement.

Ribs

There are 14–15 pairs (some individuals may have 14 ribs on one side and 15 on the other). Ten pairs are attached to the sternum, with four to five pairs unattached, ending in the flank muscles. The first 11 pairs articulate between vertebrae. The remainder only articulate with one vertebral body.

Appendicular skeleton

This is unremarkable and similar to that of the cat. The feet each possess five digits, with the first digit being much shorter than the others. Ferrets have a plantigrade stance.

Muscular system

Superficial musculature is depicted in Figure 17.6. Limb muscles are similar to those in the dog or cat and a full description is given in Fox (1998).

Gastrointestinal tract

Oral cavity

The teeth have been described above.

There are five pairs of salivary glands: parotid, mandibular, sublingual, molar and zygomatic glands. The parotid is seromucous and the mandibular and sublingual glands are mucous. The molar and zygomatic are primarily mucous but partly serous.

The tongue is long and freely mobile. It is covered in four types of papillae:

- Filiform (rostral three-quarters)
- Fungiform (in the same area but fewer in number)
- Vallate (arranged in a V-shape at the base of the tongue)
- Foliate (in elongated groups in the fold just rostral to the tonsillar fossa, which contains the palatine tonsil).

Oesophagus

The oesophagus is long. When not dilated, the mucous membranes lie in longitudinal folds. There are three points of constriction: the origin; where the

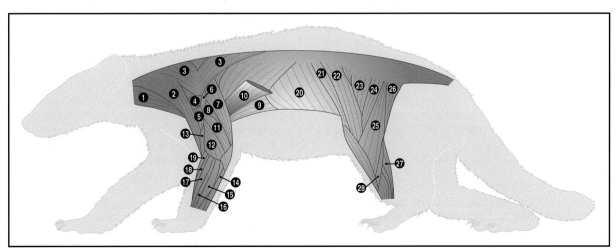

17.6 Superficial musculature of the ferret: (1) sternocephalicus; (2) brachiocephalicus; (3) trapezius; (4) omotransversarius; (5) deltoideus; (6) teres major; (7) triceps (angular head); (8) latissimus dorsi; (9) deep pectoral; (10) cutaneous trunci (cut); (11) triceps (long head); (12) triceps (lateral head); (13) brachialis; (14) flexor carpi ulnaris; (15) ulnaris lateralis; (16) lateral digital extensor; (17) common digital extensor; (18) external carpi radialis; (19) brachioradialis; (20) external abdominal oblique; (21) sartorius; (22) tensor fasciae latae; (23) superficial gluteal; (24) caudofemoralis; (25) biceps femoris; (26) semitendinosus; (27) lateral gastrocnemius; (28) abductor cruris caudalis.

left bronchus crosses; and just cranial to the diaphragm. The oesophagus consists entirely of striated muscle.

Stomach

The stomach is simple (Figure 17.7) and similar in shape to the human stomach. It is relatively large and can thus allow gorging of food. Stomach glands and secretions have been well studied as they are so similar to those of humans, with production of hydrochloric acid and proteolytic enzymes. The natural infection of the ferret stomach with *Helicobacter pylori* also increases the volume of study of this organ in the ferret (see Chapter 25).

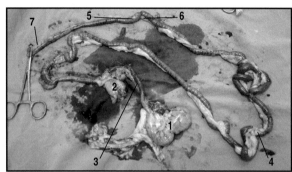

17.7 Gastrointestinal tract of the ferret: (1) stomach (simple monogastric structure); (2) pancreas (partly obscured by pancreatic tumour); (3) duodenum; (4) jejunum; (5) colon; (6) ileocolic junction; (7) rectum.

Small intestine

The small intestine is very short, which is typical of an obligate carnivore. Its length is approximately 190 cm (ratio small intestine to body length approximately 5:1) and it is divided into duodenum, jejunum and ileum.

Pancreas

The pancreas is a long lobulated pink V-shaped structure that is divided into two limbs by a body lying close to the pylorus. The right limb is the more extensive, lying dorsomedial to the duodenum, and follows the descending part of the duodenum.

The left limb extends dorsal to the stomach and medial to the spleen. The ducts from both limbs connect to form a common pancreatic duct that joins the bile duct.

The pancreas has both exocrine and endocrine functions (see also Chapter 30). Insulin is produced in the cells of the islets of Langerhans. Interestingly, blood flow appears to be from the islets *to* the exocrine tissue, which may indicate that the endocrine tissue influences the exocrine.

Large intestine

This is very short (approximately 10 cm) and is divided into colon, rectum and anus. There is no caecum and the ileocolic junction is hard to identify grossly.

The anus is closed by two sphincters: an internal smooth muscle sphincter, and an external striated muscle sphincter that encloses the openings of the ducts of the anal sacs. These paired sacs sit at the 4 o'clock and 8 o'clock positions of the anal canal. They are very large (1.5–2 cm long) and contain the foul scent that is released when the animal is frightened.

Liver

The liver is relatively large in the ferret at approximately 4.3% of body weight (compared with 3.4% in the dog). It has six lobes, with the left lateral lobe being largest. There are cavities in the visceral surface of the caudate lobe for the right kidney and the descending duodenum.

The gall bladder is well developed with a volume of 0.5–1 ml. The cystic duct is joined by three hepatic ducts (left, right and central) to form the common bile duct. The pancreatic duct joins this and the combined duct opens into the duodenum at the major duodenal papillae.

Spleen

The spleen is a large crescent-shaped organ firmly attached to the stomach and liver by the gastrosplenic ligament. In older ferrets the spleen may become very large indeed. While this may reflect a pathological process, even extreme enlargement may simply reflect extramedullary erythropoiesis and be a normal event in the older animal.

Respiratory system

The nasal cavity is comparatively short and is connected to the nasopharynx via the nasopharyngeal opening. The larynx protects the opening of the trachea and contains the vocal cords. The trachea consists of 60–70 C-shaped cartilages extending from the larynx to the bifurcation of the bronchi.

The thoracic cavity is long and narrow but it does widen caudally, effectively forming a tube. The inlet is particularly restricted as the first ribs are very short.

The lungs extend from the 1st to 10th/11th intercostal spaces (see Figure 17.3). The left lung has two lobes (cranial and caudal) and the right has four (cranial, caudal, middle and accessory).

Heart

The heart is placed relatively caudally in the thorax, from 6th to 9th/10th ribs. Its structure is similar to that of other mammals.

Thymus

In young animals a thymus gland is present in the cranial part of the thorax. In older animals it may be replaced by fat (see Figure 17.3).

Urogenital system

The kidneys are smooth bean-shaped structures located in the cranial abdomen, surrounded by fat lying retroperitoneally in the sublumbar region (Figure 17.8). The right kidney is more cranial and is closely related to the caudate lobe of the liver. Ureters pass from the kidneys to the urinary bladder. The bladder is relatively large and, when full, may extend a long way cranially. Urine is voided via the urethra.

Male reproductive tract

Paired testes are located in an external scrotum and vary in size and position according to season (see later). The penis contains an os penis and the end of the penis has a distinctive J-shape (see Chapter 18). There is a distinct prostate gland at the base of the bladder, surrounding the urethra.

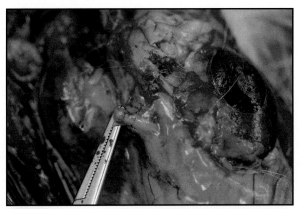

17.8 Kidneys. The right kidney is still contained in its capsule. The left kidney has been exposed, showing the normal slightly pitted surface.

Female reproductive tract

The paired ovaries are located caudal to the kidneys (Figure 17.9). The uterine horns are long and join into a short uterine body with a single cervix. The vagina is relatively short but highly dilatable.

The vulva consists of the vestibule, clitoris and labia. The clitoris is well developed in the ferret. The vulva is covered in hair when out of season but becomes greatly enlarged when in season, under the influence of oestrogen.

The urethra opens at the vaginovestibular junction.

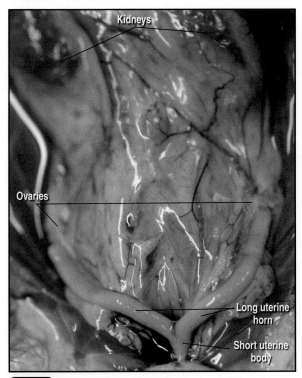

17.9 Female reproductive system.

Adrenal glands

The adrenal glands lie craniomedial to the kidneys (Figure 17.10.) The right gland is closely applied to the caudal vena cava while the left gland is further away. The glands vary in shape from nodular to elongate. The right gland is generally more elongate

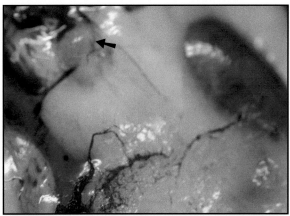

17.10 This enlarged left adrenal gland (arrowed) is clearly visible craniomedial to the kidney. Note the venous drainage of the caudal pole to the vena cava (as an exception to the norm).

than the left. The blood supply to the adrenal glands is very variable and may differ between individuals. However, in general the cranial pole receives blood from the aorta and the caudal pole from the renal artery. Blood drains to the renal vein.

Blood

There is no evidence for blood groups in ferrets, i.e. cross-matching is not essential before transfusing. It should be noted that haematocrit and red blood cell counts are relatively high in ferrets (see Chapter 20). Blood cells are manufactured in bone marrow, but disease or loss of the bone marrow or age-related changes may mean that red blood cell production is switched to the spleen.

There is an extensive system of lymph glands (Figure 17.11) where antigen may be presented to the immune system. Lymphadenopathy is common in systemic or localized infection. Similarly, the spleen may also be involved in such reactions, with splenomegaly sometimes being a feature of systemic infection.

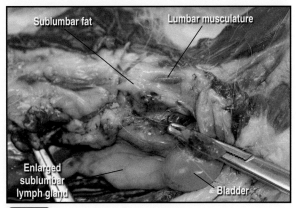

17.11 Position of sublumbar lymph gland(s).

Skin and fur

While dermal structure in ferrets is very similar to that of other furred mammals it is exceptionally thick, especially around the neck area. There are extensive fat deposits within the skin.

The fur is dense with both guard hairs and underfur, though Rex varieties are now being bred. While the basic polecat is dark and the traditional ferret is an albino, there are many different colour varieties and the rarer ones are much prized at shows (Figure 17.12).

There are extensive sebaceous glands associated with the hair follicles and it is these that are responsible for the musky odour of ferrets. There is hormone-associated proliferation of skin glands when in season (hobs more than jills), resulting in an increase in the general odour of ferrets. However, even neutered ferrets have some glandular activity and a musky odour, though much reduced compared with an entire hob. It is important to note that it is not the *anal* glands that are responsible for this smell: 'de-scenting' by surgical removal of the anal glands will have no effect on the skin glands. Routine de-scenting is prohibited in the UK.

Nervous system

The cranium of the ferret is large and the brain, accordingly, is quite large. The olfactory lobes are particularly well developed. Otherwise the structure of the nervous system is similar to that of other mammals (see Chapter 28).

Senses

Ferrets have relatively poor eyesight compared with their senses of smell, taste, and hearing. The eyes, therefore, are relatively small. This poor eyesight accounts for the tendency of ferrets to nip at objects that suddenly loom towards them. Chapter 29 describes the anatomy and physiology of the eye.

The external ears are small and generally held close to the head unless the ferret is excited and aroused. Their size does not indicate poor hearing. Rather, the relatively large tympanic bullae indicate excellent hearing.

The nasal turbinate system of ferrets is extensive (in spite of a relatively short nose) and may assist in providing increased surface area for olfactory receptors. The vomeronasal apparatus is well developed.

Reproductive biology

Ferrets are seasonally monoestrous. Females (jills) come into oestrus (evidenced by marked vulval swelling; Figure 17.13) as day length increases in spring and they will stay in oestrus until they are mated or until day length shortens again. The prolonged high levels of oestrogen mean that many unmated jills die from oestrogen-associated anaemia unless they are artificially brought out of oestrus.

The jill is an induced ovulator and mating is a rough process, with the male (hob) grabbing the female by the scruff before and during mating. There is frequently a lot of noise and mating may be repeated until the jill goes out of oestrus with pregnancy or pseudopregnancy. Both these strategies are adaptations to life as a solitary hunter.

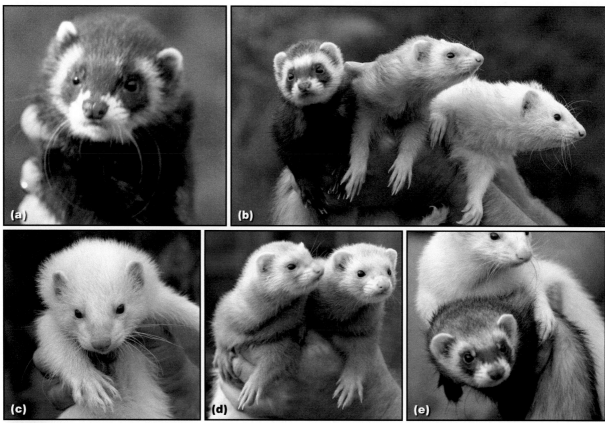

17.12 Colour variations. **(a)** Polecat: note the very dark mask typical of the European polecat from which ferrets were domesticated. **(b)** Colour varieties; from left: polecat-ferret, sandy, silver mink. **(c)** The classic albino ferret. Note the all-white fur and red eyes compared with the silver mink in (b). **(d)** Sandy ferrets. There can be a great range in colours. **(e)** Polecat-ferret and albino.

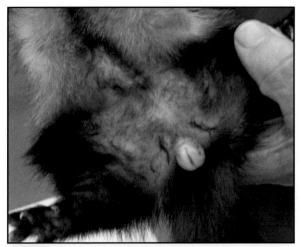

17.13 Swollen vulva of the in-season jill. This animal has been in season for a while, hence the ventral alopecia.

The male also shows seasonality, with the testes being withdrawn into the abdomen during winter before descending and becoming enlarged as day length increases. At this time increased testosterone levels will result in greatly increased body weight and increased activity of the skin glands, such that the hob becomes odorous and has a sticky fur coat. Castrated hobs are known as 'hobbles'.

Both male and female ferrets become sexually mature in their first spring (i.e. when they are approximately 9 months old), but some females will show signs of oestrus in their first autumn if they were born early in that season and the weather conditions are suitable.

Mated jills come out of oestrus in a few days (some authors feel it is quicker if they are pregnant than if they are not).

Gestation is approximately 42 days and the average litter size is six. Fetuses are usually palpable from around 14 days and ultrasonography can also be used in pregnancy diagnosis. The teats start to enlarge in the last few days of pregnancy.

The pregnant jill should be separated from the male. Towards term she should be provided with an insulated whelping box full of hay or shredded paper or towelling. Whelping is rarely problematic (with dystocia being rare in non-laboratory ferrets) but may take several hours. Tarry diarrhoea in the jill is not unusual after whelping, following ingestion of the placentae.

The kits are born hairless and blind and weigh 8–10 g. Teeth start erupting from 2 weeks of age. Eyes open at around 4 weeks, when the kits become more active and start taking solid food, which should be offered *ad libitum*. They are usually completely weaned by 8 weeks, though early weaning is possible from 6 weeks. Kits should be handled regularly from the time they emerge so that they become used to human contact.

Artificial rearing is sometimes necessary. Ferret milk is higher in fat than that of the dog or cat, therefore the addition of egg yolk to cat milk formulae is recommended. Feeds should be given every 2 hours, using a kitten-feeding bottle.

Behaviour

Ferrets maintain many of the characteristics of the European polecat from which they are descended. They are capable of being kept as solitary animals, but they can also live in small family groups. These may be related or unrelated ferrets, or may be an extended family that includes other pets and humans.

Contrary to popular belief, ferrets are not aggressive to each other or to humans. While mating certainly can be violent and males will become more aggressive to each other during the breeding season (especially if an in-oestrus jill can be scented), ferrets are capable of living peacefully in large groups provided that food is plentiful. When new ferrets are added to the group there is usually vigorous sorting of social position, but this normally calms down in a few days. Bite wounds and abscesses are not unknown, but are the exception rather than the rule in a stable colony (see Chapter 24).

As expected in an active hunter, ferrets are exceptionally inquisitive. They will test out most objects by biting them, which is where their reputation as biters comes from. Few bites stem from overt aggression; most are the result of tempting fingers or noses being placed within reach of the mouth of an animal that has poor eyesight. Hands should not be inserted into boxes or sleeping quarters to remove ferrets; instead, they should be picked up as they emerge.

The domestic ferret is much less aggressive and a less active hunter than its wild counterpart, with the result that some ferreters deliberately mate polecats with their ferrets in order to produce more aggressive F1 hybrids.

Ferrets are either very active or fast asleep, which is typical behaviour for a small carnivore. This sleep may be very deep and many owners become concerned at the lack of response from their sleeping ferret.

Ferrets seem to enjoy play activity and interact readily with their owners (Figure 17.14). Care must be taken that playing does not become too rough – human skin is not as thick as ferret skin. Regular confident handling from an early age is the key to avoiding such problems.

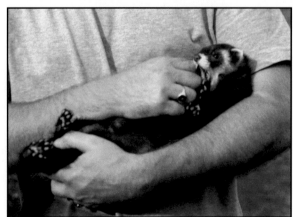

17.14 Ferrets are not vicious. This polecat-ferret is enjoying being handled and mouthing the hand of the handler.

Ferrets are relatively silent but do emit a range of squeaks and whimpers during play or courtship, and when scared they may hiss or scream.

When a ferret is emotionally aroused (especially if scared), its tail is often held straight with the hair on end, known as a 'bottlebrush' tail. If very alarmed the ferret may release the foul-smelling contents of its anal sacs. However, this is an extremely unusual event and certainly does not warrant the prophylactic removal of these glands.

Husbandry

> **WARNING**
> **In some US states it is illegal to keep ferrets, even as pets.**

Traditionally ferrets have been kept outdoors and many owners continue to do this as the basic body odour of ferrets can be deemed offensive or overwhelming, especially if they are kept in small under-ventilated rooms. However, with the growth in popularity of ferrets as pets, there is also a growth in desire to keep ferrets indoors. Many owners will house the ferret outside and then bring it inside to play and 'socialize'. Others will house their pet inside, especially if they have large basements or utility rooms.

Outdoor keeping

The traditional outdoor system was a ferret 'pit' or 'court': a sunken walled enclosure in which a group of ferrets could be kept, with access to a house or box containing bedding materials. Usually the floor of the pit was underwired, as ferrets are not averse to exploratory digging. Ferrets are great escape artists and any enclosure must be secure; even the smallest hole is a potential problem. Enclosure wire must be such that the ferret's head cannot be pushed through. The wire does not have to be thick gauge as ferrets are not great chewers. It is now more usual to house ferrets in purpose-built wooden units. Some of these are large with a play space as well as enclosed sleeping quarters (Figure 17.15).

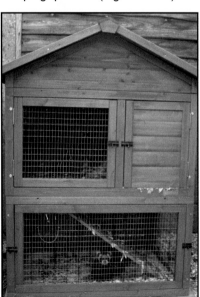

17.15 Basic ferret unit with sleeping quarters (upstairs) and play area.

Working ferrets, or those regularly let out (or brought into the house to play), may be kept in a basic hutch as used for rabbits or guinea pigs. The hutch should be raised off the ground (Figure 17.16), partly to give underfloor ventilation against damp and partly for the convenience of the owner. Where wooden hutches or enclosures are used, they should be regularly checked for lifting panels that could enable a ferret to squeeze through.

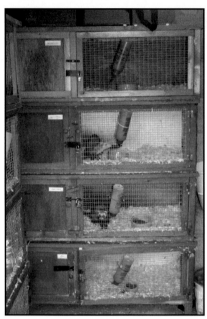

17.16 Hutches for ferrets. Many keepers will stack hutches.

Ferret enclosures should *never* be sited in direct sunlight as the animals are susceptible to overheating, especially if temperatures rise above 30°C.

Sleeping quarters should be well insulated and waterproof. Reflective materials can be placed over the sleeping quarters on hot days to reduce the chances of hyperthermia. The access need not be large (e.g. via a tube or tunnel) and must be sited in such a way that the prevailing wind does not drive in the rain. Suspended hammocks make excellent sleeping areas during the day (Figure 17.17).

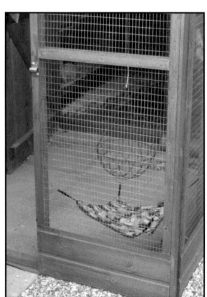

17.17 Two types of sleeping hammock for ferrets. Importantly, they are suspended above ground level.

Bedding

Hay and straw make excellent bedding material, but poor quality bedding may result in respiratory or eye problems. Torn paper is equally effective and does not cause dust-related problems. Either newspaper or shredded paper may be used, though newsprint may rub off and give albino or pale fur a grey tinge.

Towelling or synthetic fleece may also be used as bedding but care must be taken with loose fibres, which may cause problems following ingestion or tangling.

Whatever the bedding material, the floor should be covered with layers of newspaper or sawdust/shavings. Sand should not be used as dropped food may become covered, leading to gut problems following sand ingestion.

Latrines

Ferrets are extremely clean and generally choose one particular area as a latrine. It is best to allow them to choose their own site initially as they rarely just toilet where the litter tray or material is put by the owner. The latrine area is normally in a corner. In a pit or court it is usual for the latrine area to be a soil or sanded area.

Ferret litter trays are normally corner-shaped and have two high sides (ferrets will normally defecate by lifting their tails and squirting soft faeces upwards). Litter material can be placed inside; either soil (or soil–sand mixes), sawdust/wood shavings or cat litter may be used. If the latter, non-scented varieties are best, to avoid chances of chemical reaction and discomfort for the ferret. Rather than litter trays, thick layers of newspaper are useful, but the paper should be folded and placed so that the wall is covered.

If ferrets start changing their toilet habits the reasons for this should be investigated, rather than just moving the litter tray.

Hygiene

The latrine area should be cleaned at least once daily. The rest of the enclosure can be cleaned out on a weekly basis unless it becomes wet or contaminated.

When cleaning out, it is important to check for food stashes (especially if giving fresh food). If stashes are found they should be removed immediately and a note made to reduce daily feeding amounts. Ferrets will usually stash in the same place, making checking easier, but if food is regularly removed ferrets will learn to find new hiding places, which will increase the chances of problems from spoiled food in the enclosure. It is simpler to tailor feeding to the level where there is not sufficient to stash.

Bathing: Ferrets rarely require bathing, though access to fresh water baths may be provided each week. If cleaning is required, warm clean water should suffice. Where indicated, shampoos suitable for cats may be used.

Enrichment

Ferrets are active and inquisitive animals and it is essential to give some form of environmental enrichment (Figure 17.18). As a minimum, a variety of tubes (drainpipes are ideal) and climbing shelves should be provided.

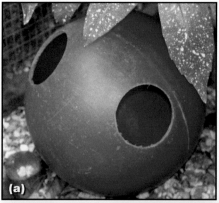

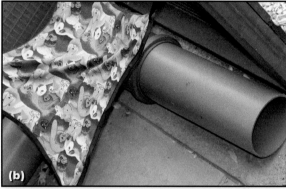

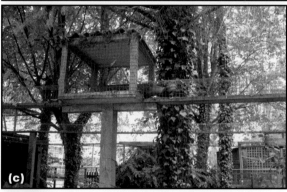

17.18 Environmental enrichment. **(a)** Playball for ferrets. Food can be hidden inside so smaller animals can enter, or larger ones can roll the ball to remove the food. **(b)** A drainpipe provides an excellent enrichment device for ferrets; food can be hidden inside, or ferrets will simply play by running through it. **(c)** Overhead runs for displaying ferrets to the public in a zoo. Ferrets are very active along these runs, even though they have ample sleeping quarters and a basic enclosure.

In addition, food may be hidden in boxes or toys so that the ferret must break in to get access to it. Care must be taken with these toys to ensure that the ferret cannot break off sections and injure itself or ingest pieces. Scatter feeding may also be practised, especially if dry food is given.

Indoor keeping

Hutches and runs (similar to those used outdoors) may be used for indoor keeping. Tall wire cages similar to those used for chinchillas are also suitable.

Cages should not be placed in direct sunlight, nor should they be too close to fires or radiators. Weatherproofing is not needed, but escape-proofing most certainly is.

If space allows, whole rooms can be given over to ferrets, allowing placement of tubes and other enrichment devices. Ferret rooms or areas where ferrets are let out to play must have any potentially harmful object removed and, preferably, the ferrets should be closely supervised when out. They are not particularly destructive chewers, but they do interact with their environment by eating it. Foreign body ingestion, therefore, is very common and particular care must be taken with rubber objects and toys. The spongy filling material of soft furnishing is commonly found as a gastric foreign body. Electrical wires should always be placed out of reach.

The major drawback to keeping ferrets indoors is the smell. The use of air fresheners and deodorants is not recommended as these can cause respiratory irritation. However, smells can be minimized by changing all bedding material regularly (every few days). In an indoor setting, paper is far cleaner and easier to manage as bedding than hay or straw.

Toileting can provide another problem. Ferrets are not easily house-trained as they have such a rapid gut transit time, but they can be trained to recognize a litter tray (see above). Therefore litter trays should be placed in every room to which the ferret is allowed access. Latrine areas should be cleaned whenever they become soiled.

Exercise

Ferrets should be given daily exercise (unless they are kept in groups and their run or court is large enough to allow vigorous play). This may be in the garden or the house and may involve toys or tunnels, or may simply involve direct play with owners. Many ferrets can be easily trained to accept a lead and harness and be taken out for walks.

Diet

Ferrets are obligate carnivores. Their dietary needs (Figure 17.19) can be summarised as follows:

- Protein is the primary metabolite
- Fat is the major source of energy
- Carbohydrate is hardly utilized and the short gut cannot digest any fibre with ease.

In the wild, dietary needs are fulfilled by eating fresh whole carcasses, with rodents and rabbits being the principal prey items. In captivity there are two choices: fresh carcass feeding or prepared diets.

Protein	Levels should be high: 35–40% is recommended Ideally protein should be animal-sourced rather than plant-based Essential amino acids, including taurine, must be included
Fat	High (> 20%)
Fibre	Low (< 2.5%)
Carbohydrate	< 25%
Calcium: phosphorus	Approx 1.1–1.5 (calcium content approx. 1.2 %)

17.19 Constituents of the ferret diet.

Fresh carcass feeding

Care must be taken not simply to feed pure muscle meat or similarly imbalanced diets. Some keepers like to give day-old chicks, though this can be very messy. Frozen rodents are available for feeding but are extremely high in fat, necessitating careful management of the ferret's body weight. Hunting ferrets are often given occasional feeds of fresh rabbit, especially after successful hunting trips; many feel this motivates the ferrets.

Certainly if fresh carcass is given there is a much greater emphasis on monitoring of hygiene. Food spoilage must be avoided when defrosting and preparing feed. Uneaten or stashed food must be removed quickly, especially in summer. Processed meats (e.g. sausage, bacon) must be avoided.

Prepared diets

The advent of good quality dried diets has revolutionized ferret keeping and greatly contributed to increased longevity. It should be remembered that, before these diets, many ferreters fed bread and milk as staple for these obligate carnivores.

There are many diets now available. When selecting the diet, careful analysis of the ingredients and nutrient breakdown should be done and the criteria in Figure 17.19 must be considered.

The major problems with dry diets are:

- Increased need for fresh water – this must be provided at all times
- Obesity – it is easy for ferrets to get fat on these diets and so feeding quantities and ferret body condition must be monitored closely
- Quality – dried diet must be purchased in sealed packets/sacks. While it may seem more economical to buy large bags, failure to use the food quickly will result in spoilage and loss of vitamin content
- Boredom factor – dried diets do not provide much stimulation for the ferret. This can be increased by:
  - Scatter feeding
  - Hiding food in enrichment devices to make the ferret work to obtain the food
  - Provision of occasional treats, e.g. raw bone or raw eggs (in shell). The latter is an excellent method of enriching the diet; ferrets love eggs and will spend hours breaking into one.

Supplements

Many ferreters ask if vitamin supplements should be used. Certainly they are unnecessary when giving a good quality dry diet. Defrosted frozen carcasses, however, may suffer some loss of vitamins and so a general supplement might be useful. When feeding fresh or defrosted carcass, pregnant jills should be given a calcium/vitamin D3 supplement.

Probiotics are not generally believed to have a role in the ferret diet as the gut is short and food undergoes little or no fermentation.

Emergency feeding

Critical nutrition is discussed in Chapter 18. Clinics will sometimes unexpectedly receive rescued or found ferrets and in these cases a dry cat diet (adult maintenance or kitten-type diets) can be fed where proprietary ferret food is not available. Dog food is higher in carbohydrate and may result in diarrhoea.

Treats

In general treats should be avoided (other than as part of a positive reinforcement training regime), otherwise obesity easily develops.

Ferrets are extremely fond of high-fat vitamin gels (e.g. 'NutriPlus', Virbac) and these are ideal treats. Small pieces of the usual ferret kibble may also be used.

Ferrets often show interest in high-carbohydrate human foods such as cakes or fruit. Presumably this is due to novel taste and sweetness. However, they are indigestible for the ferret and should be avoided.

Water

Fresh water must always be provided. Ferrets should be trained to use drinker bottles as they can make a mess with bowls (they seem to enjoy turning these over) or use them as latrines.

Where water bowls are used they should be heavy ones (stones may be placed in them to increase the difficulty in turning them over) and should not be placed near the latrine area.

Identification

Polecat-ferrets often have very distinctive markings and owners are advised to photograph their pets for reference.

Microchips can be placed and are essential if the pet is to be moved under the Pet Travel Scheme (PETS) in Europe. The microchip should be inserted subcutaneously between the shoulder blades. The skin is very thick here and ferrets may wriggle during placement; some vets may therefore choose to anaesthetize the ferret for this procedure.

Collars can be placed, but are readily lost and may also become a hazard for an escaped ferret. Name tags are easily lost or eaten by the ferret.

There is sometimes a reluctance to identify working ferrets individually, in spite of the large numbers lost while working. Many ferreters feel that they might be blamed if the lost ferret kills any domestic stock and therefore do not even advertise that they have lost a ferret.

Even responsible pet owners will have the occasional escape. In these instances it is essential that they secure their own at-risk pets (e.g. rabbits, guinea pigs) and warn neighbours.

Health care

Routine preventive care

An annual health check is recommended and this may coincide with vaccination (see later). While a full physical examination is always advisable, it is important to pay attention to the teeth as dental disease can be common (see also Chapter 18).

Aleutian disease

Some ferret clubs still insist on annual blood or saliva testing of ferrets for Aleutian disease virus (ADV)

antibodies (see Chapter 31). Blood testing relies on the countercurrent electrophoresis test, which is quite insensitive and so results in many false negatives – not ideal as a screening test. The small volume of blood is normally taken by means of a toenail clip, though this is deemed cruel by the National Ferret Welfare Society in the UK. Saliva testing seems better but practically is very hard to perform without the ferret eating the swab. It does not seem to be much more sensitive than blood testing and has the similar disadvantage of being an antibody rather than an antigen test.

Disease due to ADV is rare in ferrets and the screening tests are relatively insensitive and may cause harm. Therefore many clubs are now abandoning their compulsory testing policies. In the author's experience this has not resulted in any increase in disease due to ADV and has had the added advantage that ferreters at shows have become more vigorous in their approach to biosecurity, thus reducing the chances of contracting more common diseases.

Neutering

There have been many changes in this advice over recent years, particularly in respect of an improved understanding of the pathogenesis of adrenal gland disease and the commercial availability of GnRH analogue implants (deslorelin (Suprelorin), Virbac). As of June 2008 this author's advice is as follows.

- Jills:
  - DO NOT SPEY unless there is obvious uterine disease
  - Instead, she should be allowed to come into season in the Spring before being given a 'jill jab'. Typically this is proligestone given at 50 mg/ferret s.c. The injection may sting and cause a reaction but this is normally transient. Occasionally more chronic reactions are seen in the skin and pyometra is a rare complication. The injection is normally given only once each year, with the jill staying out of season after a single dose. However, in years where ferrets come into season early, or where there is a long spell of fine weather in the autumn, or where weather patterns are very changeable, it may be necessary to give additional doses as the jill comes back into season. The owner needs to observe closely for the signs of vulval swelling, etc. as prolonged seasons may result in oestrogen-associated anaemia
  - Where the owner wishes to breed from the jill later that year, buserelin is given at 0.25 ml/ferret i.m. This will induce ovulation and a false pregnancy – the jill will come back into season after 1–2 months
  - Alternatively, GnRH implants may be given subcutaneously every 18–24 months
  - Working ferreters with many jills may elect to have a hob vasectomized as a 'teaser' to mate with the jills and take them out of season. However, as mentioned earlier, ferret mating is violent and repeated matings through the

season may result in damage to the skin at the back of the jill's neck. This is unacceptable to pet owners and in show ferrets. Certainly the practice of sharing teaser hobs between ferreters is to be discouraged, due to the risk of disease transmission.

- Hobs:
  - This is a more difficult issue, as the entire male is extremely large and smelly, with a 'sticky' unattractive feel to the coat. Therefore it is very hard to keep them indoors, or to let them come inside at all. If maintained alone outside then it may be possible to keep them entire. However, owners are often reluctant to handle them, which does make for a less than desirable lifestyle
  - GnRH analogue implants are effective and can be given subcutaneously every 18–24 months
  - If castration must be performed, and the owner is aware of the attendant increased risk of adrenal disease, it should not be done until after puberty – to delay the possible onset of adrenal disease.
- If a ferret has already been surgically neutered and is showing no signs of adrenal disease, then there is a very strong argument to implant GnRH analogue every 18–24 months in order to prevent adrenal disease.

Vaccination
See also Chapter 31.

Rabies
The UK is currently free from rabies and so rabies vaccination is not recommended unless the ferret is travelling within the EU as part of the PETS scheme. There are no vaccines currently licensed in the UK for use in ferrets, but the three vaccines available for use in dogs and cats ('Nobivac Rabies', Intervet; 'Rabisin', Merial; 'Quantum Rabies', Schering-Plough) have been used successfully in ferrets. Whichever vaccine is used, the same protocol is followed, with a single primary vaccination given from 3 months of age and annual booster vaccination. In each case a 1 ml dose is given subcutaneously. Owners should be warned that none of these products is licensed in the UK for ferrets and that adverse reaction is possible.

In other countries where rabies is endemic, vaccination is more to be recommended. However, the basic advice is to consult the drug company before using an unlicensed vaccine in a ferret.

Distemper
In the UK this is recommended for all working ferrets or for those taken out in public for walks. Canine distemper virus is endemic in UK foxes as well as dogs in some areas. There are no licensed distemper vaccines for ferrets in the UK and so drug companies

should always be consulted before off-label use; many have excellent field data for use of their vaccines. In the US a canary-pox adjuvanted vaccine is licensed for use in ferrets ('Purevax Ferret Distemper', Mérial).

Parasite control

Ectoparasites

Fleas: Fleas can be a problem in ferrets and the cat flea is found regularly. When ferrets are housed indoors, they should be included in the overall household flea control programme. Outdoor ferrets rarely require prophylactic control unless fleas prove a persistent problem. In these cases it should be remembered that both on-ferret and environmental control are important. No products are licensed for this purpose in the UK and so drug companies should be contacted before using their products on ferrets.

Ticks: Ticks are a major problem in working ferrets, especially when mature female ticks are inadvertently picked up during hunting trips. They may then lay eggs in the enclosure, resulting in continuing problems.

It is important that ferreters carry tick hooks for removal of ticks. Fipronil spray may be used for on-ferret control of ticks (both treatment and limited prophylaxis). Care must be taken when using the spray that the ferret is kept warm (but not near a naked flame), to avoid hypothermia from cooling effects of the alcohol spray; and that the ferret is not placed in an enclosed area until after the spray has dried, to avoid intoxication from the alcohol vapour.

Endoparasites
Routine endoparasite control is rarely indicated as ferrets are rarely affected. One exception is travelling on the PETS travel scheme in the EU, where anti-tapeworm therapy is compulsory 24–48 hours before returning to the UK. In these instances, praziquantel at 5–12.5 mg/kg s.c. is recommended.

Routine heartworm prophylaxis with ivermectin is indicated where infection is endemic (USA). For further details see Chapter 26.

References and further reading

Fox JG (1998) *Biology and Diseases of the Ferret, 2nd edn.* Williams and Wilkins, Baltimore
Lewington JH (2007) *Ferret Husbandry, Medicine and Surgery, 2nd edn.* Saunders Elsevier, Oxford
Porter V and Brown N (1993) *The Complete Book of Ferrets, rev. edn.* D& M Publications, Bedford

Useful addresses
National Ferret Welfare Society homepage.ntlworld.com/ferreter/index.htm
The Vincent Wildlife Trust, 10 Lovat Lane, London EC3R 8DN

18

Ferrets: physical examination and emergency care

John Chitty

Introduction

The word triage is derived from the French *trier* (to sort) and was originally used in the medical context during the Napoleonic wars. It is still a concept of importance today when assessing the needs and timing of seeing and treating a case. In the practice setting it involves all members of staff, from the receptionist taking the initial call and seeing the ferret as it arrives at the clinic, to the clinician on making an immediate assessment on examination, and to the nursing staff assessing how the needs of the hospitalized patient are changing.

'The call'

The receptionist is the client's first contact with the practice. A well informed and interested receptionist who understands the ferreter's jargon or requests and who appreciates what is an emergency will be a positive boon. It is up to the ferret-interested veterinary surgeon to provide the necessary training.

Receptionists need to be aware of who in the practice works with ferrets and of the correct procedure (who else in the practice should be approached, or where to send difficult cases) when the ferret veterinary surgeon is not available. The following information should be provided:

- Practice neutering policy – time of year, whether the practice approves neutering, minimum ages, preanaesthetic preparation, operating days, timing of preanaesthetic checks, time of discharge, aftercare, etc.
- The difference between vasectomy and castration and why these are performed (this seems obvious but there is a often confusion in the owner's mind)
- 'Jill jabs' – what they are, when done, etc.
- Practice vaccination policies – which vaccines against which diseases, which ferrets need them, when they should be given and when repeated
- Routine anti-parasite treatments – what is needed and when (this is important with many parasiticides being available from other sources; what sets the veterinary clinic apart is the quality of information that comes with the treatment)
- Basic dietary needs – will the practice stock ferret diets and will it order them in specially?

- When to ask for advice or to take a message for the veterinary surgeon to speak with the client
- How to transport the ferret and how to deal with the ferret on arrival (see later)
- Instructions to the client to bring food and usual bowls or drinkers in case the ferret has to be hospitalized
- Triage – what is a routine non-urgent appointment *versus* an urgent appointment *versus* an emergency.

The last point is one of the most difficult and certainly one of the most important. As a basic rule when dealing with smaller exotics, everything should be treated at least as an urgent case, especially if the animal has already been ill for a while. Clinical signs requiring urgent attention are given in Figure 18.1. In all cases, the owner's perceptions have to be taken into account. While some may need persuading that their ferret is an emergency case, the opposite situation will also occur. In these cases it is unwise to dismiss out of hand the owner's opinion that it is an emergency; instead the earliest appointment at mutual convenience should be offered.

Collapse
Hyperthermia
Dyspnoea
Hindlimb paralysis/paresis
Hypersalivation and pawing at the mouth
Seizures/syncope
Vomition
Abdominal swelling
Dysuria
Diarrhoea if associated with ill health
Discharge from eyes, nose or vulva if associated with ill health

---

18.1 Clinical signs that should be regarded as requiring urgent attention.

Transport

Ferrets are small and easily transported. Working ferreters and some owners have special ferret travelling boxes, which tend to be wooden with lift-up tops (Figure 18.2a). Many are made to carry more than one ferret, each in an individual compartment. Otherwise picnic baskets and cat carriers are ideal (Figure 18.2b,c); top-opening baskets are better than front-opening carriers. The carrier can be covered with a towel or blanket, which may help to calm the ferret.

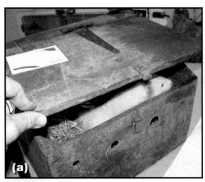
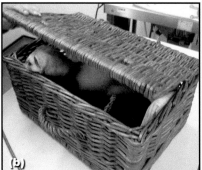
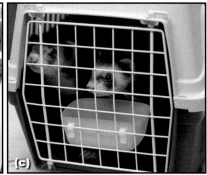

18.2   **(a)** Ferreter's transport box. **(b,c)** Alternative transport boxes. Note the water/food carrier on the door of the plastic carrier.

Ferrets should be transported individually unless they are used to living together, in which case two or three may be brought in the same carrier. The transport box should be lined with paper, hay or straw. Paper is ideal as it is absorbent and creates less mess in the consulting room when the ferret is removed.

Water drinkers may be attached to the front of the carrier if it is to be a long journey, but it is important to make sure these do not drip. Bowls are inappropriate. It is rarely necessary to provide food for the journey.

It is vital to avoid overheating, so ferrets should never be left in the car on a hot day. Hypothermia is much less likely. However, if in doubt (on a cold day), the car should be pre-warmed before placing the ferret in it.

Collapsed ferrets will become hypothermic very quickly due to their high surface area to volume ratio. They should therefore be wrapped in towels and placed on a hot-water bottle (or hand warmer) during transportation.

Ferrets should not be carried loose unless collapsed. Very calm ferrets may be brought in on harness and lead, but it is important that the owner maintains full control at all times.

Arrival at the clinic

If the practice has been correctly informed, the emergency case should be seen immediately by the veterinary surgeon. Where an emergency has not been expected or where a ferret has worsened or destabilized since the clinic was contacted, the animal should be seen immediately and admitted straight away to where it can receive instant attention. A veterinary surgeon should be located as soon as possible. Meanwhile some basic care (warmth, oxygen) may be administered by a veterinary nurse. History taking and full examination may have to wait until after stabilization.

The waiting time should always be kept as short as possible to reduce the stress on a patient that may well be fearful in a situation with many strange scents or sounds. However, working ferrets often work in tandem with dogs so being in a general waiting area may not be a problem for these animals. Pet ferrets that are not used to dogs should be admitted to a separate quiet area. Waiting areas used for rabbits or rodents should not be used for ferrets: the scent of predator will cause undue stress to these other patients.

Handling

The vast majority of ferrets are not vicious and are easy to handle. Correct handling, as in any species, is vital to reduce patient stress and to facilitate a proper examination. It also creates an excellent impression on the owner. Gloves are necessary in some cases, but should be reserved only for vicious animals. Gloves reduce handling sensation and once the ferret is secured the gloves should be removed and the animal held with bare hands.

Once secured, difficult animals can also be tightly towel-wrapped (as for a cat or rabbit) for injections or for certain more invasive examinations (Figure 18.3), but these situations are rare.

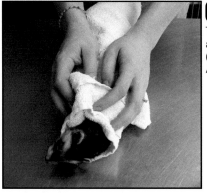

18.3
Towel-wrapping a ferret. (Courtesy of Angela Lennox.)

Most bites occur on removing the ferret from its box. This occurs partly through fear (ferrets have comparatively poor eyesight and may well be stressed by the strange environment and the car journey to the clinic). Ferreters will usually tell you if the ferret is a known biter. In these cases it is appropriate to ask the ferreter to pick up their own animal. Otherwise, it is important to follow two rules:

- Look at the ferret. If it appears excited (very bright expression; moving in an agitated fashion), or is vocalizing or has the classic 'bottlebrush' tail, do not simply reach for the ferret. It is showing signs of fear and excitement and is much more likely to bite
- *Never* reach into the travelling box. Instead, open the door and lid and wait for the ferret to emerge. It can then easily be grasped around the shoulders (Figure 18.4a,b).

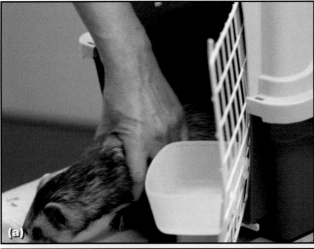

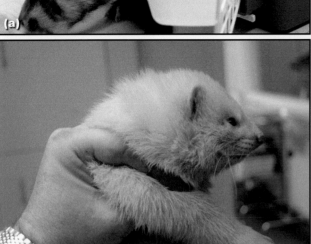

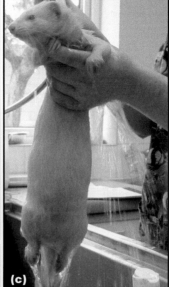

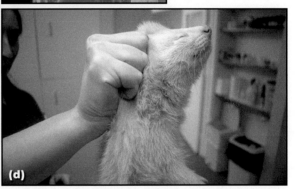

18.4

Handling. **(a)** Never reach into a box to catch a ferret. Allow its natural curiosity to bring it out, then grasp it around the shoulders from above. **(b)** Ferret grasped around the shoulders. **(c)** If allowed to dangle, ferrets appear to relax and allow many procedures – in this case bathing. **(d)** Scruffing a ferret.

Once grasped around the shoulders, the ferret can be held upright, allowing the hindlegs to dangle (Figure 18.4c). Most ferrets appear relaxed in this position and will allow the majority of a clinical examination to be performed while suspended. However, if the animal is gravid, its weight should be supported with the other hand.

More awkward animals may be restrained by scruffing (Figure 18.4d). Again the hindlegs are allowed to dangle, though these may be loosely held by an assistant if the ferret struggles. Scruffing is a particularly useful hold when giving subcutaneous injections, such as 'jill jabs'. In these cases, the injected solution (usually proligestone) is highly irritant and the ferret may immediately try to turn or struggle. The injector can hold the ferret just above its transport box so that, should the ferret react, it can immediately and rapidly be lowered into its box, the grip released and the hand withdrawn quickly.

The more usual way of holding pet animals on the examination table (restrained at top and tail ends) is not particularly suitable for ferrets and can cause distress. Relaxed pet ferrets can be scooped up with a hand placed under the ventrum. However, even these animals often tolerate more when held as described above.

More invasive examinations, sample taking or injections can be facilitated by an assistant giving a small quantity of a high-fat high-protein nutritional gel (e.g. 'NutriPlus', Virbac) while the ferret is being held.

History and physical examination

In general, the history is taken before the examination (Figure 18.5). This also gives an ideal opportunity to observe the ferret from a distance, either through the wire of the carrying basket or loose on the consulting room floor. In an emergency the history may be taken after initial stabilization of the patient.

Subject	Points and questions
Signalment	Age and sex Breed (in this author's experience there do not appear to be any breed-related conditions, but as more unusual breeds are being produced, it is fair to presume that levels of inbreeding and line-breeding are increasing) Neutering: is the ferret neutered? If so, at what age and what time of year? Jill jabs?
Source, and how long owned	
Recent mixing with other ferrets	New animals, shows, etc.
Vaccination history	
Use of parasiticides, etc.	

18.5 History taking. (continues) ▶

Subject	Points and questions
Diet	Any recent changes? Is the ferret drinking more, or less? Is it drinking from unusual sources (e.g. puddles)?
Recent changes in body weight or condition	Are these normal for this ferret at this time of year?
Clinical signs as reported by the owner	How long present? Initial signs and how they have progressed Any other ferrets affected? Other species (including people) in contact, and are these affected? Medications given
Changes in faeces/ urine	Volume, form, colour, etc. Difficulty passing urine or faeces Is this painful? Is blood present?
Blood loss	

18.5 (continued) History taking.

It is essential to note that ferrets are very susceptible to infection with human influenza viruses, especially if already weak and run-down. As part of the history, it is important to find out whether anyone in the owner's family has been suffering from influenza recently, especially if the ferret is showing signs of respiratory disease or submandibular lymphadeno-pathy. In the clinic, it is advisable that anyone with influenza (or even severe 'cold-like' viral infections) should not treat ferrets. If there is no choice, those in contact with the ferret should wear a facemask and gloves.

Clinical examination

The principles of examination are similar for all species; this section will dwell on features unique to ferrets and special considerations that pertain to them. Observations before handling are outlined in Figure 18.6.

The next step is to pick up the ferret (as described above) and assess its responses to being handled:

- Does it become distressed?
- Is it particularly fearful?
- Does handling appear to cause pain?

Demeanour	Bright? Interested? Aware of surroundings? Are the eyes wide open and ears pricked? Does it appear fearful? Vocalization?
Coat	'Bright' and shiny, or dull and staring? Alopecia?
Gait	In particular, look for hindlimb paresis
Breathing	Rate, type, noise, etc.

18.6 Observations before handling.

Body condition and weight

Body condition should be checked and the ferret should be weighed. Ferrets should not be fat, though many are when given dry diets, in particular during the winter months when they lay down extra body fat reserves (see Chapter 17). It is normal for ferrets to lose this body fat in the spring and summer and they may then appear slightly thin. This is not necessarily a concern, but becoming emaciated is abnormal and it is important to check musculature over fore- and hindquarters, as well as checking condition over the ribs and the lumbar spine. A finding of reasonable or good condition over the forequarters and lumbar area combined with muscle loss over the pelvis and hips indicates problems in this area.

The situation is further confused in entire hobs that 'weight up' in spring as testosterone levels rise. The difference is that this is muscle-related, not fat, and tends to be laid down over the neck and fore-quarters. The smell and coat quality of an in-season hob should make its hormonal state obvious.

Some basic steps regarding body condition are as follows:

- Ask the owner what is normal for that particular ferret
- Assess whether the changes seen are normal, considering age, sex and season
- Assess body condition, not just body weight
- Assess condition over several points – forequarters, ribs, spine, pelvis/hips
- The ribs should be covered in a thin layer of fat. In summer (when fat reserves are reduced and the coat thinner) it can be normal to be able to just see the ribs through the skin
- The lateral and dorsal processes of the lumbar vertebrae should just be palpable.

Lymph glands should be checked, especially submandibular (see below), axillary, inguinal and popliteal.

Skin should be picked up and 'dropped' to assess hydration and protein status. Ferrets are very like cats in that skin tenting may indicate either dehydration or protein loss/deficiency (often the result of anorexia or malabsorption). The mucous membranes of the mouth should also be checked: if 'wet' and there is saliva present, the ferret is unlikely to be dehydrated.

Ancillary aids such as urinalysis and serum biochemistry will also assist in diagnosis of these conditions.

Body temperature

Rectal temperature probes or thermometers may be used but with care. The normal body temperature of the ferret is 37.8–40°C (100–104°F). This may be slightly raised if the ferret is stressed or excessively fearful. It is unusual for rectal temperature to provide much additional clinical information and so it should only be taken if the ferret is fairly tolerant. If it struggles, the figure gained is likely to be excessively high and it is doubtful whether it is worth the ordeal, especially as there is some risk of rectal damage.

Skin

The coat should be checked for general character: colour, density, sheen and cleanliness. A dull staring coat is often a sign of general debility or illness. The density of the coat will vary through the year, being thinnest in summer. The coat of a pale ferret may have been discoloured by newspaper being used as bedding.

Alopecia is common and the skin should be examined for any changes, such as areas of excoriation indicating pruritus. Even if no skin changes are obvious, it is still important to check for pruritus with the owner, who may have noticed that the ferret is scratching or grooming more than normal. Changes such as polyuria or polydipsia may be significant in the alopecic ferret. Alopecia can be cyclical in ferrets and the owner should be questioned as to whether hair loss is normal for that ferret – many entire males lose hair from their tails each autumn (known as 'rat-tail'). This appears similar to signs of adrenal disease, but 'rat-tail' cases are non-progressive and the hair will generally grow back in a month or two.

Where hair appears broken off, a trichogram should be performed to see if the hair has been bitten off or has broken off. The hair should be parted to look for parasites and the skin surface should be examined for crusts, scabs and other lesions (e.g. papules, masses, discoloration). These lesions may be sampled (see Chapter 24).

Limbs and spine

These are readily palpated while the ferret is restrained. The spine is more mobile than in dogs and cats. The limbs are short and fractures are uncommon. Regions of muscle loss or wastage should provoke further investigation of the joints in that region. The feet should be checked; masses are common on the distal limbs and claw loss or damage may also be a cause of lameness.

Head

Some ferrets resent excessive handling around the head and many will give a 'curiosity nip' if not handled carefully. Discharges from the eyes or nares, signs of hypersalivation and any swellings (particularly around the cheek areas, typical of malar abscesses) should be noted. Figure 18.7 outlines checks that should be made for the ears, eyes, mouth and submandibular lymph glands.

Ears: Many ferrets, if they are handled properly, will tolerate gentle auriscopic examination using a small cone. However, if signs of ear disease are present, anaesthesia is often necessary to allow full (ideally endoscopic) examination and to clean the ears. While the ferret is conscious, small samples of cerumen can be taken for cytological and parasitological examination.

Eyes: It is very hard to perform a full ophthalmological examination of such a small eye. In addition, use of a direct ophthalmoscope will mean that the examiner has to put their face very close to the ferret, increasing the chances of a bite. Use of an indirect ophthalmoscope may help. If ocular disease is suspected,

Area	What to note	Comments
Ears	Position; excessive cerumen; signs of excoriation or hair loss around the ears	
Eyes	Brightness; discharges; colour; colour changes or obvious lesions within the eyes; periocular or ocular swelling	Be aware of colour difference between albino and non-albino forms. If cataracts are obvious, check how long they have been present, i.e. sudden or slow onset; also check age of ferret and whether it is drinking more
Mouth	Teeth Gums	
Submandibular lymph glands	Size, firmness and regularity Abscesses	Enlarged (often massively so), firm or irregular glands should warrant further investigation. Abscess: fine-needle aspiration for fluid or cell sample for cytology

18.7 Physical checks around the head.

full examination under anaesthesia may be necessary. See Chapter 29 for full discussion of ophthalmological examination.

Mouth: This can be very difficult to examine. Ensure that the ferret is well secured and then carefully elevate its lips to allow a basic examination of the teeth and gums (Figure 18.8). Use of a speculum to open the mouth is not recommend as it may cause damage or distress. Relaxed ferrets often yawn during examination, allowing a cursory inspection, but more detailed examination may require anaesthesia.

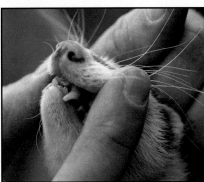

18.8
Careful examination of the teeth in an older ferret.

Chest

The initial examination of the chest should include palpation and gentle percussion. The chest should feel springy and not solid (the latter may increase suspicion of an intrathoracic mass). Percussion should not produce 'solid' sounds; instead the chest should sound as if it is full of air. This may be performed with or without a stethoscope

Full examination should always be made with a stethoscope, as in the cat. Due to the small size of the ferret, a paediatric stethoscope is recommended.

Lungs: At most, soft air sounds should be audible. Crackles and fluid sounds are abnormal and should warrant further investigation. Areas of 'silence' are similarly suspicious, especially if combined with a thorax that feels solid. Both sides should be auscultated and in various positions, which should correspond with the position of each lung lobe (see Chapter 17). Sounds referred from the upper respiratory region may also be heard.

Heart: The heart, if very enlarged, can also be palpated, but auscultation is the main tool in the cardiac examination. It is important to remember that the heart is positioned more caudally than in other pet species. Both sides of the heart should be auscultated as well as the apex and base.

It is wise to listen to the heart while determining pulse rate and character. As in the dog or cat the femoral pulse can be used, though sometimes this can be difficult to identify. If so, an 8 MHz Doppler probe can be used to auscultate the femoral artery. However, use of this device precludes simultaneous assessment of pulse and heart. See Chapter 26 for further details of cardiac examination and detectable abnormalities.

Abdomen

Abdominal masses and organomegaly are common, therefore abdominal palpation is an essential part of the examination. Ferrets rarely resent this, but it should be done with great care as organs may have fragile walls, especially a distended bladder. No attempt should be made to express the bladder in a conscious ferret.

In cases of abdominal distension, the abdomen should be percussed to see whether there is fluid present. If so, this can be tapped and a sample taken for analysis.

It should be relatively easy to identify kidneys, the spleen and the gastrointestinal tract. The kidneys may be palpated as irregular or shrunken, but this can be very hard to assess given their normal position in retroperitoneal fat pads.

The spleen is often large (it can be massive) in older ferrets. This is not necessarily abnormal even if the surface is irregular. It is very close to the skin and needle aspirates can easily be taken from the conscious ferret for cytological examination. If the ferret is not calm and relaxed, sedation may be required. Some clinicians prefer to perform this procedure under ultrasound guidance.

In some cases of adrenal disease the enlarged gland(s) may be palpated slightly cranial to the kidneys, but the absence of this finding does not rule out adrenal disease. The liver is rarely palpable unless enlarged. The intestines may feel thickened in chronic diarrhoea cases and gas-filled loops may be found in foreign body obstruction cases.

Sublumbar and mesenteric lymph nodes should be assessed. They should not normally be palpable, but chains of masses may be found in some cases of lymphoma. In male ferrets with adrenal disease an enlarged prostate may be palpable in the caudal abdomen. If the bladder is distended, this region should be palpated with great care. Rectal palpation should not be performed in the conscious ferret, even in large hobs.

Clinical techniques

Nail trim

Nail trimming is a common request from pet owners. The ferret's feet are long, as are the claws, which can scratch owners or get caught in carpets. Declawing is not an ethical procedure in the UK. Claws are simple to cut and any clippers suitable for cats or birds may be used. The claws are normally white so the quick is normally visible (Figure 18.9). The clippers should be applied 1–2 mm below the end of the visible quick and the nail squeezed side-to-side to minimize bleeding should the quick accidentally be cut. If the quick is cut, it may be cauterized with potassium permanganate or silver nitrate.

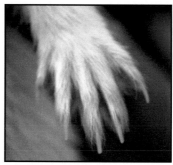

18.9 Normal foot and claws of an albino ferret.

Injection techniques

Subcutaneous injection technique

Subcutaneous injection is suitable for most drugs and for fluid therapy (see below).

The usual area for subcutaneous injection of drugs is the loose skin (scruff) between the shoulder blades. The ferret is scruffed and the scruffing hand is used to tent up the skin. The needle is inserted caudally to this (Figure 18.10a). The ferret may be more easily restrained by holding the scruff so that the hind limbs dangle (Figure 18.10b). If an irritant injection is to be given, the ferret can be given some nutrient jelly as a distraction.

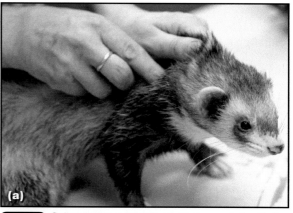

(a)

18.10 Subcutaneous injection techniques: **(a)** with the ferret restrained on the table. (continues) ▶

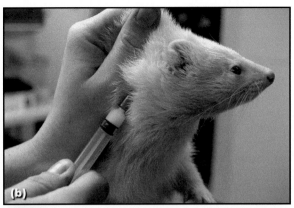

18.10 (continued) Subcutaneous injection techniques: **(b)** with the ferret restrained dangling from the scruff.

Microchip transponders: Microchips should be inserted subcutaneously between the shoulder blades. A bleb of tissue glue may be used to close the insertion hole. Once inserted, the microchip should be palpated and manoeuvred manually so that it is no longer aligned with the insertion hole. This reduces the risk of the ferret grooming out the microchip.

Intramuscular injection technique
Few drugs need to be given intramuscularly. The muscle masses are relatively small in ferrets and large volumes should not be given into them. Intramuscular injections frequently cause pain and the ferret needs to be well restrained with the hind limbs also held. Nutrient jelly should be given to distract the ferret.

Two muscle groups are suitable for injection:

- Biceps femoris – cranial thigh (avoid caudal thigh as there is a risk of irritant injections causing a neuropathy due to interaction with the sciatic nerve)
- Epaxial muscles – either the lumbar group (for very small volumes, 0.25 ml or less) or the cervical group. The latter is a good choice in hobs; less so in jills, due to the smaller bulk of muscle. There is some risk of injection into fat pads, which may delay drug absorption.

Intraperitoneal injection technique
The intraperitoneal route (Figure 18.11) is suitable for fluid therapy or for concentrated dextrose injections. This route is described in the Fluid therapy section (see Figure 18.19).

Blood sampling and intravenous injection techniques

Toenail: A toenail clip has been commonly used in the UK for collecting small volumes of blood into capillary tubes for, say, Aleutian disease serology. It is not appropriate for biochemical or haematological analysis, due to contamination and tissue fluid dilution. The ease of collection (the nail is clipped at 90 degrees to the method for nail clipping described above, and done below the quick) is balanced by the pain it causes. Multiple clips (e.g. for annual

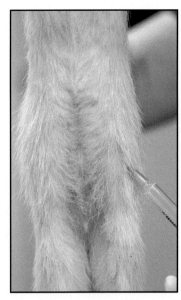

18.11 Intraperitoneal injection technique, using the line of the hind leg to guide the needle into the caudal abdomen. Negative pressure should be applied to the syringe before injecting (in case the needle has been placed into a viscus).

Aleutian testing) will result in nail deformities. For these reasons, coupled with the lack of evidence in favour of testing, the National Ferret Welfare Society in the UK condemns the practice of obtaining samples in this manner.

Jugular vein and cranial vena cava: The jugular vein is the most common site for blood collection (Figure 18.12). In tractable ferrets either the left or right jugular may be used, with a method similar to that in cats and dogs. However, the majority of ferrets have extremely thick skin in this region, making jugular venipuncture difficult. For this reason the author recommends the following:

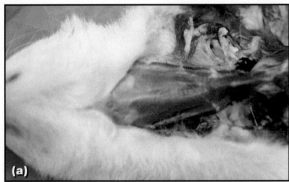

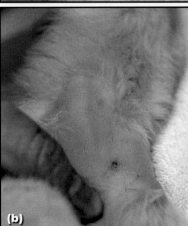

18.12 **(a)** Dissection showing position of left and right jugular veins. **(b)** In the live anaesthetized ferret, the jugular vein can be seen as it is raised.

- Venipuncture under isoflurane anaesthesia. The laboratory should be alerted to this method as there may be alteration of some parameters associated with isoflurane anaesthesia. All materials should be prepared beforehand and the blood taken without delay, otherwise there may some changes in electrolytes
- Use of small gauge needles (23 gauge or less). Thicker needles tend to blunt as they pass through the skin then simply bounce off the vein. A small stab incision in the skin overlying the vein may also make insertion easier and minimize blunting, but great care has to be taken not to incise the vein accidentally.

Where jugular venipuncture becomes difficult, the cranial vena cava may be used. This is an excellent vein and readily accessible as the heart is placed so far caudally in the thorax. Again, this is more suitable in anaesthetized ferrets, but is also possible in tractable or weak conscious ferrets (Figure 18.13). The technique is as follows:

1. Lay the ferret on its back with the head pulled ventrally (or rested over the edge of a table).
2. Insert the needle (typically 1.25 inch, 23 gauge) at 45 degrees into the left thoracic inlet (previously clipped and prepared aseptically), aiming towards the right hind leg.
3. As the needle is inserted, apply gentle negative pressure to the syringe until blood is aspirated. This will be from either the proximal jugular vein or the cranial vena cava.

4. As the needle is withdrawn, apply digital pressure to the thoracic inlet to minimize haematoma formation.

This technique is rarely used for catheterization except in very collapsed or anaesthetized animals.

Cephalic vein: The cephalic vein is suitable for drawing small volumes of blood or for insertion of catheters. The position of the vein and technique are as for dogs and cats, though the shortness of the leg does make this technique more difficult in ferrets (Figure 18.14).

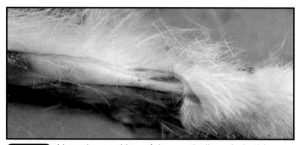

18.14 Note the position of the cephalic vein in this dissection: it lies just medial to the dorsal midline of the leg.

Lateral saphenous vein: This is a useful vein for drawing small to medium volumes of blood and is also suitable for catheterization in collapsed ferrets (Figure 18.15). The technique is as for cats and dogs.

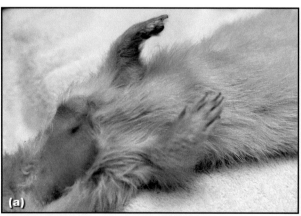

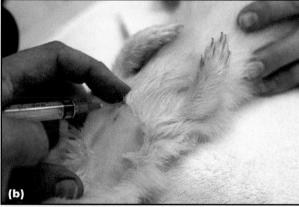

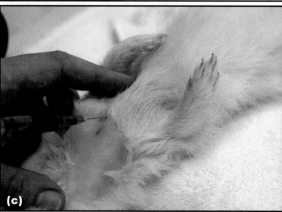

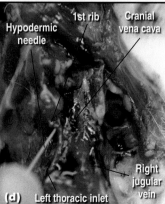

18.13

Hypodermic needle — 1st rib — Cranial vena cava — Right jugular vein — Left thoracic inlet

(a) Anaesthetized ferret positioned for cranial vena cava puncture. **(b,c)** The needle is inserted at 45 degrees into the left thoracic inlet, aiming at the opposite hind leg. As the needle is advanced negative pressure is applied until blood is aspirated. **(d)** Dissection showing the entry of the needle into the thoracic inlet and into the cranial vena cava.

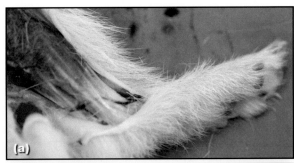

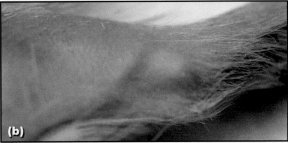

18.15 **(a)** Dissection showing the passage of the lateral saphenous vein proximal to the tarsus. **(b)** In the live animal the vein is readily seen under the clipped skin.

Intraosseous catheterization

Intraosseous catheters (typically 1–1.5 inch, 21–18 gauge hypodermic needles or spinal needles, depending on the size of ferret) can be inserted into the proximal femur (Figure 18.16). The technique is as for cats.

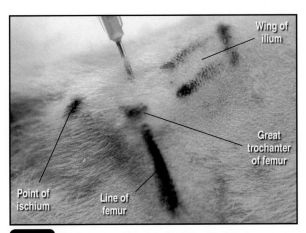

18.16 Positioning of an intraosseous needle.

A syringe pump or Springfusor™ pump is essential whether using this route for fluids or for chemotherapy. The advantage over the intravenous route is that the needles are quicker to place and easier to maintain. However, the procedure is invasive and either the ferret should be anaesthetized or local anaesthetic should be infused over the insertion site.

Ferrets appear to tolerate intraosseous catheters well and this author has not experienced problems with ferrets damaging catheters. Nonetheless, close observation is required. Should the ferret begin chewing the catheter, it may be protected with bandages/tapes or the route of fluid therapy may be reassessed (especially as the ferret improves in demeanour).

The same routes may be used for bone marrow aspiration. The technique is much the same as for dogs or cats, but the iliac crest is probably too small for this to be used safely in ferrets. The tibia or femur may be used instead (see Chapter 20).

Urine collection

While a free-catch sample may be suitable for some tests, cystocentesis is often essential for urine collection. It should be remembered that the bladder may be very fragile if over-distended. Very tractable individuals may allow samples to be taken while conscious, but most animals should be anaesthetized. The ferret is restrained by the scruff and the hind legs (extended) on its side. The bladder is palpated and fixed in position. A 23 gauge 1.25 inch needle is inserted into the ventral midline (previously prepared aseptically) and directed caudally into the bladder. Ultrasound guidance of the needle may also be useful to aid this technique.

Urethral catheterization

This is rarely used to collect urine, but is commonly required to relieve urethral obstruction. The latter is rare in females. Where female urethral catheterization is needed, endoscopic guidance is of great help. In males the situation is greatly hindered by the J-shaped end of the penis (Figure 18.17). Anaesthesia helps in exteriorizing the penis and locating the urethral opening. End-opening silicone catheters are ideal; the gauge should be dictated by the size of urethra, with the widest gauge possible being used.

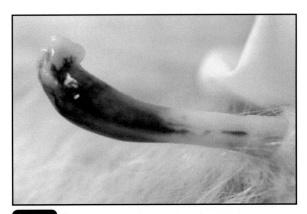

18.17 Ferret penis. Note the J-shaped end.

Blood pressure measurement

Blood pressure measurement (Figure 18.18) is becoming more important in ferrets. While there is little evidence for primary hypertension in this species, it is an invaluable technique in the evaluation and monitoring of the critical patient. The technique used provides indirect assessment of systolic pressure and is very similar to that in cats. An 8 MHz Doppler unit is essential in locating a distal artery in the foreleg (the tapering shape of the hind leg makes it harder to use for this purpose). The cuff is inflated until the pulse can no longer be auscultated. The cuff is deflated while observing the sphygmomanometer reading. Systolic pressure is the pressure recorded when the

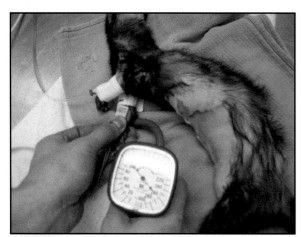

18.18 Taking ferret blood pressure using an 8 MHz Doppler and miniature cuff. Note the intravenous drip secured in the cephalic vein of the other front leg. (Courtesy of Angela Lennox.)

pulse is heard again. Normal systolic pressure is 80–120 mmHg in the ferret. The main source of inaccuracy is an incorrect cuff size. This should be no wider than 40% of leg circumference.

Cytology and biopsy

Needle aspirates may be taken from any mass or swelling. This can usually be done in a conscious ferret during initial examination. Percutaneous needle aspirate/biopsy of the spleen is also easily performed in the ferret. Open lesions may be sampled by direct smear or the taking of acetate tape strips. (See also Chapter 23.)

Cerebrospinal fluid (CSF) collection

CSF collection is indicated in many neurological diseases (see Chapter 28). Where it is to be combined with myelography, the site of collection and of injection of contrast medium should be selected on the basis of the major area required for radiography. Where CSF collection is the major interest, cisternal puncture allows easier collection of larger volumes.

Cisterna magna CSF collection technique

A 23 gauge (0.6 mm) 1.25 inch (30 mm) needle is used. Alternatively a spinal needle may be chosen; the shorter bevel means that it is less likely that there will be extradural leakage, but placement involves use of a stylet and repeated stabilization and checking for CSF during placement. With the limited space in ferrets, a conventional hypodermic needle is preferable.

1. Anaesthetize the ferret and place it in lateral recumbency with the head flexed at 90 degrees to the neck. Excessive flexion should be avoided since it may increase intracranial pressure and increase the potential for brain herniation.
2. Clip the fur on the dorsal head and neck and surgically prepare the site.
3. With the head flexed, insert the needle in the dorsal midline approximately midway between the external occipital protuberance and the craniodorsal tip of the dorsal spine of the C2

(axis) vertebra, just cranial to the cranial wings of the C1 (atlas) vertebra.
4. Slowly introduce the needle until the subarachnoid space is entered. This may be felt as a sudden loss of resistance or, more commonly, when CSF is seen within the hub of the needle.
5. CSF may then be passively collected into tubes (plain and EDTA) or a drop collected on a clean glass slide. Alternatively, gentle aspiration using a 1 ml syringe may be used to collect a larger sample.

No more than 0.25 ml CSF should be collected from an average sized ferret and this should be collected over no less than 10 seconds. Overaggressive aspiration of fluid may result in cerebellar herniation.

If aspirated, a fresh smear should be made before transferring fluid to storage tubes. As with all clinical samples, these should be submitted to a laboratory as soon as possible.

Lumbar CSF collection technique

In order to avoid damage to the spinal cord, fluid should *not* be aspirated by this route.

1. Anaesthetize the ferret and place it in ventral recumbency.
2. Clip the fur over an area cranial to the pelvis, and surgically prepare the site.
3. Introduce a 23 gauge 1.25 inch hypodermic needle almost perpendicular to the spine just cranial to the 6th lumbar vertebra (aiming for the L5–6 space).
4. Insert the needle slowly until CSF is seen in the hub.

It will probably only be possible to collect a drop or two of fluid for cytology from this site.

Saliva collection

This is used in Aleutian disease testing where ELISA methods for antibody testing of saliva have been developed. It appears to be less invasive than blood testing, especially now that toenail clipping is not encouraged. However, the tests used by the author recommend inserting a swab into the ferret's mouth for 60 seconds, which is not easy and there is considerable risk of foreign body ingestion. In a small study of 10 ferrets by this author, saliva testing appeared less sensitive than blood testing, presumably due to difficulties in sampling. Further testing was abandoned using this technique due to the physical problems encountered. Testing under anaesthetic will not necessarily provide better results, since saliva secretion may be reduced. Essentially the risks of testing must be balanced against the benefits.

Emergency support

The following is the author's initial recommended approach to common emergencies encountered in ferrets.

Dyspnoea

- Provide oxygen:
  - If collapsed: place head in facemask. If distressed: add isoflurane (only anaesthetize lightly so the animal becomes still). CHECK AIRWAYS
  - If not collapsed: provide oxygen by chamber.
- Does mucous membrane colour improve? Does breathing stabilize?
- If improved, perform physical examination:
  - If breathing worsens, immediately place back in oxygen, stabilize and re-perform examination under anaesthesia
  - If breathing does not worsen, provide antibiosis, anti-inflammatories and monitor. Look to perform further diagnostics after a few hours.
- As soon as practicable:
  - Perform chest radiography
  - If necessary, drain any pleural effusion.

Collapse

- Provide oxygen:
  - Intubate and provide isoflurane if the ferret begins to regain consciousness and becomes distressed
  - IPPV may be required.
- Check rectal temperature
- Provide warmth, via heat pad or overhead lamp. 'Hot hands' (warm water-filled rubber gloves) may also be used (if hyperthermic, see below)
- Perform physical examination
- Perform further diagnostic tests:
  - Radiography – whole body
  - Blood sampling – electrolytes, PCV, blood smear for differential count and cell morphology, glucose, ionized calcium as minimum database
  - ECG and cardiac ultrasonography if cardiac silhouette enlarged
  - Blood pressure measurement.
- Provide fluid therapy, ideally by intravenous/intraosseous routes. Choice and volume of fluids is dictated by biochemical and haematological results and blood pressure readings
- Further therapy as indicated.

Seizure/syncope

Is the animal still seizuring? If not, treat as normal 'urgent' case (see earlier).
  If it is seizuring:

- Stabilize seizure. Most will stop if general anaesthesia is induced with isoflurane. Otherwise intramuscular or rectal diazepam may be used (0.5–3.0 mg/kg as required)
- Take blood samples for glucose, ionized calcium, PCV, electrolytes as a minimum. Also urea, creatinine and liver parameters if sample size permits
- Provide glucose or calcium if indicated

- Provide fluid therapy based on blood results via intravenous, intraosseous or intraperitoneal routes, depending on perceived need and whether or not fluid is to be given continuously or as bolus
- Recover from anaesthesia. If seizuring resumes, use phenobarbital (1.5–5.0 mg/kg i.v. as required) or diazepam for longer control
- Further diagnostics as required.

Hyperthermia

The ferret will usually feel hot to the touch. Weather conditions and history will probably confirm suspicions.

- Anaesthetize (or stabilize with oxygen if collapsed)
- Measure rectal temperature. Digital units are best as the probe can be inserted rectally, allowing continuous monitoring
- Cover in wet cloths (water should not be cold, so as not to induce shock)
- Give covering antibiotic and anti-inflammatory drugs
- Monitor respiratory and cardiac function
- When rectal temperature normal, place in cool hospitalization unit. Air fans may be useful.

Hindlimb weakness and spinal damage

- Perform full neurological examination as for dog and cat (see also Chapter 28). In particular assess spinal, proprioceptive and hindlimb reflexes and consciousness and awareness of pain in hindlimbs
- Is the ferret thin (i.e. could paresis be due to weakness)?
- If reflexes are diminished or absent, perform spinal radiography (plain films) as soon as possible under anaesthesia in order to establish prognosis
- If there is a history of acute injury, ultra-short-acting corticosteroids may be of some use in the first few hours (methylprednisolone sodium succinate at 30 mg/kg i.m., i.v.). Otherwise, provide antibiotic cover, NSAIDs and further analgesia as required.

Hypersalivation and pawing at the mouth

This is very suggestive of hypoglycaemia.

- Blood glucose should be measured as soon as possible.
- If normal, check mouth for foreign body or investigate for a gastric foreign body (see below).

Acute vomition

- Consider foreign body presence.
- Stabilize with fluid therapy.
- Obtain blood sample for biochemistry and haematology and perform abdominal radiography as soon as possible – three views (left lateral, right lateral and dorsoventral) as minimum.
- Contrast studies as required.

Dysuria

If this occurs in a neutered male, consider adrenal gland disease (and prostatomegaly) as major differential. Urinary calculus is a differential in all animals.

- Examine and gently palpate the abdomen to assess bladder size.
- If bladder is empty, consider possibility of cystitis:
  - Give antibiotic and anti-inflammatory therapy and then monitor
  - Try to obtain a urine sample by free catch.
- If bladder is full, anaesthetize animal:
  - Reduce pressure by withdrawing urine by cystocentesis
  - Perform urinalysis
  - Perform radiography
  - Catheterize bladder and flush
  - Assess blood electrolytes and renal parameters and provide fluid therapy as indicated
  - Further surgical or medical intervention as required.

Hospitalization

Hospitalized ferrets have several particular needs and this can be a stressful time for them. In general, units used for cats are suitable for ferrets, but should have a solid glass or Perspex door, *not* wire or cage front. Ferrets are excellent escapologists and may escape or become stuck. They should be hospitalized in units close to the ground, since they are not a climbing species and often use the front of the cage as a latrine area.

Ferrets that are habituated to dogs and cats can be hospitalized in the same areas as these pets. However, many pets are fearful of dogs and so a separate quiet hospital ward is ideal. If this is shared with cats, they should not be able to see each other.

The hospital unit should not be too hot; it should always be below 30°C even when using a critical care unit for a collapsed animal. For critical care, any unit suitable for puppies and kittens may be used, provided that temperature regulation is in place. Alternatively, solid heating pads (ensuring that there are no exposed wires) or well padded hand warmers or hot-water bottles can be used in the short term.

The hospital unit may be lined with newspaper but towels or Vetbed should also be provided. Ferrets love curling up in these and seem more secure when they have something to hide under. Owners may wish to bring in a favourite toy for the ferret.

Nutrition in the hospital

The ferret should preferably be provided with its usual food bowls and drinkers; otherwise the clinic's own should be used, but should be of the same design as used by the keeper. Bowls should be heavy duty or they will be turned over.

The owner should be asked to bring in some of the ferret's usual diet, unless this is of the same brand stocked by the clinic. Even where dietary deficiency is suspected as a part of the disease, the ferret will probably still fare better if encouraged to eat its normal diet. Once eating, it can then be converted to a more desirable ration.

Critical nutrition may also be required in severely ill animals. The following may be used.

- Nutrient gels may be given directly to the sick ferret or may be smeared on (or mixed with) other foods to encourage eating. They are also excellent for encouraging the taking of tablets, which may simply be coated in gel or crushed into the gel to make a paste.
- Critical care diets suitable for cats are also likely to be suitable for ferrets as they will be high in protein and fat, yet low in carbohydrate and fibre. These can be given by syringe into the mouth or via nasogastric or pharyngostomy tube. Quantities to be given can be calculated in the same way as for cats.
- More specialized critical care diets are now available for ferrets (e.g. 'Emeraid Carnivore Diet', Lafeber or 'Oxbow Carnivore Care Diet', Oxbow). When a specialized diet is used, the manufacturer's instructions should always be followed.
- For short periods, more general critical care mixtures may be used (e.g. 'Critical Care Formula', Vetark). However, this should only be in the short term as many of these are more carbohydrate-based than protein/fat-based.

Fluid therapy

Fluid therapy is often the mainstay of critical care. Various routes may be used and the pros and cons are summarized in Figure 18.19. As a guide to rate, maintenance fluid needs can be estimated at 100 ml/kg/day. Additional requirements can be calculated as in the dog or cat.

Route	Site	Suggested volumes	Continuous vs. bolus	Advantages	Disadvantages
Subcutaneous	Between shoulder blades, or over lateral abdomen	Up to 30 ml/kg	Bolus	Easy and fairly atraumatic Useful for perioperative fluids	Relatively slow absorption Not suitable for the very collapsed animal. Only isotonic solutions may be used. Repeated boluses may be given but some ferrets may resent these

18.19 Fluid therapy routes. (continues) ▶

Route	Site	Suggested volumes	Continuous vs. bolus	Advantages	Disadvantages
Intraperitoneal	The ferret is held vertically and the needle inserted into the caudolateral abdomen at a 45 degree angle	Up to 30 ml/kg	Bolus	Easy and a wider range of fluid solutions (including hypertonic) may be used Also suitable for peri-/postoperative. More rapid absorption	Repeated boluses may cause resentment. Struggling may increase risks of iatrogenic damage. Not to be used where abdominal fluid or likely abdominal pathology (e.g. mass)
Intravenous	Cephalic vein Lateral saphenous vein Jugular vein (more rarely) See earlier	Adjust rate of flow to body mass and likely needs. Shock rates = 60 ml/kg for first hour before reducing to maintenance rates Syringe drivers or infusion pumps can be invaluable	Either	The ideal method for isotonic or hypertonic solutions	May be difficulties in placing and maintaining catheters Ferrets will often have to be anaesthetized for catheter placement
Intraosseous	Proximal femur (see earlier)	As for intravenous technique Syringe driver essential	Continuous	Easier to place and maintain than intravenous. Uptake rapid and a wide range of solutions can be used	More invasive than intravenous. Requires local or general anaesthesia

18.19 (continued) Fluid therapy routes.

The importance of oral fluids should never be underestimated. Ferrets should always be provided with fresh drinking water. Isotonic rehydration formulae normally used for dogs and cats will also be appropriate for ferrets and can be given by syringe or by nasogastric or pharyngostomy tube.

Choice of fluids

The choice of fluids should be based on need. A patient-side electrolyte monitor is invaluable, as is the ability to monitor haematocrit/packed cell volume and plasma proteins.

In general, any of the routine isotonic fluids used for dogs and cats may also be used via the routes outlined above. Hypertonic dextrose solutions may be required in cases of hypoglycaemia and may be given by intravenous, intraosseous or intraperitoneal routes.

Colloids and blood transfusion: Colloids should be used in cases where there is blood or plasma loss and associated hypotensive shock. They should be given by intraosseous or intravenous routes and must be carefully monitored. Regular or continuous assessment of blood pressure is essential in determining when to stop colloid use.

In cases of anaemia or blood loss where the PCV has fallen below 10%, blood transfusion or Oxyglobin™ (Biopure) may be considered. The former can be used if a suitable donor is available; however, in the absence of detailed knowledge about ferret blood groups, transfusion should be performed once only. Blood can be collected from a donor at a rate of approx 3–4% body weight into a heparinized or citrated syringe before being transfused slowly into the recipient.

In view of possible disease risks and the need to anaesthetize the donor, this author prefers the use of Oxyglobin™ in spite of the additional expense. It is important to remember that diagnostic blood samples should be taken before giving Oxyglobin™ and that this compound will affect the ability to monitor electrolytes and PCV.

Whether blood or Oxyglobin™ is used by intravenous or intraosseous routes, a syringe driver or paediatric infusion pump should always be utilized in order to control flow more accurately. Total volume is based on blood pressure measurement, with cessation of colloid when systolic pressure has returned to normal levels.

Euthanasia

While some working ferrets may be regarded as 'tools' or 'stock', many are pets and there may be a considerable bond between a ferreter or pet owner and their ferret. The veterinary surgeon should always proceed in a sympathetic manner.

The procedure may be technically difficult. The author's recommended method of euthanasia is intravenous or intracardiac injection of barbiturate. The latter should never be performed in a conscious animal. The former is not straightforward as ferret veins can be difficult to access (see above) or the owner may find handling to access these veins distressing.

It may be useful to sedate or anaesthetize the ferret first (see Chapter 22). The following may further complicate the procedure:

- Use of some sedatives may reduce blood pressure such that intravenous injection becomes more difficult
- Use of gaseous anaesthesia may reduce the ability to have the owner present, due to health and safety legislation in the UK.

In the author's clinic, ferrets are anaesthetized using isoflurane and a scavenge mask is used. The owner is invited to be with the ferret when a final intracardiac injection of pentobarbital is given. The nature of this injection is always explained to the owner before it is given. An alternative would be to insert an intravenous catheter while the ferret is anaesthetized such that this may be capped and then used for the injection of barbiturate. Some owners may find this less distressing than intra-cardiac injection.

Further reading

Ivey E and Morrissey J (1999) Ferrets: examination and preventive medicine. *Veterinary Clinics of North America: Exotic Animal Practice* **2**(2), 471–494

Lewington JH (2007) *Ferret Husbandry Medicine and Surgery, 2nd edn.* Saunders Elsevier, Oxford

Lichtenberger M (2007) Shock and cardiopulmonary-cerebral resuscitation in small mammals and birds. *Veterinary Clinics of North America: Exotic Animal Practice* **10**(2), 275–292

Pollock C (2007) Emergency medicine of the ferret. *Veterinary Clinics of North America: Exotic Animal Practice* **10**(2), 463–500

Quesenberry KE and Carpenter JW (2004) *Ferrets, Rabbits and Rodents, 2nd edn.* WB Saunders, Philadelphia

19

Ferrets: diagnostic imaging

Simon J. Girling

Radiography

Positioning

Incorrect positioning of small mammal patients such as ferrets has been quoted as the most common reason for non-diagnostic radiographs or misdiagnosis of disease (Williams, 2002). In the majority of cases it is preferable to ensure that the patient is immobilized chemically when performing radiography, either through gaseous or injectable sedation or anaesthesia (see Chapter 22). This will allow the correct anatomical positioning of the patient for standard comparable views to be taken and ensure that clinicians and support staff can vacate the immediate area, complying with any ionizing radiation Health and Safety regulations. Ferrets also tend to be uncooperative when physically restrained, therefore chemical restraint is recommended for their safety and that of the operators.

The usual two views at 90 degrees to each other are required in the majority of cases; a lateral (usually right) and ventrodorsal (VD) or dorsoventral (DV) view (Figure 19.1). Further oblique views may be useful when imaging structures such as the head, where right and left dental arcades may need to be viewed separately. In addition, rostrocaudal views of the head may be useful where visualization of the temporomandibular joint or frontal sinuses is required.

Bisecting angle radiographs are useful, as in cats and dogs, to assess the extent of periodontal disease, a common medical problem in domestic ferrets (see Chapter 25). This technique involves positioning the X-ray beam at 90 degrees to a line equally bisecting the planes of the radiographic film and the axis of the tooth to be examined (Figure 19.2). This avoids distortion of the true length of the root of the tooth, which will occur with standard DV/lateral views, and allows assessment of the periodontal alveolar socket for early abscessation and periodontal disease.

Equipment

Radiography unit

For small mammals such as ferrets, the use of a radiographic unit capable of a range of voltages from 40 to 70 kV, with a rapid exposure time of 0.008–0.16 seconds, is advisable (Silverman, 1993). The latter is useful in ferrets, due to the rapid respiration rates seen. In addition, a radiography unit that permits some variation in the focal–film distance can allow the clinician to magnify some images, which may be useful in smaller patients.

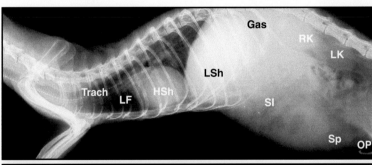
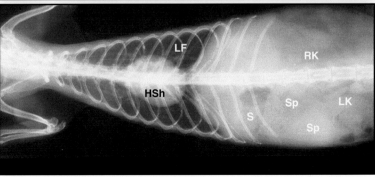

19.1 Right lateral and DV whole body radiographs of a 3-year-old male ferret. Gas = small gas pocket of fundus; HSh = heart shadow with early cardiomegaly; LF = lung field; LK = left kidney; LSh = liver shadow; OP = os penis; RK = right kidney; S = stomach; SI = small intestines; Sp = spleen; Trach = trachea.

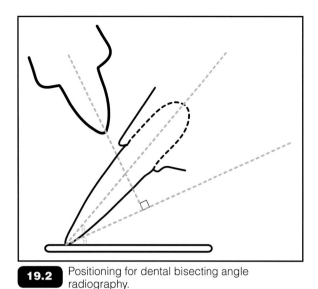

19.2 Positioning for dental bisecting angle radiography.

Smaller radiographic units, such as human dental machines, are particularly helpful. They generally operate on a fixed voltage and amperage, the only variable being the exposure time, which may be varied from 0.1 to 3 seconds on modern digital machines. This allows the fine-detail imaging of distal limbs and the head, and if combined with non-screen dental film it can provide superior imaging to standard veterinary radiography. The possibility of longer exposure times means that patients generally have to be chemically restrained to avoid motion blurring of the image.

Radiographic film and cassettes

The use of grids is rarely necessary in the majority of ferrets, due to their small size.

Non-screen dental films, such as the Kodak series (DF50 and DF75), are extremely helpful for dental and distal limb imaging. Their ability to highlight fine detail, as well as their small size (which can facilitate intra-oral views in smaller individuals), makes them an important asset in ferret radiography. Traditional non-screen mammography film can also be used to enhance imaging for soft tissue detail and distal limbs.

The incorporation of rare earth phosphors in modern cassettes has further enhanced the image produced and allows lower radiation doses to be used, benefiting patient and clinician alike.

Interpretation

Thoracic cavity

Heart: The heart in the ferret is situated rather more caudally than in the cat or dog (Figure 19.3). The thoracic cavity is narrow, which often makes the heart look slightly globoid and preternaturally large, but ferrets are prone to both dilated and hypertrophic cardiomyopathy with true cardiac enlargement (Figure 19.4). The heart normally may be slightly elevated from the sternum, due to fat deposition in the pericardiac ligament, which may be confused with findings of a pneumothorax.

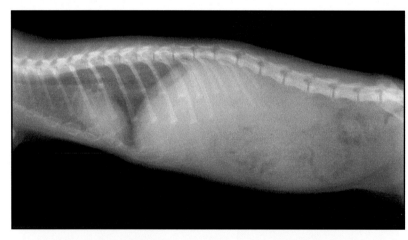

19.3 Right lateral radiograph of an immature ferret with normal heart shadow and obvious vertebral growth plates. (Courtesy of M Ward and the R(D)SVS.)

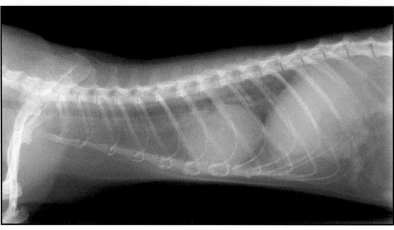

19.4 Right lateral chest radiograph of a ferret with cardiomegaly and perihilar lung oedema. (Courtesy of M Ward and the R(D)SVS.)

The size of the heart may be evaluated using the modified vertebral heart score (VHS), which compares heart length along the long axis against its width on a right lateral plain radiograph, and relating this to the length of the heart in thoracic vertebral units. In ferrets, this has been found to be more variable between the two sexes than the ratio of the right lateral cardiac silhouette long axis length (RL LA) + short axis width (RL SA) in centimetres to the length of the fifth to eighth thoracic vertebrae (T5–T8), i.e. (*RL LA* (cm) + *RL SA* (cm)) / *T5–T8* (cm) (Figure 19.5).

The latter ratio showed no significant difference between the sexes or in differing body weights and was quoted as having a mean of 1.35 (SD 0.07) for males and a mean of 1.34 (SD 0.06) for females (Stepien *et al.*, 1999).

Heartworm disease may present with a pleural effusion and cardiomegaly, with principally the right side of the heart being enlarged. In addition, the caudal vena cava is often noticeably dilated, though peripheral pulmonary artery changes seen in dogs with heartworm are not so easily seen in the ferret. This is thought to be due to the siting of the worms in the right ventricle and main pulmonary artery in the ferret (Supakorndej *et al.*, 1995).

Lungs and other organs: Pneumonia may be seen radiographically, usually starting as an interstitial pattern and then progressing to a more alveolar pattern. In severe cases marked bronchial patterns may be observed (Figure 19.6).

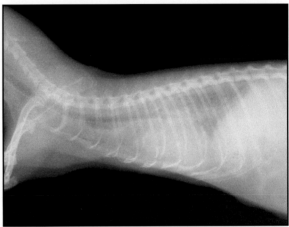
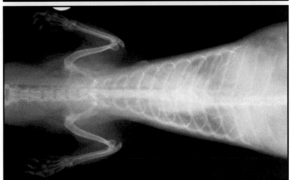

19.6 Lateral and DV chest radiographs of a ferret with pneumonia and cardiomegaly, showing alveolar and bronchial patterns.

Congestive heart failure may lead to a perihilar distribution of lung oedema (see Figure 19.4).

Pleural effusions may be seen due to a right-sided failure (as with heartworm infestation), or, more commonly in the UK, as a result of thoracic neoplasia such as lymphoma (Figure 19.7). Pleural effusions may also be seen as a result of pleurisy (associated with pneumonia or penetrating thoracic wounds) and, more rarely, chylothorax. Juvenile lymphoma in the ferret characteristically affects ferrets under 14 months of age and one of the target organs for neoplastic change is the thymus (see also Chapter 30). Primary lung neoplasia is rare in ferrets.

Calcification of the soft tissues can occur due to over-supplementation of the diet with vitamin D3 and calcium or may be found coincidentally. It may be

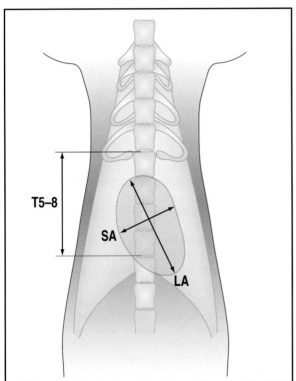
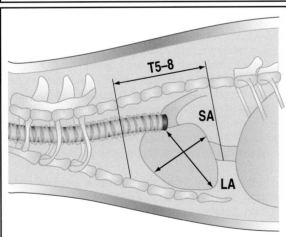

19.5 DV and lateral drawings of the thorax showing measurements of the cardiac outline, indicating thoracic vertebrae measurements (T5–T8) and the long axis (LA) and short axis (SA) of the heart. (Adapted from Stepien *et al.*, 1999, with permission).

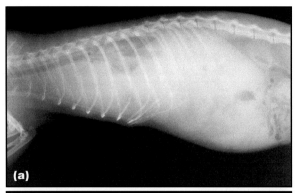

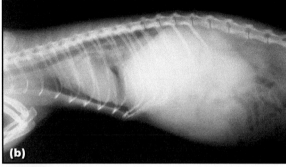

19.7 Lateral radiographs of a ferret with dyspnoea. **(a)** Extensive pleural effusion. **(b)** After removal of the effusion, showing a precardiac mass indicative of thymic neoplasia/lymphoma.

seen in a number of forms, including calcification of the major blood vessels in the thorax and lungs (Figure 19.8) as well as calcification of some of the major organs such as the kidneys.

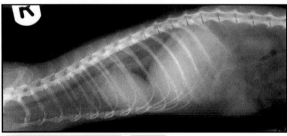

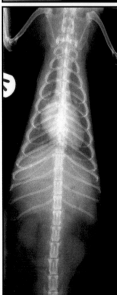

19.8 Lateral and VD radiographs of a ferret chest, showing metastatic calcification of the lungs of unknown aetiology. (Courtesy of M Ward and the R(D)SVS.)

Oesophagus: The oesophagus is not easily seen in the healthy ferret, but megaoesophagus has been reported and may be seen on plain lateral radiographs. As it may still be difficult to discern the enlarged but thin-walled oesophagus in these cases, contrast studies are preferred (see Figure 28.7a). Barium sulphate can be used at a dose of 10–15 ml/kg orally and may be made more palatable by mixing with a meat-based enteric support formula for humans or cats and dogs. Pollock (2007) reported that strawberry-flavoured barium sulphate was readily accepted by ferrets. Oesophageal strictures and motility have also been assessed using a human commercial barium sulphate paste (Esophotrast Cream®, Rhone-Poulenc Rorer Pharmaceuticals) (Stefanacci and Hoefer, 2004).

Abdominal cavity
The ferret abdomen is naturally elongate in form. The visceral organs are generally clearly delineated, due to the presence of retroperitoneal fat depots. The spleen in particular may be very obvious in adult ferrets and is normally of a large size relative to the ferret's overall mass (see Figure 19.1).

Liver: The liver resembles the shape of the liver shadow in the cat. It is normally completely covered by the caudal ribcage. Enlargement of the liver shadow has been associated with neoplasia (such as lymphoma, biliary cystadenoma, cholangiosarcomas and hepatocellular carcinomas), polycystic disease and infectious disease such as mycobacteriosis (Saunders and Thomsen, 2006).

Stomach and intestines: The stomach is situated on the left side on the DV view and immediately behind the dorsal part of the liver shadow on the lateral view. The cranial border of the stomach in a VD radiograph is at the same level as the T13 vertebra (Evans and An, 1998). It is normally devoid of gas, but a very small fundus gas cap can be present in a healthy ferret starved for anaesthesia (see Figure 19.1). Large volumes of gas in the stomach are abnormal and gastric bloat has been reported on ferret farms in recently weaned ferrets (Fox, 1988). Other causes of gas in the stomach include foreign bodies, gastritis and gastric ulcers, including those associated with *Helicobacter mustelae* infections.

Gastric foreign bodies are common in ferrets and along with gastric ulcers are one of the main reasons for performing positive contrast studies. Radiographic evidence of radiolucent gastrointestinal foreign bodies includes increased gas in the stomach and distension and ileus of the small intestine. Ferrets are also prone to gastric adenocarcinomas, which may result in obstructive disease.

In the healthy ferret, the pylorus is situated just to the right of midline on a DV view, with the pyloric opening pointing craniodorsally. The duodenal loop descends close to the right body wall and curves cranially again from mid-abdomen. The jejunum is situated (as with cats) more ventrally and in the mid-abdomen, caudal and ventral to the stomach on a lateral radiograph. It can be seen containing ingesta and small bubbles of gas on plain radiographs. The ileum and large intestine are difficult to discern on plain radiographs unless abnormally gas-filled as a result of total or partial obstructions or intestinal disease (Figure 19.9). The large intestine is short in the ferret. There is no caecum and the most obvious portion is the descending colon and rectum.

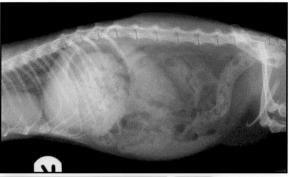

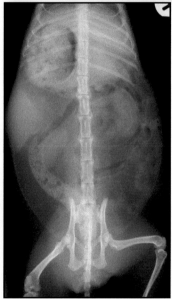

19.9 Lateral and VD radiographs of a ferret with mild gaseous distension of the small intestines due to intestinal disease. (Courtesy of M Ward and the R(D)SVS.)

Thickening of the small intestine may be detectable focally in neoplasms, such as malignant lymphoma, and proliferative ileitis caused by the bacterium *Lawsonia intracellularis*. Alternatively it may be more diffuse, as in eosinophilic enteritis and inflammatory bowel disease.

Spleen: As mentioned above, the normal spleen may appear large in the ferret and so radiographic interpretation of disease in the spleen may be difficult. Gross splenic enlargement may occur due to neoplasia such as lymphoma (Figure 19.10) or haemangiosarcomas, or may be due to extramedullary haemopoiesis.

Kidneys: The kidneys are clearly seen in most cases, due to the presence of the sublumbar fat pads. The right kidney lies cranial to the left, with usually only a little overlap between their respective radiographic shadows on a lateral view.

Renal cysts are commonly seen in ferrets and may be single or multiple. They may be found in both kidneys, enlarging the renal shadows. An often iatrogenic

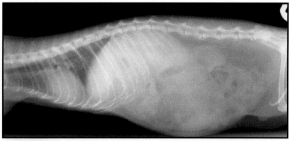

19.10 Right lateral view of a ferret with splenic enlargement due to lymphoma. (Courtesy of M Ward and the R(D)SVS.)

cause of renal shadow enlargement is hydronephrosis, which has been commonly associated with inadvertent ligation of a ureter during ovariohysterectomy.

Urinary bladder: Urolithiasis is common in ferrets (Figure 19.11). It is more frequently reported in male ferrets and urinary obstruction due to uroliths lodging behind the os penis can occur. In general they are magnesium ammonium phosphate (struvite) based and so are relatively easily visualized radiographically. Smaller calculi can be difficult to discern when trapped at the proximal os penis (see also Chapter 27).

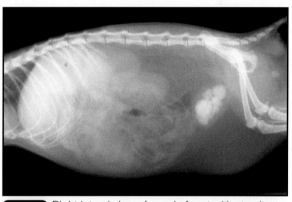

19.11 Right lateral view of a male ferret with struvite uroliths. (Courtesy of M Ward and the R(D)SVS.)

Reproductive organs: The male ferret possesses a prostate gland situated at the neck of the urinary bladder. In addition, a J-shaped os penis is present (see Figure 19.1).

In the female, radiography may be used to detect gravidity, particularly once skeletal development has started, which occurs from the last one-third of the gestation period (i.e. from around day 29–30).

Pyometra does occur in female ferrets, but is perhaps less common now due to the increased number of ovariohysterectomized females. It may be detected radiographically in the same manner as for cats and dogs.

Gastrointestinal tract – contrast studies: All ferrets undergoing contrast gastrointestinal studies should be fasted for 3–4 hours to reduce the intestinal contents. Some authors have recommended up to 6–12 hours' fasting (Oxenham, 1991) but there is a concern regarding the development of hypoglycaemia in ferrets with early or advanced insulinomas and even in otherwise medically healthy ferrets when fasted for this length of time.

Contrast radiography may be performed using 10–15 ml/kg liquid barium sulphate orally or by stomach tube. Palatability is improved by mixing with a proprietary meat-based liquid feed formula or by using strawberry-flavoured barium (see above). Stomach tubing may be performed after deep sedation, but there is a consequent risk of passive reflux and aspiration pneumonia. If there is any concern that gastrointestinal rupture or perforation has occurred, radio-opaque iodine-based products (e.g. iohexol) can be used. These should be diluted 1:1 with tap water and the mixture administered at a rate of 10–15 ml/kg orally or by stomach tube. Sequential radiographs can then be taken, with timings of 5, 10, 20, 40, 60, 90, 120 and 150 minutes after barium administration recommended (Pollock, 2007).

Gastric emptying is almost immediate after administration of barium. Final emptying times have been shown to vary from conscious ferrets (75 ± 54 minutes) to ferrets sedated with ketamine and diazepam (130 ± 40 minutes) (Schwarz et al., 2003). These transit times have considerable cross-over and are statistically not significant in their differences. The small intestines were best highlighted in the above study by the positive contrast media at around 20–40 minutes post administration, when bowel width should be assessed for signs of distension suggestive of an obstruction. Small intestinal width should not normally exceed 5–7 mm.

The large intestine is wider than the small on contrast studies, which differs from that seen in the mink. The ileum is situated near the midline in a DV or VD view. The ascending large intestine runs close to the right body wall before crossing to midline and descending just to the ferret's left of midline. Barium studies highlight the colonic longitudinal folds with filling defects in normal ferrets, which could be confused with linear foreign bodies or nematode parasites.

Urinary tract – contrast studies: Positive contrast urinary bladder studies are limited by access to the bladder. In all cases, anaesthesia of the patient is advised. Catheterization of the female ferret's bladder is possible, but difficult with the urethral opening positioned approximately 1 cm cranial to the clitoris on the ventral floor of the vestibule. The male ferret is more challenging, due to the J-shaped os penis and the small diameter of the urethra. Most cat catheters are not long enough. Orcutt (2003) recommended using a 22 gauge, 8 inch jugular catheter to catheterize male ferrets. If severe para-urethral/prostatic disease is present, the pressure on the urethra may still prevent passage of a catheter.

For this reason an intravenous pyelogram (IVP) is often used to assess the size, position and perfusion/function of the kidneys, ureters and ultimately urinary bladder. IVPs can be useful to highlight renal and ureteral calculi as well as cystic changes and neoplasia. A dose of 720 mg iodine/kg ferret of a non-ionic iodine-containing medium (e.g. iohexol) can be used intravenously to perform an excretory urogram

(Orcutt, 2003). Non-ionic iodine media are preferable to ionic as they do not induce osmotic diuresis, so making contrast studies clearer, and they induce fewer side effects. The cephalic vein is perhaps the most easily accessed vessel (see also Chapter 18). Care should be taken to rehydrate the patient adequately before administering an IVP if the patient has azotaemia.

Head
Dental disease, specifically periodontal disease, is one of the commonest radiographic abnormalities of the head of ferrets. Bisecting angle radiography aids in the detection of periodontal disease and abscess formation (see Figure 19.2). An example of the often advanced periodontal disease and alveolar bone destruction can be seen in Figure 19.12.

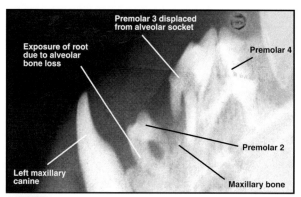

19.12 Intraoral radiograph of alveolar bone loss around premolar 2/premolar 3 of the left maxillary arcade of a 4-year-old castrated male ferret.

Osteomas of the skull have been reported in the ferret and commonly arise from the intramembranous bone of the skull or mandible. They appear as increased areas of radio-opacity, irregularly shaped and slow growing from the surface of the normal bone (Dernell et al., 2001). Faster growing locally invasive osteomas affecting the tympanic bulla have also been reported in the ferret (DeVoe et al., 2002). Other head tumours include squamous cell carcinomas of the gingiva, which may invade underlying bone, producing radiolucent bony changes on radiography.

Axial and appendicular skeleton
The skeleton of the ferret follows a similar form to that seen in most small carnivores. The overall body shape is typically an elongated torso with short limbs and small skull. Notable skeletal differences from other small mammals include the possession of vestigial clavicle bones and the J-shaped os penis in the male. The vertebral formula of the ferret is C7, T15, L5–7, S3, Cd18 (see Figure 19.1), and the dental formula is I 3/3, C 1/1, P 3/3, M 1/2 in the adult ferret. The growth plates, particularly in the pelvis and long bones, do not often close until the ferret is over 7 months of age (Figures 19.3 and 19.13).

Spinal lesions are frequently reported in ferrets, with traumatic injuries resulting in vertebral disc collapse or, more commonly, vertebral body fractures and neoplastic processes being seen.

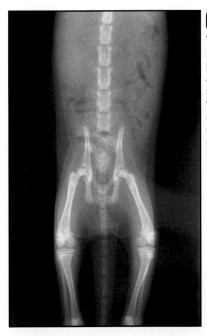

19.13

VD view of an immature ferret pelvis and abdomen showing obvious vertebral, pelvic and hindlimb growth plates. (Courtesy of M Ward and the R(D)SVS.)

Neoplasms affecting the spinal column are mainly chordomas and these chiefly affect the tail. They are benign and slow growing and so rarely produce serious clinical disease. Chordomas of the cervical region have also been reported, although uncommonly (Li and Fox, 1998). These have caused lysis of the cervical vertebrae and produced clinical paresis and paralysis due to compression of the spinal cord and adjacent tissues. Other neoplasms affecting the spine in ferrets include metastatic lymphoma and plasma cell myeloma, both of which can produce lytic lesions.

The most common reported cause of orthopaedic injury in the ferret involves traumatic injury to the long bones, joints or spine, with the most common fracture sites listed as the long bones of the fore- and hindlimbs, particularly the femur (Ritzman and Knapp, 2002). Femoral fractures are usually in the distal metaphysis, and oblique to spiral in nature. Tibial fractures are usually associated with fibular fractures and are generally seen in the mid-metaphyseal region, being oblique to transverse in nature. Femoral head fractures and olecranon fractures of the ulna appear uncommon in the ferret, with only one report documented in each case (Ritzman and Knapp, 2002).

Luxations of joints are also seen, with elbow luxation being the most commonly reported with proximal displacement of the radius and ulna.

Postoperative or traumatic osteomyelitis is not uncommon in ferrets and radiographically resembles that seen in cats and dogs with periosteal proliferation, fracture malunion and lysis being present.

Other primary tumours documented in the musculoskeletal system of ferrets include osteomas, chondromas, chondrosarcomas, fibrosarcomas, rhabdomyosarcomas and synovial cell sarcomas. Acute myelogenous leukaemia causing a cystic bone lesion of the proximal humerus and inducing non-supporting lameness has also been reported (Li and Fox, 1998).

Ultrasonograpy

Positioning

Standard views of the ferret may be obtained using similar techniques to the dog and cat. A right lateral position, using a cut-out imaging window in the table on which the animal is lying to allow access with the probe, is useful for the examination of the heart and kidneys, but it can be stressful to some patients and generally requires prior sedation or anaesthesia.

A standing or upright position, where the ferret's front end is lifted up off the table, is often better tolerated in the conscious patient and allows easier access to organs such as the liver, kidneys and bladder.

Equipment

Ultrasound unit

The ultrasound unit should have a sector probe transducer, due to its smaller footprint. This is particularly important if trying to image the heart, because of the narrow inter-rib spaces. Transducer frequencies of 5–7.5 MHz are required for most ferrets and 10 MHz probes may be useful for imaging structures such as the eye. B-mode ultrasound is mainly used to provide a two-dimensional real-time image of the organs being examined. M-mode is useful when examining the heart to assess its contractility. Pulsed wave Doppler techniques for assessing blood flow direction and the measurement of ejection volumes with continuous wave Doppler are also extremely useful in assessing cardiac disease and may be used in the ferret as with cats and dogs.

Additional equipment

The patient should be shaved and a coupling gel applied a few minutes before imaging, as with any species, to allow it to soak into the outer layers of the skin. In some cases, a stand-off is required. This is often needed where the structure to be imaged is less than 3–5 cm away from the skin or body surface, such as with the eye where a considerable amount of gel needs to be applied to the cornea after first applying local anaesthetic and chemically immobilizing the patient (see also Chapter 29). Commercial stand-offs are superior to home-made ones as they do not create attenuation, resolution or distortion artefacts. Although it is possible to image the eye of a ferret, the technique can prove challenging due to the small size of the organ being imaged.

A printer or video recording capability is also useful to retain images and build up a library of information, both to show owners and to allow reassessment of a patient's progress.

Interpretation

Thoracic cavity

Echocardiography: M-mode and colour Doppler ultrasonography of the heart has been reported in ferrets in two studies (Stepien *et al.*, 2000; Vastenburg *et al.*, 2004). Both studies used chemical restraint, with one using isoflurane and the other using ketamine with midazolam, but there was no significant statistical difference between the majority of intra-cardiac measurements made except as follows: the left ventricular internal diameter on both diastole and systole was greater under isoflurane than under ketamine with midazolam; and the left ventricular width (in both diastole and systole), left atrial appendage diameter and the aorta were smaller under iso-flurane than ketamine with midazolam.

There was no significant difference in the measurements made between males and females in these studies. In addition, the use of the pulmonary artery as opposed to the aorta to measure volume flow in ferrets was recommended, due to the difficulty in aligning the aortic outflow tract (Stepien *et al.*, 2000). See Chapter 26 for echocardiographic values.

Colour Doppler information from Vastenburg *et al.* (2004) demonstrated small regurgitant jets of the mitral and pulmonary valves in five out of 29 sampled and these were judged to be non-significant, in line with similar findings in normal dogs and horses.

Dilated cardiomyopathy is perhaps one of the commonest cardiovascular complaints of ferrets. It generally presents with either individual left or right ventricular dilation or both. Where the left ventricle is dilated, the end-diastolic and end-systolic dimensions are increased and the left atrium is also dilated. Left ventricular outflow velocities are generally reduced in these cases. Where the right ventricle is dilated, again the end-diastolic and end-systolic dimensions are increased and the right atrium is also dilated. In addition, as seen in cats and dogs, the fractional shortening percentage is decreased in both cases and atrioventricular valvular insufficiency due to annulus dilation is often seen. See also Chapter 26 for further information.

Hypertrophic cardiomyopathy has been reported in ferrets. It generally presents echocardiographically as diffuse or occasionally focal thickening of the left ventricular wall with impaired diastolic filling of the left ventricle, resulting in reduced left ventricular diastolic and systolic dimensions. Left atrial enlargement may also be present, as may septal hypertrophy. Doppler colour flow studies of the outflow of the left ventricle can show turbulence due to mitral valve regurgitation and dynamic obstruction.

Valvular insufficiency is also an increasingly commonly diagnosed heart condition in middle-aged to older ferrets. It may be seen as thickening of the affected valves on echocardiography, as with dogs. It often occurs with an increase in left ventricular diasto-lic dimensions, normal systolic dimensions and nor-mal fractional shortening in the early stages. Doppler colour flow can highlight regurgitation and turbulence of blood flow through the damaged valves, but aortic regurgitation is a common incidental finding on ferret echocardiographic examinations and is generally clinically insignificant (Petrie and Morrisey, 2004).

Heartworm disease due to *Dirofilaria immitis* produces typically a right-sided heart failure with right ventricle, right atrial and caudal vena cava enlargement on echocardiography. The adult worms may be seen in the right ventricle, right atrium and pulmonary artery. Pulmonary hypertension may be confirmed with Doppler echocardiography, as for dogs.

Abdominal cavity

Adrenal glands: Adrenal neoplasia has been repeat-edly detected using ultrasound. Normal adrenal size appears to vary according to the sex of the ferret, being greater in width in males, and according to its weight, being generally larger in the heavier individual (O'Brien *et al.*, 1996; Neuwirth *et al.*, 1997). The right adrenal gland is also larger than the left, with ultra-sound measured lengths of the left adrenal gland ranging from 5 to 10.5 mm and right adrenal gland from 7.5 to 12.7 mm. Adrenal widths of the left gland measured 3–4.8 mm and the right gland 2.9–5.1 mm. Adrenal depths of the left gland measured 2–3.8 mm and the right gland 2.2–4.1 mm (Neuwirth *et al.*, 1997). Figure 19.14 shows a normal right adrenal gland and a left adrenal gland from the same ferret but with an adenocarcinoma present.

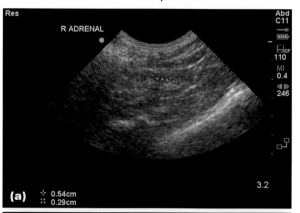

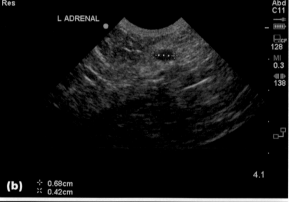

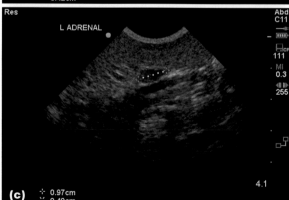

19.14 **(a)** Normal right adrenal gland in cross-section (dotted line). **(b)** Adenocarcinomatous left adrenal gland in cross-section (dotted line); **(c)** in longitudinal section, showing nodule formation at one pole (dotted line). (Courtesy of W Lewis and R Doyle.)

One review (Besso *et al.*, 2000) was unable to differentiate specific different forms of adrenal neoplasia using ultrasound but could determine whether the tumour was either non-resectable or malignant. This was based on the absence of periglandular fat in malignant/non-resectable lesions between the adrenal gland and the large vessels (caudal vena cava or aorta) or the liver, and/or deviation or compression of the large vessels by the adrenal lesion. Interestingly, malignancy could not be based on the size of the adrenal mass. The same study also determined that non-specific adrenal neoplasia could be detected before an increase in adrenal length occurred by increased echogenicity and a focal increase in the adrenal gland width/thickness creating a nodular appearance to the gland. However, the same study found in a small number of cases that ultrasonographically normal adrenal glands could still contain neoplastic (adenomatous) changes histopathologically. Other studies have suggested that the adrenal gland should not exceed 3.9 mm in width (Kuijten *et al.*, 2007).

Kidneys: The renal outline should measure 3 cm × 3 cm (Orcutt, 2003). Solitary renal cysts have been reported as a frequent incidental finding during ultrasound examinations, with 10–15% of ferrets undergoing a post-mortem examination reported as having a renal cyst (Orcutt, 2003). These tend to produce smooth-outlined discrete cysts, usually just underneath the renal capsule.

Polycystic disease, including polycystic kidneys, is unusual in ferrets and is differentiated by the presence of multiple irregular cysts. These are often deep within the renal architecture and may significantly disrupt it, though perinephric cysts may also be associated with this (Puerto *et al.*, 1998). There are also often multiple irregular cysts present in the liver of ferrets suffering from this condition.

Hydronephrosis may be easily detected using ultrasonography. The cause has usually been reported as iatrogenic ligation of the ureter when performing ovariohysterectomy.

Spleen: Splenic enlargement is common in ferrets and may be benign with no obvious cause. The spleen can also be one of the target sites, along with the thymus and liver, for juvenile lymphoblastic leukaemia, as well as less commonly haemangiosarcomas. The latter neoplasm has much the same characteristics as in the dog, with anechoic blood-filled cysts being present, often with some free peritoneal blood. Splenic lymphoma has an increased, slightly grainy echogenicity, with small hypoechoic areas, often less than 5 mm in diameter in comparison with normal splenic parenchyma.

Liver: The normal ferret liver is deeply divided into six lobes and possesses a gall bladder, which empties into the small intestine via a common duct with the pancreas.

Liver enlargement can be due to a number of causes, including mycobacteriosis, neoplasia and right-sided heart failure. Neoplasms of the liver are common in the ferret and include juvenile lymphoblastic leukaemia, biliary cystadenoma, cholangiosarcoma and hepatocellular carcinoma. Tumours of the biliary tree are generally more hyperechoic, producing linear features and hypoechoic cystic structures, whereas those of the hepatocellular lineage tend to be more anechoic in nature and may be associated with cirrhosis.

Pancreas: It may be possible to detect larger insulinomas using ultrasonography. However, they are often only 1–2 mm in diameter and therefore difficult to detect. The author has seen a greater number of insulinomas in the descending limb of the pancreas that runs parallel to the duodenal loop than in other portions of the pancreas.

Intestines: The small intestine is much the same diameter as the large intestine and differentiating the two is sometimes difficult as there is no caecum in the ferret. For this reason, separation of the two is determined more on the position of the bowel in the abdomen (see section in radiography). In addition, the mesenteric lymph node (see below) does sit roughly at the junction between small and large intestines and can also be used as a marker. Thickening of the small intestine may be detectable focally in neoplasms such as malignant lymphoma and proliferative ileitis caused by the bacterium *Lawsonia intracellularis*. Alternatively, it may be more diffuse as in eosinophilic enteritis and inflammatory bowel disease with hyperechoic areas of gas.

Urinary bladder: Cystitis is relatively common in female ferrets and in association with urolithiasis and prostatic cysts and abscesses in males. It may be detected as a diffuse thickening of the bladder wall on ultrasound examination, in conjunction with clinical signs and urinalysis. Bladder neoplasms, specifically transitional cell carcinomas, have been reported in the ferret and these appear as a focally thickened irregular area, often around the neck and dorsal surface of the bladder.

Prostate: The prostate is bilobed in the male ferret and situated as one would expect at the neck of the urinary bladder. Massive cystic enlargement of the prostate can occur, particularly associated with adrenal gland hyperplasia and neoplasia. Prostatic abscesses are also common, though again most seem to be associated with cystic changes and pre-existing adrenal gland disease. Fine-needle aspiration of anechoic structures within the prostate can be easily undertaken, due to the close association between the enlarged prostate and the ventral abdominal wall. Occasionally, prostatic neoplasia has been reported.

Para-urethral disease: Para-urethral disease is generally associated with adrenal gland hyperplasia or neoplasia and involves cystic changes in the dorsal wall of the bladder and proximal urethra. These outpouchings often form large cystic structures, which may also press on the outflow of the urinary bladder and so result in urinary obstruction clinically. Ultrasonography is extremely useful in determining the cysts' relationship with the urinary bladder and thereby aiding the diagnosis.

Uterus: The uterus may be evaluated ultrasonographically, with normal measurements of the (non-gravid) uterine body diameter being quoted as 1.1–2.5 mm (An and Evans, 1988). Conditions such as gravidity, cystic and neoplastic endometrial changes and pyometras may all be diagnosed with ultrasonography. It may also be used to detect uterine stump hypertrophy in previously ovariohysterectomized ferrets suffering from adrenal gland disease.

Mesenteric lymph node: Ferrets possess one large mesenteric lymph node located at the junction of the cranial and caudal mesenteric veins, embedded in the fat at the root of the mesentery. This may be mistaken for one of the adrenal glands, but its mobile and more ventral position should aid in differentiating it. A technique to allow fine-needle aspirate cytology of the mesenteric lymph node as an aid to detecting lymphoma has been described in the ferret (Paul-Murphy *et al.*, 1999).

Other organs

Ocular ultrasonography and biometry has been performed in ferrets under chemical restraint. B-mode images as opposed to A-mode are used, as for dogs, due to the reproducible nature of the spatial relationship amongst normal ocular and orbital structures. A 10 MHz transducer is also required, because of the short focal distances involved. Despite this, a considerable amount of contact gel is required as a stand-off pad to avoid near-field artefacts. Normal values for the anterior chamber depth, lens thickness, vitreous chamber depth and axial length of the eye have been determined (Figure 19.15).

Ocular measurement	Distance in millimetres (±SD)
Anterior chamber depth	1.31 (±0.16)
Lens thickness	3.42 (±0.15)
Vitreous chamber depth	2.26 (±0.11)
Axial length	7 (±0.24)

19.15 Biometric measurements of the globe in ferrets (adapted from Hernandez-Guerra *et al.*, 2007).

MRI and CT scanning

Magnetic resonance imaging (MRI) relies on aligning protons within the patient by subjecting it to a strong magnetic field. It is therefore more useful for assessing soft tissue structures, such as aneurysms, tumours and organ enlargement. Ferrets are prone to lymphoma and many other neoplasms, such as adrenal gland adenocarcinomas, and this modality may prove to be particularly useful in the diagnosis of these conditions. It also requires the patient to be anaesthetized and completely immobile.

Computed tomography (CT) scanning creates a cross-sectional image of the patient and is particularly good for assessing bony changes, such as those seen in cases of osteomyelitis and primary and secondary bone neoplasms such as chondromas and osteosarcomas. Anaesthesia must be used, as the patient must be completely immobile whilst a rotating X-ray beam images the patient.

References and further reading

An NQ and Evans HE (1988) Anatomy of the ferret. In: *Biology and Diseases of the Ferret*, ed. GJ Fox, pp. 15–65. Lea and Febiger, Philadelphia

Besso JG, Tidwell AS and Gliatto JM (2000) Retrospective study of the ultrasonographic features of adrenal lesions in 21 ferrets. *Veterinary Radiology and Ultrasound* 41(4), 345–352

Dernell WS, Straw RC and Withrow SJ (2001) Tumors of the skeletal system. In: *Small Animal Clinical Oncology, 3rd edn*, ed. SJ Withrow and EG MacEwen, pp. 406–454. WB Saunders, Philadelphia

DeVoe RS, Pack L and Greenacre CB (2002) Radiographic and CT imaging of a skull associated osteoma in a ferret. *Veterinary Radiology and Ultrasound* 43(4), 346–348

Evans HE and An NQ (1998) Anatomy of the ferret. In: *Biology and Diseases of the Ferret, 2nd edn*, ed. JG Fox, pp. 19–70. Williams and Wilkins, Baltimore

Fox JG (1988) Systemic diseases. In: *Biology and Diseases of the Ferret*, ed. JG Fox, pp. 258–259. Lea and Febiger, Philadelphia

Girling SJ (2002) Mammalian imaging and anatomy In: *Manual of Exotic Pets, 4th edn*, ed. A Meredith and S Redrobe, pp. 1–12. BSAVA Publications, Gloucester

Hernandez-Guerra AM, Rodilla V and Lopez-Murcia MM (2007) Ocular biometry in the adult anesthetized ferret (*Mustela putorius furo*). *Veterinary Ophthalmology* 10(1), 50–52

Jensen W, Myers R and Lin C (1985) Osteoma in a ferret. *Journal of the American Veterinary Medical Association* 187(12), 1375–1376

Kuijten AM, Schoemaker NJ and Voorhout G (2007) Ultrasonographic visualization of the adrenal glands of healthy ferrets and ferrets with hyperadrenocorticism. *Journal of the American Animal Hospital Association* 43, 78–84

Li X and Fox JG (1998) Neoplastic diseases. In: *Biology and Diseases of the Ferret, 2nd edn*, ed. JG Fox, pp. 405–447. Williams and Wilkins, Baltimore

Neuwirth L, Collins B and Calderwood-Mays M (1997) Adrenal ultrasonography correlated with histopathology in ferrets. *Veterinary Radiology and Ultrasound* 38(1), 69–74

O'Brien RT, Paul-Murphy J and Dubielzig RR (1996) Ultrasonography of adrenal glands in normal ferrets. *Veterinary Radiology and Ultrasound* 37(6), 445–448

Orcutt CJ (1998) Emergency and critical care of ferrets. *Veterinary Clinics of North America: Exotic Animal Practice* 1(1), 99–126

Orcutt CJ (2003) Ferret urogenital diseases. *Veterinary Clinics of North America: Exotic Animal Practice* 6(1), 113–138

Oxenham M (1991) Ferrets. In: *Manual of Exotic Pets, 3rd edn*, ed. PH Beynon and JE Cooper, pp. 97–110. BSAVA, Cheltenham

Paul-Murphy J, O'Brien T, Spaeth A, Sullivan L and Dubielzig RR (1999) Ultrasonography and fine needle aspirate cytology of the mesenteric lymph node in normal domestic ferrets (*Mustela putorius furo*). *Veterinary Radiology and Ultrasound* 40, 308–310

Petrie J-P and Morrisey JK (2004) Cardiovascular and other diseases. In: *Ferrets, Rabbits and Rodents: Clinical Medicine and Surgery*, ed. KE Quesenberry and JW Carpenter, pp. 58–71. WB Saunders, Philadelphia

Pollock C (2007) Emergency medicine of the ferret. *Veterinary Clinics of North America: Exotic Animal Practice* 10(2), 463–500

Puerto DA, Walker LM and Saunders M (1998) Bilateral perinephric pseudocysts and polycystic kidneys in the ferret. *Veterinary Radiology and Ultrasound* 39(4), 309–312

Ritzman TK and Knapp D (2002) Ferret orthopedics. *Veterinary Clinics of North America: Exotic Animal Practice* 5(1), 129–155

Saunders GK and Thomsen BV (2006) Lymphoma and *Mycobacterium avium* infection in a ferret (*Mustela putorius furo*). *Journal of Veterinary Diagnostic Investigation* 18(5), 513–515

Schwarz LA, Solano M, Manning A, Marini RP and Fox JG (2003) The normal upper gastrointestinal examination in the ferret. *Veterinary Radiology and Ultrasound* 44(2), 165–172

Silverman S (1993) Diagnostic imaging of exotic pets. *Veterinary Clinics of North America: Small Animal Practice* 23, 1287–1299

Stefanacci JD and Hoefer HL (2004) Radiology and ultrasound. In: *Ferrets, Rabbits and Rodents, Clinical Medicine and Surgery, 2nd edn*, ed. KE Quesenberry and JW Carpenter, pp. 395–413. WB Saunders, Philadelphia

Stepien RL, Benson KG and Forrest LJ (1999) Radiographic measurement of cardiac size in normal ferrets. *Veterinary Radiology and Ultrasound* **40**(6), 606–610

Stepien RL, Benson KG and Wenholz LJ (2000) M-mode and Doppler echocardiographic findings in normal ferrets sedated with ketamine hydrochloride and midazolam. *Veterinary Radiology and Ultrasound* **41**(5), 452–456

Supakorndej P, Lewis RE and McCall JW (1995) Radiographic and angiographic evaluations of ferrets experimentally infected with *Dirofilaria immitis. Veterinary Radiology and Ultrasound* **36**(1), 23–29

Vastenburg MHAC, Boroffka SAEB and Schoemaker NJ (2004) Echocardiographic measurements in clinically healthy ferrets anesthetized with isoflurane. *Veterinary Radiology and Ultrasound* **45**(3), 228–232

Williams J (2002) Orthopaedic radiography in exotic animal practice. *Veterinary Clinics of North America: Exotic Animal Practice* **5**(1), 1–22

20

Ferrets: clinical pathology

Angela Lennox

Introduction

The ferret is frequently used as a laboratory model and practitioners benefit from data derived from this source. In some cases, normal parameters are extrapolated from those established in other domestic carnivores.

Blood analysis

Collection of blood samples of adequate volume and quality is relatively easy, even in smaller ferrets. As in any other species, successful analysis depends on adequate sample volume and quality. It is worth practising and reviewing sample collection and handling techniques in order to minimize error due to artefact and poor sample quality (see Chapter 18).

Sample volume, handling and delivery requirements must be determined prior to submitting ferret samples to a reference laboratory. Ideally, the laboratory should be able to provide normal reference values based on results from the laboratory's own equipment. Most published values for ferrets are derived from animals maintained in a laboratory setting and may not reflect the pet ferret population. Regardless, published data can provide useful guidelines for interpretation of the ferret haemogram and chemistry panel.

Collection and sample handling

Collection techniques are described in detail in Chapter 18. The author prefers the vena cava technique in calm awake patients, or with mild sedation or brief anaesthesia (e.g. midazolam 0.25 mg/kg, with or without isoflurane administered via facemask).

Practitioners outside the US report that ferrets are frequently difficult to restrain while awake and find sedation and anaesthesia a necessity. The author can report that a number of visiting European veterinary surgeons are surprised by the relative docility of US-bred ferrets.

Isoflurane has been reported to affect haematology parameters. All haematological parameters decrease rapidly after induction of anaesthesia, then remain steady and partially recover to preanaesthetic baselines at 45 minutes post induction of anaesthesia (Marini, 1994). Ferrets apparently do not produce a 'stress haemogram' secondary to stress, fear and pain (Fudge, 2000).

Safe volume collection in a healthy animal is up to approximately 10% of blood volume, which in the ferret is 6–7% of body weight. Therefore, in a 1.0 kg ferret it is safe to collect a maximum of 6–7 ml of whole blood. For most practical purposes, however, most common diagnostic tests do not require more than 1–2 ml whole blood and sometimes even less.

Proper sample handling post collection is just as important as proper collection itself. Dilution errors have two sources: collection of samples that are too small and require dilution by the reference laboratory; and smaller samples added to collection tubes prepared with liquid anticoagulant appropriate for larger samples (Figure 20.1a). Samples intentionally or inadvertently diluted are by nature subject to inaccuracy. Haemolysis of red cells is another common source of poor quality samples and will affect both the complete blood count and chemistry panel. A common cause of haemolysis is forcing blood samples through smaller needles during collection (excessive negative pressure) or during transfer to sample tubes (Figure 20.1b).

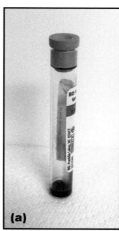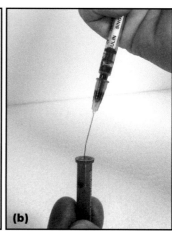

20.1 Test results are dependent upon excellent sample collection and handling techniques, which is more problematic with smaller sample sizes. **(a)** A small whole blood sample has been added to a tube containing liquid anticoagulant, which will result in dilution error. **(b)** The sample is forced through a small 25 gauge needle into a collection tube, which results in cell trauma and haemolysis.

Some in-house chemistry analysers are ideal for smaller samples (Figure 20.2). For example, the Abaxis® chemistry analyser (Abaxis, Union City,

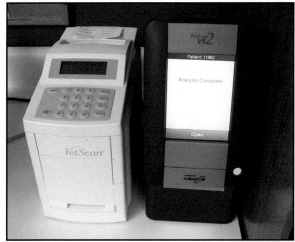

20.2 The advantage of in-house diagnostic testing is speed of results. An additional benefit of this unit is the ability to produce reliable results with at minimum 0.15 ml high quality whole blood. (Courtesy of IDEXX Abaxis, Union City, California.)

California) is capable of generating a chemistry panel with 0.13 ml high quality, whole blood. The most significant advantage of in-house diagnostic testing is rapid results.

Haematology

The ferret haemogram is similar in appearance to that of other carnivores. Red cells are anucleated and regeneration is indicated by polychromasia. The predominant white cell type in normal animals is usually the neutrophil, followed by the lymphocytes, with monocytes, eosinophils and basophils present in much lower numbers. Morphology is similar to the other carnivore species (Figure 20.3). Abnormalities in white cells include left shift and varying degrees of toxicity. White cell abnormalities have not been standardized in this species. Characteristics of the normal ferret haemogram are reported in Figure 20.4.

Earlier references note a correlation between elevated lymphocyte counts and the presence of various forms of lymphoma (Fudge, 2000). However, the author has seen numerous cases of lymphoma with a normal complete blood count.

Leucocytosis is associated with infection, inflammation and neoplasia (Figure 20.5). Leucopenia can result from overwhelming bacterial infection or inflammation, viral infection, neoplasia or any disease affecting marrow white cell lines.

Anaemia is a common clinical finding in ill ferrets and can result from a number of disease processes. Blood-loss anaemia occurs with trauma and most commonly bleeding into the urinary and gastrointestinal tracts. Other potential causes of blood-loss anaemia include aneurism and organ rupture, most commonly ruptured spleen.

Anaemia can also result from chronic infection and inflammation, marrow dysfunction and resultant decreased red cell production. Although undocumented, the author has seen a single case of an apparent immune-mediated anaemia in a ferret that appeared to respond to steroid therapy.

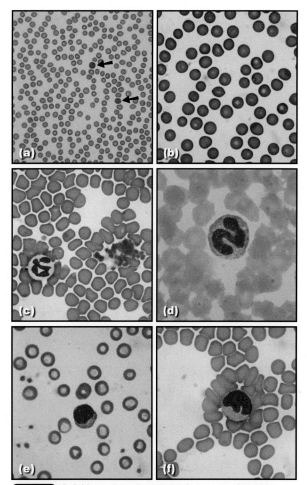

20.3 **(a)** Normal erythrocytes demonstrating polychromatophils (arrows); original magnification X40. **(b)** Normal erythrocytes; original magnification X100. **(c)** Normal segmented neutrophil with a clump of normal platelets. **(d)** Normal eosinophil. **(e)** Normal lymphocyte. **(f)** Normal monocyte. (Courtesy of Raffaella Capitelli.)

Parameter	SI units	US units
Total white blood cell count	4.3–10.7 x 10^9/l	4.3–10.7 x 10^3/µl
Neutrophils (%)	18–47	18–47
Lymphocytes (%)	41–37	41–37
Monocytes (%)	0–4	0–4
Eosinophils (%)	0–4	0–4
Basophils (%)	0–2	0–2
Platelets	200–459 x 10^9/l	200–459 x 10^3/µl
HCT (%)	36–48	36–48
RBC	7.01–9.65 x 10^{12}/l	7.01–9.65 x 10^6/µl
Hb	122–165 g/l	12.2–16.5 g/dl
MCV (fl)	50–54	50–54
MCH (pg)	15–18	15–18
MCHC	320–350 g/l	32–35 g/dl

20.4 Haematology results for the normal ferret. (Data courtesy of Carolyn Cray, University of Miami.)

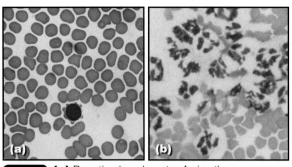

20.5 **(a)** Reactive lymphocyte. As in other mammalian species, this may indicate immune response. **(b)** Marked neutrophilia in an ill ferret, most likely indicative of an infectious or inflammatory disease process. (Courtesy of Raffaella Capitelli.)

Pancytopenia, secondary to hyperoestrogenism as a result of prolonged oestrus, is a well documented cause of anaemia, and is seen in intact females and those with ovarian remnants post ovariohysterectomy. This condition is seen only rarely in the US due to the paucity of intact females in the pet trade. Hyperadrenocorticism can produce elevated oestrogen

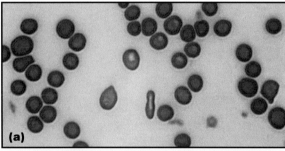

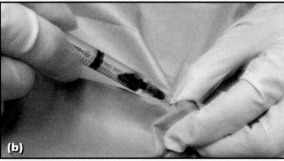

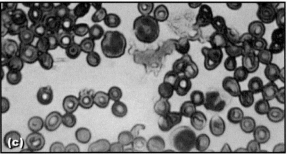

20.6 **(a)** Blood film of an ill ferret with chronic profound non-regenerative anaemia, PCV 12%. Note abnormal erythrocyte morphology and absence of polychromatophils. **(b)** Ferrets with haematological abnormalities benefit from analysis of bone marrow. Collection of bone marrow in an anaesthetized ferret via the tibia. **(c)** Bone marrow from the same patient demonstrating adequate leucocyte precursors with absence of erythroblasts suggesting red cell aplasia.

levels and similar clinical signs, such as an enlarged vulva. However, it is unclear whether hyperadrenocorticism produces anaemia. In the author's experience, most ferrets with adrenal disease are not anaemic despite elevated oestrogen levels, and most profoundly anaemic ferrets with this condition do not respond to therapy to reduce hormone levels (e.g. administration of leuprolide acetate). (See also Chapter 30.)

Evaluation of bone marrow is commonly performed in patients demonstrating abnormal complete blood count parameters, most particularly those with non-regenerative anaemia or suspected neoplasms of haematological origin (Figure 20.6). Collection of bone marrow is straightforward and similar to that in the domestic cat. The author prefers the tibia for collection of bone marrow (see also Chapter 18).

Clinical chemistry

Clinical chemistry results are very important in the diagnosis of a number of common diseases in the pet ferret. Figure 20.7 presents reference ranges reported in ferrets.

Parameter	SI units	US units
Total protein	45–62 g/l	4.5–6.2 g/dl
Albumin	25–40 g/l	2.5–4.0 g/dl
A/G ratio by machine	1.00–1.25	1.00–1.25
Glucose	4.44–6.49 mmol/l	80–117 mg/dl
Blood urea nitrogen	6.42–11.42 mmol/l	18–32 mg/dl
Creatinine	17.68–44.2 μmol/l	0.2–0.5 mg/dl
Calcium	2.02–2.37 mmol/l	8.1–9.5 mg/dl
Phosphorus	16.47–2.10 mmol/l	5.1–6.5 mg/dl
Sodium	142–148 mmol/l	142–148 mmol/l
Chloride	119–162 mmol/l	119–162 mmol/l
Potassium	4.5–6.1 mmol/l	4.5–6.1 mmol/l
Alanine aminotransferase	65–128 IU/l	65–128 IU/l
Alkaline phosphatase	25–60 IU/l	25–60 IU/l
Aspartate aminotransferase	70–100 IU/l	70–100 IU/l
CPK	55–93 IU/l	55–93 IU/l
GGT	8–34 IU/l	8–34 IU/l
LDH	200–1400 IU/l	200–1400 IU/l
Total bilirubin	3.42–8.55 μmol/l	0.2–0.5 mg/dl
Cholesterol	3.08–4.99 mmol/l	119–163 mg/dl
Triglycerides	0.03–1.4 g/l	30–140 mg/dl
Amylase	26–36 IU/l	26–36 IU/l
CO_2	22–29 mmol/l	22–29 mmol/l

20.7 Clinical chemistry values reported for normal ferrets. (Data courtesy of Carolyn Cray, University of Miami.)

Protein

Total protein, albumin, globulin and protein electrophoresis values have been reported in the ferret (Figure 20.8). Alterations from normal values have similar significance to those seen in canine/feline patients, including elevated albumin with dehydration, and elevations in globulins with inflammation. Aleutian disease tends to produce marked hyperproteinaemia in affected ferrets, with total protein levels of up to 80 g/l or higher.

Parameter	Value
Albumin	25.0–33.1 g/l
α$_1$-globulin	3.3–5.6 g/l
α$_2$-globulin	3.6–6.0 g/l
β-globulin	8.3–12.0 g/l
γ-globulin	3.1–8.1 g/l
A/G ratio	1.05–1.33

20.8 Electrophoresis reference ranges for the ferret. Divide by 10 for g/dl. (Data courtesy of Carolyn Cray, University of Miami.)

Glucose

Like other carnivores, ill or fasting ferrets are able to maintain glucose range within normal values until very late in the disease process. The most common glucose abnormality is hypoglycaemia associated with insulinoma and excessive beta cell production of insulin. Many ferrets with insulinoma are able to maintain glucose within the normal range as long as frequent consumption of high-protein meals is uninterrupted. Later in the course of the disease, however, insulinoma cannot be managed with diet alone. Another common scenario is decompensation of well regulated insulinoma secondary to another disease process, especially gastrointestinal disease where nutrient absorption is impaired or interrupted. While some texts report blood glucose below 600 mg/l as diagnostic for insulinoma, the author considers any ferret with levels below 750 mg/l (4.16 mmol/l) as within the suspicious range for this disease. As many ferrets can maintain glucose within the normal range with diet, insulinoma cannot be ruled out without a limited fast. Fasting should not exceed 6 hours and suspect animals should be monitored carefully throughout the fasting period.

Clinical signs of insulinoma include lethargy, nausea, pawing at the mouth, hindlimb weakness and drooling. The author's recommended protocol for diagnostic testing in ferrets with potential insulinoma is outlined in Figure 20.9.

Hyperglycaemia can be seen with stress, although rarely in the author's experience. True diabetes is uncommon but has been documented based on histopathological appearance of the pancreas in the suspect ferret (Benoit-Biancamano, 2005). An unusual temporary but marked hyperglycaemia has been seen by the author and reported anecdotally by others

Suspect ferrets currently exhibiting signs suggesting insulinoma	Suspect ferrets currently exhibiting no signs suggesting insulinoma
• Test immediately regardless of fasting status • Glucose below 75 mg/dl (4.16 mmol/l) confirms insulinoma • Glucose within normal range in a fasted animal suggests insulinoma is not likely the cause of current clinical signs • Glucose within normal range in a non-fasted symptomatic animal does not rule out insulinoma. The ferret may have insulinoma with another, concurrent disease process. The clinician must use clinical judgement in regard to continuing the fast while attempting to diagnose and address other disease processes	• Test after 6-hour fast, monitoring carefully for evidence of hypoglycaemia • Should symptoms suggesting insulinoma appear, proceed as in left-hand column and test immediately

20.9 Protocols for diagnostic testing of potential insulinoma in ferrets.

in ferrets previously diagnosed with insulinoma. This condition appears transitory and responds to insulin therapy and intensive care.

Hepatic enzymes

The exact activity of liver enzymes in specific tissues of the ferret is poorly documented. However, alanine aminotransferase (ALT) has been shown to be useful in assessment of hepatic damage in ferrets, as tissue activity of ALT per gram of liver is 3–10 times greater than in any other tissue in the ferret. Serum enzymes in general in the ferret are similar to those in cats (Clampitt and Hart, 1978; Kawasaki, 1994).

Numerous disease processes affect the liver, including both primary liver diseases and gastrointestinal disease. The author has observed marked elevation of ALT in ferrets with gastrointestinal inflammation. Ferrets with suspected liver disease should be evaluated with radiography, ultrasonography, and hepatic biopsy.

Blood urea nitrogen and creatinine

Renal function evaluation is similar to that in dogs and cats. BUN levels are influenced by glomerular filtration rate, dietary protein and absorption of nitrogen in the gastrointestinal tract from intestinal bleeding, hepatic function and dehydration. Therefore, as in other species, creatinine levels may be more useful in the diagnosis of kidney disease. However, a number of authors have reported poor correlation between creatinine and renal disease (Kawasaki, 1994).

Calcium and phosphorus

Few abnormalities of calcium and phosphorus are documented in the domestic ferret. Abnormalities are presumed to be similar to those in other domestic carnivores. A suspected case of pseudohypoparathyroidism demonstrated low serum calcium and high serum phosphorus with very high serum parathyroid hormone levels (Wilson, 2003). This ferret improved after treatment with dihydrotachysterol (a vitamin D analogue) and calcium carbonate.

Cytology and microbiology

Indications for cytology are similar to those in traditional pet practice. Preparations from the ear canal can be used to detect inflammatory exudate or ear mites. The author encountered a case of blastomycoses in a ferret detected in a cytological preparation of nasal exudate.

Microbiology is extremely useful in the domestic ferret. Sites commonly chosen for submission of bacterial and fungal culture and sensitivity include faeces, urine and samples from the respiratory tract.

Helicobacter mustelae

Helicobacter is a common pathogen in ferrets (see also Chapter 25) and some sources consider infection rates to approach 100% (Fox and Marini, 2001). Clinical signs of this disease vary in severity and can include melaena, diarrhoea, lethargy, muscle wasting, teeth grinding and other evidence of gastrointestinal pain. A lot remains to be learned about the pathogenesis of helicobacter in ferrets. As *H. mustelae* has been cultured from the faeces of affected ferrets, fecal/oral transmission is suspected. Prevention of reinfection may require treatment of all other in-contact ferrets.

In humans, the gold standard for diagnosis of *Helicobacter* spp. is histopathology, but a number of other diagnostic options are utilized as well. Many of these are not available or practical in pet ferrets. In veterinary medicine, practitioners often assume the diagnosis based on the clinical signs described above. Unfortunately, these can occur in other situations, such as gastric foreign body or neoplasia. Diagnosis of *H. mustelae* is also often assumed based on response to therapy.

For practical purposes, absolute confirmation of *Helicobacter*-induced lesions in ferrets is currently limited to documentation of the organisms and associated pathological changes in gastric biopsy samples. Samples are collected via full thickness surgical biopsy or endoscopy. If *Helicobacter* is indeed present in nearly 100% of pet ferrets, simple documentation of organisms may be a moot point and may not correlate with presence of gastric ulceration and disease.

For therapeutic purposes, simple identification of organisms may help to monitor response to therapy or occurrence of reinfection. Collection of gastric swabs (Figure 20.10) for submission for either immunohistochemical staining or polymerase chain reaction (PCR) is relatively easy and non-invasive. The ferret is anaesthetized and intubated, and a culture swab is introduced from the oral cavity directly into the stomach. The stomach is palpated per abdomen and essentially rubbed on to the surface of the swab (Lennox, 2004).

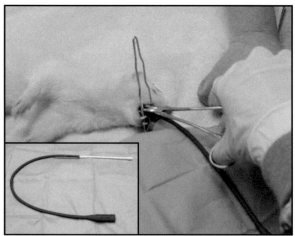

20.10 Collection of a gastric swab in an anaesthetized ferret for PCR testing for detection of *Helicobacter mustelae*. In order to reach the stomach, a sterile culture swab is fitted to the end of a red rubber catheter (inset) and advanced gently into the stomach.

Other tests

Serology

A few specialized serological tests for use in domestic carnivores may be useful in ferrets, including testing for dirofilariasis (see parasite testing below). A number of serological tests for Aleutian disease are also available.

Urinalysis

For urine sample collection techniques, see Chapter 18. Cystocentesis is preferred when considering urine culture and sensitivity. Normal urine is clear and pale to yellow in colour, depending on hydration status. Abnormal gross findings can include mucus, pus, blood and fine grit. Results of normal urinalysis in the ferret are reported in Figure 20.11.

Parameter	Normal value	Comments
Urine volume	8–140 mg/24 h (average 26–28 ml)	
Protein	0–330 mg/l (0–33 mg/dl)	Trace amounts common in normal ferrets
Glucose		Trace amounts common in normal ferrets
Blood	Negative	Infection, inflammation, neoplasia
pH	6.5–7.5	
Ketones	Negative	Prolonged anorexia, diabetes mellitus
Bilirubin	Negative	
Sediment		Struvite crystals reported in ferrets on inappropriate (grain-based) diets
Specific gravity		Not reported in the literature, but assumed to be similar to other carnivore species

20.11 Normal urinalysis results for the pet ferret. (Data from Hoefer, 2000)

Cerebrospinal fluid (CSF) analysis

Normal values for CSF samples collected from the cerebellomedullary cistern have been reported. Results are similar to those in other species; however, protein concentrations (28–68 g/l; 280–680 g/dl) are higher than those reported in dogs and cats (Morrisey and Ramer, 1999).

Parasite testing

Faecal parasites are uncommon in pet ferrets, but occasionally reported in wild and research colony animals. Coccidiosis, in particular *Isospora* spp., is the most common parasitic disease seen in ferrets in the US, particularly in young animals. Coccidiosis is most commonly diagnosed with faecal flotation.

Giardia has been reported in ferrets, and there is some evidence that ferrets acquire the infection from dogs and cats. As in other species, zinc sulphate flotation is considered the most useful in-house test for detection of cysts in faeces. Serology and other ancillary testing have not been evaluated in the ferret. Recent genotype studies indicate that zoonotic *Giardia* can occur in the ferret.

Oocytes of *Cryptosporidium* spp. can be detected in ferrets, but infection is usually inapparent and self-limiting. Fatal cases have been reported, but are more difficult to detect and commonly overlooked. Oocytes can be detected via faecal flotation, but are commonly missed as they are small and float in a higher plane than other parasites. Several laboratories in the US offer PCR for *Cryptosporidium*.

Dirofilaria immitis infections appear to be most similar to disease in the cat, with transient low-volume microfilaraemia. ELISA-based antigen tests are considered most useful in the ferret, but false negatives occur and may be related to relatively low worm burdens (McCall, 1998).

Miscellaneous testing

Specific PCR tests are available for detection of ferret coronavirus (FECV), canine distemper virus, Aleutian disease, rotavirus and *Helicobacter mustelae*; and novel PCR tests are offered for detection of *Salmonella* spp. and for *Mycobacterium* spp. (Figure 20.12)

Some gastrointestinal diseases such as *Helicobacter*-related gastric ulceration produce haematochezia. Faecal occult blood testing can help to confirm the presence of blood. As some diseases produce only intermittent bleeding, a single negative occult faecal blood test does not rule out gastrointestinal haemorrhage. In the US, the Hemoccult Fecal Occult Blood Test (Beckman Coulter, www.coulter.com) has been evaluated by the author in clinical practice for use in ferrets. Elimination of dietary haem must precede testing, and can be accomplished by feeding a non-haem-containing diet. The author has demonstrated success with the use of a carnivore critical care product (Oxbow Pet Products, Murdock, Nebraska, www.oxbowhay.com). Other occult blood-testing systems may be applicable for ferrets as well.

Measurements of plasma sex steroids can be used to aid in the confirmation of and to track management of adrenal gland disease in ferrets. It should be noted that the dexamethasone suppression test and ACTH stimulation test are not useful for diagnosis of hyperadrenocorticism in the ferret (see Chapter 30).

Test	Comments	Facility (USA)
Helicobacter mustelae	Gastric or colonic swabs	Research Associates Laboratory 1-972-960-2221
Aleutian disease	Tissue samples or blood	Department of Pathology College of Veterinary Medicine, University of Georgia 1-706-542-2919
Canine distemper	Whole blood, lymphoid tissue or nervous tissue	Michigan State University, Diagnostic Center for Population and Animal Health 1-517-353-2296
Rotavirus	Faeces, intestinal biopsy samples	Michigan State University, Diagnostic Center for Population and Animal Health 1-517-353-2296
Ferret coronavirus (ECE)	Faeces, GI biopsy samples	Michigan State University, Diagnostic Center for Population and Animal Health 1-517-353-2296
Salmonella spp.	Faecal or GI swab	University of Georgia, Infectious Diseases Laboratory 1-706-542-8092
Mycobacterium spp.	Faeces, GI swab, target tissue	Veterinary Molecular Diagnostics 1-513-576-1808
	Faeces, target tissue	Washington State University, Washington Animal Disease Diagnostic Laboratory 1-509-335-9696
	Consult laboratory for submission instructions; culture and sensitivity also available	National Jewish Medical and Research Center, Denver, CO 1-303-398-1339 Download acquisition form: www.njc.org

20.12 Specialized polymerase chain reaction (PCR) testing to aid diagnosis of gastrointestinal disease in ferrets.

Some authors have reported measurement of insulin levels and insulin/glucose ratios to support the diagnosis of insulinoma. Normal insulin concentrations for ferrets are reported as 22–311 pmol/l or 4.6–43.3 µIU/ml (Quesenberry and Rosenthal, 2004).

References and further reading

Abe N, Read C, Thompson RCA and Iseki M (2005) Zoonotic genotype of *Giardia intestinalis* detected in a ferret. *Journal of Parasitology* **91**(1), 179–182

Benoit-Biancamano MO, Morin M and Langlois I (2005) Histopathologic lesions of diabetes mellitus in a domestic ferret. *Canadian Veterinary Journal* **46**(10), 895–897

Bernard SL, Leathers CW, Brobst DF and Gorham JR (1982) Estrogen-induced bone marrow depression in ferrets. *American Journal of Veterinary Research* **44**, 657–661

Brown SA (1997) Clinical techniques in domestic ferrets. *Seminars in Avian and Exotic Pet Medicine* **6**(2), 75–85

Clampitt RB and Hart RJ (1978) The tissue activities of some diagnostic enzymes in ten mammalian species. *Journal of Comparative Pathology* **88**, 607–621

Fisher PG (2006) Exotic mammal renal disease: diagnosis and treatment. *Veterinary Clinics of North America: Exotic Pet Practice* **9**, 69–96

Fox JG and Marini RP (2001) *Helicobacter mustelae* infection in ferrets: pathogenesis, epizootiology, diagnosis and treatment. *Seminars in Avian and Exotic Pet Medicine* **10**, 36–42

Fudge AM (2000) Ferret hematology. In*: Laboratory Medicine Avian and Exotic Pets,* ed. AM Fudge, pp. 69–72. WB Saunders, Philadelphia

Hoefer HL (2000) Rabbit and ferret renal disease diagnosis. In: *Laboratory Medicine: Avian and Exotic Pets,* ed. AM Fudge, pp. 311–318. WB Saunders, Philadelphia

Jenkins J (2000) Rabbit and ferret liver and gastrointestinal testing. In: *Laboratory Medicine: Avian and Exotic Pets,* ed. AM Fudge, pp. 291–304. WB Saunders, Philadelphia

Kawasaki T (1991) Creatinine unreliable indicator of renal failure in ferrets. *Journal of Small Exotic Animal Medicine* **1**, 28–30

Kawasaki TA (1994) Normal parameters and laboratory interpretation of disease states in the domestic ferret. *Seminars in Avian and Exotic Pet Medicine* **3**(1), 41–47

Lennox AM (2004) Working up mystery anemia in the ferret. *Exotic DVM* **6**(3), 22–26

Marini RP, Jackson LR, Esteves MI *et al.* (1994) Effect of isoflurane on hematologic variables in ferrets. *American Journal of Veterinary Research* **55**(1), 1479–1483

McCall JW (1998) Microfilariasis in the domestic ferret. *Clinical Techniques in Small Animal Practice* **13**(2),109–112

Morrisey JK and Ramer JC (1999) Ferrets: clinical pathology and sample collection. *Veterinary Clinics of North America: Exotic Animal Practice* **2**(3), 553–564

Murray MJ (2000) Rabbit and ferret sampling and artifact considerations. In: *Laboratory Medicine Avian and Exotic Pets*, ed. AM Fudge, pp. 265–268. WB Saunders, Philadelphia

Patton S (2000) Rabbit and ferret parasite testing. In*: Laboratory Medicine: Avian and Exotic Pets,* ed. AM Fudge, pp. 358–365. WB Saunders, Philadelphia

Quesenberry KE and Orcutt C (2004) Basic approach to veterinary care. In: *Ferrets, Rabbits and Rodents, Clinical Medicine and Surgery, 2nd edn,* ed. KE Quesenbery and JW Carpenter, pp. 13–24. WB Saunders, Philadelphia

Quesenberry KE and Rosenthal KL (2004) Endocrine diseases. In: *Ferrets, Rabbits and Rodents, Clinical Medicine and Surgery, 2nd edn*, ed. KE Quesenberry and JW Carpenter, pp 79–90. WB Saunders, Philadelphia

Rosenthal KL, Peterson ME, Quesenberry KE *et al.* (1993) Hyperadrenocorticism associated with adrenocortical tumor or nodular hyperplasia of the adrenal gland in ferrets: 50 cases (1987–1991). *Journal of the American Veterinary Medical Association* **203**, 271–275

Sherill A and Gorham J (1995) Bone marrow hypoplasia associated with estrus in ferrets. *Laboratory Animal Science* **35**, 280–286

Wilson GH, Greene CE and Greenacre CB (2003) Suspected pseudohypoparathyroidism in a domestic ferret. *Journal of the American Veterinary Medical Association* **222**(8), 1093–1096

21

Ferrets: therapeutics

James Morrisey

Introduction

Despite the varied roles of ferrets, little specific pharmacological information is available for these animals. As small carnivores, ferrets share many pharmacological traits with the cat, such as a short gastrointestinal tract, rapid drug elimination and tolerance of similar antibiotics. Although they are similar to cats in some ways, they should not be treated as cats. Any extrapolation of drug dosages from cats or dogs to ferrets should be done cautiously, though for the most part drug dosages extrapolated from cats to ferrets are used with seemingly few disagreeable outcomes (Quesenberry and Orcutt, 2004).

Therapeutic approach

Ferrets are perhaps the easiest of 'exotic' pets to incorporate into a small animal practice, because the therapeutic approach is similar to that for cats and dogs. As with any species, the goal of therapy should be to eliminate the problems, while causing the fewest side effects. Because many drug dosages are extrapolated, there should be diligent observation to avoid the potential risks of the drug used. A solid understanding of adverse effects of the drug will help to avoid or lessen complications. For a detailed discussion of possible adverse effects of drugs mentioned in this chapter the reader is referred to other resources (e.g. Plumb, 2005). Since the use of many of these drugs is 'off-label', appropriate legislation should be followed and the owner kept fully informed.

The small size of ferrets often means very small drug doses, so the veterinary surgeon should keep U-100 insulin (100 units = 1 ml) and tuberculin syringes on hand for accurate administration of medication.

Ferrets can often be distracted from unpleasant medication techniques, such as injections, with simultaneous administration of a sweet treat or honey.

Routes and methods of medication

Oral medication

This is the most common route of drug administration to ferrets. Medications should be given in liquid form when possible as most owners find this method the easiest for at-home administration. Liquids should be flavoured to increase palatability. Several flavouring systems exist and are available to most compounding pharmacies or veterinary surgeons. Sweet flavours such as fruits, molasses and peanut butter seem to be most appealing, but savoury flavours such as liver are preferred by some ferrets. Fish flavours are poorly tolerated (Quesenberry and Orcutt, 2004). The importance of palatability cannot be underestimated: ferrets are adept at spitting out medications and can react violently to offensive tastes, with vigorous pawing at the mouth, hypersalivation, retching and vomiting.

Ferrets have small mouths, with many sharp teeth, and administration of tablets is very difficult. Some owners find it easier to crush pills in palatable liquid or pastes, such as cod liver oil, peanut butter or commercial flavouring systems. Oily substances are often more palatable than sweet liquids and may work better in this respect. The stability of the medication, especially when removed from the coated surface of the pill, may be affected by crushing it, and this can profoundly affect absorption rate and drug efficacy. Tablets may also be given whole, disguised in a small piece of the ferret's normal wet food or in a piece of chicken or ham; the animal should be closely monitored to ensure that the pill is ingested.

Parenteral medication

Parenteral administration of drugs is warranted in moderately to severely ill animals and in anorexic patients. Distracting the animal with sweet-tasting substances is helpful.

Subcutaneous injections are well tolerated in most patients, though ferrets lack sufficient subcutaneous space for large volumes. Subcutaneous injections are generally given between the shoulder blades; however, the skin may be very thick here, especially in intact hobs.

Intramuscular injections are problematic in ferrets as they lack a large muscle group for injections, so again volumes should be kept low. The cranial and caudal thigh muscles are the most useful for intramuscular injections. A 25–29 gauge needle should be used to avoid muscle damage.

Intravenous injections are often given to severely ill animals but necessitate intravenous catheter placement. Intravenous injections without a catheter are very difficult in ferrets. A vascular access port (VAP) can be inserted into the jugular vein and the hub placed under the skin around the scapulae. This can make repeated intravenous injections much easier and is used most commonly for chemotherapy. Special needles, called Huber needles, are needed for use with VAPs.

Intraosseous administration of drugs may also be a feasible option for those patients in which an intravenous catheter cannot be placed. Most intravenous drugs can be given in this manner, unless they cause bone marrow damage or suppression.

Intraperitoneal injections can be used for a few chemotherapeutic drugs (see Chapter 18).

Ophthalmic administration of drugs in ferrets is hampered by the small size of the eyes and quick head movements. It may be easier and safer to apply eye ointment to a clean finger and then place it into the ferret's eye.

Alternative routes

Nebulization of antibiotics, antifungals and bronchodilators is helpful in treating moderate to severe respiratory infections. The injectable form of a drug can be diluted in saline or water, depending on what the drug is reconstituted or dissolved in. Ferrets should be placed in a small space without food or water for 10–15 minutes before nebulization treatment.

Hunting ferrets fed whole prey can be medicated by injecting the drug into the muscles or viscera of the prey item. Although some injectable medications will not be very palatable, this may make it easier to medicate ferrets that are less amenable to repeated handling.

Agents

Antibiotics

Antibiotics should be chosen based on culture and sensitivity testing of samples from the affected area, whenever possible. The normal intestinal flora of ferrets is predominantly Gram-negative bacteria, making it similar to that of a cat, so some of the side effects of oral administration of antibiotics seen in other species (e.g. rabbits) are rare. Decreased appetite, nausea and vomiting can be seen in ferrets on oral antibiotics. Metronidazole is extremely unpalatable to ferrets and can cause severe retching or forceful pawing at the mouth. Intense flavouring may be required for compliance with the treatment regimen. Some ferrets will simply not tolerate metronidazole. Oral antibiotics are used commonly in ferrets to treat helicobacteriosis, pneumonia, enteritis and genitourinary infections. A list of antibiotics commonly used in ferrets is given in Figure 21.1.

Drug	Dosage	Uses and comments
Amikacin	8–16 mg/kg i.v., i.m., s.c. q8–24h	Single dose may be less nephrotoxic
Amoxicillin	10–35 mg/kg s.c., orally q12h	
Amoxicillin/clavulanate	12.5–25 mg/kg orally q8–12h	
Ampicillin	5–30 mg/kg i.v., i.m., s.c q8–12h	
Cefadroxil	15–20 mg/kg orally q12h	
Cefalexin	15–30 mg/kg orally q8–12h	
Chloramphenicol	30–50 mg/kg i.m., s.c. q12h	
Ciprofloxacin	10–30 mg/kg orally q12h	Tablet mixes well with water and can be flavoured
Clarithromycin	12.5 mg/kg orally q8–12h	*Helicobacter* treatment
Clindamycin	5–10 mg/kg orally q12h	
Cloxacillin	10 mg/kg i.v., i.m., orally q6h	
Enrofloxacin	10–20 mg/kg i.m, s.c. orally q12–24h	Injectable form causes inflammation and necrosis Oral suspension made from tablets in the US; oral suspension available commercially in the UK
Erythromycin	10 mg/kg orally q6h	Useful in controlling *Campylobacter* diarrhoea
Lincomycin	11 mg/kg orally q8h	
Metronidazole	15–20 mg/kg orally q12h	Used to treat many GI infections including *Helicobacter*. Very bad taste, should be heavily flavoured
Neomycin	10 mg/kg orally q6h	Avoid long use, potential nephrotoxicity and neuromuscular blockage
Netilmicin	6–8 mg/kg i.v., i.m., s.c. q24h	Severe staphylococcal infections
Penicillin G procaine	40,000 IU/kg s.c. q24h	
Trimethoprim/sulphonamide	30 mg/kg s.c., orally q12h	Renal disease possible
Tylosin	10 mg/kg s.c., orally q8–12h	

21.1 Antibiotics commonly used in ferrets. (Data from Besch-Williford, 1987; Collins, 1995; Smith and Burgmann, 1997; Fox, 1998; Brown, 1999; Marini *et al.*, 1999; Lewington, 2000; Williams, 2000; Morrisey and Carpenter, 2004)

Antifungal agents

Antifungal agents are used occasionally in ferrets to treat dermatophytosis and systemic infections, most commonly in the respiratory tract. A list of antifungals commonly used in ferrets is given in Figure 21.2.

Antiparasitic agents

Antiparasitic agents for use in the ferret are listed in Figure 21.3. Topical treatments for flea control that are safe in puppies and kitten are generally safe for ferrets. In fact, these chemicals may last longer in ferrets because of the increased amount of sebum on the skin. Intestinal parasites are less common in pet ferrets than in cats and dogs, other than coccidians in young animals. Heartworm treatment in ferrets is difficult and potentially life-threatening and

prophylaxis should be given in any area in which heartworms are endemic.

Chemotherapeutic agents and protocols

A list of chemotherapeutic agents is given in Figure 21.4. Some protocols for lymphoma are given in Figure 21.5; none of these protocols has been evaluated by controlled studies in ferrets, and alterations may need to be made based on results of diagnostic testing, patient condition and logistics. Additionally, there may be some confusion in the literature, as protocols attributed to the same authors were found to have three different doses for vincristine in three separate references (Lewington, 2000; Williams, 2000; Carpenter, 2005). For these reasons, the reader is strongly encouraged to discuss each case with an oncologist. For further information, see Chapter 30.

Drug	Dosage	Uses and comments
Amphotericin B	0.4–0.8 mg/kg i.v. once weekly to total dose of 7–25 mg	Blastomycosis and other severe fungal infections. Monitor BUN/creatinine closely
Fluconazole	50 mg/kg orally q12h for 2–6 months	For CNS fungal infections
Griseofulvin	25 mg/kg orally q12h	Dermatophytosis
Itraconazole	15 mg/kg orally q24h	
Ketoconazole	10–30 mg/kg orally q12–24h	Systemic mycoses
Lime sulphur	Dip q7d	Use with griseofulvin for refractory cases of dermatomycosis

21.2 Antifungal agents commonly used in ferrets. (Data from Hillyer and Brown, 2000; Lewington, 2000; Williams, 2000; Morrisey and Carpenter, 2004; Hanley *et al.*, 2006)

Drug	Dosage	Uses and comments
Amitraz	0.3% solution topically q7d	Demodicosis: use full strength for small areas
Carbaryl 5% powder	Apply topically q7d	
Diethylcarbamazine	5–11 m/kg orally q24h	Heartworm preventive, used rarely
Fenbendazole	20 mg/kg orally q24h x 5d	Nematodes
Fipronil	0.2–0.4 ml topically q30d	
Imidacloprid	0.1–1 ml topically q30d	
Ivermectin	0.2–0.4 mg/kg s.c., orally repeat in 14d	Mange and most nematode infections
	0.5–1.0 mg/kg topically in ears q14d	
	0.05 mg/kg s.c., orally q30d	Heartworm prevention and preferred heartworm treatment
Melarsamine	2.5 mg/kg i.m. repeat in 30d and then 24h later	Heartworm adulticide (see also Chapter 26)
Metronidazole	20 mg/kg orally q12h	Protozoal disease
Milbemycin oxime	1.15–2.33 mg/kg orally q30d	Heartworm preventive
Praziquantel	5–10 mg/kg s.c., orally repeat in 10d	Cestodes
Pyrethrins	Topical q7d	Fleas
Selamectin	6–10 mg/kg topically q30d	Fleas, lice, most mites (except *Demodex*)
Sulfadimethoxine	50 mg/kg once then 25 mg/kg orally q24h x 9d	Coccidial infections
Thiacetarsemide	2.2 m/kg i.v. q12h x 2d	Heartworm adulticide. May need to follow with ivermectin

21.3 Antiparasitic drugs commonly used in ferrets. (Data from Smith and Burgmann, 1997; Morrisey, 1998; Brown, 1999; Morrisey, 1999; Hillyer and Brown, 2000; Lewington, 2000; Williams, 2000; Morrisey and Carpenter, 2004)

Drug	Dosage	Uses and comments
Bleomycin	10 IU/m² s.c.	Treatment for squamous cell carcinoma
Chlorambucil	1 mg/kg orally	
Crisantaspase	400 IU/kg i.m., s.c.	
Cyclophosphamide	200 mg/m² s.c., orally 10 mg/kg orally	High dose used for salvage
Doxorubicin	1 mg/kg i.v. q21d for 4 treatments	Salvage protocol for lymphoma. Used also as primary treatment for lymphoma
Methotrexate	0.5 mg/kg i.v.	
Prednisolone	1–5 mg/kg orally q12–24h	Used in combinations or alone (palliative, higher dosages) for lymphoma
Vincristine	0.75 mg/m² i.v. 2.0 mg/m² i.v. 0.12 mg/kg i.v. 0.2 mg/kg i.v.	Minimal myelosuppression. See Rescue protocol (Figure 21.5d)

21.4 Chemotherapy agents used in ferrets. (Data from Williams, 2000; Antinoff and Hahn, 2004; Carpenter, 2005)

(a) From Brown (1993).

Week	Day	Agents	Dosage
1	1	Prednisolone Vincristine	1–2 mg/kg orally q12h continued throughout therapy 0.025 mg/kg i.v.
1	3	Cyclophosphamide	10 mg/kg orally, s.c.
2	8	Vincristine	0.025 mg/kg i.v.
3	15	Vincristine	0.025 mg/kg i.v.
4	22	Vincristine Cyclophosphamide	0.025 mg/kg i.v. 10 mg/kg orally, s.c.
7	46	Cyclophosphamide	10 mg/kg orally, s.c.
9	63	Prednisolone	Gradually decrease dose to 0 (zero) over next 4 weeks

NOTES
- Monitor CBC weekly
- Stop the vincristine if WBC count is <2000 cells/ml (0.002 × 10⁹ cells/l) or haematocrit is <25%

(b) From Rosenthal (1994).

Week	Drug	Dosage
1	Vincristine Crisantaspase Prednisolone	0.025 mg/kg i.v. 400 IU/kg i.p. 1 mg/kg orally q24h throughout protocol
2	Cyclophosphamide	10 mg/kg s.c.
3	Doxorubicin	1 mg/kg i.v.
4–6	Repeat weeks 1–3 without crisantaspase	
7	Rest; go to every other week	
8	Vincristine	0.025 mg/kg i.v.
10	Cyclophosphamide	10 mg/kg s.c.
12	Vincristine	0.025 mg/kg i.v.
14	Methotrexate	0.5 mg/kg i.v.

NOTES
- Continue protocol biweekly until remission
- Monitor CBC weekly
- Stop the vincristine if WBC count is <2000 cells/ml (0.002 × 109 cells/l) or haematocrit is <25%

21.5 Some lymphoma protocols for ferrets. (continues) ▶

(c) From J Mayer (personal communication).

Week	Drug	Dosage
1	Crisantaspase Cyclophosphamide Prednisolone	10,000 IU/kg s.c. 250 mg/m² s.c., orally in 50 ml/kg of NaCl s.c. 2 mg/kg orally daily for 7d then q48h
2	Crisantaspase Perform CBC	10,000 IU/kg s.c.
3	Crisantaspase Cytarabine	10,000 IU/kg s.c. 300 mg/m² s.c. × 2 days (dilute 100 mg with 1 ml H₂0)
4	Perform CBC	
5	Cyclophosphamide	250 mg/m² s.c., orally in 50 ml/kg of NaCl s.c.
7	Methotrexate Perform CBC	0.8 mg/kg i.m.
8	Perform CBC	
9	Cyclophosphamide	250 mg/m² s.c., orally in 50 ml/kg of NaCl s.c.
11	Cytarabine Chlorambucil	300 mg/m² s.c. × 2 days (dilute 100 mg with 1 ml H₂0) 1 tablet/animal orally
12	Perform CBC	
13	Cyclosphosphamide	250 mg/m² s.c., orally in 50ml/kg of NaCl s.c.
15	Procarbazine	50 mg/m² orally q24h × 14d
16	Perform CBC	
17	Perform CBC	
18	Cyclophosphamide	300 mg/m² s.c. × 2 days (dilute 100 mg with 1 ml H₂0)
20	Cytarabine Chlorambucil	300 mg/m² s.c. × 2 days (dilute 100 mg with 1 ml H₂0) 1 tablet/animal orally
23	Cyclophosphamide	250 mg/m² s.c., orally in 50 ml/kg of NaCl s.c.
26	Procarbazine	50 mg/m² orally q24h × 14d
27	Perform CBC and chemistry panel	IF NOT IN REMISSION, CONTINUE WEEKS 20–26 FOR 3 CYCLES

NOTES
If CBC indicates severe myelosuppression, reduce dosage by 25% for **all** subsequent treatments of the previously used myelosuppressive drug

(d) From Antinoff and Hahn (2004).

Week	Drug	Dosage
3 days	Crisantaspase	400 IU/kg s.c. (premedicate with diphenhydramine at 2 mg/kg)
1	Vincristine Prednisolone Cyclophosphamide	0.12 mg/kg i.v. 1 mg/kg orally q24h continue throughout therapy 10 mg/kg orally
2	Vincristine	0.12 mg/kg i.v.
3	Vincristine	0.12 mg/kg i.v.
4	Vincristine Cyclophosphamide	0.12 mg/kg i.v. 10 mg/kg orally
7, 10, 13 etc.	Vincristine Cyclophosphamide	0.12 mg/kg i.v. 10 mg/kg orally

Continue therapy every 3 weeks for one year, then decrease to every 4–6 weeks

| **Rescue treatment** | Doxorubicin | 1–2 mg/kg i.v. (over 20 minutes) |

21.5 (continued) Some lymphoma protocols for ferrets.

Cardiopulmonary agents

Dilated cardiomyopathy is a common finding in ferrets older than 4 or 5 years. Other cardiac conditions occur, such as hypertrophic cardiomyopathy, congenital malformations, non-pathological murmurs and thrombus formation, but are much less common. Pulmonary diseases in ferrets are less common, but include pneumonia, influenza and neoplasia. Intrathoracic neoplasia, such as thymic lymphoma, can mimic or cause pulmonary disease (see Chapter 26). A list of cardiopulmonary agents is given in Figure 21.6.

Topical agents

Topical agents used in the ferret are listed in Figure 21.7. (Topical agents used for flea and tick control are listed in Figure 21.3.)

Miscellaneous agents

Miscellaneous agents used in ferrets are listed in Figure 21.8. The most commonly used agents in this category are the gastrointestinal protectants, as any stressed or sick ferret is susceptible to gastric ulceration.

Drug	Dosage	Uses and comments
Adrenaline	0.02 mg/kg i.v., intratracheally prn	Cardiac arrest. Can give i.m. for anaphylaxis
Aminophylline	4 mg/kg i.v., i.m., orally q12h	Bronchodilation
Atenolol	3.125–6.25 mg/kg orally q24h	Beta-adrenergic blocker for HCM
Atropine	0.02–0.04 mg/kg i.m., s.c. prn	Bradycardia
	0.1 mg/kg intratracheally	Bradycardia
Benazepril	0.25–0.5 mg/kg orally q24h	Vasodilator for DCM. Less nephrotoxic than enalapril
Digoxin	0.005–0.01 mg/kg orally q12–24h	Positive inotrope for DCM
Diltiazem	1.5–7.5 mg/kg orally q12h	Calcium channel blocker for HCM
Doxapram	1.2 mg/kg i.v.	Respiratory stimulant
Enalapril	0.25–0.5 mg/kg orally q24–48h	Vasodilator for DCM. Do not use in renal disease
Furosemide	1–4 mg/kg i.v., i.m., s.c., orally q8–12h	Diuretic
Lanoxin	1/8 of 0.125mg tablet q48h	Mix tablet into solution
Nitroglycerine 2% ointment	1–6 mm strip topically q12–24h	Vasodilator. Apply to shaved inner thigh or pinna
Pimobendan	0.625–1.25 mg/kg orally q12h	Phosphodiesterase inhibitor, increases heart contractility
Theophylline	4.25 mg/kg orally q8–12h	Bronchodilator. May suppress appetite

21.6 Cardiopulmonary agents for use in the ferret. (Data from Flecknell, 1987; Rosenthal, 1994; Stamoulis, 1995; Quesenberry, 1997; Orcutt,1998; Brown, 1999; Lewington, 2000; Petrie and Morrisey, 2004)

Drug	Dosage	Uses and comments
Clotrimazole	Apply to affected area	Topical fungal infections
Lidocaine (2.5%) and prilocaine (2.5%)	Apply thin layer, cover if possible, wait 15 minutes	Topical anaesthetic, e.g. prior to catheter placement or for minor skin wounds
Miconazole	Apply thin layer q24h	Topical fungal infections
Chlorhexidine gluconate	Dilute to 10% solution	Use to cleanse wounds
Povidone–iodine	Apply topically or dip feet	Nail bed infections secondary to pedal form of mange
Silver sulfadiazine	Apply thin layer to skin wounds and burns	Good cover against Gram-negatives; promotes epithelialization

21.7 Topical agents for use in ferrets.

Agent	Dosage	Uses and comments
Adrenaline (epinephrine)	0.02 mg/kg i.v., i.m.	Severe vaccine reaction
Amantadine	6 mg/kg as aerosol q12h	Influenza; experimental antiviral
Atropine	5–10 mg/kg i.m., s.c.	Organophosphate toxicity
Bismuth subsalicylate	0.5–1.0 ml/kg orally q6–8h	GI protectant; may help prevent *Helicobacter* colonization

21.8 Miscellaneous agents used in ferrets. (Data from Brown, 1993; Quesenberry, 1996; Fox, 1997; Quesenberry, 1997; Rosenthal, 1997; Fox, 1998; Brown, 1999; Lightfoot, 1999; Hillyer and Brown, 2000; Lewington, 2000; Williams, 2000; Burgess and Garner, 2002; Antinoff, 2004; Morrisey and Carpenter, 2004; Pollock, 2004; Carpenter, 2005) ▶
(continues)

Agent	Dosage	Uses and comments
Chlorphenamine	1–2 mg/kg orally q8–12h	Antihistamine
Cimetidine	5–10 mg/kg orally, s.c., i.m., i.v. (slowly) q8h	H2-blocker. GI ulcers
Cisapride	0.5 mg/kg orally q8–12h	Antiemetic. Motility enhancer
Dexamethasone	1 mg/kg s.c., i.m.	Post adrenalectomy
Diazoxide	5–30 mg/kg orally q12h	Insulinoma treatment
Diphenhydramine	0.5–2.0 mg/kg i.v., i.m., s.c. orally	Antihistamine. Vaccine reactions
Edetate calcium disodium	20–30 mg/kg s.c. q12h	Heavy metal toxicity
Erythropoietin alfa	50–150 IU/kg i.m. q48h	Stimulates erythropoiesis. Use weekly once desired PCV has been reached
Famotidine	0.25–0.50 mg/kg i.v., s.c., orally q24h	GI ulcers
Flunixin meglumine	1 mg/kg i.m., s.c. i.v? orally?	Prevention of prostaglandin-mediated hypotension of endotoxaemia
Gonadotropin-releasing hormone (GnRH)	20 µg/animal i.m., s.c.	Termination of oestrus after 10th day; repeat in 2 weeks
Human chorionic gonadotrophin (hCG)	100 IU/animal i.m.	Use 10 or more days after onset of oestrus to induce ovulation. Repeat in 1–2 weeks prn
Hydroxyzine	2 mg/kg orally q8h	Antihistamine
Iron dextran	10 mg/animal i.m. once	Iron-deficiency anaemia. Haemorrhage
Kaolin/pectin	1–2 ml/kg orally q2–6h	GI protectant
Leuprolide acetate	100 µg i.m. for ferrets <1 kg, 200 µg i.m. for ferrets >1 kg q4–6wk	Adrenal gland disease/hyperadrenocorticism
Loperamide	0.2 mg/kg orally q12h	Antidiarrhoeal; useful in treatment of coronaviral enteritis (ECE)
Mannitol	0.5–1.0 g/kg i.v. prn	Cerebral oedema. Head trauma. Anuric renal failure. Give over 20 minutes for all indications
Metoclopramide	0.2–1.0 mg/kg i.m., s.c., orally, i.v? q6–12h	Antiemetic
Misoprostol	1–5 µg/kg orally q8h	Prostaglandin E1 analogue. Treatment of gastric ulcers. Works in face of NSAID administration. Causes abortion in pregnant jills
Omeprazole	0.7 mg/kg orally q24h	Proton pump inhibitor; decreases gastric acid production. Used for ulcers and as part of *Helicobacter* treatment
Oxytocin	0.2–3.0 IU/kg i.m., s.c.	Expels retained fetus. Stimulates lactation
Phenobarbital	1–2 mg/kg orally q8–12h	Seizure control
Phenoxybenzamine	3.75–7.50 mg/animal orally q24–72h	Smooth muscle relaxant for urethral obstruction. Possible GI or cardiovascular side-effects
Potassium bromide	22–30 mg/kg/day orally 70–80 mg/kg/day orally	Lower dose if used with phenobarbital
Prednisolone	0.25–2.2 mg/kg orally q12h	Anti-inflammatory; immunosuppressive. Treatment of insulinoma. Use lower doses for insulinoma, higher doses for immunosuppression
Prostaglandin F_2-α	0.1–0.5 mg/animal i.m. prn	Metritis
Proligestone 100 mg/ml	0.5 ml per jill s.c, repeat at 0.25 ml in 7 days if no response	For oestrus suppression 10 days into heat
Ranitidine	3.5 mg/kg orally, s.c, i.v q12h	GI ulcers
Stanozolol	0.5 mg/kg s.c., orally q12h	Anabolic steroid. Use with caution in hepatic disease
Sucralfate	25 mg/kg orally q8–12h	GI protectant. Tablet suspends well in water. Give before meal or after other medications
Ursodiol	15 mg/kg orally q12h	Chronic hepatic disease
Vitamin B complex	1–2 mg/kg i.m. or mixed with i.v. fluids	Supplement
Vitamin K	1–3 mg/kg s.c., orally divided q12h	Rodenticide toxicity. Treat for 1–6 weeks depending on agent

21.8 (continued) Miscellaneous agents used in ferrets. (Data from Brown, 1993; Quesenberry, 1996; Fox and Lee, 1997; Quesenberry, 1997; Rosenthal, 1997; Fox, 1998; Brown, 1999; Lightfoot, 1999; Hillyer and Brown, 2000; Lewington, 2000; Williams, 2000; Burgess and Garner, 2002; Antinoff, 2004; Morrisey and Carpenter, 2004; Pollock, 2004; Carpenter, 2005)

References and further reading

Antinoff N (2004) Musculoskeletal and neurologic diseases. In: *Ferrets, Rabbits and Rodents: Clinical Medicine and Surgery, 2nd edition,* ed KE Quesenberry and JE Carpenter, pp.115–120. WB Saunders, St Louis

Antinoff N and Hahn K (2004) Ferret oncology: diseases, diagnostics and therapeutics. *Veterinary Clinics of North America: Exotic Animal Practice* **7**, 579–626

Bartlett LW (2002) Ferret soft tissue surgery. *Seminars in Avian and Exotic Pet Medicine* **11**, 221–230

Besch-Williford CL (1987) Biology and medicine of the ferret. *Veterinary Clinics of North America: Small Animal Practice* **17**, 1155–1183

Brown SA (1993) Ferrets. In: *A Practitioner's Guide to Rabbits and Ferrets,* ed. JR Jenkins and SA Brown, pp. 43–111. American Animal Hospital Association, Lakewood, Colorado

Brown SA (1999) Ferret drug dosages. In: *Exotic Formulary, 2nd edn,* ed. N Antinoff *et al.,* pp. 43–61. American Animal Hospital Association, Lakewood, Colorado

Burgess M and Garner M (2002) Clinical aspects of inflammatory bowel disease in ferrets. *Exotic DVM* **4**, 29–34

Carpenter JW (2005) *Exotic Animal Formulary.* Elsevier Saunders, St Louis

Collins BR (1995) Antimicrobial drug use in rabbits, rodents, and other small mammals. In: *Antimicrobial Therapy in Caged Birds and Exotic Pets,* pp. 3–10. Veterinary Learning Systems, Trenton, New Jersey

Flecknell PA (1987) *Laboratory Animal Anesthesia.* Academic Press, San Diego

Fox JG (1998) *Biology and Diseases of the Ferret.* Williams & Wilkins, Philadelphia

Fox JG and Lee A (1997) The role of *Helicobacter* species in newly recognized gastrointestinal diseases of animals. *Laboratory Animal Science* **47**, 222–227

Hanley CS, MacWilliams P, Giles S and Paré J (2006) Diagnosis and successful treatment of *Cryptococcus neoformans* variety *grubii* in a domestic ferret. *Canadian Veterinary Journal* **47**(10), 1015–1017

Hillyer EV (1992) Gastrointestinal diseases of ferrets (*Mustela putorius furo*). *Journal of Small Exotic Animal Medicine* **2**, 44–45

Hillyer EV and Brown SA (2000) Ferrets. In: *Saunders Manual of Small Animal Practice,* ed. SJ Birchard and RG Sherding RG, pp.1464–1492. WB Saunders, Philadelphia

Lewington JH (2000) *Ferret Husbandry, Medicine and Surgery.* Butterworth-Heinemann, Oxford

Lightfoot TL (1999) Common ferret syndromes. In: *Proceedings of North American Veterinary Conference,* pp. 839–842. NAVC, Gainesville, Florida

Marini RP, Fox JG, Taylor NS *et al.* (1999) Ranitidine bismuth citrate and clarithromycin, alone or in combination, for eradication of *Helicobacter mustelae* infection in ferrets. *American Journal of Veterinary Research* **60**, 1280–1286

Morrisey JK (1998) Ectoparasites of ferrets and rabbits. In: *Proceedings of North American Veterinary Conference,* pp. 844–845. NAVC, Gainesville, Florida

Morrisey JK (1999) Parasites of ferrets, rabbits and rodents. *Seminars in Avian and Exotic Pet Medicine* **5**, 106–114

Morrisey JK and Carpenter JW (2004) Formulary. In: *Ferrets, Rabbits, and Rodents: Clinical Medicine and Surgery,* ed. KE Quesenberry and JW Carpenter, pp. 436–444. WB Saunders, St Louis

Orcutt CJ (1998) Emergency and critical care of ferrets. *Veterinary Clinics of North America: Exotic Animal Practice* **1**, 99–126

Petrie JP and Morrisey JK (2004) Cardiovascular and other diseases. In: *Ferrets, Rabbits, and Rodents: Clinical Medicine and Surgery,* ed. KE Quesenberry and JW Carpenter, pp. 58–71. WB Saunders, St Louis

Plumb DC (2005) *Veterinary Drug Handbook, 5th edn.* Blackwell Publishing, Ames, Iowa

Pollock CG (2004) Urogenital diseases. In: *Ferrets, Rabbits, and Rodents: Clinical Medicine and Surgery,* ed. KE Quesenberry and JW Carpenter, pp. 41–49. WB Saunders, St Louis

Quesenberry KE (1996) Gastrointestinal disorders of ferrets. In: *Proceedings of North American Veterinary Conference,* pp. 870–871. NAVC, Gainesville, Florida

Quesenberry KE (1997) Basic approach to veterinary care. In: *Ferrets, Rabbits and Rodents: Clinical Medicine and Surgery,* ed EV Hillyer and KE Quesenberry, pp.14–25. WB Saunders, Philadelphia

Quesenberry KE and Orcutt C (2004) Basic approach to veterinary care. In: *Ferrets, Rabbits, and Rodents: Clinical Medicine and Surgery,* ed. KE Quesenberry and JW Carpenter, pp. 13–24. WB Saunders, St Louis

Rosenthal K (1994) Ferrets. *Veterinary Clinics of North America: Small Animal Practice* **24**, 1–23

Rosenthal KL (1997) Respiratory diseases. In: *Ferrets, Rabbits, and Rodents: Clinical Medicine and Surgery,* ed. EV Hillyer and KE Quesenberry, pp. 77–84. WB Saunders, Philadelphia

Smith DA and Burgmann PM (1997) Formulary. In: *Ferrets, Rabbits, and Rodents: Clinical Medicine and Surgery,* ed. EV Hillyer and KE Quesenberry, pp. 394–395. WB Saunders, Philadelphia

Stamoulis ME (1995) Cardiac disease in ferrets. *Seminars in Avian and Exotic Pet Medicine* **4**, 43–48

Williams BH (2000) Therapeutics in ferrets. *Veterinary Clinics of North America: Exotic Animal Practice* **3**, 131–153

22

Ferrets: anaesthesia and analgesia

Cathy A. Johnson-Delaney

Introduction

Ferrets exhibit signs of pain (Figures 22.1 and 22.2) in a different way to dogs and cats and for this reason it is frequently reported in the literature that they are stoical and not very sensitive to pain. Practitioners experienced with ferrets find just the opposite: ferrets are extremely sensitive to pain and stress, with the consequence often being haemorrhage and ulceration of the gastrointestinal (GI) tract. Pain also contributes to anorexia and dehydration that may exacerbate endocrine disorders such as islet cell neoplasia (insulin-producing), renal disease and cardiomyopathy.

Analgesia

Choice of analgesic involves consideration of the type of pain being treated, route of administration, formulation, duration of action (frequency of administration), owner compliance and side effects or

- Abnormal emotional behaviours including biting in a previously very gentle ferret, or wanting cuddling and burrowing into owner's clothing while being held
- Anaemia (due to gastrointestinal haemorrhage)
- Anorexia, weight loss
- Bruxism, hypersalivation, pawing at mouth
- Changes in gait
- Collapse
- Lack of play behaviour
- Ignoring favourite toys or treats, withdrawal from other ferrets or humans, refusal to eat unless hand-fed
- Feeling cool to the touch
- Lack of grooming
- Cringing when touched
- Dehydration
- Facial expression: dull look in the eyes, glassy eyes, seeming 'far away' although conscious
- Refusal/reluctance to move, reluctance to wake
- Tarry faeces (due to haemorrhage in the gastrointestinal tract)
- Tension in the forehead skin, 'looking pitiful'
- Trembling
- Vocalizations when touched or moved

22.2 Signs and consequences of pain in ferrets.

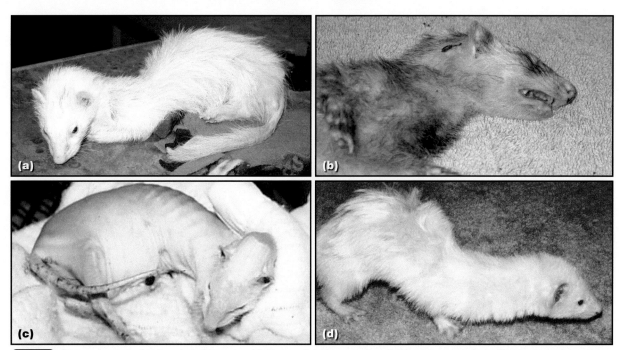

22.1 Signs of pain in the ferret. **(a)** Ferret exhibiting weight loss, pallor, dull facial expression with glassy look to eyes, hunched abdomen and reluctance to move. **(b)** This ferret is moribund and emaciated and had been suffering for one month before the owner presented it for euthanasia. The ferret was periodically screaming. **(c)** This ferret had end-stage adrenal gland disease and would occasionally whimper. **(d)** This animal had gastrointestinal pain and shows a hunched position.

contraindications from other medications or medical conditions. Acute pain such as that from trauma or post surgery can be treated with local anaesthetics, opiates for 1–3 days, coupled with a non-steroidal anti-inflammatory drug for up to 7 days, depending on severity of injury or surgical incision. Chronic pain, as seen with neoplasia, may need long-term pain control that the owner may need to administer based on clinical signs. The clinician needs to educate the owner on signs of pain in their ferret and what the different medications will do, as well as work out dosage and frequency schedules. Many owners are in tune with their ferrets and can become astute in recognizing the subtle signs of pain. They are very willing to provide pain control to keep their ferret comfortable.

Ferrets have a propensity to develop GI ulcers (Figure 22.3) and acid reflux disease, and so GI protectant and antihistamine/anti-acid therapy should accompany administration of NSAIDs. The author encourages treatment of all ill, stressed or post-surgical ferrets with one of the GI antihistamines for the duration of the medical problem.

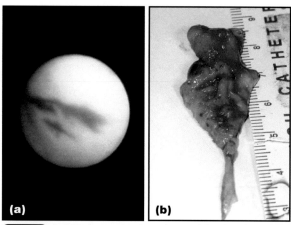

(a) **(b)**

22.3 **(a)** Endoscopic view of a gastric ulcer in a ferret. (Courtesy of Angela Lennox.) **(b)** Gastric ulceration in a ferret that had undergone adrenal gland surgery 3 weeks previously. The cause of death was haemorrhage from the ulcer.

Medications, dosages, routes and usages of analgesics and adjunctive GI medications are listed in Figure 22.4.

Drug	Dosage and route	Frequency	Action and comments
Analgesics			
Aspirin	10–20 mg/kg orally	q24h	Analgesic, anti-inflammatory, antipyretic. Give with food, use with H2 blocker
Bupivacaine	1–1.5 mg/kg local delivery, s.c., area of incision	Once	Local anaesthetic, effects may last several hours, caution when using it for oral surgery
	1.1 mg/kg epidural	Once	Can be combined with morphine for more complete analgesia, may alter hindlimb motor function for up to 12 hours
Buprenorphine	0.01 mg/kg s.c., i.m., i.v.	q8–12h	Minimal sedative effect. Can be used concurrently with NSAID
Butorphanol	0.2–0.4 mg/kg s.c., i.m.	q6–8h	Has some sedative effect, can be used as part of preanaesthetic regimen when sedation needed
Carprofen	1 mg/kg orally	q12–24h	NSAID; use with H2 blocker
Fentanyl	20–30 μg/kg/hour i.v.	Continuous rate infusion	During surgery/anaesthesia, reduces inhalant anaesthetic used. Monitor blood pressure
Flunixin	0.3 mg/kg orally, s.c.	q24h	NSAID, not recommended due to potential for renal damage, use for less than 3 days, use with H2 blocker
Hydromorphone	0.1–0.2 mg/kg s.c., i.m., i.v.	q6–8 h	Opioid
Ketamine	0.5 mg/kg i.v. pre-surgery; 10 μg/kg/minute i.v. CRI during surgery, 2 μg/kg/minute i.v. CRI for 24 h postoperatively	CRI: constant rate infusion	At this low dose may provide some analgesia if ferret has indwelling catheter, on a fluid pump. Additional analgesics and/or an NSAID may still be necessary
Ketoprofen	0.5–1 mg/kg orally, s.c.	q24h	NSAID, use with caution, H2 blocker, use for less than 5 days
Lidocaine	1–2 mg/kg total, volume delivered in local area infiltrate or ring block	Once	Local anaesthetic, use either 1% or 2%; duration of action approximately 15–30 minutes
	4.4 mg/kg epidural	Once	Epidural block, can be added to morphine for more immediate and complete analgesia

22.4 Analgesics and adjunctive medications. (Data from Allen *et al.*, 1993; Gamble and Morrisey, 2005; Johnson-Delaney, 2005a; Johnston, 2005) (continues) ▶

Drug	Dosage and route	Frequency	Action and comments
Analgesics continued			
Meloxicam	0.2 mg/kg orally, s.c., i.m.	q24h	NSAID, use H2 blocker, can be used long-term, monitor liver parameters
Meperidine	5–10 mg/kg s.c., i.m., i.v.	q2–4h	Analgesic, short duration of action, causes drowsiness in some animals
Morphine	0.1 mg/kg epidural	Once, effects last 12–24h	Epidural for surgical anaesthesia/analgesia. Can combine with either lidocaine or bupivacaine for immediate and more complete analgesia
	0.5-5.0 mg/kg s.c., i.m.	q2–6h	Analgesic. Short duration of action. Usually just one preoperative dose
Nalbuphine	0.5–1.5 mg/kg i.m., i.v.	q2–3h	Analgesic. Short duration of action
Oxymorphone	0.05–0.2 mg/kg s.c., i.m., i.v.	q8–12h	Analgesic
Pentazocine	5–10 mg/kg i.m.	q4h	Analgesic, parenteral, short duration of action
Tramadol	5 mg/kg orally	q12–24 h	Analgesic, mild to severe pain, can be used with NSAID. Can be used long term q12h for pain associated with neoplasia
Adjunctive gastrointestinal medications			
Cimetidine	10 mg/kg orally, s.c., i.m., i.v. (slow)	q8h	H2 blocker, inhibits stomach acid secretions. Oral form unpalatable
Famotidine	2.5 mg per ferret orally, s.c., i.v.	q24h	H2 blocker, inhibits stomach acid secretions. Non-prescription tablet palatable
Omeprazole	4 mg/kg orally	q24h	Protein pump inhibitor, decreases gastric acid secretion
Ranitidine	3.5 mg/kg orally	q12h	H2 blocker, inhibits stomach acid secretions. Oral form unpalatable
Sucralfate	25 mg/kg orally	q8h	Give before meals, requires acid pH, oesophageal, gastric protectant

22.4 (continued) Analgesics and adjunctive medications. (Data from Allen *et al.*, 1993; Gamble and Morrisey, 2005; Johnson-Delaney, 2005a; Johnston, 2005)

Local and epidural analgesia and anaesthesia

The use of local anaesthetic agents such as lidocaine or bupivacaine can decrease operative pain. They can be delivered as ring blocks around a specific anatomical structure or lesion as well as administered at major nerve areas exiting from bony foramina. Local agents are particularly useful for dental surgeries and tooth extractions.

Dental nerve blocks
Dental nerve blocks can be done either by individual tooth or by region (Figure 22.5). The author recommends that the clinician becomes familiar with the skull landmarks and practises on a cadaver using India ink to perfect the technique. All dental nerve blocks can be done using a 25 or 27 gauge needle. The volume of local anaesthetic can be infiltrated into the approximate area of the nerve, at a depth of a few millimetres lateral to the bone.

Infraorbital and zygomatic nerves
The approximate exit of the infraorbital nerve through the infraorbital foramen on the lateral aspect of the face is indicated in Figure 22.5 by an oval. The

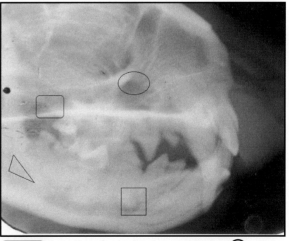

22.5 Locations for regional nerve blocks. ◯ = the approximate exit of the infraorbital nerve through the infraorbital foramen on the lateral aspect of the face. The zygomatic nerve also exits this foramen. ▷ = the mandibular nerve blocking area. It lies on the medial aspect of the mandible and is approached from inside the oral cavity. ☐ = the approximate location on the lateral surface of the mandible of the exit of the mental nerve from the mental foramen. ☐ = represents the approximate area for the maxillary nerve block. See text for further details.

zygomatic nerve also exits this foramen. It is sometimes palpable but can be approximated just anterior to the zygomatic arch, rostral of the orbit, and in the area of maxillary premolars 2 and 3. These nerves supply sensory fibres to the maxillary incisors, canines, upper lip and adjacent facial tissues (Figure 22.6).

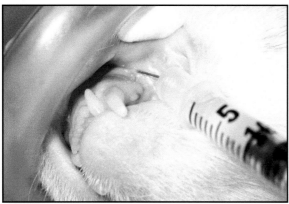

22.6 Infraorbital nerve block, showing the location of the infraorbital foramen. The ferret has not yet been intubated, as it is often advantageous to put the blocks in first before intubation, giving the local anaesthetic a few minutes to work before proceeding with dentistry. The site is first swabbed with 2% chlorhexidine rinse.

Mandibular nerve
The mandibular nerve blocking area is represented in Figure 22.5 by a triangle symbol. This nerve provides sensory fibres to the mandibular molars, premolars and adjacent soft tissues. It lies on the medial aspect of the mandible and is approached from inside the oral cavity. It is approximately midway between the molar and the ventral aspect of the mandible, and 2–5 mm distal to the molar. An infusion needle of appropriate length can be 'walked along' the medial aspect of the mandible for infusion in the general area.

Mental nerve
The approximate location on the lateral surface of the mandible of the exit of the mental nerve from the mental foramen is indicated in Figure 22.5 by a square symbol. This nerve supplies sensory fibres to the ventral and lateral aspect of the mandible, lip, lower incisors and canine teeth, and motor fibres to local muscles. It is usually 2–4 mm rostral to mandibular premolar 2 or 3.

Maxillary nerve
The approximate area for the maxillary nerve block is indicated in Figure 22.5 by a blunt-cornered rectangle symbol. The maxillary nerve lies in the infraorbital canal, and it may be difficult to insert a needle in the canal in small ferrets from the oral cavity. The syringe must be aspirated to ensure that the needle is not in a blood vessel. It is recommended that firm digital pressure be applied to the rostral end of the canal while slowly infusing the local anaesthetic. If the canal cannot be entered, the needle can be inserted at the rostral entrance to the canal; firm digital pressure is applied to that locale and the anaesthetic is infused in the area just caudal to the finger.

Seizures induced by local anaesthetics
In the author's experience, bupivacaine at a calculated dosage of 1 mg/kg administered to block maxillary teeth or mandibular canine tooth innervation causes mild seizures in some ferrets. This reaction has not been seen with either 1% or 2% lidocaine administration at 1–2 mg/kg. Nor have these mild seizures been seen with bupivacaine administered elsewhere in the body for local anaesthesia.

Local anaesthesia in cardiomyopathy
The use of a local anaesthetic coupled with a parenteral analgesic and a benzodiazepine relaxant may be adequate to remove small masses in ferrets with cardiomyopathy that are considered anaesthetic risks. Local infiltration as a line block can be used in a planned area for incision.

Epidural administration
Epidural administration of morphine (Figure 22.7) decreases postoperative pain responses, especially for abdominal surgeries. The combination of morphine epidural formulation at 0.1 mg/kg with either lidocaine 2% at 4.4 mg/kg or bupivacaine at 1.1 mg/kg increases the effectiveness of the analgesia/anaesthesia provided and becomes effective within a few minutes. The analgesic effects of morphine last approximately 12–24 hours (Johnston, 2005).

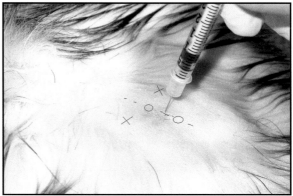

22.7 Epidural analgesia. X = wings of ileum, O = dorsal spines of the last lumbar vertebra (usually L6 but in some ferrets it may be L5 or L7) and of the sacral vertebrae. Small lines are the midline and other dorsal prominences of vertebrae. Entry site for the needle is in the midline between the vertebrae at the level of the wings of the ileum. It helps to flex the lumbar/pelvic area to open the vertebral spaces. The head of the ferret is to the left.

The ferret should be anaesthetized prior to the epidural administration. The procedure for lumbosacral epidural puncture is essentially the same as in dogs and cats. The ferret should have the lower back in a flexed position, which allows for the maximal opening of the lumbosacral space. The skin should receive a surgical preparation and the technique should be performed as aseptically as possible. The author usually uses a 25 gauge needle and does not experience the 'pop' during puncture of the intervertebral ligaments as is felt in other small animals with epidural puncture. A small amount of cerebrospinal fluid may be seen in the needle hub.

Sedation and anaesthesia

Most of the agents for sedation and anaesthesia used in small animal practice can be used in ferrets. In all cases, agents that have the least cardiovascular depression are preferable as many ferrets have subclinical cardiomyopathy. Short-acting sedatives without analgesic properties are usually adequate for diagnostic imaging and blood sampling. Combinations of drugs to provide both sedation and analgesia may

be necessary for short diagnostic procedures such as fine-needle aspiration of a mass. A balanced approach to sedation and anaesthesia is preferable for dental procedures and surgeries. This includes pre-emptive pain control: systemic analgesia, local anaesthetics and, for abdominal or hindquarters surgery, epidural anaesthetic and analgesia.

Figure 22.8 lists sedatives and anaesthetics used in ferrets as well as preoperative adjunctive medications.

Drug	Dosage, route	Frequency	Action, comments
Atipamezole	0.4–1 mg/kg s.c., i.m., i.p., i.v.	Once: volume will be the same as the dosed medetomidine	Medetomidine reversal
Atropine	0.05 mg/kg s.c., i.m., i.v.	Once	Preanaesthetic drug; reduces salivation, bradycardia
Diazepam	0.5–2 mg/kg i.m., i.v.; can be used with combination anaesthetics	Once; effects may last 4–6 hours	Benzodiazepine, sedative-hypnotic, anxiolytic, muscle-relaxant, anticonvulsant. Excessive sedation may occur if used with cimetidine, barbiturates, narcotics, anaesthetics
Diphenhydramine	1.25 mg/kg orally, s.c.	Once	Antihistamine to counter histamine release during surgery, stress, may have slight sedative effect
Etomidate	1 mg/kg i.v.	Once approximately 15–20 minutes after midazolam at 0.25–0.3 mg/kg i.m., i.v.	Induction, usually sufficient for intubation, no depression of cardiopulmonary parameters, excellent for ill, critical animals
Fentanyl/fluanisone	0.3 ml/kg i.m.	Once	Anaesthetic
Fentanyl/droperidol	0.15 ml/kg i.m.	Once	Deep sedation, minor surgical procedures, some analgesia
Glycopyrrolate	0.02 mg/kg i.m.	Once	Preanaesthetic drug; reduces salivation, bradycardia
Isoflurane	Induce at higher concentration, maintenance 1–3%	–	Inhalant anaesthetic. Has hypotensive effects
Ketamine	10–20 mg/kg i.m.	Once	Mild sedation, no muscle relaxation, alone causes sneezing reflex; rarely used alone
	0.5 mg/kg i.v. pre-surgery; 10 µg/kg/minute i.v. CRI during surgery, 2 µg/kg/minute i.v. CRI for 24 h postoperatively	CRI: constant rate infusion	At this low dose may provide some analgesia if ferret has indwelling catheter, on a fluid pump. Additional analgesics and/or an NSAID may still be necessary
Ketamine (K) + Diazepam (D)	10–20 mg/kg (K) + 1–2 mg/kg (D) i.m.	Once	Light anaesthesia, poor analgesia
	25–35 mg/kg (K) + 2–3 mg/kg (D) i.m.	Once	Moderate anaesthesia, poor analgesia
Ketamine (K) + Medetomidine (M)	5–8 mg/kg (K) + 0.08–0.1 mg/kg (M) i.m.	Once	Light anaesthesia, analgesia; hypotensive, respiratory depression: have oxygen ready, atipamezole for reversal of (M)
Ketamine (K) + Midazolam (Mi)	5–10 mg/kg (K) + 0.25 mg/kg (Mi) i.m.: give Mi 10 minutes before K	Once	Heavy sedation–induction, follow with inhalant anaesthetic
Medetomidine	0.08–0.1 mg/kg s.c., i.m.	Once	Light sedation, rarely used alone, may cause hypotension, bradycardia: have oxygen ready, atipamezole for reversal
Medetomidine (M) + Butorphanol (B)	0.08 mg/kg (M) + 0.1 mg/kg (B) i.m.	Once	Anaesthesia, hypotensive and respiration depression: have oxygen ready, atipamezole for reversal (M)
Midazolam	0.25–0.3 mg/kg i.m., i.v.; can be used with combination anaesthetics	Once; effects may last 2–4 hours	Benzodiazepine, sedative-hypnotic, anxiolytic, muscle-relaxant, amnesiac, anticonvulsant. Hypotensive if used with meperidine

22.8 Sedatives, anaesthetics and premedications. (Data from Allen *et al.*, 1993; Gamble and Morrisey, 2005; Johnson-Delaney, 2005a; Johnston, 2005) (continues)

Drug	Dosage, route	Frequency	Action, comments
Morphine	0.1 mg/kg epidural	Once	Epidural anaesthetic/analgesic; combine with either lidocaine at 4.4 mg/kg or bupivacaine at 1.1 mg/kg for faster and more complete action
Naloxone	0.02–0.04 mg/kg s.c., i.m., i.v.	Once	Reversal of opioids
Propofol	5 mg/kg i.v. to effect	Once	Induction, titrate to effect
Sevoflurane	Induce at higher concentrations, maintenance at lower %	Depending on sedation from premedications, induction may be obtained using 2.5–4.0%. If no premedications are used, induction is usually done with the maximum concentration (5% most vaporizers)	Inhalant anaesthetic
Thiopental 2%	8–12 mg/kg i.v. to effect	Once	Induction
Tiletamine/zolazepam	12–22 mg/kg i.m.	Once	Lower doses sedation, higher light anaesthesia, recovery prolonged with higher doses; rarely used in ferrets
Xylazine	0.5–1 mg/kg s.c., i.m.	Once, usually in combination with ketamine at 10–20 mg/kg i.m.	Sedation; severe hypotension, bradycardia, arrhythmias, not recommended for use in ferrets. Reverse xylazine with yohimbine
Yohimbine	0.2 mg/kg i.v. or 0.5 mg/kg i.m.	Once	Xylazine reversal

22.8 (continued) Sedatives, anaesthetics and premedications. (Data from Allen *et al.*, 1993; Gamble and Morrisey, 2005; Johnson-Delaney, 2005a; Johnston, 2005)

In the author's opinion, xylazine or acepromazine should not be used for ferret anaesthesia or sedation, due to the vasodilatory effects and depression of cardiac functions (xylazine). Blood pressure can be severely depressed with xylazine even in a normal healthy ferret. In a ferret with heart disease it can lead to fatalities. A balanced anaesthesia approach that includes anti-anxiety drugs, relaxants, analgesics and anaesthetics can reduce the depression in cardiac parameters seen with using just anaesthetic agents,

either injectable or inhalant. Ketamine should be used in combination with either diazepam or midazolam. Ketamine alone does not provide adequate relaxation in the ferret: it seems to trigger paroxysmal sneezing, hyperreflexiveness and salivation. Ketamine may not provide adequate analgesia by itself for surgical procedures (Gamble and Morrisey, 2005; Johnson-Delaney, 2005a). Figure 22.9 lists several pre- and postoperative medication regimens suitable for ferret procedures and surgeries.

Procedure	Preoperative	Induction	Postoperative
Abdominal – exploratory or mass removal (Ferret should have an i.v. catheter (usually cephalic) in place for continuous fluid infusion)	Famotidine 2.5 mg orally or s.c., Diphenhydramine 1.25 mg/kg orally or s.c., Buprenorphine 0.01 mg/kg s.c., Atropine 0.05 mg/kg s.c.; Midazolam 0.25 mg/kg i.m. Wait 20–30 minutes	Etomidate 1 mg/kg i.v.; Lidocaine 0.1 ml squirted on glottal area, entubate; begin Isoflurane, usually at 4% decreasing to 3%, then surgical level of 1–2%. Epidural of morphine 0.1 mg/kg with lidocaine 4 mg/kg added (note slight decrease since lidocaine used in throat). Maintain blood pressure, body temperature, also monitor ECG, respirations. [*Editor's note*: Etomidate is a human drug not widely used in the UK. The author suggests that an alternative would be to use intravenous ketamine titrated to effect (load syringe with a dose of 20 mg/kg, but this full dose is rarely required)]	Meloxicam 0.2 mg/kg s.c.; Buprenorphine at 0.01 mg/kg at 6 hours after initial administration. Continue meloxicam at 0.2 mg/kg orally q24h × 7 days with famotidine 2.5 mg/ferret orally q24h × 7 days; buprenorphine at 0.01 mg/kg s.c. q12h × 3 days. Teach owner how to administer
Cutaneous mass removal, wound repair	Famotidine 2.5 mg orally or s.c. Diphenhydramine 1.25 mg/kg orally or s.c. Atropine 0.05 mg/kg s.c.; Butorphanol 0.2 mg/kg s.c., Midazolam 0.25 mg/kg i.m. Wait 15–20 minutes.	Isoflurane via mask – induce at 4–5% then decrease until light surgical plane reached. While masked, clip, initial surgical scrub of mass, surrounding area. Local infiltration of area lidocaine 1.5 mg/kg or bupivacaine 1.25 mg/kg. If planning to intubate, then lidocaine 0.1 ml to glottal area, intubate. Subcutaneous fluids should be given while being masked, prepped. When suturing finished, meloxicam 0.2 mg/kg s.c. Monitor during surgery with ECG, blood pressure, respirations, body temperature.	Buprenorphine 0.01 mg/kg s.c. at 4–6 hours post butorphanol administration. Depending on severity of mass removal, tissue excision, may continue buprenorphine q12h × 1–2 days; Meloxicam 0.2 mg/kg orally q24h × 3–5 days. Famotidine 2.5 mg/ferret while on meloxicam

22.9 Balanced anaesthesia combinations for selected procedures suggested by the author. (continues) ▶

Procedure	Preoperative	Induction	Postoperative
Dental cleaning, extractions	Famotidine 2.5 mg orally or s.c., Diphenhydramine 1.25 mg/kg orally or s.c., Atropine 0.05 mg/kg s.c.; Butorphanol 0.2 mg/kg s.c., Midazolam 0.25 mg/kg i.m. Wait 15–20 minutes.	Isoflurane via mask – induce at 4–5% then decrease until light surgical plane reached. Lidocaine 0.1 ml to glottal area, intubate. Subcutaneous fluids should be given while being masked, prepped including eye lubricant applied, gingiva swabbed with dilute chlorhexidine oral rinse. If a tooth requires extraction, local block with lidocaine 2% at 1.5 mg/kg (can do around root, at foramina, in pulp cavity if open). May get lidocaine seepage into nasal cavity if volume too great or if there is osteolysis due to abscessation. Monitor with ECG, blood pressure, respiration, body temperature. At conclusion of procedure, discontinue isoflurane. When ferret begins to awaken, and heart rate and blood pressure return to preoperative levels, administer meloxicam at 0.2 mg/kg s.c.	Buprenorphine 0.01 mg/kg s.c. 6–8 hours after initial butorphanol and continued q12h × 2–3 days depending on severity and number of extractions. Meloxicam 0.2 mg/kg orally q24h × 5–7 days. Famotidine 2.5 mg/ferret orally q24h while on meloxicam. Usually an antibiotic is sent home for oral administration × 14 days; also have owner swab gums with dilute chlorhexidine oral rinse once a day for 3–5 days after surgery or as long as sutures are in place. Ferrets can accumulate food material in extraction sites

22.9 (continued) Balanced anaesthesia combinations for selected procedures suggested by the author.

Monitoring

A sedated or anaesthetized ferret should be supported with a heating system to maintain body temperature. This is best achieved with forced-air convective blanket systems (Figure 22.10). Circulating warm-water blankets or heated gel discs can also be used.

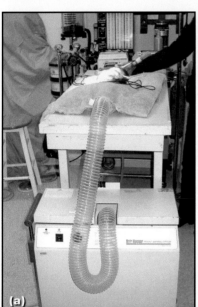

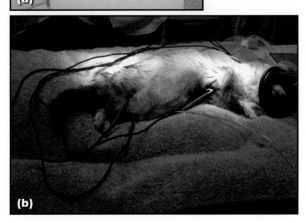

22.10 (a) Use of a Bair Hugger® forced-air convective blanket system. The unit is set at an air temperature of 38°C (100°F). (b) Anaesthetized ferret lying on a BairHugger® with ECG leads attached.

Monitoring includes blood pressure (on front leg/wrist or tail), ECG, respirations (rate and depth, character), temperature, reflexes to judge anaesthesia depth (corneal, blink, swallowing, rectal tone, toe pinch) and degree of muscle relaxation.

Capnography can be used when the ferret is intubated and is preferable to pulse oximetry as an indicator of perfusion and gas exchange. Pulse oximetry can be used, but instruments designed for cats and dogs are frequently too large to attach to the ferret's tongue, cheek or ear.

Fluid therapy

Warm isotonic fluids should be provided. Subcutaneous administration is usually sufficient for surgeries lasting 30 minutes or less or for those with minimal expected blood loss. Intravenous fluid therapy should be instigated for longer surgeries or those with potential for significant blood loss. Except for short minor procedures, a 24 gauge intravenous catheter should ideally be placed for all surgical procedures. The cephalic vein is the most common site for placement, but lateral saphenous, jugular and intraosseous catheters can also be used.

When a jugular catheter is necessary, a 22 gauge venous catheter can be placed in the jugular vein. In many ferrets a cut-down to expose the jugular vein for catheter placement may be necessary, as the neck can be muscular with thick subcutaneous fat and tough skin.

Blood transfusion therapy may be necessary if there is major blood loss, preoperative anaemia or splenectomy and the ferret cannot maintain a haematocrit greater than 25%. See also Chapter 18.

Premedication

Ferrets have a strong vagal reflex and may also demonstrate arrhythmias and apnoea in response to gaseous anaesthesia. In addition, because of strong oesophageal reflux during stress and gastric irritation and subsequent histamine release, and in many ferrets pre-existing GI ulceration, the author has found that premedication with both famotidine and diphenhydramine along with atropine minimizes intraoperative and postoperative complications due to these physiological responses. Ferrets should be fasted for 1–4 hours prior to surgery, except those with islet cell neoplasia for which the fast must be monitored and should be under 2 hours.

Anaesthetic induction by mask alone should be avoided as the increased anxiety, panic and subsequent increases in heart rate, blood pressure and other stress-related physiological changes can make it difficult to maintain homeostasis during surgery and postoperatively. Pre-emptive analgesia before any surgery is necessary and may also serve as the preoperative sedative that allows for smoother induction. Butorphanol at 0.2 mg/kg s.c. 20–30 minutes prior to gas induction provides this function. Use of a benzodiazepine decreases anxiety and increases muscle relaxation, both of which contribute to a smooth induction. Midazolam at 0.25–0.3 mg/kg i.m. or i.v. can be given 15–20 minutes prior to induction with an inhalant anaesthetic. Diazepam at 1–3 mg/kg i.m. or i.v. could be used as an alternative to midazolam.

Restraint (physical and chemical)

Ferrets can be masked until they are sufficiently anaesthetized to allow endotracheal intubation. An aggressive ferret can be restrained using thick leather gloves (e.g. leather primate handling gloves or thick gardening gloves) and administered midazolam at 0.5 mg/kg along with butorphanol at 0.4 mg/kg i.m. This will sufficiently sedate the ferret so that further handling and induction proceed safely and smoothly. An agitated or frightened ferret will have elevated blood pressure and heart rate that can complicate anaesthesia.

If an induction chamber is used, it is still preferable to administer midazolam to decrease the anxiety and keep blood pressure and heart rate at physiologically normal levels. It is often necessary to use a small amount of lidocaine (0.1 ml) to paralyse the larynx and accomplish intubation, as in the feline species. With sufficient premedication, this can usually be accomplished with a flow rate of 2 litres per minute and a 4–5% isoflurane concentration. The animal relaxes in 2–5 minutes. Because struggling or excitement is minimal, chamber induction is not usually necessary.

Intubation

All ferrets are intubated except for the most minor procedures (Figure 22.11). Use of 1.5 to 4.5 French endotracheal tubes is sufficient for most ferrets. If the tubes are allowed to become cold in a refrigerator, they will become stiff and more easily introduced into the trachea. A stylet may be used to provide rigidity.

Because ferrets vary in body size, several tube sizes should be available. European ferrets, which are generally larger than the American breeds and can weigh up to 2.5 kg, need slightly larger endotracheal tubes. Whenever possible, a cuffed tube is recommended. The endotracheal tube can be secured by tying it with gauze bandage material cinched around the tube as it exits the mouth and a length looped around each foreleg above the elbow. If

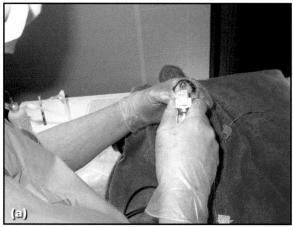
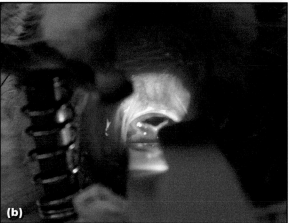

22.11 **(a)** Positioning for intubation. **(b)** View of the ferret glottis, using a size 0 Miller laryngoscope blade. The mouth is propped open with a 'Nazzy Ferret Mouth Gag' (designed by the author and manufactured for Universal Surgical Instruments, Glen Cove, New York).

a cephalic catheter is in place, the gauze loop on that leg should be placed distal to the catheter. This method of securing the endotracheal tube works well with the ferret in dorsal recumbency, as ferrets have such a short muzzle and elongated skull and neck that methods used to secure the tube in dogs or cats do not work well in the ferret.

Ventilation

A non-rebreathing system is used with a flow rate of 0.6–1.0 l/minute once intubated. If apnoea occurs, doxapram (2–5 mg/kg i.v., i.m.) may be administered as needed to stabilize respiration. If a mechanical ventilator is used, it should be adjusted according to estimated lung volume with frequency of respirations set between 40 and 70 breaths per minute. Because ventilators allow for better aeration and regular chest excursions, the percentage of inhalant anaesthetic used is less than in the patient allowed to respire spontaneously. An electrocardiograph with respiratory monitor capabilities including capnography and pulse oximetry is extremely useful to monitor the ferret, particularly if throat and neck manipulation have triggered the vagal response and the heart rate has markedly decreased or become irregular. The ferret should be stabilized with a regular heart rate, ECG and respiration rate prior to the initial incision.

Postoperative procedures

Isoflurane or sevoflurane should be discontinued upon the surgeon's determination of the conclusion of the surgery. The ferret can be maintained on oxygen until it is breathing spontaneously (ventilator off) and blood pressure, heart and respiratory rate approximate to the preanaesthetic level. The ferret will usually begin moving or gagging, signalling readiness for endotracheal tube removal and disconnection from ECG and other probes. Temperature as well as reflexes should continue to be monitored until the ferret begins to move about. Generally ferrets will then curl up into their usual sleep position and sleep postoperatively. Heat and plenty of cloths or towels for burrowing into for rest should be provided.

Postoperative anaesthetic complications

It is not uncommon for ferrets to awaken and then have a massive drop in blood pressure and succumb several hours after surgery. This has been seen particularly following surgeries that have manipulated the upper GI tract or have significant blood loss, such as a splenectomy when the spleen is massively enlarged. The hypothesis for this is histamine release and the triggering of the vagal reflex (Johnson-Delaney, 2005a). Death after apparent recovery may also be a consequence of low blood pressure, depressed cardiovascular function (although heart and respiratory rates seemed acceptable) coupled with mild to moderate hypothermia during the surgery.

Blood pressure drops can be minimized using drugs with minimal cardiovascular depressive effects such as midazolam and etomidate as induction medications, then lowered percentages of inhalant anaesthetics. Intravenous fluid therapy can be used intraoperatively to increase intravascular volumes. Fluids should be warmed to body temperature before infusion.

The author has successfully reversed this effect when it was noted during induction or surgery by administering additional diphenhydramine, atropine and, in rare cases, adrenaline intravenously, titrated to effect. If this happens during induction, the ferret is recovered and the surgery is aborted. If it happens during the surgery, the procedure is halted as the ferret is stabilized, then finished as quickly as possible. The recovery period is closely monitored for 12–24 hours, with continued intravenous access available. Postoperative analgesia should be administered at time points to coincide with the expected end of analgesia provided by the preoperative butorphanol (usually 1–3 hours post surgery, or 8–10 hours post surgery if buprenorphine was used). NSAIDs such as meloxicam can be given at the conclusion of the surgery when the blood pressure and body temperature have returned to preanaesthetic levels. The author routinely combines the use of an opioid and an NSAID, along with continued famotidine administration postoperatively, for most surgeries requiring general anaesthesia.

Acknowledgements

The author would like to acknowledge Dr Angela Lennox, Dr Marla Lichtenberger, the volunteers and ferrets of the Washington Ferret Rescue & Shelter, staff of Eastside Avian & Exotic Animal Medical Center, and all my ferret family for helping me to understand ferret pain and a better way to take care of them.

References

Allen DG, Pringle JK, Smith DA *et al.* (1993) Small animals. In: *Handbook of Veterinary Drugs*, ed. DG Allen *et al.*, pp. 1–289. JB Lippincott, Philadelphia

Gamble C and Morrisey JK (2005) Ferrets. In: *Exotic Animal Formulary*, 3rd edn, ed. JW Carpenter, pp. 445–476. Elsevier Saunders, St Louis

Johnson-Delaney CA (2005a) Ferret cardiopulmonary resuscitation. *Seminars in Avian and Exotic Pet Medicine* **14**(2), 135–142

Johnson-Delaney CA (2005b) The ferret GI tract and *Helicobacter mustelae* infection. *Veterinary Clinics of North America: Exotic Animals* **8**, 197–212

Johnston MS (2005) Clinical approaches to analgesia in ferrets and rabbits. *Seminars in Avian and Exotic Pet Medicine* **14**(4), 229–235

23

Ferrets: common surgical procedures

Vittorio Capello

General principles of surgery

Equipment

Anatomical and physiological features important for anaesthesia and surgery in the ferret are not that different from those of more common pets like dogs and cats (see Chapter 17). Standard equipment for anaesthesia is described in Chapter 22. Surgical instruments for ferrets include those most commonly used in general surgery of dogs and cats, but their size has to be smaller. Smaller finer instruments and a few specialized items that can be useful are described below.

With few exceptions, microsurgical instruments are rarely needed for general surgery, but in some cases these instruments can greatly simplify certain procedures. Microsurgical instruments are delicate and expensive, and require special skill and care. Magnification (2.5X up to 5X) is often useful, and can help to improve the ergonomics and reduce strain. Magnifying loupes are most commonly utilized (see Chapter 7).

In addition to surgical instruments, other supplies and equipment must be appropriately sized, including scalpel blades (no.11 and no.15), suture material (2 to 0.4 metric; 3/0 to 8/0 USP) and intravenous catheters (25 gauge). A small-volume paediatric infusion pump is recommended for careful regulation of fluid administration (see Chapter 18 for more details).

Gelatin sponge haemostatic material is very useful in helping to control bleeding during splenic and liver biopsies, and during pancreatic and adrenal surgery.

The author prefers the use of a unique lightweight ergonomic retractor, particularly for exploratory laparotomy. The use of this retractor is described below.

A radiosurgical, rather than electrosurgical, unit can be useful for certain procedures. The higher frequency radio waves used in radiosurgery (4.0 MHz) as compared with the lower frequency (1.0–1.3 MHz) of traditional electrosurgery provides a micro-smooth incision and much less heat, with the least amount of tissue alteration.

Patient preparation and monitoring

Standard optimal aseptic technique is essential in the ferret, as in any other surgical patient. While ferret skin is not as delicate as other exotic mammal species, care must be taken not to damage it during shaving. As the body surface/volume ratio is high in these small patients, heat loss and hypothermia are a concern during long surgical procedures; therefore the area clipped should be minimized. Alcohol rinses should be avoided during surgical preparation, to avoid excessive cooling, and supplemental heat sources are extremely important.

Transparent (adhesive) drapes are recommended both for the anaesthetist and for the surgeon, allowing better visualization and improved monitoring of the surgical patient.

A number of devices that are easily adapted to the ferret are extremely useful for monitoring the surgical patient. These include ECG, ultrasonic Doppler, pulse oximeter and capnograph. Measurement of indirect blood pressure and core body temperature is also important. (See also Chapter 22.)

Diagnostic surgical procedures

Exploratory laparotomy

Despite the utility of non-invasive diagnostic procedures (radiography, CT scan, ultrasonography) and less invasive procedures (laparoscopy), laparotomy still remains an important diagnostic tool.

The skin incision is performed on the ventral midline and its length depends on the goal of laparotomy. In case of exploratory laparotomy both skin and abdominal incision must be maximized, from the xyphoid cranially to the pubic area caudally. In the male, it is usually extended just cranial to the prepuce, but special surgical indications or intraoperative findings might require extension up to the parapreputial region. Subcutaneous fat is usually minimal in the ferret, and the linea alba is easily identified as a wide thin aponeurosis; it even appears semi-transparent in patients neutered very young. The linea alba is grasped with a forceps or a haemostat at the level of the umbilical scar, and carefully elevated before the incision in order to prevent damage to underlying organs. A small incision is performed with the tip of the scalpel blade. The linea alba is then elevated and protected with a haemostat before extending the incision cranially and caudally with rounded-tip scissors. Cranial extension of the laparotomy incision must avoid incision of the diaphragm. Thorough examination of the abdominal cavity is made easier by the use of proper retraction. The Lone Star Retractor is a light, autoclavable plastic retractor. Its rubber bands with small stay hooks make it very effective and easy to use (Figure 23.1).

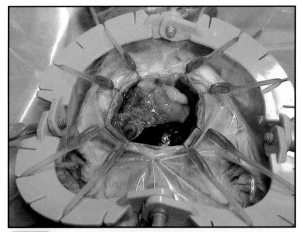

23.1 The Lone Star Retractor is very effective in providing wide access to the abdominal cavity with minimal soft tissue stress. The ability to change the configuration of this retractor makes it useful for many purposes beyond laparotomy. (© Vittorio Capello)

After the surgical procedure has been completed, the abdominal wall is sutured with 2 to 3 metric (3/0 or 2/0 USP) monofilament absorbable material (e.g. polydioxanone/PDS or polyglecaprone/Monocryl) in an interrupted pattern. Ideally, the suture material should be as small as possible, with more single stitches for a better distribution of the pressure over the tissues and the suture material. A simple continuous pattern is feasible but it is not recommended considering the wide laparotomic incision and the bright and dynamic behaviour of ferrets. The subcutaneous suture can be omitted if a superficial suture of the skin is performed with 2 metric (3/0 USP) non-absorbable suture material (polypropylene or nylon) in an interrupted pattern; otherwise 1.5 to 1 metric (4/0 or 5/0 USP) absorbable monofilament can be used to perform an intradermal suture in a simple continuous pattern.

Ferrets frequently develop wide ecchymotic areas in the abdominal skin 24–48 hours after laparotomy (Figure 23.2). This may be due to microvascular damage from the handling of the abdominal wall, but it does not represent a complication and disappears in a few days.

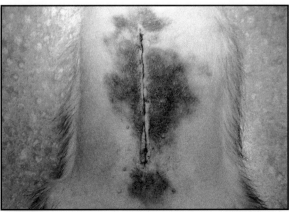

23.2 'Bruises' on the abdominal skin of a ferret two days after laparotomy. Exact aetiology is unknown, but this occurs commonly and without consequence. (© Vittorio Capello)

Biopsy of abdominal organs

Some organs can be sampled during exploratory laparotomy. In ferrets the most common tissues sampled are the liver, gastrointestinal lymph nodes and the pancreas. Gastrointestinal tract, spleen and kidney can be safely sampled as well.

Liver biopsy

Liver biopsy is performed whenever laparotomy reveals a lesion, or when diagnostic testing suggests liver disease. Metastatic neoplasia is common, as are hepatic cysts and 'steroid hepatopathy' secondary to adrenal disease. Surgical methods for liver biopsy include the guillotine technique, the haemostatic clamp technique and the punch technique.

The guillotine technique can be performed at the margin of the liver lobe by placing absorbable suture material around the tip of the lobe and tightening it slowly and gently. The ligature should be used for haemostasis and not to cut the hepatic tissue. The liver specimen is resected distal to the suture.

The haemostatic clamp technique is similar to the guillotine and also allows biopsy of the edge of the liver (Figure 23.3). Two haemostatic clamps are simply closed delimiting a small triangular area of tissue. In this case, clamps both provide haemostasis and resect the tissue. If additional haemostasis is required, haemostatic gelatin can be applied or the defect can be sutured.

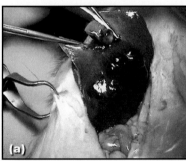
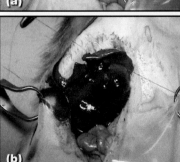
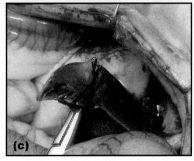

23.3 Haemostatic clamp techniques for biopsy of the liver with visible hepatic cysts. **(a)** A small rectangular sample, including a small cyst, is dissected from the edge of the liver lobe using two small haemostatic clamps. **(b)** The defect is sutured with 1 metric (5/0 USP) Monocryl. **(c)** In this case, the biopsy specimen is removed just with the haemostatic clamp, and bleeding is controlled with pressure or absorbable haemostatic gelatin sponge. (© Vittorio Capello)

The punch biopsy technique is preferred when the desired sample is not at the liver margin. A small sterile skin biopsy punch is pressed in a circular motion into the liver parenchyma. The sample is gently dissected free from the liver with small scissors and extracted. Bleeding is controlled with digital pressure, application of gelatin haemostatic sponge or suturing the liver capsule with 1 metric (5/0 USP) absorbable material.

Splenic biopsy

Splenomegaly is a common finding in ferrets. The most common histopathological diagnosis is extra-medullary haemopoiesis, but neoplasia and other pathological conditions are possible as well. Splen-ectomy should be avoided unless medically necessary (for example, in splenic neoplasia). Splenic biopsy, therefore, is of critical importance. The preferred method is the punch biopsy technique (Figure 23.4). Placement of sutures is easier than in the liver due to the relatively thick capsule.

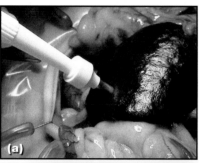
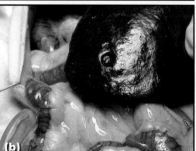
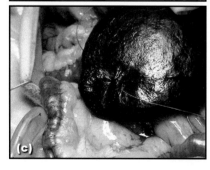

23.4 Punch biopsy technique for biopsy of the spleen. **(a)** The biopsy punch is pushed into the spleen using gentle circular motions. **(b)** Appearance of the splenic parenchyma after removal of the biopsy specimen. **(c)** Suture of the capsule with 1 metric (5/0 USP) Monocryl for better control of haemorrhage. (© Vittorio Capello)

Pancreatic biopsy

As pancreatic tissue is very soft and delicate, the punch technique is not recommended. Pancreatic biopsy is the same as small partial pancreatectomy described later in this chapter. Biopsy of small nodules is easily accomplished using gentle blunt dissection of the mass followed by digital pressure to control bleeding.

Lymph node biopsy

Biopsy of lymph nodes is indicated in cases of unresolved gastrointestinal disease other than foreign body obstruction. Common pathological findings include neoplasia and inflammation. Two or three different samples among gastric and duodenal nodes and the single mesenteric lymph node should be taken. The technique is complete excision of the lymph node from the surrounding fat (Figure 23.5). Partial excision of very large, firm mesenteric lymph node is another option. Control of haemostasis is routine and is not usually a concern.

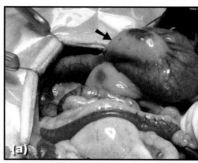
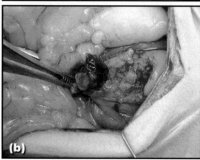

23.5 **(a)** Enlarged gastric lymph node (arrowed) in a ferret with chronic gastritis. **(b)** Excision of the lymph node from the surrounding fat. (© Vittorio Capello)

Gastric and intestinal biopsy

A number of diseases affecting the gastrointestinal tract require biopsy for confirmation and to direct treatment. A surgical approach via exploratory lap-arotomy is preferred to endoscopic biopsy because it allows collection of a full thickness rather than simple mucosal sample. An additional benefit is inspection of the entire gastrointestinal tract and abdominal cavity. A small gastrotomy site is sutured in two layers: one for the mucosal and one for the mus-cular and serosal layers, with simple interrupted pat-terns, using 1.5 to 1 metric (4/0 or 5/0 USP) monofilament absorbable suture material. The enter-otomy site is closed in a single layer (Figure 23.6).

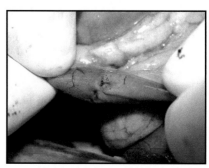

23.6 Suture of an intestinal loop with 1.5 metric (4/0 USP) Monocryl after full-thickness biopsy of the wall. (© Vittorio Capello)

Elective surgical procedures

Orchidectomy

Indications for bilateral orchidectomy include control of unwanted births, reduction of dominant or aggressive behaviour, and reduction of the secretion of the sebaceous glands. Orchidectomy is generally performed around the onset of puberty (12 weeks of age). Some large producers of pet ferrets in the US perform surgical neutering much earlier.

The anatomy of the testicles and related vascularization is similar to that of cats. Both open and closed techniques are reported, following a single incision of the scrotal skin on the midline (Ludwig and Aiken, 1997). After exteriorization of each testicle, the spermatic cord is double clamped and ligated with 2 or 1.5 metric (3/0 or 4/0 USP) absorbable suture material, or haemostatic clips. Suturing of the scrotal incision is optional. Suture of the inguinal ring is not necessary.

Deferentectomy (vasectomy)

Functional (non-hormonal) neutering is primarily performed to obtain a male for the interruption of oestrus in intact females, but without the burden of pregnancy. It should be kept in mind that this procedure will not improve the objectionable musky odour of the intact male ferret.

The surgical approach to the deferent ducts is through a prescrotal incision, slightly lateral to the ventral midline of the penis. Soft tissues are bluntly dissected until the vaginal process is identified and isolated from the surrounding tissues. The parietal tunica of the vaginal process is incised in order to expose the spermatic cord and identify the white deferent duct. The spermatic cord may be deeply embedded in fat, which makes identification challenging. A short portion (about 1 cm) of the deferent duct is separated from the spermatic cord, taking care to avoid damage to the blood supply of the testicle. It is double ligated at a distance of about 0.5 cm apart. To ensure complete interruption of the deferent ducts, the small tract is excised, resulting in a true deferentectomy rather than simple double ligation. Submission of the tissue for histopathology can confirm proper excision. Suture of the parietal tunica with absorbable 1.5 to 1 metric (4/0 or 5/0 USP) suture material is recommended, in order to protect the vascular structures of the spermatic cord. Subcutaneous tissue and skin are closed as routine.

Swelling of the scrotal area may occur postoperatively, but resolves after 2–3 days. Vasectomized hobs should not be used for 6 weeks after surgery, to allow any live semen in the spermatic cord to degenerate.

Ovariohysterectomy

The surgical technique for ovariohysterectomy (OVH) is similar to the midline abdominal approach in the domestic cat. The skin is incised starting from the umbilical scar (or about 1 cm caudal to the umbilicus) in a caudal direction for a few centimetres. The incision of the linea alba is performed as described above. The uterus of the ferret is bicornuate and the body is very short. It is often very small in the

prepubescent jill, therefore the dorsal side of the urinary bladder can be a helpful landmark. The ovaries are located by gentle cranial retraction of the thin uterine horns. The ovaries can have a dark appearance and lie inside a fold (bursa) of fat tissue. Ligation of the ovarian and uterine arteries is performed with haemoclips or with 1.5 metric (4/0 USP) absorbable monofilament suture material. Suture of the cervix is performed just distal to the junction of the two uterine bodies. Clipping, transfixing and circumferential suturing are all good options (Figure 23.7).

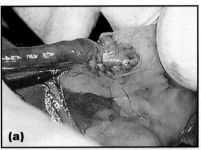
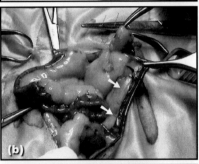
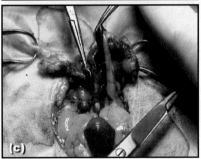

23.7   Ovariohysterectomy. **(a)** Appearance of the ovarian bursa, the salpinx and the proximal uterine horn in a jill at puberty. **(b)** Uterine vessels (white arrows) lie parallel to the uterine horn (yellow arrow), here shown in a 1-year-old ferret. The exteriorized urinary bladder is visible. **(c)** Circumferential ligation of the cervix with 2 metric (3/0 USP) Monocryl is performed just distal to the junction of the uterine horns with the short uterine body. (© Vittorio Capello)

Relatively common complications following improper OVH are: incomplete removal of both ovaries, leading to ovarian remnant; and hysterectomy performed too cranially, predisposing to uterine disease of the stump.

As with castration, OVH is not a common procedure in the US for practitioners as most jills in the pet trade arrive in the pet store already spayed. The converse situation occurs in the UK, where OVH, castration and vasectomy of ferrets are common procedures in veterinary practice. [Editors' note: Recent research indicates that surgical neutering plays a role in the development of hyperadrenocorticism (see also Chapters 17 and 30).]

Anal sacculectomy

Similar to other members of Mustelidae, a unique anatomical feature of ferrets is the presence of well developed anal sacs, located in the perianal space lateral to the distal rectum. They are very large relative to the size of the animal. The oily yellowish secretion stored in the sacs from the perianal glands has a very musky and pungent odour, which can be a concern when ferrets are kept as pets. The primary indication for bilateral anal sacculectomy is to eliminate the odour when secretions are expressed, especially indoors. Anal sac abscessation occasionally occurs in ferrets that have not been de-scented; therefore this represents a therapeutic procedure as well.

However, this preventive surgery is considered unethical and is not permitted in the UK or in The Netherlands. It is rarely done in general practice in the US, as anal sacculectomy is usually performed with surgical neutering prior to arrival at pet stores. In other countries, it is a common procedure performed at the age of puberty, concurrently with neutering or spaying. Neutering or spaying will not cause atrophy of the anal glands or the anal sacs and the tendency of ferrets to express the anal sac secretion is related to behavioural and environmental factors.

Two different surgical techniques are reported for preventive anal sacculectomy of the ferret. For both techniques the ferret can be placed in ventral or dorsal recumbency, with the pelvis slightly elevated. The most traditional is the ductal technique. In this case the opening of the duct of the anal sac is grasped with the tip of haemostat forceps. A circumferential incision of the mucosa around the duct opening is performed with a no.11 or no.15 scalpel blade, and the duct is exteriorized by retracting it with the forceps, while the mucosa is reflected from the sac with gentle scraping using a scalpel blade in a transverse fashion, or by careful blunt dissection with haemostats. When the anal sac is completely exteriorized, the caudal end is dissected free from the retractor muscle of the anal sac (Figure 23.8a). Bleeding and damage to the anal sphincter are minimal if dissection is performed close to the sac. Nevertheless, a frequent complication of ductal sacculectomy can be mild to severe lesions involving the anal sphincter, predisposing to rectal prolapse.

The extraductal technique provides an important advantage in preventing damage to the anal sphincter, as the initial skin incision is made 1 cm lateral to the opening of the anal sac (Figure 23.8b). Also, it greatly reduces the risk of iatrogenic lesions to the distal tract of the rectum, as the dissection is performed laterally. The anal sac is bluntly dissected free from the surrounding tissues and the constrictor muscle, up to the duct (Figure 23.8c). Suture of the skin at the mucocutaneous junction is performed with the apposition of single knots of 1.5 metric (4/0 USP) absorbable material in a U-shaped suture pattern.

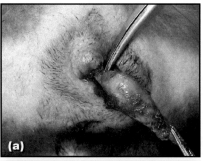

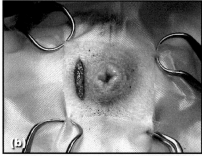

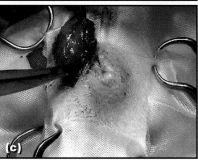

23.8 Preventive anal sacculectomy. **(a)** Ductal technique. **(b,c)** Two surgical steps of the extraductal technique. (© Vittorio Capello. Reproduced from Capello (2006b) with permission of the Zoological Education Network)

Therapeutic surgical procedures

Surgical procedures of the gastrointestinal system

Gastrotomy

Removal of ingested foreign bodies is common, especially in young ferrets. The most commonly reported location is the small intestine, with gastric foreign bodies occurring less frequently.

Trichobezoars (hairballs) are relatively common in ferrets and result from excessive grooming behaviour or are induced by underlying gastrointestinal disease and alteration of GI transit. The typical shape of bezoars is curved, resembling the curvature of the stomach, often with a small 'tail' entering the pylorus and the duodenum. Other than vomiting, which is not as frequent as in other domestic species, clinical signs may be challenging in these cases since they may typically be absent when the bezoar is positioned in the stomach and appear when it moves into the pylorus.

During any laparotomy, it is essential to explore and thoroughly palpate the entire gastrointestinal tract, because more than one foreign body can be present (Figure 23.9a).

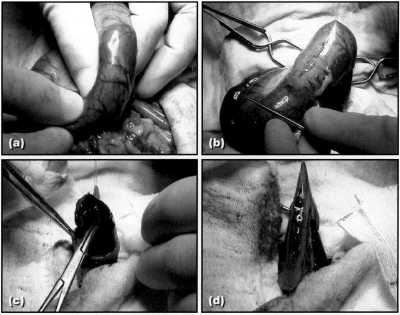

23.9 Gastrotomy for removal of a trichobezoar. **(a)** The stomach is exteriorized and palpated. The trichobezoar is visible through the gastric wall. **(b)** Stay suture and incision of the serosal and muscular layer. **(c)** The bezoar is removed through the gastrotomy incision. **(d)** Suture of the mucosal layer in a simple continuous inverting pattern. (© Vittorio Capello)

Prior to gastrotomy, the stomach is gently exteriorized and isolated with moistened sponges. The stomach is then stabilized by an assistant after passing two full-thickness stay sutures in the least vascular area of the body of the stomach, about 3–5 cm apart. Incision of the serosal layer is performed gently between the stay sutures. A second incision is made in the muscular layer, while any minimal haemorrhage is controlled with cotton-tipped applicators (Figure 23.9b). The mucosal layer pops up through the muscular incision and it is dissected while the assistant holds the tip of the aspirator ready to absorb fluids and prevent spillage of gastric contents. At this time the mucosal incision is widened with round-tipped scissors. The trichobezoar or gastric foreign body is removed (Figure 23.9c) and the stomach is closely inspected, with careful attention to the pylorus, and then flushed. The gastrotomy incision is sutured in two layers using 1.5 to 1 metric (4/0 or 5/0 USP) monofilament absorbable suture material in a simple inverting continuous pattern. The first suture layer incorporates the mucosa; the second suture layer the muscular and serosal layers (Figure 23.9d).

Soft food and fluids can be administered orally about 4–6 hours after surgery in order to prevent hypoglycaemia, especially in ferrets with concurrent insulinoma. Food is offered in small amounts every few hours for the next 2–3 days.

Enterotomy

Enterotomy can be more challenging due to the small size of the organ. The surgical procedure is similar to gastrotomy, and the intestinal tract must be well isolated from surrounding loops and other tissues with moistened sponges. If possible, the incision should be performed 1 cm distally to the location of the foreign body in order to reduce the chances of a dehiscence of the suture and of a stenosis, as the intestinal wall is already affected by the pressure from the foreign body. The foreign body is then gently pushed distally and removed. In cases of multiple foreign bodies, the number of incisions should be minimized. Suture of the enterotomy site is usually performed in one layer using 1.5 or 1 metric (4/0 or 5/0 USP) monofilament absorbable suture material. Both simple interrupted and simple continuous patterns are acceptable. Single layer is recommended to prevent excessive reduction of the lumen. For very small diameter bowel loops, a longitudinal incision is sutured transversely to prevent luminal stricture. Postoperative recommendations are similar to those described for gastrotomy.

Enterectomy

Indications for intestinal resection and anastomosis are neoplasia, severe damage of the bowel loop following obstruction from foreign bodies, and to resolve complications of pancreatic surgery and vascular damage.

The general principles of this surgery are the same as in other common pet species. The pattern of anastomosis can be termino-terminal, latero-lateral or termino-lateral. The first option carries the highest risk of stricture.

Surgical procedures of the endocrine system

Surgery of the adrenal glands

Adrenal disease is very common in ferrets, and surgical treatment is a therapeutic option, often in conjunction with medical treatment. Anatomy of the adrenal glands, as well as aetiology, pathophysiology, clinical signs, diagnostic options and therapeutic indications for adrenal disease are described in Chapter 30.

Adrenal disease often presents concurrently with other disease processes. Therefore, in addition to complete medical workup, thorough examination of the entire abdominal cavity is extremely important. Complete access to the right adrenal gland requires a surgical incision extending cranially to the xiphoid, and excellent retraction.

Inspection of adrenal glands usually begins with the left adrenal. Normal adrenal glands are about 5–8 mm long and 2–3 mm wide, resembling rice grains. They are pale pink and the surface is smooth and regular. The normal left adrenal is usually completely embedded in the fat surrounding the kidney and can be difficult to visualize. Diseased adrenal glands are often increased in size, with an irregular shape and surface; they may be more pink to yellow in colour, more round or more firm on palpation. Some abnormal glands have small dark foci or grossly visible cysts. In some cases, the only indication of an abnormality is increased vascularization of the gland. It is important to remember that not all diseased adrenal glands are enlarged, therefore the fat surrounding the adrenal must be carefully dissected in order to visualize the gland.

The right adrenal gland lies cranial to the right kidney, caudal to the right caudate liver lobe and medial-to-dorsal to the caudal vena cava, adherent to the wall of the vena cava itself. For this reason, it is not usually embedded in fat but must be gently retracted medially and ventrally for a complete and proper evaluation. Omission of this step can lead to underestimation of the size and condition of the right adrenal gland.

A number of different techniques for adrenalectomy have been reported. Clinical trials comparing survival rates associated with various techniques are unavailable.

Complete excision represents the only chance for complete cure. However, subtotal excision is commonly performed and can be considered in cases of right adrenal gland disease with invasion into the vena cava, or as a strategy to prevent possible hypoadrenocorticism.

While complete adrenalectomy in any other species necessitates lifetime replacement of adrenal steroids, the requirement in ferrets is unclear. Anecdotal reports of complete excision without the need for replacement suggest failure of complete bilateral excision because of local metastasis, or the presence of ectopic adrenal tissue.

Total excision of the diseased left adrenal is straightforward. Blunt dissection of the gland from the surrounding fat tissue is performed using blunt scissors and cotton-tipped applicators. The phrenico-abdominal vein is ligated with 1 metric (5/0 USP) absorbable suture material or haemostatic clips. The adrenal gland is then dissected free from surrounding tissue and removed (Figure 23.10).

Excision of the right adrenal gland can be very challenging. In case of unilateral involvement, total excision of the gland is sometimes feasible by performing sharp and blunt dissection with extreme care. Since direct vascular connection with the caudal vena cava can be present, one or more haemostatic clips are placed tangentially to the wall of the vena cava before complete excision (Figure 23.11). When intimate connection with the wall of the vena cava is present and subtotal excision is not an option, partial phlebectomy is required. A special vascular clamp, the neonatal Satinsky tangential vascular clamp, is temporarily applied to the vena cava around the base of the adrenal gland. The wall of the vein is resected along with the diseased gland and sutured with 0.4

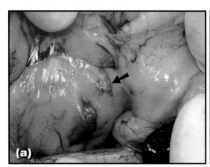 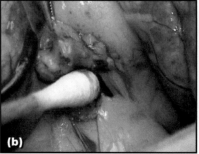 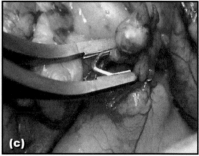

23.10   Total excision of the left adrenal gland. **(a)** The enlarged left adrenal gland (arrowed) is visible cranial to the left kidney, which can be identified protruding through surrounding fat. The size, shape and colour are abnormal. **(b)** Exteriorization of the left adrenal gland using cotton-tipped applicators. **(c)** The vascular supply of the adrenal gland is ligated with haemostatic clips. (© Vittorio Capello)

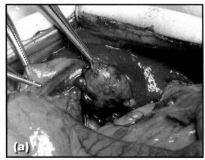 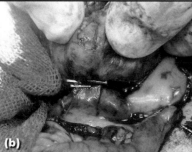 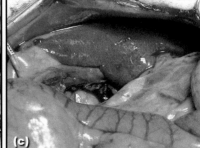

23.11   Total excision of the right adrenal gland. **(a)** A very enlarged right adrenal gland is visible medial to the caudal vena cava and caudal to the right caudate liver lobe. **(b)** The huge adrenal gland is gently dissected free from the wall of the vena cava and the vascular connections are clipped tangential to the wall itself. **(c)** Appearance of the caudal vena cava after total excision of the diseased adrenal gland. (© Vittorio Capello)

metric (8/0 USP) absorbable suture material in a simple continuous pattern. Magnifying loupes and microsurgical instruments are essential for this surgical technique. Additional haemostasis can be obtained with gelatin sponge haemostatic material. When extensive invasion of the vena cava is present, partial resection and anastomosis may be needed. Complete ligation of the vena cava is not recommended but has been reported and is apparently not uniformly harmful (Weiss *et al.*, 1999).

Subtotal excision of the right adrenal gland is performed by debulking using the haemostatic clip or the incision technique. The haemostatic clip technique (Figure 23.12) is similar to total excision with the use of clips, but in this case only part of the adrenal tissue is removed. Alternatively, a longitudinal incision of the adrenal gland can be performed and the medullary tissue shelled out and removed using small forceps or a haemostat. To prevent haemorrhage from direct vascular connection with the vena cava, tangential clips may be placed soon after the incision of the capsule (Figure 23.13).

Alternative techniques for surgical treatment of adrenal disease include laser surgery, radiosurgery, cryosurgery and injection of the gland with alcohol. These techniques do not allow tissue biopsy, and the extent of the tissue destruction may be difficult to evaluate. Thermal damage to the vena cava may also be of concern.

Surgery of the pancreas

Partial excision of neoplastic pancreatic tissue (partial pancreatectomy) or neoplastic small masses (nodulectomy) is commonly performed due to a high incidence of insulin-secreting pancreatic islet tumour in ferrets (commonly called insulinoma, or pancreatic beta cell tumour). Aetiology, pathophysiology, clinical signs, diagnostic options and therapeutic indications are described in Chapter 30. Surgical anatomy of the pancreas is shown in Figure 23.14.

During exploratory laparotomy, thorough and careful inspection of the pancreas must be performed looking for small nodules. The right and the left pancreatic lobes should be inspected and gently palpated on both the ventral and dorsal surfaces, while the body of the pancreas can be inspected only on the ventral surface. Magnifying loupes can help inspection, but very small nodules can be completely embedded into the glandular tissue and detected only with patient and gentle palpation. Multiple nodules are common. When a large nodule or multiple masses are present on one lobe, pancreatectomy is indicated.

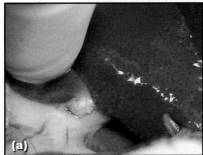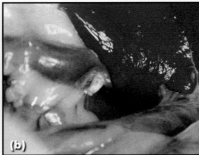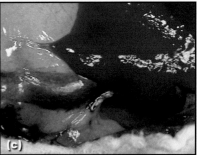

23.12 Subtotal excision by debulking the right adrenal gland with the haemostatic clip technique. **(a)** An abnormal right adrenal gland is visible cranial to the surrounding fat of the kidney, medial to the caudal vena cava and caudal to the right caudate liver lobe. **(b)** A haemoclip is placed tangential to the wall of the vena cava at the base of the adrenal gland. **(c)** Most of the right adrenal gland is removed after clipping. Part of the adrenal tissue is still visible between the clip and the caudal vena cava. (© Vittorio Capello)

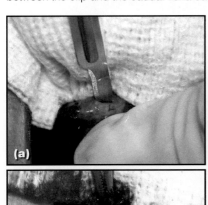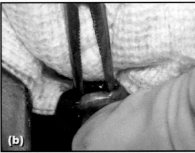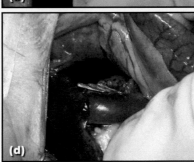

23.13 Subtotal excision by debulking the right adrenal gland with the incision technique. **(a)** The abnormal right adrenal gland is exteriorized and longitudinally incised with the tip of a scalpel blade. **(b)** Most of the medullary tissue of the adrenal gland is removed using a small haemostat. **(c)** Appearance of the adrenal gland after debulking. **(d)** The base of the adrenal gland is clipped and more adrenal tissue is removed. (© Vittorio Capello)

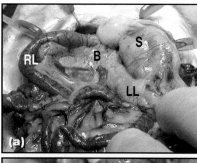

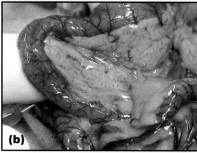

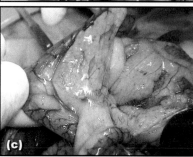

23.14 Anatomy of the pancreas in ferrets. **(a)** The entire pancreas is shown. B = body of the pancreas; LL = left lobe of the pancreas; RL = right limb of the pancreas; S = stomach. **(b)** Right limb and cranial pancreaticoduodenal artery (arrowed). **(c)** Right limb and caudal pancreaticoduodenal artery (arrowed). (© Vittorio Capello)

Before ligation and dissection of the pancreatic tissue to be removed, special attention must be paid to the blood supply shared between the right lobe and the duodenum, and between the left lobe and the spleen. The right lobe is supplied by the cranial and caudal pancreaticoduodenal vessels (Figure 23.14b,c). Damage to these vessels may result in avascular necrosis of the duodenum. The left pancreatic limb is supplied by a branch of the splenic artery.

The mesentery surrounding a limb of the pancreas is carefully dissected with blunt scissors or with a haemostatic clamp, creating a fenestration. Cotton-tipped applicators can be used to separate the pancreatic tissue from the blood vessels. The end of the pancreatic lobe is then ligated with a circumferential 1.5 metric (4/0 USP) monofilament absorbable suture material and dissected distal to the ligature (Figure 23.15). Haemorrhage is usually minimal.

Single or multiple nodulectomy can be performed with careful blunt dissection of the glandular tissue around the nodule, which usually shells out easily (Figure 23.16). In case of nodulectomy, haemorrhage can be controlled with direct pressure or a haemostatic sponge.

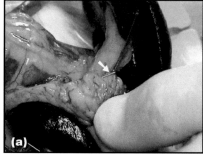

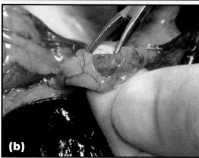

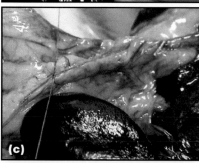

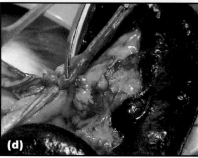

23.15 Partial pancreatectomy of the left limb with the guillotine suture technique. **(a)** The pancreatic vascular branch from the splenic artery has been ligated with a haemostatic clip (white arrow). A neoplastic nodule is also visible (yellow arrow). **(b)** The omentum is carefully dissected with a haemostat creating a window for the suture. **(c)** The guillotine suture is tied proximally to the margin of the left lobe of the pancreas. **(d)** The distal part of the left limb of the pancreas is dissected and removed. (© Vittorio Capello)

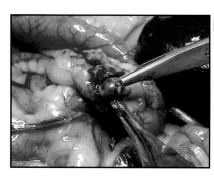

23.16 Nodulectomy for removal of a beta cell tumour of the pancreas (insulinoma). (© Vittorio Capello)

Splenectomy

Total splenectomy is similar to that in dogs and cats and is performed by ligation of all the blood vessels (splenic artery and vein) supplying the spleen under the visceral side. Attention must be paid to avoid damaging the left lobe of the pancreas. Ligature can be performed with either absorbable suture material or haemoclips.

Surgical procedures of the reproductive system

Ovariectomy/Ovariohysterectomy

Besides elective surgery described above, specific indications for selective ovariectomy or hysterectomy are occasionally encountered in pet ferrets.

Unilateral or bilateral ovarian remnants occur more frequently when jills are spayed very young. Clinical signs include evidence of persistent oestrus, which can also be seen in cases of adrenal disease. Prior to exploratory surgery, the patient must be carefully evaluated from the clinical standpoint for possible pancytopenia related to hyperoestrogenism.

Uterine horns are usually not present, therefore they are not a landmark during surgery. The ovarian remnant, normal or cystic, is usually found caudal to the kidney. More than one ovarian remnant can be present and so both sides must be thoroughly inspected. It should be kept in mind that a remnant lost or dropped during elective surgery can be lodged in any part of the abdominal cavity (Figure 23.17). Surgical excision of the remnant ovary is performed by ligation of the ovarian artery or the newly formed vascular supply. Indications for therapeutic ovario-hysterectomy include uterine disease in non-spayed jills or infection of the uterine stump in case of incomplete hysterectomy.

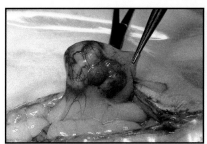

23.17 Cystic ovarian remnant in a 5-year-old ferret. (© Vittorio Capello)

Surgical treatment of prostatic cysts

Prostatic disease usually occurs concurrently with adrenal disease due to hormonal stimulation of the prostate gland. Common presentation is related to stranguria and urinary obstruction. When catheterization is unsuccessful, especially when paraurethral cysts are also present, cystocentesis is performed. Ideally, it should be done under ultrasonographic guidance in order to prevent centesis of the potentially infected prostatic cyst(s) and consequent peritonitis. Surgical treatment includes thorough exploratory laparotomy and adrenalectomy.

Prostatic cysts (Figure 23.18), usually filled with septic fluid and therefore actually prostatic abscesses, can be approached with three different techniques, depending on their number and size.

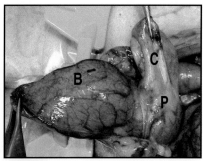

23.18 Bacterial prostatic infection and prostatic cyst in a 3½-year-old ferret with concurrent adrenal disease. B = urinary bladder; C = prostatic cyst; P = prostate gland. (© Vittorio Capello)

- When cysts are small, simple drainage can be performed using a 21 or even 18 gauge needle, as the fluid or pus is usually dense. The fluid should be submitted for culture and sensitivity testing.
- If cysts are bigger than 1.5–2 cm a portion of the cyst wall is removed and omentalization or marsupialization is performed to allow complete drainage and reabsorption. Omentalization allows continuous drainage and enhances adhesions. The cyst cavity is filled with a portion of the omentum which is sutured to the cyst wall with absorbable suture material.
- When the prostatic cyst is very large or when a communication between the urinary bladder and the cyst is present and uroperitoneum may be a concern, marsupialization of the cyst is performed. A small circular opening including the cyst wall, the abdominal wall, the subcutaneous fascia and the skin is sutured with absorbable or non-absorbable material in a simple interrupted pattern. Alternatively, marsupialization is performed with a paramedian incision of the abdominal wall, while the linea alba is closed routinely. The marsupialization suture will be removed about a week later and the surgical opening of the abdominal wall and the skin will be surgically addressed or often heals by secondary intention.

The prostate gland and the prostatic cysts usually regress in a few days after adrenalectomy and antibiotic treatment.

Surgical treatment of preputial masses and penile amputation

Preputial neoplasms are reported in ferrets as malignant apocrine gland adenocarcinomas. Depending on size and involvement of adjacent tissues, they may require simple surgical excision or penile amputation. Simple excision is preferred in cases of small neoplastic masses and the technique is routine.

Prior to penile amputation, a urinary catheter is placed in order to identify and preserve the urethra. The skin incision is U-shaped with a border cranial to the prepuce and a two borders parallel to the penis. The subcutaneous tissue and the muscular fascia are bluntly dissected. The neoplastic mass, a portion of the abdominal wall including the penis and the os penis are dissected and removed. The urethra is resected at the base of the penis. The abdominal wall, the subcutaneous tissue and the skin are sutured as described above for exploratory laparotomy. The resected urethra is sutured as described for urethrostomy (see below).

Surgical procedures of the urinary system

Nephrectomy
Indications for nephrectomy include unilateral hydronephrosis and neoplasia. Surgical technique is similar to that performed in dogs and cats. During laparotomy, the spleen (in the case of left nephrectomy) and intestinal loops are properly retracted in order to expose the kidney fully. Incision of the dorsal peritoneum is performed in order to access the retroperitoneal space, and the kidney is dissected free from the abundant surrounding fat. Renal vessels are carefully isolated at the hilus and double ligated separately. The ureter is dissected up to the urinary bladder, ligated and resected distally close to the bladder.

Cystotomy and urethrotomy
The most common indication for cystotomy is urolithiasis of the urinary bladder. Urolithiasis can also cause obstruction of the urethra in male ferrets.

Surgical technique is similar to that performed in dogs. Incision of the skin and laparotomy access is performed at the caudal abdominal midline in females and on the caudal abdominal midline/parapreputial area in males.

Once the bladder has been located, it is exteriorized by placing two stay sutures a few centimetres apart using 1.5 metric (4/0 USP) suture material. The incision is made between the stay sutures and an assistant holds the tip of the aspirator ready to adsorb urine and prevent spillage. The cystic calculi are removed and the urinary bladder is carefully inspected and flushed. The urethra is also flushed to make sure that no small uroliths are still present. The cystotomy site is sutured with 1 metric (5/0 USP) monofilament absorbable material in a simple continuous inverting pattern, taking care to avoid the mucosal layer. In cases of thickened bladder wall, a simple interrupted pattern is preferred. After suturing, the urinary bladder is checked carefully for leakage by filling it with saline using a 25 gauge needle.

Urethrotomy is possible in male ferrets with urethrolithiasis, but the risk of urethral stricture makes this technique a less common surgical option. Urethrostomy appears to be a more effective surgical technique (see below).

Cystostomy
The most common indication for temporary cystostomy may be severe urogenital complications of adrenal disease in male ferrets, such as concurrent prostatic disease, multiple prostatic cysts or paraurethral cysts where catheterization is not feasible, and when regression is not expected to occur quickly post surgical or medical therapy for adrenal disease.

Cystostomy may be performed by placing a cystostomy tube (a Foley catheter) or with true marsupialization of the urinary bladder through a paramedian/parapreputial incision of the abdominal wall. In the first case, a minilaparotomy incision approximately 1 cm in length is made on the midline, or paramedian. The bladder is exteriorized through the small abdominal incision with two retention sutures and incised, and a Foley catheter is placed. The catheter is sutured to the abdominal wall using the retention sutures. With either technique a second surgical treatment to address the cystostomy site is required.

Urethrostomy
Permanent urethrostomy may be indicated in the male ferret with urethral obstruction secondary to recurrent urethrolithiasis or with complications from adrenal disease (paraurethral cysts).

The urethrostomy site should be caudal (proximal) to the os penis and is better located just proximally to the obstruction site. The most common site is a few centimetres ventral to the anus. As for anal sacculectomy, the patient can be placed in ventral recumbency or in dorsal recumbency with the pelvic area slightly elevated, according to the surgeon's preference. Urinary catheterization is helpful if possible. A longitudinal incision is performed 1 or 2 cm ventrally to the anus directly over the urethra, which is isolated with sharp and blunt dissection. The ventral midline of the urethra is incised, whilst ensuring that the cavernous well vascularized tissue lateral to the urethra is avoided. The urethral incision is enlarged, keeping in mind that complete healing will reduce the finished urethrostomy site by up to 50%. The urethral mucosa is sutured to the skin with 1 metric (5/0 USP) or thinner material, with a simple interrupted pattern. The use of both absorbable and non-absorbable material is reported. A urinary catheter can be passed and kept in place to help to maintain the stoma, but it not always necessary. The surgical site is better protected with the use of an Elizabethan collar. Sutures are removed about 2 weeks after surgery under anaesthesia, otherwise absorbable material can be left in place to dissolve.

Urethrostomy may be performed concurrently with penile amputation in selected cases, as described above.

Basics of orthopaedics and fracture repair

Orthopaedic lesions are common in ferrets, most of them as a result of improper handling or restraint, falls from a height or from a terrace, or attacks from other animals. The most commonly encountered fractures are those of the long bones.

Evaluation of the orthopaedic patient
If the injury is recent, the ferret must be considered a trauma patient. Shock, concurrent thoracic or abdominal trauma, potential haemorrhage and central neurological lesions must be addressed immediately. Most bone and articular lesions do not represent true

emergencies: repair may be delayed until the patient is stabilized and possibly until resolution of soft tissue swelling and/or haematoma.

Fractures of distal limbs are sometimes open due to lack of significant overlying soft tissue. Open fractures (especially grade I and grade II) are often hidden by fur, which necessitates careful examination. Open fractures must be managed with strict aseptic technique and aseptically bandaged and splinted until primary repair can be performed.

Methods of fixation

Methods of fixations are not technically different from those performed on dogs and cats. Definitive fracture repair may be achieved through external coaptation, intramedullary pinning, wiring, plating and external fixation. Sometimes combined techniques can be used.

Only a few fracture types heal well with external coaptation which may not be well tolerated by the ferret. Intramedullary pinning may not offer enough stability; bone plating is often not feasible due to the patient size. External fixation is feasible in most cases, provides excellent stability and is usually well tolerated (Figure 23.19). Cost is often reasonable and affordable to most owners.

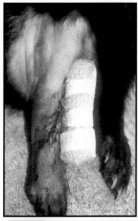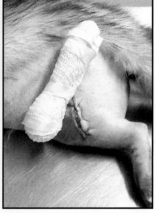

23.19 External fixation devices are usually well tolerated by ferrets, but they have to be carefully bandaged. An Elizabethan collar is not usually necessary. (© Vittorio Capello)

The basic principles of orthopaedics in ferrets are the same as in other mammal species and surgical anatomy is similar as well. Nevertheless, the clinician must be familiar with surgical anatomy and with the differences presented by patient behaviour and smaller size.

External fixation

The main indications for external fixation are open fractures, comminuted or highly comminuted fractures, or fractures of bone segments where anatomy does not allow intramedullary pinning. This method of fixation allows proper stabilization against all forces acting on bone fragments in all three dimensions, without involving the fracture site. These advantages are particularly important in the ferret, where postoperative control of excessive movement is much more difficult than in dogs and cats.

Depending on the bones affected and the features of the fracture, closed or open reduction can be performed.

Basic principles of pin insertion and external fixation

Basic principles of pin insertions and external fixation are not different from those applied in larger species.

1. Pins should be inserted through at least two bone cortices, ideally at an angle of 70 degrees relative to the longitudinal axis of the bone.
2. Proper pin size should not exceed 30% of the bone diameter, which necessitates the use of pins as small as 0.8–1.5 mm in diameter. Kirschner wires can be smooth or threaded. Threaded pins are more secure and unlikely to loosen during the postoperative period.
3. Pin insertion should be accomplished using a low-speed power drill rather than a hand chuck, because hand-driven pins tend to produce an oval-shaped insertion site, which increases the risk of pin loosening.
4. Pins should be inserted along a single plane to allow connection to a single external rod. Polymethylmethacrylate can be used to connect pins to bars. Alternatively, systems of lightweight clamps and/or bars are commercially available.
5. A minimum of two pins should be inserted in each bone fragment.
6. Maximum stability is accomplished by inserting pins proximally and distally in each fragment while avoiding the fracture site.
7. External fixation can be used in conjunction with other methods of fixation (intramedullary pins, screws or cerclage wires).

The most common combined technique is external fixation with intramedullary pinning. Since in this configuration the goal of the external fixator is to provide anti-rotational stability, a single pin per fragment is adequate (Figures 23.20 and 23.21).

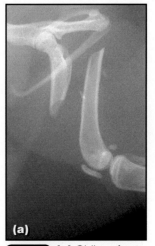

(a)

23.20 **(a)** Oblique fracture of the femoral shaft in a 1.6 kg 11-month-old male ferret. (© Vittorio Capello. Reprinted from Capello 2006a with the permission of the Zoological Education Network) (continues) ▶

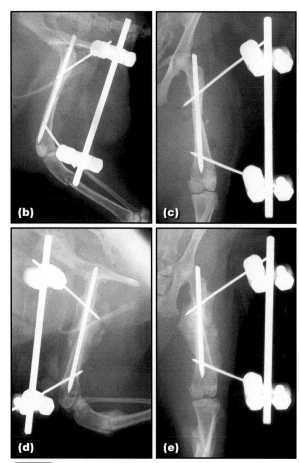

23.20 (continued) **(b,c)** Osteosynthesis of the fracture shown in (a) using a 2-pin monoplanar configuration of external fixation in conjunction with intramedullary pinning. Lateral and anteroposterior views immediately post surgery. **(d,e)** Bone healing is clearly visible 5 weeks after surgery. (© Vittorio Capello. Reprinted from Capello 2006a with the permission of the Zoological Education Network)

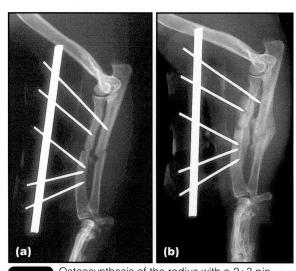

23.21 Osteosynthesis of the radius with a 2+3 pin monolateral external fixation device. **(a)** Stabilization of the radius is adequate for proper stabilization of the ulna. The most proximal pin has been inserted too deeply and appears to cross the ulnar shaft, but actually does not. **(b)** Follow-up after 4 weeks demonstrating adequate bone healing. (© Vittorio Capello)

Common orthopaedic lesions in pet ferrets

The most common fractures involve the limbs. Fractures of the radius and ulna are more frequent than humeral fractures. A very common fracture involving the ulnar epiphysis is the transverse fracture of the olecranon process. In this case, osteosynthesis by pin and tension-band wiring may be challenging due to the small size. Fracture of the scapular neck has been reported (Johnson-Delaney, in Capello and Lennox, 2008).

Fractures of the femur (including fracture of the femoral neck) and of the tibia and fibula are very common. Fractures of the pelvis have been reported (Johnson-Delaney, in Capello and Lennox, 2008).

Less commonly reported fractures include those of the mandible, the spine and even the os penis.

Elbow luxation, both unilateral and bilateral, is a common orthopaedic condition encountered in ferrets. Definitive reduction may be challenging as these tend to re-luxate. Different methods of stabilization have been reported, including: simple splinting; a transarticular pin through the joint, usually with splinting support; and an external fixation device.

Ferrets adapt very well to amputation of a single limb. Surgical technique for amputation is as in dogs and cats.

Miscellaneous procedures

Dental procedures

Ferrets are prone to dental and periodontal diseases such as calculus, gingivitis, excessive dental abrasions, fractures, caries, periapical infection, bone loss (reabsorption) and osteomyelitis. Basic principles of dentistry in ferrets do not differ from those in dogs and cats. Minimal equipment is required, including a very small mouth gag (Figure 23.22) and small elevators. A dental unit for dogs and cats can also work for ferrets.

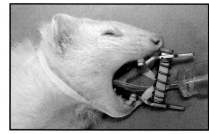

23.22 Small mouth gag for ferrets. (© Vittorio Capello)

Before any dental procedure involving extraction of teeth, a thorough radiographic examination should be performed including lateral, lateral open mouth, ventrodorsal, right and left oblique, and right and left oblique open mouth projections.

Ablation of calculus is the most common dental procedure (Figure 23.23) and can be performed with a dental scaler and polisher for dogs and cats. Special attention must be paid during this procedure because exposed roots due both to severe periodontal disease and bone reabsorption may fracture, leading to periapical infections (Figure 23.24).

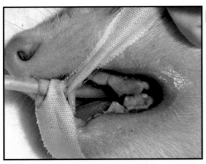

23.23
Severe calculus and periodontal disease in a 5-year-old male ferret. (© Vittorio Capello)

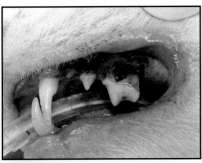

23.24 Severe gingivitis and gingival retraction in the same patient after scaling of calculus. The exposure of the roots of the maxillary third premolar is due both to gingival retraction and bone reabsorption. The maxillary third premolar is the largest cheek tooth; it is called carnassial and it is the only tooth with three roots. (© Vittorio Capello)

Oesophagostomy feeding tube placement

The placement of an oesophagostomy tube may be of great benefit for severely debilitated ferrets both for long-term oral supportive nutrition and for long-term administration of oral drugs.

The ferret is anesthetized and a 10 French rubber feeding tube length is measured from the pharynx to the stomach (9th–11th intercostal space). Curved forceps are inserted through the mouth into the proximal oesophagus and the tip is palpated through the skin. Incision of the skin, subcutaneous tissue and the wall of the oesophagus are performed, and the tip of the forceps is pushed through the incision. The tip of the feeding tube is grasped with the forceps and pulled into the mouth from the oesophagostomy incision. The tip is then directed down through the oesophagus. The external end of the tube is sutured to the skin, reflected caudally over the neck and secured with a bandage. An Elizabethan collar is usually unnecessary. The oesophagostomy feeding tube can be left in place for up to 6 weeks. The most common complication is local infection at the entry site of the tube.

Enucleation of the globe

Various severe lesions of the eye can occasionally require enucleation of the globe (see also Chapter 29). The surgical approaches are the same as performed in dogs and cats: transpalpebral or transconjunctival. Due to the small size of the ferret, the transconjunctival is the preferred technique. Special attention must be paid to the insertion of a small, curved haemostat behind the eye globe to clamp the optic nerve and the ciliary arteries supplying the globe. The stump is carefully ligated with 2 or 1.5 metric (3/0 or 4/0 USP) absorbable suture material and dissected. The extraocular muscles and the orbital fascia are sutured over the defect in order to partially fill the orbital space.

The margins of the eyelids are dissected and removed, and the skin is apposed and sutured to achieve the best aesthetic appearance.

Surgical treatment of salivary mucocele

The anatomy of salivary glands in the ferret is well reported in the literature (Fox, 1998). Among the five pairs of salivary glands (in craniocaudal direction: zygomatic, buccal, sublingual, parotid, mandibular), some can occasionally be affected by salivary mucocele (Figure 23.25). Pathophysiology is often related to trauma involving the duct of the salivary gland. Typical presentation is a large unilateral cold and non-painful swelling located at the lateroventral side of the face, unless the zygomatic gland is involved. Differential diagnosis includes abscessation (possibly related to dental disease) and a fine-needle aspirate is very helpful for diagnosis. In the case of mucocele, the aspirate often appears as a transparent mucoid fluid, very similar to egg white but even thicker. Sometimes it is so dense that it cannot be collected with a needle smaller than 18 gauge. Aspiration or incision and drainage may temporarily reduce the swelling, but the elective surgical procedure is thorough excision of all involved glandular material. Exploratory surgery may be challenging, due to the important anatomical structures present in the parotid region. Because of the density of the secretion, marsupialization is the preferred surgical option rather than application of a drain in order to prevent a relapse.

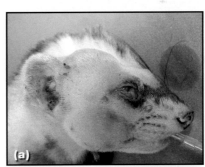

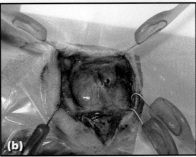

23.25 **(a)** Salivary mucocele of the parotid gland in a 5-year-old male ferret, presumably following a trauma that caused a severe lesion to the right eye globe. **(b)** Surgical excision of the salivary mucocele. Note the very dense transparent secretion protruding out of the small incision of the cyst. (© Vittorio Capello) (continues) ▶

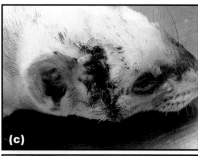

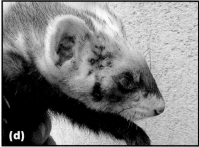

23.25 (continued) **(c)** Marsupialization of the surgical site. **(d)** Follow-up 2 weeks after surgery showing complete resolution of the mucocele and proper healing of marsupialization. (© Vittorio Capello)

Excision of cutaneous neoplasia

Excision of cutaneous neoplasia is relatively common in ferrets, especially removal of mast cell tumours. These are benign in ferrets and discomfort is mostly related to histamine production and subsequent pruritus. Ferrets typically scratch them, causing mild bleeding and scab formation. Excision is straight-forward, and it is not necessary to remove abundant tissue around the neoplastic lesion. One single stitch with absorbable or non-absorbable monofilament suture material is enough to achieve proper healing. Another option for excision is the use of a radiosurgery unit, with a round loop electrode being ideal for the excision (Figure 23.26).

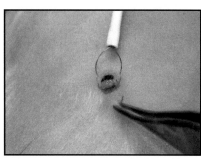

23.26 Excision of a mast cell tumour from the flank using a radiosurgical unit with a round loop electrode. (© Vittorio Capello)

References and further reading

Antinoff N and Hahn K (2004) Ferret oncology: diseases, diagnostics, and therapeutics. *Veterinary Clinics of North America: Exotic Animal Practice* **7**, 579–625

Beeber NL (1998) Surgery of pet ferrets. In: *Current Techniques in Small Animal Surgery, 4th edn*, ed. MJ Bojrab, pp. 763–769. WB Saunders, Philadelphia

Bennet A (1999) Ferret adrenal removal using temporary occlusion of the caudal vena cava. *Exotic DVM* **1**(3), 71–74

Burgess M and Garner M (2002) Clinical aspects of inflammatory bowel disease in ferrets. *Exotic DVM* **4**(2), 29–34

Capello V (2006a) External fixation for fracture repair in small exotic mammals. *Exotic DVM* **7**(6), 21–37

Capello V (2006b) Sacculectomy in the pet ferret and skunk. *Exotic DVM* **8**(2), 15–24

Capello V and Lennox A (2008) *Clinical Radiology of Exotic Companion Mammals*, Blackwell Publishing, Ames, IA

Creed JE (1998) Anal sac resection in the ferret. In: *Current Techniques in Small Animal Surgery, 4th edn*, ed. MJ Bojrab, pp. 769–771. WB Saunders, Philadelphia

Fisher P (2001) Esophagostomy feeding tube placement in the ferret. *Exotic DVM* **2**(6), 23–25

Fisher P (2002) Urethrostomy and penile amputation to treat urethral obstruction and preputial masses in male ferrets. *Exotic DVM* **3**(6), 21–25

Fisher PG (2006) Exotic mammal renal disease: diagnosis and treatment *Veterinary Clinics of North America: Exotic Animal Practice* **9**, 69–96

Fox JG (1998) *Biology and Diseases of the Ferret, 2nd edn*. Blackwell, Oxford

Johnson D (2002) Clinical use of cryosurgery for ferret adrenal gland removal. *Exotic DVM* **4**(3), 71–73

Kapatkin A (2004) Orthopedics in small mammals. In: *Ferrets, Rabbits and Rodents. Clinical Medicine and Surgery, 2nd edn*, ed. KE Quesenberry and JW Carpenter, pp. 383–391. WB Saunders, Philadelphia

Ludwig L and Aiken S (1997) Soft tissue surgery. In: *Ferrets, Rabbits and Rodents. Clinical Medicine and Surgery, 2nd edn*, ed. KE Quesenberry and JW Carpenter, pp. 121–134. WB Saunders, Philadelphia

Mehler SJ and Bennet RA (2004) Surgical oncology of exotic animals *Veterinary Clinics of North America: Exotic Animal Practice* **7**, 783–805

Murray MJ (2001) Ergonomics in avian and exotic practice. *Exotic DVM* **3**(3), 11–14

Murray MJ (2002) Laparoscopy in the domestic ferret. *Exotic DVM* **4**(3), 65–69

Orcutt C (2001) Treatment of urogenital disease in ferrets. *Exotic DVM* **3**(3), 31–37

Orcutt C (2003) Ferret urogenital diseases. *Veterinary Clinics of North America: Exotic Animal Practice* **6**, 113–138

Randolph RW (1990a) Anal sacculectomy in the pet ferret. In: *Current Techniques in Small Animal Surgery, 3rd ed*, ed. MJ Bojrab, pp. 569–572. WB Saunders, Philadelphia

Randolph RW (1990b) Ovariohysterectomy and orchiectomy in the pet ferret. In: *Current Techniques in Small Animal Surgery, 3rd edn*, ed. MJ Bojrab, pp. 572–576. WB Saunders, Philadelphia

Rosenthal KL, Petersen ME, Quesenberry KE *et al.* (1993) Hyperadrenocorticism associated with adrenocortical tumor or nodular hyperplasia of the adrenal gland in ferrets: 50 cases (1987–1991). *Journal of the American Veterinary Medical Association* **203**, 271–275

Weiss C (1999) Cryosurgery of the ferret adrenal gland. *Exotic DVM* **1**(5), 27–28

Weiss CA, Williams BH, Scott JB *et al.* (1999) Surgical treatment and long-term outcome of ferrets with bilateral adrenal tumors or adrenal hyperplasia: 56 cases (1994–1997). *Journal of the American Veterinary Medical Association* **215**, 820–823

24

Ferrets: dermatoses

Anna Meredith

Introduction

Ferret skin is thick, especially around the head and neck, and has a deep subcutis. This can make venipuncture and subcutaneous injections problematical (see Chapters 18 and 21). The skin contains numerous sebaceous glands, causing the hair coat to feel normally slightly greasy and have a characteristic musky odour. In albino animals, sebaceous secretions may cause yellowing of the hair coat with age, especially in intact males. Ferrets also have two prominent perianal scent glands, the contents of which are expelled when the animal is excited or agitated, or in oestrus. Normal ferrets may often have comedones present on the skin of the tail.

The hair coat consists of a thick, usually cream-coloured undercoat and coarse guard hairs that determine coat colour. Ferrets moult in the spring and autumn in response to changing photoperiod and their hair colour may change to a lighter shade in winter. If the coat is clipped or shaved during periods of seasonal hair loss, it may not regrow for several weeks or even months. As hair does regrow in a clipped area, or after specific treatment for alopecic disease, the skin can appear bluish. This is normal but can be mistaken for cyanosis or bruising.

Ferrets do not have well developed sweat glands and this, combined with the thick coat, makes them susceptible to heat stress and heat stroke.

The foot pads are similar to those in dogs and the jill has four pairs of mammary glands and nipples.

Approach to the skin case

The general principles of diagnosing skin disease in cats and dogs are equally applicable to ferrets, and all of the same diagnostic techniques may be used. The diagnostic approach consists of:

- Obtaining a history – general and presenting complaint
- General clinical examination
- Skin examination
- Differential diagnosis
- Specific diagnostic tests
- Definitive diagnosis and appropriate treatment.

History
Important details to obtain are:

- Source and length of time owned
- Source and sex of any companions
- Husbandry – working or pet ferret, outdoor or house ferret, type of housing, flooring, bedding and cleaning regimes
- Diet
- Water presentation – bottle or bowl
- Reproductive status – neutered or intact, in oestrus or not
- Vaccination status (distemper, rabies)
- Ectoparasitic control measures
- Presence of other pets
- General health and previous problems.

For the presenting problem:

- How long has it been present?
- Initial distribution and progression of lesions
- Are any other ferrets affected?
- Are any other pets or the owner affected?
- Is pruritus present?
- Have any parasites been seen?

Clinical examination and diagnostic testing
A thorough clinical examination should always be undertaken (see Chapter 18) before concentrating on the skin lesions. The skin should be carefully examined, visually and by palpation, from head to tail and dorsum to ventrum, including the genitalia. Pinnae and external ear canals can also be examined with an otoscope.

Alopecia is a common presenting sign in the ferret and its distribution should be noted. Examination of the bulbs of plucked hairs can give an indication as to whether anagen (active growth) or telogen (resting phase) hairs are present. Hairs in anagen have a well developed bulb, whereas those in telogen have a club-shaped bulb of solid dry material.

Any lesions should be examined in detail and described in terms of distribution, arrangement, configuration, depth, consistency, quality and colour. The morphology of the lesions should be described as either primary (macule, patch, wheal, vesicle, papule, pustule, nodule, tumour) or secondary (scale crust, hyperkeratosis, excoriation, ulcer, scar, lichenification, hyperpigmentation, fissure, comedo). Diagnostic procedures for dermatoses are listed in Figure 24.1.

Procedure	Purpose
Blood sampling (see also Chapters 18 and 30)	General health, hormone levels
Direct or magnified observation (hand lens, otoscope)	Larger ectoparasites (ticks, fleas, lice and some mites, e.g. *Otodectes*)
Bacterial sampling and culture/sensitivity testing	Intact pustules
Ultraviolet (Wood's) light	Dermatophyte detection (some isolates of *Microsporum canis* may fluoresce)
Direct microscopy of hairs (in 5% KOH)	Dermatophyte detection, trauma, stage of growth cycle
Fungal culture	
Coat brushings	Fleas
Adhesive tape collection and microscopy	Surface-living mites
Skin scraping (KOH or liquid paraffin and direct microscopy)	Superficial (surface-living mites) or deep (burrowing and follicular mites)
Impression smear	Exudative leasions or after a scrape to identify a cellular infiltrate
Fine-needle aspiration	Nodular lesions
Biopsy	Especially for neoplasia, mite infestation, fungal infection, immune-mediated conditions and endocrine disease. Excisional biopsy often indicated for discrete lesions

24.1 Diagnostic procedures for dermatoses.

Parasitic skin disease

Mites

Sarcoptes scabiei
Sarcoptes scabiei can occasionally infest ferrets, and causes either generalized alopecia and intense pruritus, or localized lesions of the toes and feet (colloquially known as foot rot). Nails can become deformed and slough. Diagnosis is by skin scrapings but false negative results are common. Treatment is with ivermectin at 0.2–0.4 mg/kg s.c. repeated every 7–14 days for three doses. Affected and in-contact animals should be treated and the environment thoroughly cleaned. As in dogs, the zoonotic aspect is important.

Otodectes cyanotis
The ear mite *Otodectes cyanotis* can affect ferrets as well as cats and dogs, and causes chronic irritation and secondary bacterial and yeast infections. The mite can be identified directly via an otoscope or rigid endoscope, or by examining aural debris obtained by a swab, mixed with mineral oil under 40–100X magnification (Figure 24.2). The life cycle of *Otodectes* takes 3 weeks and the mite can persist for 12 days off the host. Systemic ivermectin is very effective.

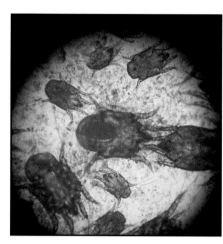

24.2 Ear mites (*Otodectes cyanotis*) viewed at 100X magnification. (Courtesy of C Johnson-Delaney.)

Selamectin spot-on treatment at 45 mg (a 0.75 ml single-dose tube), applied between the scapulae, has been reported as efficacious and safe in ferrets (Miller and Eage, 2006). Aural topical treatments are often ineffective in ferrets because the ear canal is so small that medication may not penetrate.

Demodex spp.
Demodex spp. have been reported as a cause of local alopecia and pruritus in two ferrets (Noli *et al.*, 1996) and treatment with amitraz (0.05%) was effective, with no noticeable side effects.

Lynxacarus mustelae
The fur mite *Lynxacarus mustelae* has been associated with ulcerative lesions on the face of ferret kits (Schoemaker,1999). Treatment was successful with permethrin powder, both of the affected animal and of the environment.

Fleas
Cat and dog fleas (*Ctenocephalides* spp.) and *Pulex irritans* can infest ferrets. Mild to intense pruritus can be seen, generally around the neck. Occasionally alopecia occurs on the neck and thorax. Signs of flea-bite hypersensitivity may also be seen in some animals, such as papulocrustous dermatitis over the tail base, ventral abdomen and caudomedial thighs (Fox, 1998). The affected ferret and any in-contact cats and dogs should be treated, along with the environment. Products approved for cats can be used in ferrets. Spray or pump products such as fipronil should be measured carefully and applied to a cloth that is then applied to the ferret, to avoid overdose. Imidacloprid has been used safely and effectively and lufenuron appears to be effective when given at cat dosages (Orcutt, 2004).

Ticks
Ticks can also affect ferrets, especially those used for outdoor hunting. Lyme disease has not been reported. Ticks should be removed manually.

Myiasis
Cuterebra larvae can cause subdermal cysts in ferrets and *Hypoderma bovis* larvae can cause

granulomatous masses in the cervical area, but these are both uncommon. Flystrike is also uncommon in pet ferrets, but has been reported in farmed ferrets and mink, caused by the flesh fly *Wohlfahrtia vigil* (Fox, 1988).

Bacterial disease

Bite wounds in ferrets are common, resulting from playing, mating or true fighting. They generally occur in the thick skin around the neck and often become infected with *Staphylococcus*, *Streptococcus*, *Corynebacterium*, *Pasteurella* and *Actinomyces* spp. and *Escherichia coli*, resulting in abscesses, deep pyoderma or cellulitis. Bacterial pyoderma can also be secondary to pruritus and self-trauma due to ectoparasite infection. Treatment is by debridement and appropriate antibiosis based on culture and sensitivity. Abscesses may be lanced and flushed, and drains may be placed, or wet to dry dressings employed.

Actinomyces spp. can cause 'lumpy jaw' lesions in ferrets. Affected animals have nodules or abscesses in the neck that can discharge green–yellow pus. Treatment is by curettage and drainage plus antibiosis. The lesions can respond to high dose penicillin (40,000 IU/kg s.c. q24h) or tetracycline (25 mg/kg orally q24h).

Fungal disease

Ringworm
Microsporum canis is the more common cause of ringworm in ferrets, but *Trichophyton mentagrophytes* is also seen. Young or immunosuppressed animals are generally affected, with typical non-pruritic annular lesions of alopecia, broken hair and scale. Transmission is often from co-housed domestic cats. Diagnosis and treatment are as for other species, with shaving of the affected hair, topical keratolytic shampoos and antifungals such as enilconazole (0.2% solution) usually being effective. Systemic griseofulvin is rarely needed but can be used at 25 mg/kg/day for 21–30 days (Collins, 1987). Orcutt (1997) recommended that complete blood counts are monitored every 2 weeks during treatment. The environment should also be decontaminated if possible by vigorous vacuuming, steam cleaning or the application of dilute bleach or chlorhexidine solution. Spontaneous remission is also reported.

Other fungal diseases
Blastomyces dermatitidis has been reported in one ferret with pneumonia and an ulcerated footpad (Lenhard, 1985). Treatment included oral ketoconazole at 8 mg/kg and intravenous amphotericin B at 0.4–0.8 mg/kg for approximately 1 month. Histoplasmosis and coccidioidomycosis have been diagnosed as the cause of subcutaneous nodules (Scott *et al.*, 2001). Cryptococcosis can cause a wide spectrum of clinical signs (rhinitis, lymphadenitis, pneumonia, pleurisy) but can also cause localized lesions of distal limbs (Malik *et al.*, 2002) (Figure 24.3).

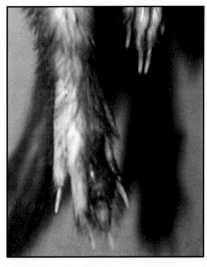

24.3
Fungal pododermatitis in a ferret with lymphosarcoma. (Courtesy of C Orcutt.)

Viral disease

Canine distemper virus
The ferret is acutely susceptible to canine distemper virus, and mortality reaches 100% (see Chapter 31 for further details). A characteristic rash under the chin (Figure 24.4a) and in the inguinal area is typically seen at 10–15 days post-infection. Foot pads and nasal pads often undergo swelling and hyperkeratosis (Figure 24.4b). Diagnosis can be made by serum antibody titres and fluorescent antibody tests for viral antigen on blood or conjunctival smears. There is no treatment and prevention is by vaccination.

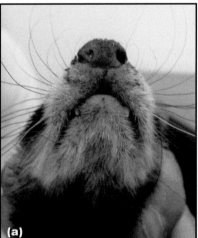

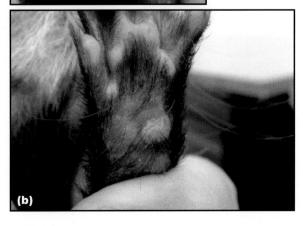

24.4
Typical skin lesions in a ferret with distemper virus. **(a)** A chin rash is a typical early presentation. **(b)** Swelling and crusting of the foot pads. (Courtesy of O Contreras and B Portillo Lopez.)

Endocrine disease

Hyperadrenocorticism

This condition occurs commonly in middle-aged ferrets in the USA, associated with adrenocortical hyperplasia, adenoma or adenocarcinoma. Pituitary-dependent hyperadrenocorticism has not been recognized in ferrets. Cutaneous signs include bilateral symmetrical alopecia (Figure 24.5) and vulval swelling in females, which should be differentiated from hyperoestrogenism. Hair is easily epilated and is lost progressively over the perineum, tail, flanks, sides and back. Over 30% of cases may be pruritic. On physical examination, adrenal gland enlargement may be palpated. The aetiology, diagnosis and treatment of adrenal gland disease is described in detail in Chapter 30.

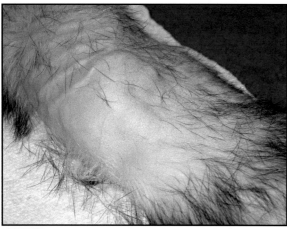

24.5 Alopecia in a ferret with hyperadrenocorticism. (Courtesy of C Johnson-Delaney.)

Hyperoestrogenism

This is probably the most common endocrine condition encountered in practice in ferrets in the UK. In these latitudes the normal breeding season for ferrets is between March and September, during which time females are seasonally polyoestrous with induced ovulation. Ovulation occurs approximately 30–40 hours following mating. If unmated or not stimulated to ovulate, as many as 50% of females may develop aplastic anaemia after prolonged oestrus (up to 6 months). High levels of oestrogen lead to oestrogen suppression of the bone marrow and resulting anaemia with pancytopenia. Other causes of hyperoestrogenism include an ovarian remnant following ovariohysterectomy or adrenal neoplasia. Pseudopregnancy following a sterile mating has been recorded in ferrets.

The main cutaneous sign is alopecia, usually starting over the tail base and progressing cranially. Diagnosis, treatment and prevention of hyper-oestrogenism are described in detail in Chapter 30.

Neoplasia

Cutaneous neoplasia is relatively common in ferrets and is reported as the third most common form of neoplasia (Li *et al.*, 1995).

Basal cell tumours have been reported at an incidence of 58% in a study of 57 cutaneous neoplasms submitted from ferrets over a 5-year period (Parker and Picut, 1993). Average age at diagnosis was 5.2 years and 70% of affected animals were female. The appearance is usually of a pedunculated or plaque-like minimally invasive mass that can become ulcerated. Complete excision is usually curative.

Mast cell tumours commonly involve the skin in ferrets and are usually benign. Parker and Picut (1993) reported that mast cell tumours represented 16% of all cutaneous neoplasms submitted from ferrets over a 5-year period. The appearance is usually of single or multiple well circumscribed raised hairless nodules (Figure 24.6) that can become ulcerated and crusted with a black exudate. Some are pruritic, and oral or topical antihistamines can be used to obtain temporary relief. Surgical excision (Figure 24.7) is generally curative, and premedication with antihistamines or wide surgical margins are not required (Antinoff and Hahn, 2004).

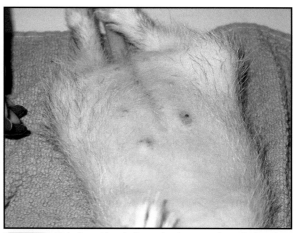

24.6 This ferret had alopecia due to adrenal gland disease and several mast cell tumours on the abdomen. (Courtesy of C Johnson-Delaney.)

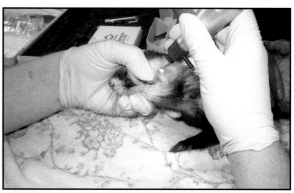

24.7 Use of cryosurgery (cryopen) for removal of small skin tumours. The ferret was given butorphanol 0.2 mg/kg as a sedative, and the lesion was blocked locally with 0.1 ml 2% lidocaine. (Courtesy of C Johnson-Delaney.)

Squamous cell carcinoma, adenoma, adenocarcinoma, epitheliotropic cutaneous lymphoma, haem-angiosarcoma and fibroma are among other rarer skin tumours reported in this species (Figure 24.8). Perianal apocrine gland adenocarcinoma may also

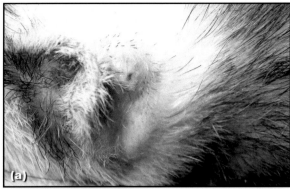

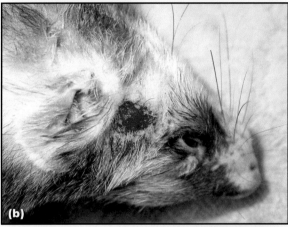

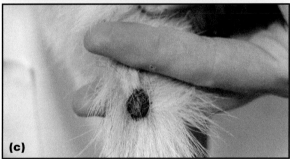

24.8 Skin tumours. **(a)** Fibrosarcoma adjacent to the ear of a ferret. **(b)** Squamous cell carcinoma on the face of a ferret. (Courtesy of C Johnson-Delaney.) **(c)** Sebaceous gland adenoma on the tail. (Courtesy of C Orcutt.)

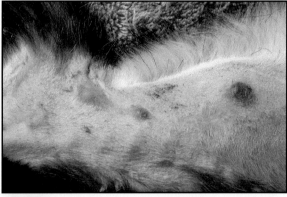

24.9 Injection site fibrosarcoma following vaccination for distemper. In this ferret there was one major fibrosarcoma at the injection site which was removed surgically and over the course of the next 1.5 years seven more tumours were removed. One tumour eventually penetrated the thoracic wall and spread into the chest. (Courtesy of C Johnson-Delaney.)

be seen. Diagnosis is based on fine-needle aspirates or biopsy. Squamous cell carcinoma is best treated by excision with wide surgical margins, but the use of bleomycin (20 IU/m² once a week) has been reported as temporarily reducing tumour size (Hamilton and Morrison, 1991). Isoretinoin may be useful in the palliative treatment of epitheliotropic lymphoma (Rosenbaum et al., 1996), and prednisolone at 2.5 mg/kg orally twice daily has also been reported as giving symptomatic relief for 6 months post diagnosis in one case (Kelleher, 2001). Radiation therapy can play a role in postoperative management of some cutaneous tumours.

Vaccination site fibrosarcomas

Vaccination site fibrosarcomas (Figure 24.9) have been reported in the ferret. In one study 7 out of 10 dermal or subcutaneous fibrosarcomas were from the interscapular region, dorsal neck or dorsal thorax (Munday et al., 2003). This is of interest as, until this study, vaccination had not previously been associated with oncogenesis in non-feline species. Wide and deep surgical excision, possibly followed by local radiation, is indicated (Antinoff and Hahn, 2004).

The convention is still to administer vaccines subcutaneously in the interscapular region. Although the number of reports of sarcomas is very small, it may be more prudent to give vaccines subcutaneously in the rear limb, or at least to note on the animal's records where the vaccine was given. If a mass is still apparent at the inoculation site more than 2 months after vaccination, a recommendation in cats is that it should be removed with wide margins and submitted for histopathology (Professor Danielle Gunn-Moore, personal communication) and this could also be applicable to ferrets.

Chordoma

Ferrets appear to have a relatively high incidence of developing chordoma, mostly at the tip of the tail (see Chapter 30, Figure 30.7), but thoracic, cervical and tail base locations have also been reported. Although not a cutaneous neoplasm, coccygeal chordoma presents as a very slowly expanding mass, usually of the tail tip. Metastasis is rare but has been reported. Treatment is by surgical excision of the affected tail tip, but no treatment is possible if the tumour is located elsewhere along the vertebral column.

Miscellaneous conditions

Musky odour

Ferret skin naturally contains numerous sebaceous glands, which cause the natural musky odour and sometimes greasy feel of the coat. It is not possible to de-scent a ferret, but neutering and feeding of a commercial pelleted diet will help to minimize offensive odours. There is some debate on the regular shampooing of ferrets, with some veterinary surgeons, owners and breeders maintaining that this strips away the sebaceous secretions and stimulates their increased production, while others insist that it is highly effective at reducing odour. Excessive bathing can cause dry pruritic skin and, if required, a bathing frequency of not more than once a month is generally recommended by the author. A mild cat or specific ferret shampoo should be used. Male ferrets are always more odiferous and secretions can be so profuse that the coat of albino animals appears yellow and dirty.

Seasonal alopecia

Normal thinning of the coat occurs in both intact and neutered ferrets as days lengthen and the weather warms, and a bilaterally symmetrical alopecia of the tail, perineum and inguinal area can often occur during the breeding season. This effect is usually most pronounced in intact jills and should be distinguished from endocrine disease (see Chapter 30).

Stress

Telogen defluxion can sometimes be seen 2–3 months after a stressful event.

Atopy

Presumptive atopy has been reported (Scott *et al.*, 2001), presenting as symmetrical non-lesional pruritus over the thorax, dorsal tail area and paws and responding to glucocorticoids or chlorphenamine (1–2 mg/kg orally q8–12h). Fleas were absent and hypoallergenic diets ineffective.

Food hypersensitivity

One case of food hypersensitivity has been noted and responded well to feeding a commercial hypoallergenic diet for cats (Scott *et al.*, 2001).

Blue ferret syndrome

This is an idiopathic syndrome reported by Burgmann (1991). Ferrets of either sex, neutered or intact, present with a bluish discoloration of the abdominal skin, but are otherwise asymptomatic. The coloration disappears within a few weeks. It is often seen in ferrets clipped for surgery during catagen. The clipped skin area remains hairless and then turns blue and it seems that the hair follicles are manufacturing melanin to be incorporated into growing hairs. Hair regrowth begins within 1–2 weeks after the blue colour appears (Scott *et al.*, 2001).

References and further reading

Antinoff N and Hahn K (2004) Ferret oncology: disease, diagnostics and therapeutics. *Veterinary Clinics of North America: Exotic Animal Practice* **7**(3), 579–625

Burgmann P (1991) Dermatology of rabbits, rodents and ferrets. In: *Dermatology for the Small Animal Practitioner*, ed. GH Nesbitt and LJ Ackerman, p. 205. Veterinary Learning Systems, Trenton, New Jersey

Collins BR (1987) Dermatologic disorders of common small nondomestic animals. In: *Contemporary Issues in Small Animal Practice: Dermatology*, ed. GH Nesbitt. Churchill Livingstone, New York

Fisher MA, Jacobs DE, Hutchinson MJ *et al.* (2001) Efficacy of imidocloprid on ferrets experimentally infested with the cat flea, *Ctenocephalides felis. Compendium on Continuing Education, Practitioners Veterinary Supplement* **23**(4A), 8–10

Fox JG (1998) Parasitic diseases. In: *Biology and Diseases of the Ferret, 2nd edn.* Williams & Wilkins, Baltimore

Graham JE, Roberts, RE, Wilson GH *et al.* (2001) Perianal apocrine gland adenocarcinoma in a ferret. *Compendium on Continuing Education for the Practicing Veterinarian* **23**(4), 359–362

Hamilton TA and Morrison WB (1991) Bleomycin chemotherapy for metastatic squamous cell carcinoma in a ferret. *Journal of the American Veterinary Medical Association* **198**(1), 107–108

Kelleher SA (2001) Skin diseases of ferrets. In: *Veterinary Clinics of North America: Exotic Animal Practice: Dermatology* **4**(2), 565–572

Lenhard A (1985) Blastomycosis in a ferret. *Journal of the American Veterinary Medical Association* **186**, 70–72

Li X, Fox JG and Padrid PA (1995) Neoplastic diseases in ferrets: 574 cases (1968–1997). *Journal of the American Veterinary Medicine Association* **212**, 1402

Malik R, Alderton B, Finlaison D *et al.* (2002) Cryptococcosis in ferrets: a diverse spectrum of clinical disease. *Australian Veterinary Journal* **80**(12), 749–755

Miller D and Eage RP (2006) Efficacy and safety of selamectin in the treatment of *Otodectes cynotis* infestation in domestic ferrets. *Veterinary Record* **159**(22), 748

Munday JS, Stedman NL and Richie LJ (2003) Histology and immunohistochemistry of seven ferret vaccination-site fibrosarcomas. *Veterinary Pathology* **40**, 288–293

Noli C, van der Horst HH and Willemse T (1996) Demodicosis in ferrets (*Mustela putorius furo*). *Veterinary Quarterly* **18**(1), 28–31

Orcutt C (1997) Dermatologic diseases. In: *Ferrets, Rabbits and Rodents: Clinical Medicine and Surgery*, ed. EV Hillyer and KE Quesenberry, pp. 115–125. WB Saunders, Philadelphia

Parker GA and Picut CA (1993) Histopathologic features and post-surgical sequelae of 57 cutaneous neoplasms in ferrets (*Mustela putorius furo L.*). *Veterinary Pathology* **30**(6), 499–504

Patterson MM and Kirchain SM (1999) Comparison of three treatments for control of ear mites in ferrets. *Laboratory Animal Science* **49**(6), 655–657

Rosenbaum MR, Affolter VK, Usbourne AL and Beeber NL (1996) Cutaneous epitheliotropic lymphoma in a ferret. *Journal of the American Veterinary Medical Association* **209**(8), 1441–1444

Schoemaker NJ (1999) Selected dermatological conditions in exotic pets. *Exotic DVM* **1**, 5

Scott DW, Miller WH and Griffin CE (2001) Dermatoses of pet rodents, rabbits and ferrets. In: *Muller and Kirk's Small Animal Dermatology* pp. 1415–1458. WB Saunders, Philadelphia

Timm KI (1988) Pruritus in rabbits, rodents, and ferrets. *Veterinary Clinics of North America: Small Animal Practice* **18**(5), 1077–1091

Tunev SS and Wells MG (2002) Cutaneous melanoma in a ferret (*Mustela putorius furo*). *Veterinary Pathology* **39**(1), 141–143

25

Ferrets: digestive system disorders

Cathy A. Johnson-Delaney

Introduction

The gastrointestinal (GI) tract of the domestic ferret has been studied extensively as a model for several human GI tract diseases, including spontaneous gastric and duodenal ulcers, gastro-oesophageal reflux, gastric carcinoma and lymphoma, the lack of acid mucosubstances (similar to humans), and *Helicobacter mustelae* infection. The clinician must also be aware of GI pain and hydration status accompanying most GI disease.

Anatomy and physiology

The ferret has a short transit time of 148–219 minutes when fed a meat-based diet. The digestive system is under vagal and sacral innervation and is spontaneously active, even under anaesthesia. Motility can be moderated with atropine. The stomach spontaneously produces acids and proteolytic enzymes, and histamine and vagal stimulation provoke increased secretions. Histamine H2 receptor antagonists abolish the acid secretion response to exogenous histamine or exogenous stimulation with pentagastrin. Atropine only reduces acid secretion by 30%.

Stomach

The ferret has a simple stomach, similar in shape to that of the dog. There is prominent vasculature of the stomach as well as a prominent lymph node lying in the lesser curvature.

Because of the similarity to human anatomical and physiological mechanisms, the ferret is used as an emesis model as well as a model for acid reflux disease in humans.

Hypoglycaemia induced by insulin produces a sustained stimulation of acid secretion. This is particularly relevant to ferrets with insulinomas: therapy needs to include medications that decrease acid secretion.

Intestine

The ferret intestine consists of three sections. Villi and goblet cells are present in all sections.

The duodenum is the proximal segment. It is innervated by vagal preganglionic parasympathic neurons originating in the dorsal motor nucleus of the vagal nerve in the brainstem. The major duodenal papilla contains the common opening for the bile and pancreatic ducts. This is located about 3 cm from the pylorus. The minor papilla may be absent. Brunner's glands are present in the submucosa of the duodenum proximal to bile duct.

The jejunal and ileal segments cannot be distinguished and may be referred to as the jejunoileum, which ends at the ascending colon. The small intestine is innervated by the vagus nerve and the sympathetic trunks arise from the coeliac and cranial mesenteric plexus.

Cervical (mechanical) vagus stimulation will affect motility. This has significant implications for the clinician who, during intubation, may manipulate the neck and thorax and inadvertently stimulate the vagus nerve and intestinal motility at the beginning of surgery.

The large intestine is composed of the colon and rectum. There is no caecum and no ileocolic junction. The junction is inferred by the presence of the anastomosis of the jejunal artery with the ileocolic artery. The colon consists of the ascending, transverse and descending colon, with the largest being the descending. The colon is innervated by autonomic fibres from the vagus, and the cranial and caudal mesenteric plexus.

There are tubular glands and goblet cells in the colon. The motility of the colon resembles that of a dog ileum. Motility is vagus dependent and mediated by cholinergic and non-cholinergic fibres. Sacral innervation is excitatory. Retroperistalsis begins in the colon, which may be the genesis of vomiting in the ferret.

Exocrine pancreas and biliary system

The exocrine pancreas and biliary system are also under vagal stimulation. There is a trophic relationship with capillary connections between the islets and the exocrine pancreatic tissue. A bile salt-dependent lipase is produced; if lipase elevations are present in the blood, pancreatic inflammation or disease should be considered. The pancreas lies adjacent and adherent to the greater curvature of the stomach, and extends along the proximal 6–10 cm of the duodenum. It then has a lobe curving cranially towards the stomach, forming a C-shaped formation with loose connective tissue and fat attached in the middle of the C.

The gallbladder contracts in response to cholecystokinin, which is found throughout the GI tract. This contraction inhibits gastric emptying and stimulates small intestine and colonic motility.

Diseases of the GI tract

Ferrets are used as animal models for emesis as they have a low tolerance for many chemicals and the vagal reflex is strong, with a simple stomach for propulsion. They are also used as models of *Helicobacter* gastritis, gastric carcinoma, pyloric and intestinal ulceration, inflammatory bowel disease, colitis and GI neoplasia.

Although *H. mustelae* is found in most adult ferrets, it is not always implicated in clinical gastritis or ulcers. It does play a role as an opportunist and exacerbates ulceration of the stomach and intestines. It appears to be involved in the development of gastric neoplasia and may play a role in inflammatory bowel disease and colitis. As *H. mustelae* is a model for human *H. pylori* infection, further knowledge of clinical implications and improvements in diagnosis and treatment will be forthcoming.

In addition, ferrets are prone to stress-induced GI ulcers with associated haemorrhage and hypermotility. All of the above conditions may result in varying degrees of diarrhoea: acute, chronic or intermittent; with or without visible haemorrhage; and with or without secondary bacterial or viral involvement.

Inflammatory bowel disease (usually lymphoplastic) probably has multiple causes and may have an underlying genetic component, particularly considering its progression to neoplasia in many ferrets. Food allergies have yet to be explored other than some clinical trials in some cases involving alternative protein feline diets. The grain carbohydrates used in commercial food formulations may be a problem: allergy testing as done in dogs and cats should be pursued. Immunomodulating medications such as prednisolone at 0.5–2.0 mg/kg orally q12–24h, azathioprine at 0.9 mg/kg orally q24h and metronidazole at 25 mg/kg orally q24h have been used, based on therapies for other species

Ferrets groom themselves similarly to cats and can develop trichobezoars, particularly in the spring and autumn during coat changes. Trichobezoars can become large enough to block the pyloric outflow and fill the stomach (Figure 25.1). Signs include a slow decrease in appetite and weight loss. Occasionally there will be increased hair in the faeces. Ferrets usually do not vomit hair like cats, but seem to pass it through the faeces. Prevention includes diligent owners assisting the ferret with hair removal, bathing and grooming, as well as administration of a petrolatum-based flavoured feline laxative during coat change.

Figure 25.2 lists GI diseases of ferrets, their diagnosis and treatment.

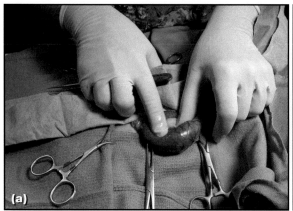 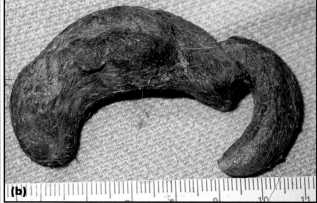

25.1 **(a)** Gastrotomy in a ferret with a trichobezoar. **(b)** Trichobezoar after surgical removal (see Chapter 23 for technique). Recovery was uneventful.

Disease	Clinical signs	Diagnosis	Treatment	Age grouping
Bacterial, primary or secondary: 1. *Helicobacter mustelae* 2. *Lawsonia intracellularis/ Desulfovibrio* 3. *Campylobacter jejuni*	1. Anorexia, dehydration, condition loss, diarrhoea, abdominal pain, emesis, GI haemorrhage and/or ulceration, tarry faeces, gastric neoplasia, enlargement of lymph nodes surrounding stomach 2. Anorexia, dehydration, diarrhoea, weight loss 3. Diarrhoea with dehydration, possibly anorexia, weight loss	Culture and sensitivity 1. *Helicobacter* PCR, histopathology 2. Biopsy, histopathology 3. Culture difficult, human laboratories	Appropriate antimicrobial therapy, adjunctive	Any. 2. Usually younger
Bacterial, uncommon: Mycobacteriosis	Enlargement of lymph nodes, possibly organomegaly (liver) depending on location of granulomas; unthriftiness, condition and weight loss despite appetite, elevated WBC, liver enzymes if liver infiltrated; may see diarrhoea depending on location of granulomas	Histopathology PCR	Zoonotic risks should be considered and may make treatment inadvisable. Euthanasia may be indicated. Successful treatment of *M. genavense* has been reported. Practitioners should be aware of local public health regulations concerning mycobacteriosis reporting and animal treatments	> 2 years

25.2 GI disease in ferrets. (continues) ▶

Disease	Clinical signs	Diagnosis	Treatment	Age grouping
Viral: 1. Ferret enteric coronavirus (FECV) 2. Rotavirus 3. Canine distemper virus 4. Ferret infectious peritonitis virus (FeIPV) (variant of FEVC)	Diarrhoea, usually mucoid, often bile-tinged green, undigested or poorly digested food passage. Rotavirus is usually in young ferrets	Coronavirus isolation, PCR 4. Immuno-histochemistry	Supportive care	1. Any, usually following stressful event, ferret gathering 2. Neonate, weanlings 3. Ferrets that did not complete their primary series of vaccinations, unvaccinated ferret
Parasitic: coccidiosis (Figure 25.3); giardiasis; cryptosporidiosis (Figure 25.4)	Diarrhoea, secondary dehydration	Faecal flotation, direct smear	Anti-coccidial drugs; metronidazole for *Giardia*; no effective treatment for cryptosporidiosis; symptomatic care, especially fluids as needed	Usually < 1 year; frequently ferrets in shelters
Inflammatory bowel disease	Chronic, usually intermittent diarrhoea (Figure 25.5) with gradual weight/condition loss. Usually palpable mesenteric lymph nodes, may be unresponsive to symptomatic anti-diarrhoeal treatments; usually older ferrets	Histopathology, ultrasonography, check lymph nodes. History and previous treatments as rule-outs	Some suggest anti-inflammatory drugs such as azathioprine; caution in ferrets with possible *Helicobacter*, symptomatic, supportive treatment	Usually > 2 years, history of intermittent diarrhoea. Will progress to lymphoma (Figure 25.6)
GI neoplasia: primary, metastatic, localized/ segmental or diffuse (Figures 25.6 and 25.7)	Emesis, anorexia, weight loss, diarrhoea, pain, nausea, enlarged mesenteric, pyloric, gastric lymph nodes, masses, thickening or irregularities in intestinal walls	Histopathology, ultrasonography, radiology with contrast; exploratory surgery. Check lymph nodes	Surgical excision. Chemotherapy. Mainly supportive and symptomatic care	Usually > 3 years
Foreign body ingestion	Usually acute loss of appetite or change of appetite, may see change in stool, gradual loss of weight/condition. Depending on the foreign body and if it causes full or partial obstruction, degree of anorexia, dehydration, pain, faecal consistency will vary	Physical examination, radiographs, ultrasonography, exploratory surgery	Surgery	Usually < 2 years
Rectal prolapse (Figure 25.8), rectal tissue swelling	Recent surgery in the area (demusking, tumour removal); tenesmus upon defecation	Seen in young ferrets where anal sac removal may have damaged large amount of tissue; also seen in young, stressed ferrets secondary to hypermotility, may also see in severe coccidiosis with explosive diarrhoea irritating the mucosa	Preparation H in mild cases for several days may resolve; reduction of prolapse if tissue more than 0.2 cm or ulcerating or drying; may need to reconstruct rectal area as ferret grows if damage to rectal innervation. Perform faecal examination to rule out intestinal parasites as a cause	Ferrets < 3 months of age, especially after shipping
Stress – medical or psychological (anorexia, emesis, diarrhoea)	Anorexia, emesis, diarrhoea, abdominal pain	History. Detection of underlying medical condition	Correction of underlying medical disorder or psychological stress	Any
Trichobezoar (see Figure 25.1)	See foreign body clinical signs; more likely during seasonal coat changes or in a ferret which does a lot of social grooming of other ferrets; or subsequent to GI motility changes due to diet change, other illness	Radiographs, palpation, pain, weight loss history	Surgery, then preventive care	Any, especially spring/autumn at coat change
Idiopathic megaoesophagus	Frequent vomiting, whole food; constantly hungry, weight and condition loss. Often can keep small amounts of liquid food and water down, particularly if fed with chest and head elevated	Radiology, including contrast studies	Unrewarding, may try therapies based on canine megaoesophagus treatment	Any

25.2 (continued) GI disease in ferrets.

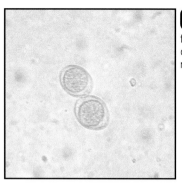

25.3 Coccidia isolated from a ferret with diarrhoea. (Original magnification x 100.)

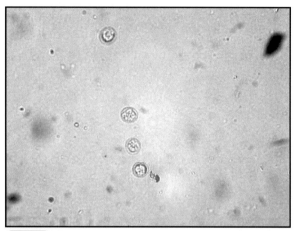

25.4 Cryptosporidia from a ferret with severe chronic diarrhoea at a ferret shelter. (Original magnification x 40.)

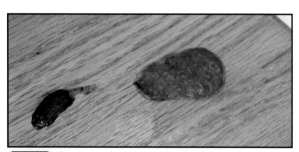

25.5 Diarrhoea from a ferret with inflammatory bowel disease.

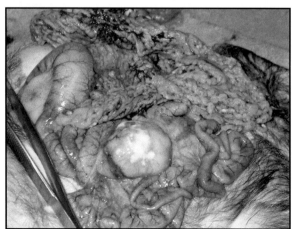

25.6 Necropsy photograph showing disseminated lymphosarcoma following inflammatory bowel disease. Note enlarged mesenteric, pyloric lymph nodes (including large mass).

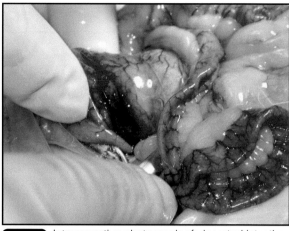

25.7 Intraoperative photograph of ulcerated intestine in a ferret. It was found to have segmental lymphoma, with several lymph nodes involved as well. The area of ulceration was not considered neoplastic.

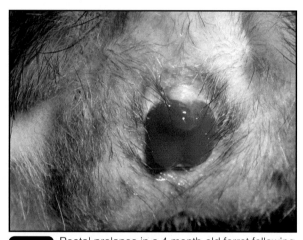

25.8 Rectal prolapse in a 4-month-old ferret following poor anal sacculectomy done at 4 weeks of age. The prolapse was unresponsive to repeated topical treatments. Surgical repair was required.

Diagnosis of GI disease

Clinical history

A detailed history is needed to determine a course of action. This includes volume, colour, consistency and frequency of faeces, and the duration for which the client has seen diarrhoea. The source of the ferret, including breeder, may play a significant role in the priority of aetiologies. Other information should include how long the ferret has been in the household, other ferrets and pets present, as well as human family members – are any symptomatic with diarrhoea? The type of litter used and sanitation programme may be of importance. Diet fed (including treats), toys available and incidental environmental information (such as access to showers or sinks) should be recorded. Ferrets are notorious for licking soaps, chewing on stuffing dug out of furniture, shoes and shoe liners, and even perfume or shampoo bottles. Correlation with activity should also be figured into the evaluation. For example, does it occur round the clock or is it only after intense playtime? Does it only occur after the vacuum cleaner is run near the ferret's cage? Tenesmus or vocalization, or accompanying borborygmus or flatulence, should be recorded. Teeth grinding may indicate pain, and anorexia may be a sequel to the pain. The clinical history should also indicate if this is an acute or chronic problem, continuous or intermittent.

Clinical examination

A physical examination of the ferret should be thorough and include auscultation of the abdomen and examination of the anal area. A full dental examination should also be done as severe dental disease may be part of the clinical presentation. An important physical finding is loss of weight and coat/muscle condition, which would indicate a more chronic problem even if the owner has only noted occasional GI signs such as intermittent diarrhoea.

Diagnostic tests

A faecal examination should include flotation and direct smear of fresh material, as well as staining to look at bacterial levels and presence of blood cells. A rectal culture and cytology may be indicated. Blood analysis should include lipase, which has been shown to be elevated in many cases of inflammatory bowel disease. Lipase may also be elevated with pancreatitis. Anaemia is not an uncommon finding and may indicate GI haemorrhage. Faecal occult blood can be tested, but the ferret should be placed on a diet that does not contain meat for at least 24–36 hours prior to testing, as normal ferret foods contain meat and blood products that result in positive test results (see

also Chapter 20).

Radiographs including a contrast study are frequently useful (see Chapter 19) (Figure 25.9).

Ultrasonography can be used to look at motility of the stomach including the pyloric area. Ultrasonography of the abdomen may also uncover other pathological conditions, including enlarged or necrotic lymph nodes. The gall bladder and duct can be visualized as bile is ejected into the duodenum. Intestinal mucosa may appear thickened (in inflammatory bowel disease) or irregular, as is seen with ulceration or neoplasia (see Figures 25.6 and 25.7). The ferret should be fasted for at least 4 hours prior to ultrasonography, particularly when the GI tract is the primary system for examination. With a relatively empty tract, a sweet treat substance such as Nutrical® gel (Evsco, Buena, New Jersey) can be given. The passage of this gel can be viewed with ultrasonography, which is useful to assess motility.

Endoscopy is useful for examination of the stomach, pylorus and colon. It can also be used abdominally (laparoscopy). Biopsies can be taken endoscopically or via laparotomy. A PCR test for gastric *Helicobacter mustelae* is available in the US. The author uses a sterile length of infusion set tubing measured for the particular ferret. Using a sterile haemostat, the culturette swab can be inserted into the tubing and pushed in until it is firmly seated. The tube is then passed into the sedated ferret's stomach and the stomach is manually massaged around the culturette. (See also Chapter 20 for diagnostic tests and sample collection technique.)

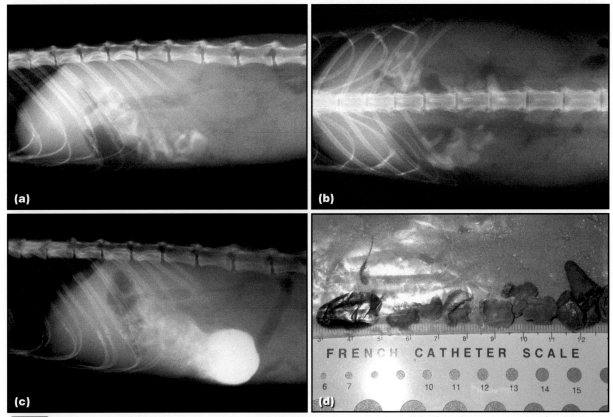

25.9 **(a)** Lateral radiograph of a ferret with multiple palpable foreign bodies. **(b)** VD radiograph showing foreign bodies. **(c)** Contrast (barium) study in the same ferret. **(d)** Material removed (owners identified it as part of a favourite toy).

Treatment of GI disease

Hydration should first be assessed and corrected (see Chapter 18). If abdominal pain is noted during the examination, the author usually administers either butorphanol at 0.4 mg/kg i.m. or buprenorphine at 0.01–0.03 mg/kg s.c., and midazolam at 0.25–0.5 mg/kg i.m., before proceeding with additional diagnostic testing. With the ferret's pain diminished, abdominal palpation can often detect organomegaly, enlarged lymph nodes, masses, and degree of abdominal fat. Fluid or gas in the intestines may also be assessed, though survey radiographs may be more definitive. Auscultation of the abdomen is useful to assess borborygmus.

Diagnostic tests include faecal examination for parasites, faecal and/or rectal culture for enteric bacteria, radiographs and, if indicated, a contrast series after the ferret is hydrated, ultrasonography to assess abdominal organs and lymph nodes, haematology and serum chemistries, including lipase. Additional diagnostic tests may include serum protein electrophoresis to assess the immunological response, *Helicobacter mustelae* PCR, endoscopic examination, exploratory laparotomy and biopsy. Symptomatic and supportive care should be instigated until the definitive diagnosis is made. In many cases, the problem may be one of managing the disease for a good quality of life rather than curing it.

Figure 25.10 lists treatments published for *H. mustelae* infection. Figure 25.11 lists adjunctive therapies for gastroenteritis.

Effective combinations
Amoxicillin (30 mg/kg q8h × 21–28d)
Metronidazole (20 mg/kg q8h × 21–28d)
Bismuth subsalicylate (7.5 mg/kg q8h × 21–28d)
Enrofloxacin (8.5 mg/kg/day divided q12h) × 14d
Bismuth subcitrate [a] (12 mg/kg divided q12h) × 14d
Clarithromycin (12.5 mg/kg q12h × 14d)
Ranitidine bismuth citrate [a] (24 mg/kg q12h × 14d)
Clarithromycin (12.5 mg/kg q 8 h × 14d)
Ranitidine bismuth citrate [a] (24 mg/kg q8h × 14d)
This is also a published dosage

Unsuccessful medications
Amoxicillin alone. May not be effective at q12h even in combinations
Metronidazole alone. May not be effective with amoxicillin if given at 12h intervals
Chloramphenicol alone
Enrofloxacin alone
Tetracycline
Bismuth subsalicylate alone
Omeprazole and amoxicillin
Omeprazole alone

25.10 Treatment regimens for *Helicobacter mustelae* infection, based on clinical trials (Johnson-Delaney, 2005; Lennox, 2005). [a] Not commercially available in the US; can be compounded.

Drug	Dosage	Comments
Azathioprine	0.9 mg/kg orally q24–72h	Used in IBD if other treatment ineffective. Immunosuppressive
Bismuth subsalicylate	5–7.5 mg/kg orally q8–12h	Symptomatic use for diarrhoea, cherry flavour preferred, refrigerate to increase palatability
Buprenorphine	0.01 mg/kg s.c. q10–12h as needed	Analgesic for severe GI pain and/or if bleeding ulcers suspected. Has very slight constipating effect with continued use. Ferret should receive intravenous or subcutaneous fluids and assisted feeding as drug may cause some sedation
Famotidine	0.25–0.5 mg/kg orally, i.m., i.v. q24h	Histamine antagonist; available over the counter; decreases gastric acid; provides pain relief. Oral over the counter non-prescription tablets can be crushed, mixed with flavoured gel, palatable
Meloxicam	0.1–0.2 mg/kg orally q24h	Use with protectant and/or histamine antagonist for pain, cramping
Metoclopramide	0.2–1.0 mg/kg orally, s.c., i.m. q6–8h	Anti-emetic, anti-gastric reflux; motility enhancer without stimulation of gastric, bile or pancreatic secretions
Metronidazole	50 mg/kg orally q24h	IBD, some immunosuppressive effects; usually effective for *Giardia* using divided dosage q12h; use benzoate formulation to increase palatability
Omeprazole	0.7 mg/kg orally q24h	Protein pump inhibitor, short-term usage only
Prednisolone	1–2.5 mg/kg orally q24h	Anti-inflammatory. Used in eosinophilic gastroenteritis, IBD, palliative in lymphoma/lymphosarcoma. Monitor liver, kidney, cardiac parameters and GI ulceration, faecal occult blood
Preparation-H	About 0.25 cm dab, topical, q6–8h	Used on inflamed rectal tissue, post-rectal prolapse to decrease swelling, shrink
Ranitidine USP	24 mg/kg orally q8h × 14d	Histamine inhibitor; decreases gastric acid; provides pain relief. Tablet form available over the counter, must be compounded as human formulation unpalatable
Sucralfate	25 mg/kg orally q8h	Coats oesophageal and gastric mucosa, local effect only. Syrup palatable

25.11 Medications used as adjunctive therapy of GI tract disease (Johnson-Delaney, 2005; Lennox, 2005).

In summary, the ferret GI tract is designed to be excitatory, have rapid motility and be highly secretory. Exogenous stressors and chemical and neurological stimulations further increase motility and secretion. During any hypoglycaemic episode the clinician needs to be aware of the pancreatic and gastric physiology and treat the nausea and secretions in addition to the hypoglycaemia. It may also be prudent to administer medication to inhibit acid secretions prior to surgeries and in any stressed, ill ferrets.

Acknowledgements

The author would like to acknowledge Dr Angela Lennox, Ernie Coliazzi, the Washington Ferret Rescue & Shelter ferrets and volunteers, and the Farscape Kids.

References and further reading

Blackshaw LA, Staunton E, Dent J *et al.* (1998) Mechanisms of gastro-oesophageal reflux in the ferret. *Neurogastroenterology and Motility* **10**, 49–56

Evans HE and An NQ (1998) Anatomy of the ferret. In: *Biology and Diseases of the Ferret, 2nd edn*, ed. JG Fox, pp. 19–69. Williams & Wilkins, Baltimore

Johnson-Delaney CA (2004) A clinician's perspective on ferret diarrhea. *Exotic DVM* **6**(3), 27–28

Johnson-Delaney CA (2005) The ferret GI tract and *Helicobacter mustelae* infection. *Veterinary Clinics of North America: Exotic Animal Practice* **8**, 197–212

Lennox AM (2004) Working up mystery anemia in ferrets. *Exotic DVM* **6**(3), 22–26

Lennox AM (2005) GI diseases of the ferret. *Veterinary Clinics of North America: Exotic Animal Practice* **8**, 213–226

26

Ferrets: cardiovascular and respiratory system disorders

Connie Orcutt and Rebecca Malakoff

Introduction

Primary cardiac disease is a relatively common finding in pet ferrets, therefore it is important for practitioners who work with this species to be able to recognize pertinent historical clues and physical examination findings as well as understand diagnostic and therapeutic options. Heart disease is most commonly diagnosed in middle-aged to older ferrets and presentations are similar to those seen in other species. In contrast, primary respiratory disease, with the exception of influenza, is uncommon in clinical practice and can affect ferrets of any age. A number of respiratory abnormalities are the result of primary cardiac disease, trauma, neoplasia, or space-occupying lesions. Even profound weakness (e.g. secondary to hypoglycaemia or systemic disease) can manifest as a respiratory abnormality. Cardiovascular and respiratory signs are intimately connected and the clinician should include diagnostic tests that will evaluate both systems in reaching a definitive diagnosis.

Anatomy and physiology

The ferret has a long thoracic cavity bordered by 14–15 ribs (as opposed to 13 ribs in dogs and cats). The heart, located farther caudally in the thorax compared with dogs or cats, lies roughly between the 6th and 9th–10th ribs.

In the authors' experience the ferret's normal heart rate is 180–250 beats per minute (but see also Chapter 17). It is not uncommon to auscultate a normal sinus arrhythmia during routine examination of the unsedated ferret. Short pauses may also be auscultated, which are often the result of second-degree atrioventricular block.

Ferrets have a large lung volume relative to their body weight. This anatomical feature, along with other characteristics similar to those of human lungs, is one of the reasons ferrets are used as experimental models for respiratory physiology and disease in people. The normal respiratory rate for an unsedated ferret is approximately 33–36 breaths per minute.

General approach to the cardiorespiratory case

While upper respiratory signs may be readily apparent to the owner, signs of lower respiratory disease or cardiac disease may be considerably more subtle. The history is important in helping to narrow down the differential diagnosis (Figure 26.1). The client should be questioned about the ferret's contact with other ferrets or with people who are ill, the home environment and travel history, the ferret's vaccination status, and any episodes of trauma, collapse or exercise intolerance.

Clinical sign	Differential diagnoses	Further investigations
Upper respiratory signs (nasal discharge or crusting, increased inspiratory effort or sounds, coughing, nasal swelling)	Primary upper respiratory disease (viral, bacterial, fungal, neoplasia, foreign body, hypersensitivity) Space-occupying masses compressing respiratory tract (e.g. abscess, lymphadenopathy, neoplasia) Congestive heart failure	History, vaccination status, concurrent clinical signs (e.g. dermatopathy, lymphadenopathy), CBC, serum biochemistry, radiography, echocardiography, ECG, tracheal wash for bacterial and fungal culture/sensitivity and cytological analysis, CT scan
Dyspnoea/collapse	Pneumonia (viral, bacterial, fungal, aspiration) Primary or metastatic neoplasia Congestive heart failure (CHF) Arrhythmia/syncope Pleural effusion (neoplasia, CHF, heartworm disease) Pneumothorax – usually secondary to trauma Diaphragmatic hernia Hypoglycaemia Metabolic acidosis Anaemia Compressive lesions (abscesses, neoplastic masses)	Radiography, blood glucose, CBC, serum biochemistry, blood gas/electrolytes, echocardiography, ECG, thoracic ultrasonography (if suspect intrathoracic mass)

26.1 Differential diagnosis based on cardiorespiratory signs. (continues) ▶

Clinical sign	Differential diagnoses	Further investigations
Abdominal distension/ascites	Right-sided congestive heart failure Neoplasia Haemoabdomen (trauma, neoplasia) Hypoalbuminaemia (GI disease, liver disease) Polycystic disease (liver, renal)	Radiography, echocardiography, abdominal ultrasonography

26.1 (continued) Differential diagnosis based on cardiorespiratory signs.

Signs of upper respiratory disease include increased inspiratory effort or sounds, nasal or ocular discharge, coughing or gagging, sneezing, squinting and fever. In contrast, lethargy, decreased appetite and/or fever may be the only apparent abnormalities in the ferret with lower airway disease or cardiac disease. Expiratory dyspnoea may be subtle. Likewise, pulmonary pathology may not be evident on auscultation. Muffled heart and respiratory sounds are usually appreciated in ferrets with pneumothorax or pleural effusion. The ferret's thorax should be auscultated in all areas for murmurs and arrhythmias, both of which are usually readily evident. Because respiratory sinus arrhythmia is very common, the clinician should evaluate auscultation in concert with the respiratory pattern. Cyanosis may be evident with pneumonia or heart disease, and pallor is usually obvious in cases of significant anaemia. Ascites, which can be seen in some cases of right-sided heart failure, is generally easy to palpate.

If upper respiratory signs do not resolve within several days (as one would expect with influenza or contact inflammation), the authors' further workup includes radiographs, a complete blood count (CBC), serum biochemistry and a tracheal wash. If signs persist, computerized tomography (CT) may provide useful information. Rhinoscopy is difficult to perform in ferrets because of the narrow nasal cavity.

If the ferret is presented collapsed, a packed cell volume (PCV) as well as total protein and blood glucose levels should be evaluated immediately. An analysis of blood gases and electrolytes may also provide valuable information. Survey radiographs, a CBC and serum biochemistry are indicated if the following abnormalities are noted in the history or physical examination:

- Persistent lethargy/inappetence/weakness
- Tachypnoea/dyspnoea
- Fever
- Muffled heart or lung sounds
- Abnormal heart rhythm
- Heart murmur
- Ascites.

Radiographic findings of cardiomegaly, ascites, pleural effusion or perihilar oedema concurrent with an arrhythmia or murmur should be further evaluated with an echocardiogram. Significant pneumothorax or pleural effusion may require thoracocentesis; the effusion can then be submitted for further analysis. Pneumonia is sometimes treated empirically with antibiotic therapy, but a tracheal wash for cytological analysis and bacterial ± fungal culture may be helpful if signs persist. An electrocardiogram is important in characterizing arrhythmias. Anterior mediastinal widening (usually the result of a mass) or pleural effusion are indications for thoracic ultrasonography. In rare cases, CT may provide further useful information.

Tracheal lavage: Tracheal lavage for collection of samples to submit for cytological analysis and culture is indicated in persistent cases of upper and lower respiratory disease. The procedure is performed through a sterile endotracheal tube using a technique similar to that used in cats. Sterile saline is instilled at a dose of 1 ml/kg and the sample is aspirated back into the syringe. Sample size can be maximized by using a mucus trap attached to wall suction and a sterile paediatric suction catheter.

Cardiac disease

Clinical signs
Ferrets with heart disease may show clinical signs of dyspnoea, tachypnoea, lethargy, inappetence, weight loss and exercise intolerance. Owners may also note ascites, which can manifest as a 'pot-belly', or hindlimb weakness (not associated with thromboembolic disease). Coughing may be noted as 'gagging'. Abnormalities can sometimes be detected on auscultation of the asymptomatic ferret during routine examination.

Physical examination findings consistent with heart disease include heart murmurs, arrhythmias, gallop sounds, muffled heart or lung sounds and harsh lung sounds or crackles, which may indicate pulmonary oedema. Clinicians should check for cyanotic mucous membranes and prolonged capillary refill time. Jugular venous distension may be noted with right-sided heart disease, and femoral pulse deficits may occur with arrhythmias or poor cardiac output. Ferrets with heart disease may have ascites and/or hepatomegaly. Splenomegaly may also be noted on physical examination, though this is a common non-specific finding, particularly in older ferrets.

Diagnostic tests
Thoracic radiographs are a useful tool for detection of cardiomegaly, pulmonary vasculature changes and congestive heart failure (CHF), manifested by pulmonary oedema (Figure 26.2) or pleural effusion. As previously mentioned, the ferret's heart is located in a relatively caudal position and appears more globoid than a feline or canine heart. See Chapter 19 for more information on thoracic radiography in ferrets.

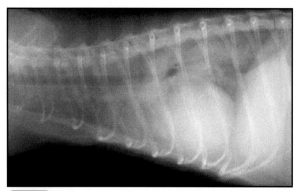

26.2 Pulmonary oedema in a ferret with valvular heart disease. This ferret had severe regurgitation of the aortic valve, moderate regurgitation of the mitral valve and mild tricuspid regurgitation.

An electrocardiogram may be obtained by placing the ferret in lateral recumbency or by scruffing the animal vertically if lateral positioning is resisted. The

teeth on the ECG clamps should be filed smooth and moistened gauze squares used to further cushion the clamps. Normal ECG findings compiled from ferrets sedated with ketamine and diazepam and positioned in either right lateral or sternal recumbency (Bublot *et al.*, 2006) are presented in Figure 26.3 and examples of ECGs showing normal sinus rhythm as well as second- and third-degree atrioventricular block are shown in Figure 26.4.

An echocardiogram obtained by a skilled sonographer will aid in the definitive diagnosis of heart disease by providing detailed information about the size of cardiac chambers, degree of wall motion and valvular function. Standard views described for dogs and cats can be easily obtained in most ferrets with or without sedation. Normal echocardiographic values from a study performed on sedated ferrets (Stepien *et al.*, 2000) are shown in Figure 26.5 and echocardiographic images of a normal ferret heart are shown in Figure 26.6. See also Chapter 19 for further details.

Parameter	Right lateral position	Sternal position
Heart rate	250 bpm → 430 bpm	
Mean electrical axis	+75 degrees → +100 degrees	+65 degrees → +90 degrees
P wave amplitude (lead II)	≤ +0.2 mV	≤ +0.3 mV
P wave duration	0.01 s → 0.03 s	
PR interval duration	0.03 s → 0.06 s	
Q(S) wave amplitude (lead I)	−0.4 mV → 0 mV	0 mV
Q wave amplitude (lead II)	−0.05 mV → 0 mV	
R wave amplitude (lead I)	≤ +0.9 mV	≤ +1.25 mV
R wave amplitude (lead II)	1 mV → 2.8 mV	1 mV → 3.1 mV
R wave amplitude (lead aVF)	1 mV → 3.1 mV	
S wave amplitude (lead II)	0 mV	
QRS complex duration (lead II)	0.02 s → 0.05 s	
T wave amplitude (lead II)	−0.4 mV → +0.4 mV Most often > 0	>0 or <0
QT interval duration	0.06 s → 0.16 s	

26.3 Expected electrocardiographic values recorded in the right lateral and sternal positions for clinically normal ferrets sedated with ketamine and diazepam. (Data from Bublet *et al.*, 2006.)

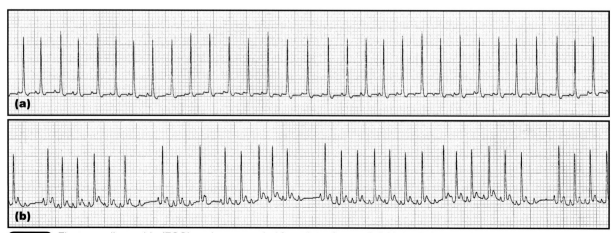

(a)

(b)

26.4 Electrocardiographic (ECG) tracings recorded from three ferrets. **(a)** Normal sinus rhythm at a heart rate of 260 bpm. Note that R waves appear tall, similar to a canine ECG tracing. **(b)** Low-grade second-degree atrioventricular (AV) block with a normal heart on echocardiography. Note the four non-conducted P waves in this tracing. (continues) ▶

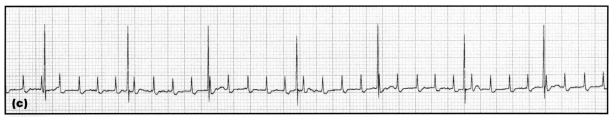

26.4 (continued) Electrocardiographic (ECG) tracings recorded from three ferrets. **(c)** Third-degree AV block. Although there are regular R–R and P–P intervals, note that there is no association between the R and P waves

Variable	N	Mean (SD)	Median	Range
IVSd (cm)	30	0.36 (0.07)	0.33	0.20–0.50
IVSs (cm)	30	0.48 (0.11)	0.47	0.27–0.77
LVIDd (cm)	30	0.88 (0.15)	0.86	0.63–1.20
LVIDs (cm)	30	0.59 (0.15)	0.60	0.27–0.87
LVWd (cm)	30	0.42 (0.11)	0.40	0.30–0.70
LVWs (cm)	30	0.58 (0.99)	0.57	0.43–0.80
FS (%)	30	33 (14)	36	0–57
RVWd (cm)	27	0.12 (0.03)	0.10	0.10–0.20
RVIDd (cm)	28	0.38 (0.10)	0.39	0.20–0.57
LA diameter (cm)	26	0.71 (0.18)	0.67	0.47–1.20
Ao diameter (cm)	25	0.53 (0.10)	0.53	0.30–0.73
LA:Ao ratio	26	1.33 (0.27)	1.35	0.80–2.0
Ao max (m/s)	25	0.89 (0.20)	0.87	0.58–1.34
PA max (m/s)	29	1.10 (0.14)	1.09	0.78–1.3

26.5 M-mode and Doppler echocardiographic values obtained from 30 normal adult ferrets sedated with an intramuscular combination of ketamine (25 mg/kg) and midazolam (0.2 mg/kg). Ao = aorta; FS = fractional shortening; IVSd and IVSs = thickness of interventricular septum in diastole and systole, respectively; LA = left atrium; LVIDd and LVIDs = left ventricular internal diameter in diastole and systole, respectively; LVWd and LVWs = thickness of left ventricular free wall in diastole and systole, respectively; PA = pulmonary artery; RVWd = right ventricular wall thickness in diastole; RVIDd = right ventricular internal diameter in diastole; SD = standard deviation. (Data from Stepien *et al.*, 2000.)

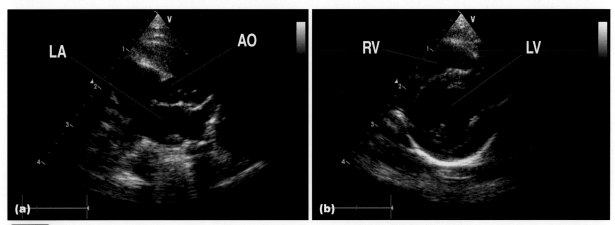

26.6 Two-dimensional echocardiogram from a ferret with a normal heart. **(a)** Right parasternal short-axis view at the level of the heart base. AO = aorta; LA = left atrium. **(b)** Right parasternal short-axis view at the level of the ventricles. LV = left ventricle; RV = right ventricle.

Dilated cardiomyopathy

Dilated cardiomyopathy (DCM) has been described as the most commonly reported form of heart disease in ferrets (Stamoulis *et al.*, 1997). This is not the case in the authors' practice, where valvular heart disease and hypertrophic cardiomyopathy are more commonly diagnosed in asymptomatic ferrets with heart murmurs. There is some thought that the prevalence of DCM in ferrets may be decreasing in the United States. Dilated cardiomyopathy remains, however, an important and common cause of CHF in ferrets.

DCM should be suspected in any ferret with cardiomegaly on radiography or evidence of CHF, such as pulmonary oedema or pleural effusion. A definitive diagnosis is based on echocardiographic findings. Ferrets with DCM have a large and often spherical left ventricular chamber with thin walls and depressed wall motion. The left atrium may be enlarged (one would expect significant enlargement with CHF), and the right atrium and ventricle may be affected as well.

A histopathological study of a ferret with DCM showed multifocal myocardial degeneration, myocardial necrosis and replacement fibrosis (Lipman *et al.*, 1987). Taurine deficiency related to DCM has not been reported in ferrets, though this is a known cause in some cats and dogs with the disease.

Hypertrophic cardiomyopathy

In the authors' experience, hypertrophic cardiomyopathy (HCM) may be diagnosed in ferrets with or without signs of CHF, although no case reports of HCM in ferrets have been published to date and the characteristics and prognosis are not well described. Diagnosis is based on echocardiographic findings, which show thickening of the left ventricular walls. The left ventricular chamber may be normal in size or small, and wall motion may be normal or hyperdynamic. The left atrium may be enlarged. Secondary hypertrophy of the left ventricle caused by hyperthyroidism or systemic hypertension (known causes in cats) has not been reported in ferrets. CHF may occur with HCM, though this is uncommon in the authors' practice. No thromboembolic complications secondary to HCM (or any cardiac disease in a ferret) have been reported.

Restrictive cardiomyopathy

Although seen less commonly in ferrets, restrictive cardiomyopathy may be diagnosed if an echocardiogram shows significant atrial enlargement with relatively normal ventricular wall thickness and motion.

Valvular heart disease

Valvular heart disease is one of the most common forms of cardiac disease in ferrets seen in the authors' practice. Most affected ferrets are middle-aged to older. Ferrets with valvular heart disease may be asymptomatic (typically diagnosed when a murmur is detected on auscultation) or may develop CHF (see Figure 26.2).

In the authors' experience, the aortic valve appears to be affected most commonly. It is very common to see a trivial to mild aortic insufficiency in ferrets during echocardiographic studies and it is possible that a trivial leakage of this valve may be a normal variation for this species. The authors have also seen aortic valve thickening associated with moderate to severe regurgitation, but it is rare to be able to auscultate the diastolic murmur of aortic insufficiency (Figure 26.7). The mitral valve may also be thickened and incompetent, followed less commonly by the tricuspid or pulmonic valve. Non-bacterial thrombotic endocarditis affecting the aortic valve has recently been reported in a ferret treated for a bite wound (Kottwitz *et al.*,

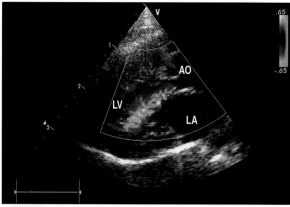

26.7 Two-dimensional echocardiogram from a ferret with severe aortic insufficiency. Right parasternal long-axis view. Note the blue–green jet of regurgitant blood flow from the aortic valve, extending back beyond the mid-left ventricular region. AO = aorta; LA = left atrium; LV = left ventricle.

2006). This ferret showed both myxomatous degeneration of the valve (a typical finding in dogs with endocardiosis) and inflammatory changes, which may represent two separate pathological processes.

Heartworm disease

Although not endemic in the United Kingdom, heartworm (*Dirofilaria immitis*) disease has been recognized as a clinical problem for ferrets in the United States, particularly in the southeast. Clinicians working in endemic areas or seeing ferrets with a travel history should be familiar with this disease. Because of their small body size, ferrets infected with *D. immitis* may present with significant and life-threatening cardiac disease even if only infected by a single worm; this is similar to the disease in cats. Heartworm infection may cause a physical obstruction to blood flow, resulting in clinical signs of right-sided CHF (e.g. pleural effusion or ascites). Ferrets may present with lethargy, coughing, cyanosis, dyspnoea or a distended abdomen and some may suffer sudden death.

Enzyme-linked immunosorbent assay (ELISA) antigen testing for heartworm disease in ferrets may provide false negative results if there is an infection by only male worms or by only one female worm, similar to test results in cats (see also Chapter 20). Thoracic radiographs most commonly show pleural effusion and may show cardiomegaly. It is common to see enlargement of the right atrium, caudal vena cava and right ventricle, though changes to the peripheral pulmonary arteries (commonly seen in dogs with heartworm disease) are typically less severe. Echocardiography may reveal the presence of heartworms, typically seen as double-lined structures within the pulmonary artery, right ventricle or right atrium. Structural changes to the heart include right atrial and ventricular enlargement and tricuspid regurgitation. Evidence of pulmonary hypertension, such as a high-velocity tricuspid or pulmonic regurgitation jet or right-sided chamber enlargement, may also be present.

If a ferret is heartworm-positive (preferably diagnosed by ultrasonography), adulticide treatment may be undertaken with melarsamine given in a two-staged protocol: 2.5 mg/kg as a deep intramuscular injection administered to the patient under isoflurane anaesthesia followed 30 days later by two doses of 2.5 mg/kg 24 hours apart (Antinoff, 2002). This protocol recommends concurrent treatment with prednisolone (1 mg/kg orally q24h) and a microfilaricidal dose of ivermectin (50 µg/kg orally q30d) until clinical signs resolve completely. Ferrets should also be treated with cardiac medications when indicated by the clinical signs. The ivermectin is a slow adulticide and renders the worms unable to reproduce. Because of the risk of potentially fatal thromboembolic complications, strict cage rest must be enforced until the ferret is deemed no longer heartworm-positive.

Anaphylaxis is a potential complication of treatment with melarsomine; so in some cases heartworm-positive ferrets have been treated only with ivermectin (at the dosage listed above) and prednisolone. However, for those ferrets that tolerate melarsomine the kill is faster, thus reducing the risk of permanent changes that can occur with the long-term presence of worms in the heart. If a ferret has an adverse reaction to melarsomine, it should not be administered again.

Heartworm prevention is recommended for all ferrets in endemic areas as well as for any ferret with a history of heartworm disease. Ivermectin is typically administered as a quarter of a 68 µg ivermectin/pyrantel tablet per ferret q30d. The drug deteriorates once the tablet is broken, so owners should be instructed to discard the remaining three quarters of the tablet.

Arrhythmias

Various arrhythmias have been diagnosed in ferrets with cardiac disease. Atrioventricular (AV) block is particularly common and low-grade second-degree AV block has been commonly seen by the authors in many ferrets with normal cardiac anatomy and function on echocardiograms (see Figure 26.4). Third-degree AV block may also be seen, with one case report of a pacemaker being used to treat this arrhythmia in a ferret (Guzman et al., 2006). Both ventricular and supraventricular arrhythmias have been seen in ferrets (usually in those with valvular heart disease or cardiomyopathy).

Other forms of heart disease

To the authors' knowledge, congenital heart disease has not been reported in ferrets. Although lymphoma is common in ferrets, including tumours affecting the cranial mediastinum, there have been no reports of neoplasia involving the myocardium or pericardium. Although pericardial effusion may be seen as part of right-sided CHF, there have been no reports of primary pericardial disease and effusion in ferrets.

Myocarditis may be suspected in ferrets with significant ventricular arrhythmias without evidence of significant primary cardiac disease on echocardiogram or with arrhythmias and acute myocardial dysfunction concurrent with a multisystemic illness. Causes of myocarditis may include parasitic disease, autoimmune disease, and bacterial or viral infections.

Acute myocardial necrosis was reported in a young ferret that received large overdoses of adrenaline and diphenhydramine while suffering a vaccine reaction. The myocardial damage was presumably the result of catecholamine toxicity and illustrates the importance of careful and appropriate drug dosing in this small animal (Orcutt and Donnelly, 2001).

Treatment options

Many of the medications used in cats and dogs with cardiac disease can be used in ferrets; in fact, if published drug dosages for a ferret are not available for a cardiac medication, the feline dose is often used by the authors. However, because of the ferret's small size, particular attention must be paid to dosing based on body weight. Administration of small dosages is facilitated by compounding tablets or capsules into a liquid suspension; ferrets should not be 'pilled'. See Chapter 21 for specific drug dosages.

Congestive heart failure in ferrets, regardless of cause, should be treated with diuretics (most commonly the loop diuretic furosemide) and supplemental oxygen in the emergency setting. If pleural effusion is significant, thoracocentesis should be performed. The optimal location for thoracocentesis should be determined using radiographic or ultrasound guidance and the best location may actually be cranial to the heart. Detailed instructions on how to perform the procedure have been recently described (Wyre and Hess, 2005).

Angiotensin-converting enzyme (ACE) inhibitors, such as enalapril, have also commonly been used in ferrets with CHF to blunt the harmful effects of the renin–angiotensin–aldosterone system. Caution with dosing should be used, as ferrets can be sensitive to the hypotensive effects of ACE inhibitors; clinical signs of hypotension include lethargy and anorexia. Nitroglycerin paste may be used for ferrets with acute CHF, but similar caution must be used in dosing to avoid hypotensive effects.

Digoxin may be considered for ferrets with DCM or those with significant supraventricular arrhythmias, though there are no data regarding the pharmacokinetics of this drug in ferrets. Cautious dosing should be used along with close monitoring for signs of toxicity (anorexia, vomiting, diarrhoea). The elixir form should be used in ferrets.

Pimobendan has recently become available for treatment of CHF caused by DCM or chronic valvular disease in dogs. Pimobendan is a phosphodiesterase-inhibiting calcium-sensitizing inodilator, which provides inotropic support and vasodilation. Some practitioners have described extra-label use in ferrets with DCM with some anecdotal success (Gaztanaga et al., 2006). To date, this drug has been used infrequently in ferrets but anecdotal dosages have included 0.25 mg/kg daily (ideally divided into two doses q12h), or 0.625 mg per ferret q12h.

Although its use is not well documented in ferrets, a beta-blocker such as atenolol may be used for the treatment of supraventricular or ventricular arrhythmias or in cases of hypertrophic cardiomyopathy. A calcium-channel blocker such as diltiazem may also be considered for supraventricular arrhythmias.

Respiratory disease

Upper respiratory disease

Viral disease

Influenza: Influenza is the main cause of upper respiratory disease seen in ferrets in the authors' practice. Ferrets are very susceptible to infection with influenza strains that affect humans and the primary source of infection is contact with a sick person. Clinical signs in ferrets are similar to those in people with colds: lethargy, inappetence, fever, sneezing, nasal discharge, epiphora and conjunctivitis. Fever is common and generally lasts 48–72 hours. Uncomplicated disease generally resolves in 4–5 days, but secondary bacterial infections can prolong the course. Disease is usually mild in adults but can be fatal in ferret kits. Infrequently, the disease can progress to pneumonia. Presumptive diagnosis is based on history and clinical signs.

Treatment of influenza primarily involves supportive care until the ferret is eating and drinking well; care is usually limited to fluid therapy and supportive feeding. Antihistamines (e.g. chlorpheniramine or diphenhydramine) may provide palliative therapy. Most ferrets can be treated at home, but dehydration, persistent fever and prolonged refusal to eat are reasons to hospitalize the animal. Transmission is by aerosol exposure and hospitalized ferrets should be quarantined. Similarly, people with colds or flu are cautioned not to have contact with ferrets, and any members of the medical team with symptoms of a cold or flu should wear a surgical mask when working with ferrets.

Ferrets have been used extensively as animal models for the study of influenza in humans, since the physiological response to the virus is very similar. Although ferrets have been used in the development of influenza vaccines, no vaccines are clinically approved for use in this species.

Canine distemper virus: Canine distemper virus is a rare cause of upper respiratory disease or pneumonia in the authors' practice. The disease progresses rapidly from the upper respiratory tract, which is the site of infection, to the skin and often the lungs. Neurological signs are common prior to death, which occurs in virtually 100% of affected ferrets. This disease can relatively easily be distinguished from influenza on the basis of exposure, vaccination status and the severity and duration of clinical signs. Refer to Chapter 31 for a more detailed description of canine distemper virus.

Contact irritation/inflammation

Ferrets spend a lot of time low to the ground and sniffing their environment or burrowing, which makes them prone to inhalation of particulate debris with the subsequent development of upper airway inflammation. Typical clinical signs include sneezing, epiphora and serous nasal discharge. To date, specific allergens have not been reported in ferrets; however, these animals seem to have the mechanisms in place to respond to them.

Environmental modification is one of the first steps in treating presumptive hypersensitivity. Some offending agents include clay cat litter (ferrets like to burrow in it), perfumed detergents or fabric softeners, carpet cleaners or other cleaning agents, new carpeting, feather dander, dust, and pollen-producing plants. Poor ventilation can exacerbate the problem. Affected ferrets may respond to treatment with chlorpheniramine or diphenhydramine.

Other causes of upper respiratory abnormalities

Ferrets on dry commercial diets infrequently develop severe dental disease. However, tooth root abscesses can sometimes affect the nasal cavity. Oronasal fistulation from any cause can also result in upper respiratory signs (see the section below on fungal disease). Occasionally, foreign bodies can become entrapped in the nasal cavity. Abscesses or enlarged lymph nodes in the cervical or pharyngeal area can compress the larynx or trachea and result in dyspnoea.

Pneumonia

Pneumonia, in general, is uncommon in ferrets. Clinical signs of pneumonia are similar to those in other animals; similarly, diagnosis is based on physical examination findings, radiographic lesions and results of CBC, cytology and cultures. Tracheal lavage may be useful in obtaining samples for testing.

Bacterial infection is an uncommon cause of upper or lower respiratory disease in ferrets and is often secondary to another disease process (e.g. infection with influenza or canine distemper virus). Bacterial pathogens reported to cause primary pneumonia in ferrets include *Streptococcus zooepidemicus*, *S. pneumoniae* and groups C and G streptococci; Gram-negative species have also been isolated. Other bacteria isolated from lungs in ferrets include *Bordetella bronchiseptica* and *Listeria monocytogenes*. Empirical choices of antibiotics pending, or in the absence of, culture results include amoxicillin/clavulanate, cephalosporins or fluoroquinolones. For dose rates see Chapter 21.

Aspiration is not a common cause of pneumonia in the authors' practice. Megaoesophagus, an idiopathic syndrome seen infrequently among ferrets, is often complicated by aspiration pneumonia (see Chapter 25). Aspiration pneumonia is also seen in some ferrets being treated with oral medications or receiving force feeding. The caudal portion of the left cranial lung lobe and the right middle lobe are the usual sites affected by inhalation pneumonia, but dependent areas of the caudal lobes can also be involved. Affected ferrets usually receive antibiotic treatment until clinical and radiographic signs resolve.

Fungal disease

Mycotic disease is uncommon in ferrets. Disease is usually confined to geographical areas with a high concentration of fungal organisms. Respiratory abnormalities are part of the usual disseminated nature of these diseases. Clinical signs may be primarily respiratory (coughing, nasal or ocular discharge, sneezing) or referable to systemic disease (lethargy, anorexia, weight loss, lymphadenopathy, draining tracts, lameness). Susceptibility to disease is enhanced during periods of immunosuppression or corticosteroid treatment. Diagnosis is based on history (travel to an endemic area), clinical signs, cytological isolation of fungal organisms, fungal culture and, in some cases, serology.

Disease with *Blastomyces dermatitidis* occurs most often in the central and southeastern USA, Canada, Africa and occasionally in Central America. Coccidioidomycosis (*Coccidioides immitis*) is endemic to the southwestern USA and parts of Latin America. *Histoplasma capsulatum* is commonly isolated from soil in the midwestern USA and is generally transmitted via aerosolization.

Cryptococcus neoformans can be a significant cause of rhinitis in ferrets. Clinical signs may include upper respiratory stertor, dyspnoea, nasal swelling, nasal discharge and crusting, deep mucosal ulceration and oronasal fistulation (Figure 26.8). Manifestations of systemic cryptococcosis can also include subacute or chronic meningoencephalitis and pneumonia. This organism is a relatively universal inhabitant of the soil and appears to have a higher incidence in excrement of pigeons and other birds. Diagnosis is often based on the classic appearance of encapsulated budding forms of the organism on cytological or histopathological analysis (Figure 26.9).

Treatment regimens most often include long-term treatment with ketoconazole, fluconazole or amphotericin B. Adequate hydration must be ensured and renal function monitored closely with the use of amphotericin B. See Chapter 21 for dose rates and treatment regimes. In general, systemic mycotic disease in ferrets carries a poor prognosis.

Mycobacteriosis

Ferrets are reportedly to be highly susceptible to several species of *Mycobacterium* (Fox, 1998). Most cases have involved ferrets on breeding farms or in research facilities. However, scattered cases involving pet ferrets have been reported in the literature and anecdotally.

Clinical signs are varied, depending on the site involved. A 5-year-old female ovariohysterectomized ferret presented to the authors' clinic for increased upper respiratory effort and sounds slowly progressing over the course of nearly 2 years. Results of radiography, CBC and serum biochemistry were unremarkable. Samples obtained by tracheal lavage showed a mixed inflammatory response with no evidence of microorganisms, so anti-inflammatory treatment with prednisolone was initiated. After the ferret's condition worsened significantly, a CT scan of the skull and neck was performed. Abnormalities included a soft tissue mass in the left nasal cavity, extending into the right nasal cavity and nasopharynx, as well as an enlarged retropharyngeal lymph node. Cytological and histopathological analysis of a lymph node aspirate and nasal turbinate biopsy, respectively, showed granulomatous inflammation and the presence of intrahistiocytic acid-fast bacilli. Subsequent tissue analysis using a DNA–RNA probe revealed infection with *Mycobacterium avium*. Treatment with clarithromycin and rifampin was unsuccessful, and the ferret was

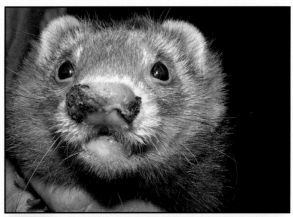

26.8 This male ferret presented with increased upper respiratory effort and sounds, nasal swelling and deep mucosal and dermal ulcerations progressing to oronasal fistulation. The aetiological agent was *Cryptococcus neoformans*. (Courtesy of Jennifer Graham, Angell Animal Medical Center.)

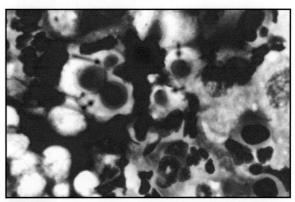

26.9 Impression smear of an intranasal mass from a ferret showing pyogranulomatous inflammation and 10–40 μm spherical yeast-like organisms surrounded by a thick clear capsule (short arrows). Some of the organisms demonstrate narrow-based budding (long arrow). The morphology of the fungal organisms is consistent with *Cryptococcus* (Diff-Quik stain; original magnification x1000). (Case submitted by Kimberly Mickley; photomicrograph provided by Patty Ewing, Angell Animal Medical Center.)

euthanased. At necropsy, acid-fast bacilli were found in the right and left retropharyngeal lymph nodes, perihilar lymph node and gall bladder.

Trauma

Because of the ferret's inquisitive nature, falls and compression injuries are common sources of traumatic damage. Pulmonary contusions and pneumothorax are abnormalities that may be seen on radiographs. Diaphragmatic hernias have also been diagnosed in ferrets.

Significant pneumothorax can be treated with thoracocentesis using a dorsal approach. In cases of persistent pneumothorax, the authors have used an indwelling chest drain fashioned from a sterile 8 French red rubber tube and placed using a Kirschner wire as a stylet. The technique used to place and secure the tube is similar to that used in other small animals. Continuous suction can be applied using a negative pressure of 13–15 cmH$_2$O.

Neoplasia

Primary neoplasia involving the respiratory tract is very rare in ferrets. Pulmonary metastases are most commonly seen with lymphosarcoma. Anterior mediastinal masses (lymphoma or thymoma) can cause lethargy and respiratory signs (e.g. coughing and respiratory distress) secondary to compression of the trachea and lungs. Osteomas, slow-growing bone tumours primarily involving the skull in ferrets, can result in compression of vital organs and subsequent respiratory abnormalities. In one case, a mass involving the occipital bone in a ferret compressed the larynx and trachea, resulting in respiratory distress (Jensen *et al.*, 1987). A 5-year-old male castrated ferret was referred to the authors' practice with moist upper airway sounds and chronic neurological deficits. The ferret exhibited significant respiratory instability under anaesthesia for imaging of the skull. A CT scan showed a proliferative bony lesion extending from the left osseous bulla to the occipital region and encroaching on the brainstem. Compression of vital central nervous system tissue was felt to be the reason for the respiratory abnormalities. The lesion was not biopsied, but its appearance was consistent with osteoma.

References and further reading

Antinoff N (2002) Clinical observations in ferrets with naturally occurring heartworm disease, and preliminary evaluation of treatment with ivermectin with and without melarsomine. *Recent Advances in Heartworm Disease: Symposium*, 45–55

Bublot I, Randolph RW, Chalvet-Monfray K *et al.* (2006) The surface electrocardiogram in domestic ferrets. *Journal of Veterinary Cardiology* **8**, 87–93

Fox JG (ed.) (1998) *Biology and Diseases of the Ferret, 2nd edn.* Lippincott Williams & Wilkins, Baltimore

Gaztanaga R, Riera A, Cabrero M *et al.* (2006) Clinical case: dilated cardiomyopathy in a ferret. *Proceedings of 41th AVEPA Congress Madrid*, 26th–29th October

Guzman DSM, Mayer J, Melidone R *et al.* (2006) Pacemaker implantation in a ferret (*Mustela putorius furo*) with third-degree AV block. *Veterinary Clinics of North America: Exotic Animal Practice* **9**, 677–687

Jensen WA, Myers RK and Merkley DF (1987) A bony growth of the skull in a ferret. *Laboratory Animal Science* **37**, 780

Kottwitz JJ, Luis-Fuentes V and Micheal B (2006) Nonbacterial thrombotic endocarditis in a ferret (*Mustela putorius furo*). *Journal of Zoo and Wildlife Medicine* **37**, 197–201

Lipman NS, Murphy JC and Fox JG (1987) Clinical, functional and pathologic changes associated with a case of dilatative cardiomyopathy in a ferret. *Laboratory Animal Science* **37**, 210–212

Orcutt C and Donnelly T (2001) Acute ataxia in a young ferret following distemper vaccination. *Laboratory Animal* **30**, 25–27

Petrie JP and Morrisey JK (2004) Cardiovascular and other diseases. In: *Ferrets, Rabbits, and Rodents, 2nd edn*, ed. KE Quesenberry and JW Carpenter, pp 58–71. WB Saunders, Philadelphia

Schultheiss PC and Dolginow SZ (1994) Granulomatous enteritis caused by *Mycobacterium avium* in a ferret. *Journal of the American Veterinary Medical Association* **204**, 1217

Stamoulis ME, Miller MS and Hillyer EV (1997) Cardiovascular diseases. In: *Ferrets, Rabbits, and Rodents*, ed. EV Hillyer and KE Quesenberry, pp. 63–76. WB Saunders, Philadelphia

Stepien RL, Benson KG and Wenholz LJ (2000) M-mode and doppler echocardiographic findings in normal ferrets sedated with ketamine hydrochloride and midazolam. *Veterinary Radiology and Ultrasound* **41**, 452–456

Whary MT and Andrews PLR (1998) Physiology of the ferret. In: *Biology and Diseases of the Ferret, 2nd edn*, ed. JG Fox, pp. 103–148. Lippincott Williams & Wilkins, Baltimore

Wyre NR and Hess L (2005) Clinical technique: ferret thoracocentesis. *Seminars in Avian and Exotic Pet Medicine* **14**, 22–25

27

Ferrets: urogenital and reproductive system disorders

Peter G. Fisher

Introduction

Urogenital disease is not uncommon in the ferret, with degenerative, infectious (bacterial, viral), metabolic, nutritional, neoplastic, anatomical and toxic causes all being represented. Primary reproductive tract disease is uncommon in countries where ferrets are routinely surgically neutered before the age of 1 year; however, as these ferrets age they are more predisposed to adrenal disease and its secondary hormonal influence on prostatic and remaining uterine tissue. Intact and periparturient jills have their own subset of disease conditions and knowledge of the pathophysiology associated with conditions such as pregnancy toxaemia, mastitis and pyometra will aid in their prevention and diagnosis. Early recognition of neonatal disease and knowledge of the normal characteristics of newborn kits will allow the veterinary surgeon to improve kit survival.

Reproductive disease

Reproductive behaviour and physiology

Most reproductive behaviour in the pet ferret is suppressed because of surgical sterilization and exposure to artificial indoor lighting for consistent periods of time (averaging 15 hours per day). An understanding of normal reproductive behaviour is important when interpreting behavioural and physio-logical changes associated with reproductive tract and adrenal disease (see Chapter 17).

Ferrets are seasonal breeders and photoperiod is the environmental stimulus that has the greatest effect on cyclical reproductive activity. The male breeding season is slightly longer than that of the female, with plasma testosterone levels increasing at the end of January (in the northern hemisphere). They then maintain a peak plateau from the end of February until the end of July, then they begin to fall off suddenly after the summer solstice, when the photoperiod is starting to decrease. Testis length similarly shows a steady increase from the end of January to a peak length reached in April.

In the female ferret, pro-oestrus, as indicated by an increase in vulvar size, usually occurs in January or February and lasts approximately 2–3 weeks. Dramatic oedematous vulvar swelling in response to oestrogen secretion by the ovaries is a clear signal that full oestrus has occurred (Figure 27.1). Being an

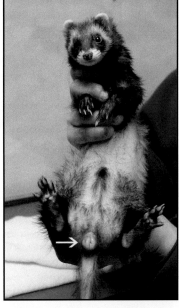

Dramatic vulvar swelling in the intact female ferret is indicative of full oestrus, but neutered ferrets with adrenal disease may also present clinically with a swollen vulva as a result of over-secretion of sex hormones.

induced ovulator, the jill may remain in oestrus for extended periods if not bred. If breeding does not occur, the vulvar tissue will remain swollen and hyperoestrogenism may occur (see Chapter 30). Cystic ovarian remnants resulting from incomplete ovariohysterectomy may also cause a clinical oestrus and hyperoestrogenism.

With the onset of full oestrus, food intake may decrease and jills may sleep less and become irrita-ble. At this time there will be anal, genital and neck sniffing, nose poking and attempts by the male to grab the female by the neck. Some jills may show evidence of being more excitable and nervous, whereas most show no behavioural changes at all. When ready to breed, the female becomes flaccid and submissive and mounting by the hob is allowed. During the mount, the male grabs the nape of the jill's neck with his teeth and will grip her body by wrapping his forelegs around her ribcage. Pelvic thrusts last variable lengths of time up to 3 minutes. Between pelvic thrust bursts, there are periods of rest where the male simply lies over the female and holds on with the neck grip. At the point of penetration the male will increase the arch of his back anteriorly, causing his foreleg grip to slip behind the female's rib cage. Holding this position for a variable but usually pro-longed period of time is the best indication of pene-tration, at which time pelvic thrusting ceases and coupled ferrets can be lifted without being disturbed. In one study (Miller and Anderson, 1989) mating times recorded in 10 pairs of ferrets lasted from 34 to 172 minutes. Abrasions and cellulitis of the vulva may be observed as a result of this aggressive mating.

Ferrets are typically born in the spring. The testes usually descend into the scrotum during fetal development, but complete descent may be delayed for several months after birth. Cryptorchidism is uncommon, with one clinical study of 1597 male ferrets showing an incidence of < 1 % (Bodri, 2000).

Vaginal cytology and vaginitis

Domestic ferret vaginal epithelial cells are morphologically and dynamically similar to those in dogs, with the percentage of highly keratinized superficial cells in vaginal lavages during oestrus usually ≥ 90% (Williams *et al.*, 1992). Vaginal cytology can be used to monitor the reproductive status of females and may serve as a tool in jills that are difficult to breed. The cytology is similar in domestic ferrets and wild species and has been used as an aid in the successful breeding in captivity of the black-footed ferret, *Mustela nigripes* (which is not a colour variant of the domestic ferret but is a wild species native to North America). Within several days following copulation or induced ovulation, superficial cells in vaginal lavages declined in number to anoestrous levels. Therefore vaginal cytology along with a reduction in vulvar size and turgidity can be used as indicators of reproductive recrudesence in oestrous females where a vasectomized male or human chorionic gonadotrophin (hCG) has been used to induce ovulation in females not intended for breeding. It should be noted that the presence of neutrophils in vaginal lavages is normal in the ferret, and *in the absence of bacteria* within neutrophils and other signs of inflammation, does not indicate vaginitis (Williams *et al.*, 1992).

Pyometra

It is generally believed that pyometra is the result of an ascending infection from the vagina or vulva. Jills are predisposed to these infections during oestrus when conditions such as poor husbandry and sanitation and aggressive hob behaviour may cause vulvar cellulitis and vaginitis. Bacteria gain access to the uterus via an open cervix and pyometra may develop when the ferret cycles out of oestrus. Infections may also develop as a sequel to pseudopregnancy in older jills (Lewington, 2007).

Diagnosis and treatment of pyometra in the intact ferret is similar to the dog and cat. A haemogram showing an elevated white blood cell count with neutrophilia and radiographic or ultrasonographic evidence of an enlarged fluid-filled tubular abdominal mass is suggestive of pyometra versus vaginitis in a ferret showing signs of lethargy and inappetence. A purulent vaginal or vulvar discharge may be present and noted after examination and palpation in the case of an open pyometra. *Escherichia coli*, *Staphylococcus*, *Streptococcus* and *Corynebacterium* spp. have all been cultured from infected uteri (Pollock, 2004). Vulvar infection is differentiated from the swelling associated with oestrus by history and vaginal cytology. Treatment of pyometra involves parenteral fluid therapy (to correct dehydration, electrolyte imbalances and any concurrent hypoglycaemia), systemic antibiotics and surgical ovariohysterectomy.

Uterine stump pyometra is seen occasionally in the spayed ferret and occurs most commonly in association with elevated sex hormones as the result of adrenal disease (Figure 27.2). Treatment involves medical and surgical therapy for adrenal disease (see Chapter 30) as well as surgical excision of the infected stump, antibiotic therapy and supportive care.

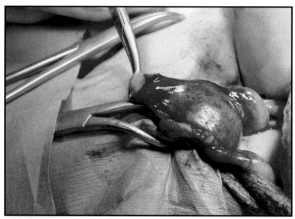

27.2 A uterine stump pyometra, seen occasionally in the spayed ferret and occurring most commonly in association with elevated sex hormones as the result of adrenal disease.

Pregnancy toxaemia

Pregnancy toxaemia is a metabolic disease that develops sporadically in the ferret during late gestation, with increased prevalence in young primiparous jills, or jills with a heavy fetal load, or in association with environmental or dietary stresses. The primary aetiological factor in the disease is development of a relative energy deficiency, either from excess demand or from inadequate dietary intake. The pathogenesis is similar to that of several periparturient metabolic diseases in ruminants, camelids, rodents and mink as well as feline idiopathic hepatic lipidosis (Batchelder *et al.*, 1999). These diseases are characterized by abnormal energy metabolism, which leads to variable degrees of hyperlipidaemia, hypoglycaemia, ketosis and hepatic lipidosis. Lack of nutritional intake with its resulting hypoglycaemia, protein deficiency and energy imbalance also adds to the shift in the physiological balance away from fatty acid metabolism in favour of pathological ketosis and hepatic lipidosis. Lipid accumulation is not directly toxic to the liver but is a marker for underlying metabolic disease.

Toxaemia is most likely to develop when an accidental fast occurs during the last week of gestation. This may happen when an owner tries to replace the ferret's normal diet with a higher quality diet that the jill refuses to eat. Pregnancy toxaemia may also occur in well fed mature jills with exceptionally large litters of 15–20 kits. The onset of toxaemia is acute and clinical signs of disease often include severe lethargy, dehydration, anorexia, weight loss and diarrhoea with or without melaena, with affected jills often shedding excess hair. Sudden death is not uncommon.

Haematological, biochemical and urine analyses are used as diagnostic and prognostic indicators. Anaemia, hypoproteinaemia, azotaemia, hypocalcaemia, and elevated liver enzymes are all common findings, with survival more likely in those ferrets with less pronounced clinical pathology. Other disease entities to consider in the differential diagnosis include septicaemia, metritis, pyometra, dystocia, renal failure and unrelated gastrointestinal or other metabolic disease.

Treatment for pregnancy toxaemia needs to be aggressive and includes Caesarean section, correction of fluid and electrolyte imbalances, reversal of nutritional deficits and treatment of concurrent metabolic disease. The survival of the jill depends on her condition prior to surgery and on intensive peri- and postoperative supportive care (see Chapter 18). Parenteral administration of intravenous fluids with glucose and balanced electrolytes, thermoregulation and addressing any ECG abnormalities are all critical. Supplementation with a high-energy high-protein diet is essential and placement of an oesophagostomy tube to aid in the nutritional reversal of associated hepatic lipidosis is recommended. A gastric antacid such as famotidine is recommended due to the high incidence of gastric ulcers in stressed ferrets (see Chapter 21 for dose rate). Agalactia is common, particularly after Caesarean section, and often necessitates cross-fostering of any surviving kits as handrearing of ferret kits from birth can be difficult.

Prevention of pregnancy toxaemia is the preferred goal. Client education about the prenatal ferret should include a discussion of the ferret's tendency towards olfactory imprinting (which determines food preferences at an early age) and the need to stay consistent with an excellent diet and observant of appetite and body condition during the last half of gestation. Ultrasonography is an effective way to determine pregnancy, gestational age, fetal number and viability in ferrets.

Reproductive tract neoplasia

In a retrospective study of 4774 ferrets (1968–1997) only 2.3% of the 639 tumours recorded involved the reproductive system (Li and Fox, 1998). Williams and Weiss (2004) identified a total of 13 primary tumours of the ovary (three Leydig cell tumours, four granulosa cell tumours, four teratomas and two sex-cord stromal tumours). Most neoplasms of the ovary and uterus were of smooth muscle origin with 72% considered malignant; however, metastasis was not seen and surgical excision was curative. Most ovarian tumours did not produce clinical signs and were incidental findings at the time of ovariohysterectomy.

Alopecia with concurrent elevations in androstenedione and 17-hydroxyprogesterone was seen in two spayed female ferrets in association with sex-cord stromal tumors found at the site of the ovarian pedicle (Patterson *et al.*, 2003); and alopecia, vulvar swelling, hydrometra and elevated oestradiol and progesterone levels were seen in another spayed female ferret diagnosed with an ovarian pedicle leiomyoma (Jekl *et al.*, 2006). Other tumours attributed to the ovarian pedicle in neutered female ferrets include granulosa cell tumour and fibrosarcoma (Brown, 1997). These cases emphasize the need for complete ovariohysterectomy when neutering and offer an additional differential for alopecia.

Williams and Weiss (2004) identified 17 testicular tumours (most commonly in cryptorchid testes): seven Leydig (interstitial) cell tumours, five seminomas, four Sertoli cell tumours (Figure 27.3) and one carcinoma of the rete testis. Of these only one Leydig cell tumour metastasized (to the liver). Affected males may show signs associated with elevated circulating sex hormones such as increased sexual behaviour and aggression, and increased dermal sebaceous gland activity, resulting in a greasy hair coat and distinctive musky odour.

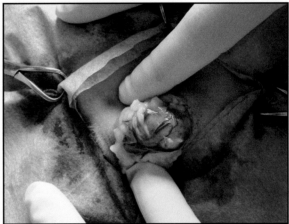
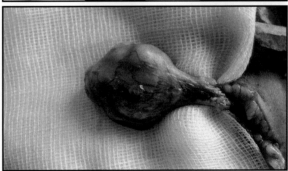

27.3 This 5-year-old 'neutered' male ferret was presented with haematuria and a palpable inguinal mass. Surgical exploration of the abdomen revealed a cryptorchid testis, which was surgically removed and identified as a Sertoli cell tumour on histopathology. The ferret recovered uneventfully and clinical signs resolved. (Courtesy of Veronique Mentre.)

The preputial gland is a specialized apocrine gland. In one study of nine preputial gland neoplasms, one was an adenoma and eight were adenocarcinomas (Li and Fox, 1998). Williams and Weiss (2004) reported that, of 13 preputial masses, nine were adenocarcinomas of the apocrine gland, three were apocrine cysts (Figure 27.4) and one was an apocrine adenoma (Figure 27.5).

Periparturient care and disease

Experienced jills rarely reject their kits but it is not uncommon for primiparous jills to lack maternal instinct and savage or abandon their litters. Ferrets are solitary animals by nature and crowded breeding facilities should be avoided.

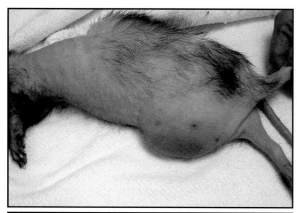

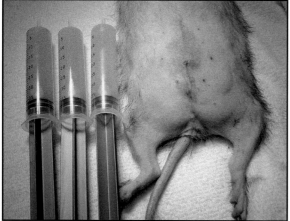

27.4 This very large preputial apocrine cyst was benign but required intermittent drainage for patient comfort and mobility.

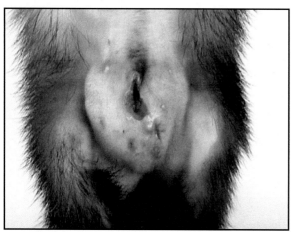

27.5 An advanced preputial apocrine gland adenocarcinoma. Unless diagnosed and resected in their early stage of development, these tumours become so extensive that complete resection requires penile amputation and urethrostomy for urine diversion.

Proper nutrition is of primary importance in maximizing successful breeding of ferrets and in preventing the most common periparturient and neonatal diseases. Ideally the diet should be 36–40% protein and 18–20% fat, with an animal-based protein, preferably meat or poultry meal, listed as the first ingredient (Bell, 1999; see also Chapter 17 for further details on ferret nutrition). This will maximize conception rates and litter size, improve lactation and decrease the susceptibility to pregnancy toxaemia. Litter size has an important effect on both parturition and lactation, with jills carrying smaller litters of less than five kits being more likely to have whelping problems and a propensity to agalactia. It is ideal to breed jills in pairs so that one may serve as a foster mother if the other has a problem with lactation or a primiparous jill rejects her kits, as newborn kits have voracious appetites and are difficult to hand rear. Elevated environmental temperatures may also have an impact on fertility, parturition and a jill's mothering instincts. The ambient temperature in the whelping box or the nursing jill's room should not exceed 21.1°C (Bell, 2004). Lewington (2007) stated that hot climates or excessively warm whelping boxes will predispose to dystocia, poor milk production and diminished maternal instinct.

Dystocia

In addition to small litter sizes and elevated environmental temperatures, other causes of dystocia include pregnancy in older jills, kits of very large size, posterior or sideways presentation and deformed and anasarcous fetuses. Jills with kits in unusual positions in the birth canal are uncomfortable and may be restless or cry out in pain. An average parturition in ferrets occurs over a period of 2–3 hours with approximately five kits born per hour, but some jills take longer than others to whelp. Progress should be steady and there should be no signs of distress. When to intervene with a whelping ferret is always a judgement call but there should be no hesitation to induce labour with oxytocin or take the jill to surgery if her labour exceeds 12–24 hours or as soon as there are any signs of difficulty.

Agalactia

Optimum nutrition and providing a quiet, clean and comfortable environment will encourage nursing and significantly reduce the chances of litter rejection and lactation failure. The jill will not start to nurse her litter until all the kits are born, at which time she will settle into a half-curved position on her side and let the kits suckle from her eight nipples (Lewington, 2007). Any delay in nursing, such as a prolonged delivery or poorly managed nursing environment where the jill fails to settle down, will predispose to the milk drying up.

Mastitis

Mastitis can occur and is usually seen soon after whelping or after the third week of nursing, when larger kits become more aggressive feeders and create increased nursing demands on the dam. Inguinal glands are most commonly affected and, if not diagnosed and treated early, infection will spread rapidly to adjacent glands. *Staphylococcus* spp. and haemolytic *Escherichia coli,* both capable of producing haemolysins and/or toxins, are most commonly incriminated (Besch-Williford, 1987). Affected ferrets will be depressed, febrile and inappetent and show one or more firm, inflamed mammary glands. Kits should be removed and hand fed or fostered and the jill treated with systemic antibiotics, such as amoxicillin/

clavulanate, and warm compresses to encourage drainage of any purulent discharge. For dose rates see Chapter 21. If mammary tissue becomes necrotic, more aggressive treatment including nutritional support, analgesia, fluid therapy and surgical debridement as needed should be instituted. Jills that have acute mastitis may heal completely but may lose a gland or be predisposed to recurrent mastitis.

Kits nursing from jills with infectious mastitis may carry the bacterium orally and spread the organism to unaffected glands or those of a fostering dam. Kits that have reached the age of 3 weeks can do well on milk replacers and Lewington (2007) offers several recipes. At the age of 4–5 weeks a slurry of milk replacer and ground meats can be offered and the kits should be able to feed themselves. Once the kits' eyes are open at 4–5 weeks they can be fed meats along with a good quality ferret food.

Pseudopregnancy

Implantation failure due to the effects of photoperiod or lack of conception from breeding with a sterile or low sperm-count male can predispose to pseudopregnancy (Lewington, 2007). Pseudopregnancy has also been associated with the use of hCG or a vasectomized hob to terminate oestrus and has been seen in oestrous females exposed to the scent of a hob in rut. Jills in false pregnancy can show physical and behavioural changes normally associated with pregnancy, such as weight gain, mammary enlargement, nesting behaviour at the time of whelping and mothering of inanimate objects. Breeders can learn to differentiate pseudopregnancy from true pregnancy as pseudopregnant jills develop a fuller hair coat at about 1.5 weeks prior to 'whelping' whereas normal pregnant jills lose their coats and develop hairless rings around their teats at this time. After the 'whelping' stage occurs the jill will cycle back to normal and return to oestrus if early in the breeding cycle or become quiescent if pseudopregnancy occurs late in the breeding season, and no treatment is required. Adjusting the photoperiod by ensuring maximum lighting intensity in breeding units in the spring and artificially extending light hours in the late summer, as well as using mature sperm-tested hobs, will aid in the prevention of pseudopregnancy.

Neonatal care

Ferret kits weigh approximately 6–12 g at birth and are altricial. They are completely dependent on the jill for homeostasis and nutrition for the first 3 weeks of life. The jill will stimulate urination and defecation by licking the perianal area from birth up until the time of weaning at 6–8 weeks of age. Kits show an interest in food at about 2 weeks but will not eat exclusively on their own until weaned.

The ear canals of ferrets do not open until approximately 32 days of age (compared with 6 days in the cat), which coincides with the appearance of a startle response to loud hand claps and the recording of acoustically activated neurons in the midbrain (Fisher, 2006). This late onset of hearing may explain why kits produce exceptionally loud piercing sounds during their first 4 weeks of life.

Early neonatal mortality, ranging from 8% to 10% of the litter, is greatest within the first 4 days post partum (Besch-Williford, 1987). Neonatal mortality or delivery of small litters of fewer than six kits may result in postpartum or lactational oestrus; and jills with kits should be bred in this oestrus in order to maintain lactation (McLain *et al.*, 1985). Common causes of early death in kits include cannibalism, stillbirths and congenital defects with agenesis of limbs, anencephaly, hemivertebrae, scoliosis, gastroschisis and cranioschisis, and cleft lip and palate all being reported (McLain *et al.*, 1985). After the kits reach 5 days of age the death rate drops dramatically, with lactation failure, maternal neglect, dirty or overheated nest boxes and infectious disease all being incriminated in older kits (Besch-Williford, 1987).

Kits may develop ophthalmia neonatorum secondary to nursing a dam with mastitis or minute eyelid punctures acquired as the result of being dragged around in the nursing box by an unsettled jill. Purulent discharge collects behind the unopened eyelids, resulting in a painful bulge that discourages nursing. Affected lids are treated by forcing the lids open with a 15 scalpel blade or 0.50 mm needle and flushing away debris followed by broad-spectrum topical ophthalmic antibiotic for several days. See also Chapter 29.

Bell (2004) reports a life-threatening neonatal diarrhoea caused by a rotavirus and/or bacterium. Kits 1–7 days old are at greatest risk of dying from weakness, anorexia and dehydration. Treatment involves subcutaneous fluids and systemic antibiotics to prevent secondary bacterial endotoxaemia.

'Swimmer' or splay-legged kits have been reported, with affected kits lacking strength in all four limbs so that they lie sternally with subsequent rib compression and potentially fatal breathing problems (Lewington, 2007). The underlying cause may be genetic or related to rapidly growing kits placing excessive weight on immature limbs and a nursery with smooth flooring that does not allow purchase of feet for standing.

Urinary tract disease

Clinical pathology

Renal function

Because the BUN can be influenced by non-renal factors, creatinine generally serves as a better indicator of renal function. However, ferrets are unique in that normal creatinine levels (17.7–46.2 µmol/l) are considerably lower than in other mammals. As a result, serum creatinine levels that can be considered high in ferrets could still be within the normal range for other species (Morrisey and Ramer, 1999). Mechanisms of creatinine excretion other than free glomerular filtration, such as renal tubular secretion or greater enteric degradation, may have a larger role in the excretion of creatinine in this species (Esteves *et al.*, 1994). Consequently, elevations in the concentration of BUN associated with renal failure are not always accompanied by increases in the concentration of serum creatinine and any increase in serum creatinine above normal should be considered significant.

Circulating levels of phosphorus are largely controlled by the kidneys, and consistent elevations in phosphorus in the face of isosthenuria and azotaemia are not uncommon in animals with renal failure. The hyperphosphataemia that occurs in chronic renal failure is closely related to dietary protein intake inasmuch as protein-rich diets are also high in phosphorus. Therefore one can assume that carnivores such as the ferret would most likely develop the hyperphosphataemia and renal secondary hyperparathyroidism seen in canine and feline chronic renal failure.

Figure 27.6 gives reference serum chemistry values for parameters associated with renal disease.

Parameter	Value
BUN (mmol/l)	3.5–16.1
Creatinine (µmol/l)	35.3–79.6
Phosphorus (mmol/l)	1.3–2.9
Calcium (mmol/l)	2.0–3.0

27.6 Ferret reference values for parameters associated with renal disease. (Data from Quesenberry and Orcutt, 2004)

Other clinicopathological abnormalities associated with renal failure may include RBC suppression, acidosis, hyperkalaemia and hypo- or hypercalcaemia. Anaemia of chronic renal failure is a common entity and results from reduced erythropoietin production by damaged kidneys, uraemic inhibition of RBC production and increased red blood cell haemolysis.

Urinalysis

Urinalysis offers practitioners an excellent tool for assessing urinary tract health and should be performed in any ferret with suspected urogenital disease. Normal results are shown in Figure 27.7. The specific gravity can help differentiate pre-renal versus renal azotaemia. Urine protein can be elevated with urinary tract inflammation, haemorrhage and infection or be an indication of renal damage. Protein levels in the urine must be interpreted along with the urine specific gravity and sediment analysis. Healthy adult domestic ferrets may have trace to small amounts of proteinuria. Proteinuria has been associated with amyloidosis occurring in black-footed ferrets (*Mustela nigripes*) having serum chemistries consistent with chronic renal disease (Garner *et al.*, 2007). Haematuria can result from upper or lower urinary tract disease or be of uterine origin in intact females.

Parameter	Value
Specific gravity	n/a
Protein (mg/dl)	0–33
pH	6.5–7.5
Urine volume (ml/24h)	26–140

27.7 Normal urinalysis results. (Data from Morrisey and Ramer, 1999)

Urine sediment analysis can offer information on urinary tract haemorrhage, inflammation and bacteria. Bacteriuria can be an indication of upper or lower urinary tract infection but is more commonly associated with lower urinary tract disease. Bacteriuria may also be associated with prostatic or uterine infections.

Renal disease

Renal pathology is not uncommon in the ferret and many ferrets older than 4 years have varying degrees of chronic interstitial nephritis. A review of 61 cases showed that the most prevalent causes of ferret renal pathology included acute nephritis (22%), renal cysts (15%), glomerulonephritis (14%), pyelonephritis (6%), glomerulosclerosis (4%), congestion (4%) and tubular atrophy (4%) (Kawasaki, 1994). Other causes of ferret renal pathology include Aleutian disease, toxic nephropathies and renal disease associated with urinary tract calculi and neoplasia.

Aleutian disease

Aleutian disease parvovirus usually presents as a chronic latent infection in ferrets. While the parvovirus itself causes little or no harm to the ferret, the marked inflammatory response generated by the host results in production of a large number of antigen–antibody complexes. These circulate in the body and with time cause systemic vasculitis, most notably in the glomerular capillaries. As the disease progresses, a marked membranous glomerulonephritis and tubular interstitial nephritis may result in eventual renal failure and death. For further details see Chapter 31.

Chronic interstitial nephritis

Varying degrees of chronic interstitial nephritis are commonly found on necropsy of geriatric ferrets. Chronic interstitial nephritis is a progressive disease with lesions seen as early as 2 years and advanced cases resulting in renal failure as early as 4.5 years (Williams, 2004). Clinical signs vary with severity of kidney pathology. Polydipsia and polyuria may be associated with early kidney failure, with progression to anorexia, weight loss and lethargy as chronic interstitial nephritis and the uraemia of chronic renal failure progress.

Kidneys with significant disease are generally grossly pitted and large focal depressions may be seen in the outer cortex as a result of scarring. Severely affected kidneys may be asymmetrical with respect to size. The pattern of microscopic changes associated with chronic interstitial nephritis in the ferret is unique and pathologists with little ferret tissue experience may be tempted to diagnose chronic infarction. As the disease progresses, there is a diffuse glomerulosclerosis throughout the cortex and fibrosis may progress so that large areas are devoid of functional glomeruli and tubules.

Depending on the progression of renal failure and uraemia, the ferret will present in varying states of lethargy, gastrointestinal upset, decreased appetite or total anorexia, increased or decreased water intake, dehydration and general malaise. Once a diagnosis is made, general treatment guidelines for animals of any species (including ferrets) with chronic renal failure include the following:

- Discontinue any potentially nephrotoxic drugs
- Identify and treat any pre-renal or post-renal abnormalities
- Identify any treatable conditions such as urolithiasis or pyelonephritis
- Initiate intravenous fluid therapy to reduce azotaemia. Follow up with maintenance subcutaneous fluid therapy (owners can be taught to do this at home). Volumes given vary with patient size; in ferrets, 50–60 ml per injection site. Normal daily water intake in ferrets is estimated to be 100 ml/kg
- Dietary management: studies have shown that cats that consume a prescription kidney-failure diet have increased survival compared with cats that do not (or will not) eat this type of diet (Plotnick, 2007). Many food manufacturers offer feline prescription renal failure diets, but benefits of their long-term use in ferrets have not been published. Renal-friendly dietary changes may be difficult to incorporate in the ferret as a result of specific high-protein requirements and the olfactory imprinting that determines dietary preference at an early age
- If hyperphosphataemic, initiate enteric phosphate binders
- Treat increased gastric acidity with H2 blockers and its associated gastroenteritis with metaclopramide or maropitant
- Multivitamin supplementation is recommended as the excessive amount of urine produced by failing kidneys commonly results in loss of water-soluble vitamins
- Human recombinant erythropoietin may be used to reverse the anaemia associated with renal failure, but the author does not have personal experience with use of this product and no published studies of its use in ferrets could be found
- Consider use of omega-3 fatty acid supplements based on studies showing their beneficial effects in other species (Plotnick, 1996)

- Depending on response to therapy, quality of life issues and euthanasia should be discussed with the owner of any patient with renal failure.

See Chapter 21 for more specific information on drug dosing and frequency.

Toxic nephropathy

Ferrets are naturally curious and are very skilful at accessing storage areas, where they may be exposed to a variety of toxins such as chemicals, cleaning agents, medications and pest control products. Unsupervised ferrets can readily pry the tops off child-resistant bottles or chew through plastic containers to access potentially toxic medications. Iatrogenic drug toxicities are also common. Potential nephrotoxic agents as reported by the National Animal Poison Control Center of the American Society for the Prevention of Cruelty to Animals (Richardson and Balabuszko, 2000) include cadmium, cholecalciferol, diquat herbicides, ethylene glycol, mercury, nephrotoxic antibacterials (polymyxin-B, gentamicin, neomycin), ibuprofen and other non-steroidal anti-inflammatory drugs (NSAIDs), oxalic acid, phenolics, rhubarb, and zinc, copper and mercury. Pharmacological agents that have nephrotoxic potential in dogs and cats (e.g. aminoglycosides) can also adversely affect ferrets.

Hydronephrosis

Hydronephrosis (Figure 27.8) is an uncommon finding in the ferret. The author has seen two cases that resulted from inadvertent ligation of the ureter during ovariohysterectomy. Presurgical biochemical renal parameters were normal, indicating a functional contralateral kidney, and both cases were treated via unilateral nephrectomy.

Hydronephrosis in the ferret has also been reported secondary to obstruction with ureteral calculi (Orcutt, 2003) and has been reported in association with a carcinoma of undetermined origin involving the renal pelvis (Bell and Moeller, 1990).

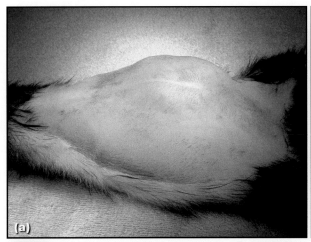
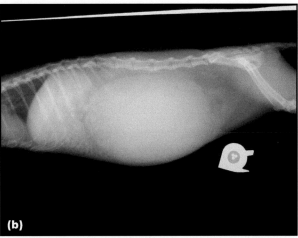

27.8 **(a)** This ferret presented for an obvious abdominal swelling, most noticeable when the ferret was laid on its back. **(b)** Abdominal palpation revealed a mid-abdominal mass, approximately 6 × 10 cm, which was confirmed radiographically as a large radiopaque mass of uniform fluid density consistent with an enlarged kidney. (continues) ▶

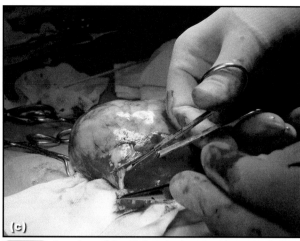
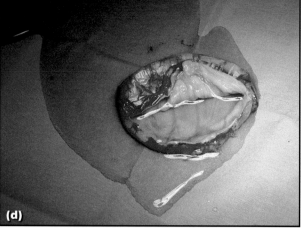

27.8 (continued) **(c,d)** Surgical exploration revealed severe hydronephrosis, which was successfully treated by unilateral nephrectomy.

Diagnosis of hydronephrosis is made by abdominal palpation of an enlarged kidney or abdominal mass and confirmed radiographically as a uniformly radiopaque unilateral mid-abdominal mass. Ultrasonography or intravenous pyelography will help to confirm the diagnosis and confirm the presence of hydroureter and underlying causes of ureteral blockage. Analysis of fluid removed from the hydronephrotic kidney via a fine-needle aspirate usually reveals a transudate, unless secondary bacterial infection is present. Unilateral nephrectomy carries a good prognosis if the remaining kidney function is normal.

Pyelonephritis

Pyelonephritis is uncommon in the ferret and when present is usually associated with an ascending bacterial urinary tract infection or septicaemia. Adrenal-associated prostatic disease and cystitis are the most common causes of urinary tract infection in the author's practice, with *Escherichia coli* and *Staphylococcus aureus* being the most common causative agents. Severe suppurative pyelonephritis progressing to end-stage chronic renal failure was reported in a ferret being treated for cutaneous epitheliotropic lymphoma (Rosenbaum *et al.*, 1996). In this case, the authors theorized that immunosuppression from long-term corticosteroid administration could have led to bacterial cystitis and subsequent pyelonephritis.

Clinical signs of pyelonephritis include pyrexia, lethargy, anorexia and pain on palpation of the kidneys. Chronic untreated pyelonephritis can result in renal failure manifested clinically as profound anorexia and lethargy with subsequent weight loss and declining condition. Differentiating cystitis and lower urinary tract disease from pyelonephritis can be difficult and is based on history, physical examination findings and diagnostic workup. Ultrasonography or an intravenous pyelogram may help to confirm pyelonephritis.

In addition to appropriate treatment for chronic renal failure as outlined above, nutritional support and 3–6 weeks of antibacterial therapy based on urine culture and antibacterial susceptibility results should be instituted. Length of therapy depends on clinical improvement, underlying disease and follow-up cultures and clinical pathology.

Urogenital cystic disease

Renal cysts: Renal cysts are not uncommon in ferrets, with the incidence being reported as high as 10–15% of necropsied ferrets (Pollock, 2004). Renal cysts may be hereditary, developmental or acquired. Hereditary conditions include polycystic disease; developmental conditions include renal dysplasia and renal cortical cysts; and acquired conditions include medullary cystic disease, post-necrotic cyst formation, endometriosis and neoplasia. The precise aetiology of cystic renal disease in the ferret is unknown, with one source presuming they are congenital in origin (Fox *et al.*, 1998) and another stating that there is some speculation that chronic urinary tract infection leads to low-grade nephritis that predisposes the kidneys to cysts (Williams, 2004).

Most renal cysts do not cause clinical disease and are found incidentally during routine surgery (Figure 27.9), necropsy or ultrasonography (as one or more hypoechoic areas). Cysts are usually present singly or in small numbers and are most commonly found in the cortices of one or both kidneys.

Polycystic kidney disease (PKD) has been reported in ferrets but is rare. Polycystic kidneys are grossly enlarged and may be palpable as a slightly irregular firm oval mass or masses in the mid-abdomen. Renal

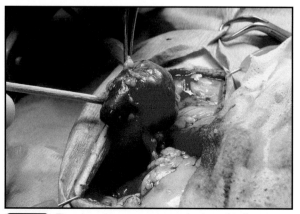

27.9 Renal cysts may range up to 1 cm in diameter and when viewed from the capsule surface are thin, bulge slightly and are fluid-filled.

failure with uraemic encephalopathy was suspected in one case of bilateral polycystic kidney disease where the cortex and medulla contained numerous fluid-filled cysts of various sizes (Dillberger, 1985). See also Chapter 19 for diagnosis.

Bladder cysts: Single or multiple semi-spherical to bilobulated fluid-filled cystic structures of variable size were observed on the dorsal aspects of the urinary bladders of four male and two female ferrets (Li *et al.*, 1996). The cysts were palpated as caudal abdominal masses and three of the six ferrets presented with dysuria and/or haematuria. The cysts were attached to the trigone or neck of the bladder, with variable intra-luminal communication with the bladder and/or ure-thra. Cystic urogenital anomalies were diagnosed based on history, clinical presentation, cystograms, involvement of both sexes and pathological findings. It was theorized that the location of the cysts on the dor-sal aspect of the urinary bladder and/or proximal ure-thra in ferrets of both sexes suggested that the cysts might have originated from the mesonephric or para-mesonephric duct remnant. Three of the six ferrets showed signs of adrenal disease, with alopecia in two and vulvar swelling in one ferret; and adrenal histologi-cal examination performed post mortem in five of the ferrets showed evidence of either adrenal hyperplasia or neoplasia. These findings support the close associa-tion of adrenal disease with various paraprostatic and urogenital cysts in the ferret. If identified, diagnosis and treatment for adrenal disease should be pursued.

Urolithiasis

Urolithiasis in the ferret may be characterized by single or multiple calculi found anywhere throughout the urinary tract. Magnesium ammonium phosphate (MAP) or struvite uroliths unassociated with concurrent urease-positive microbial infections are most commonly reported (Orcutt, 2003), but cystine bladder calculi have been reported (Dutton, 1996) and the author has seen two cases of cystine urolithiasis in mature males. The incidence of urolithiasis has lessened as ferret-specific commercial diets have improved nutritionally and gained acceptance among ferret owners. One study alluded to an association between increased protein intake and its effect in lowering urine pH as a factor in decreasing urine struvite crystalluria (Palmore and Bartos, 1987), while Bell (1999) showed an association between ferret urolithiasis and diets containing poor-quality meat protein or too high a proportion of cereal protein. It is interesting to note that, in cats (another species where non-infectious associated struvite urolithiasis occurs), diets formulated to contain higher fat and lower protein and potassium content and with increased urinary acidifying potential may minimize formation of MAP uroliths (Lekcharoensuk *et al.*, 2001). Therefore the increased fat content of modern commercial ferret foods, as well as the increase in animal-based protein and its effect on acidifying urine, may play a role in the decreased incidence of MAP uroliths in ferrets.

The recommendation for preventing recurrence of cystine urolithiasis in dogs and cats is to utilize protein-restrictive urine-alkalinizing diets. This is in direct contrast to the high-protein urine-acidifying diet recommended for prevention of MAP uroliths. The question becomes: will feeding the ferret a diet lower in protein then predispose to MAP calculi, much as diet changes recommended in the 1990s for cats with struvite stones resulted in urine pH changes that then encouraged the formation of more calcium oxalate calculi?

Alteration of the diet in the mature ferret may be difficult, due to the animal's predilection for olfactory imprinting on certain diets at a young age. In addition, it must be asked whether lowering dietary protein may predispose the ferret to muscle wasting. In the author's experience with cystine calculi, in two cases the owners did not change diets for these reasons and recurrence of cystine calculi was not seen. The relatively short lifespan of the ferret may play a role in not seeing recurrent cystine calculi, as they may not have time to redevelop. In dogs cystine uroliths are most frequently a manifestation of hereditary cystin-uria associated with the *SLC3A1 (rBAT)* gene (Henthorn *et al.*, 2000) and in the field of ferret genetics the c-kit receptor tyrosine kinase gene (*KIT*) has been anecdotally associated with two ferrets that developed cystine urinary calculi while on high-protein diets (Lewington, 2007). This raises the question as to whether diet or genetics (or both) is responsible for ferret cystine uroliths.

Clinical signs depend on calculus location. The bladder is the most common site for calculi formation and affected ferrets will show varying degrees of stranguria, pollakiuria, haematuria and abdominal discomfort. Acute renal failure and post-renal azotaemia and uraemia can occur in the ferret with calculus-associated urethral obstruction. In addition, hydronephrosis secondary to obstruction with ureteral calculi and renal pelvis calculi has been reported in the ferret.

Diagnosis of urolithiasis is made based on history, physical examination findings, urinalysis and imaging (Figure 27.10). Treatment varies with stone location and severity of disease. Cystic calculi are the easiest to remove via surgical cystotomy (Figure 27.11).

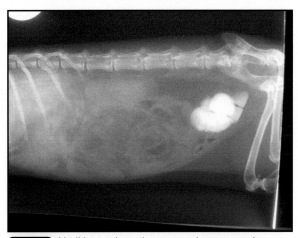

27.10 Uroliths such as the magnesium ammonium phosphate calculi seen on this radiograph are found most commonly in adult male ferrets, but an increased incidence is also reported in pregnant jills on a poor plane of nutrition.

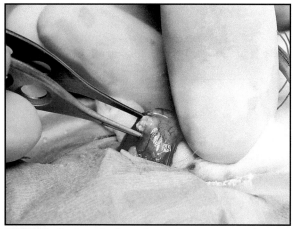

27.11   Cystic calculi are the easiest to remove via surgical cystotomy.

Urethral calculus obstruction may be relieved by anaesthetizing the patient and using a urethral catheter to flush the stone into the bladder, followed by removal via cystotomy. If unsuccessful at dislodging the calculus, perineal urethrostomy may be performed. (See also Chapter 23.)

The long-term prognosis for ferrets with bilateral renal calculi is guarded. Supportive treatment includes analgesia, appetite stimulants, antibiotics as indicated and showing owners how to administer daily or every-other-day subcutaneous fluids. Indications for surgical removal of nephroliths include obstruction of the renal pelvis and urine outflow, chronic recurrent urinary tract infection associated with nephrolithiasis, symptomatic patients where nephroliths are substantially increasing in size, or progressive deterioration of renal function. Surgical procedures vary with size and location of the nephrolith and include nephrotomy, pyelolithotomy or nephrectomy. The surgeon needs to be aware that incising renal parenchyma results in destruction of some nephrons. All animals undergoing nephrotomy should have urine production measured during and following surgery to assure normal function in the contralateral kidney. A ureterotomy can be performed for retrieval of unilateral ureteroliths but is a microsurgical technique best performed with the aid of an operating microscope and 0.7 or 0.5 metric (6/0 or 7/0 USP) absorbable suture material. Alternatively, a nephrectomy can be performed with unilateral ureteral or renal pelvic calculi causing obstruction and hydronephrosis. (See also Chapter 23.)

Calculus chemical analysis and urine bacterial culture and antimicrobial sensitivity testing is warranted in all cases of calculus-related uropathy.

Cystitis

Cystitis in the ferret may occur as a primary ascending bacterial infection similar to the canine disease. Clinical signs include haematuria, dysuria, pollakiuria and a painful abdomen. Diagnosis is based on clinical signs and urine analysis with special attention to urine sediment, where varying numbers of red and white blood cells and bacteria confirm the diagnosis. Cystitis may also be seen in association with pyelonephritis, secondary to cystic calculi, or in adrenal disease associated with prostatic cysts and/or prostatitis.

Therefore cases of recurrent cystitis warrant a further diagnostic workup including urine bacterial culture, imaging and adrenal hormone analysis.

Several antibiotic choices are appropriate for empirical treatment of uncomplicated infection, or pending bacterial culture and sensitivity results in complicated infections, and include amoxicillin, amoxicillin/clavulanate, trimethoprim/sulfadiazine and enrofloxacin. Treatment for 14 days (uncomplicated infections) or for 4 weeks (complicated infections) with follow-up urinalysis and bacterial culture as indicated is recommended.

Adrenal-associated prostatic disease

It should be noted that, according to several large private US ferret breeders, prostatic disease is rare in the intact hob and the most common problem reported in intact male ferrets is hair loss from being in season too long (Vickie McKimmey, personal communication). However, cystic prostatic disease, prostatomegaly and prostatic abscesses (Figure 27.12) are common findings in the male ferret secondary to adrenal disease.

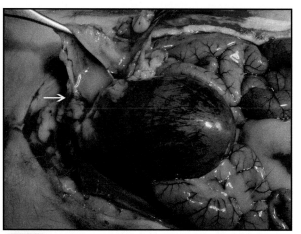

27.12   This neutered male ferret died as the result of a prostatic abscess (arrowed) that developed secondary to underlying adrenal disease.

A review of case materials at the Armed Forces Institute of Pathology identified six cases of ferret prostatitis or prostatic/periprostatic cysts (Coleman *et al.*, 1998). The review showed that a significant number of these ferrets had coexisting proliferative adrenal lesions (hyperplasia or neoplasia). Microscopic examination of prostate tissue revealed multiple cysts of various sizes lined by keratinizing squamous epithelium frequently filled by lamellated keratin admixed with numerous neutrophils. These are common histopathological changes associated with excess circulating androgen levels in many mammalian species.

Ferrets with adrenal disease commonly present with varying degrees of alopecia, pruritus, increased sexual behaviour or a more pronounced musky odour associated with dermal sebaceous gland hyperplasia. However, some male ferrets with adrenal disease present with prostatic enlargement alone (Figure 27.13). These ferrets usually show varying degrees of dysuria and pollakiuria as a result of partial or complete urethral obstruction, and, depending on the duration and degree of obstruction, may show urinary incontinence or dribbling, with wet fur and excessive licking of the prepuce or perineum. Within 24 hours, renal failure as a result of obstructive disease occurs and ferrets will demonstrate behaviours consistent with abdominal pain, including depression, grinding of the teeth (bruxism), walking with an arched back and vocalizing when urinating. Ultrasonography can be performed to confirm adrenal disease and to rule out urolithiasis.

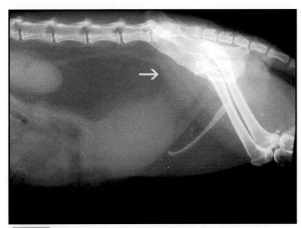

27.13 Prostatomegaly or periprostatic cysts may cause urethral compression and bladder distension. Ferrets present with two or more firm to fluctuant masses palpable in the caudal abdomen and confirmed radiographically (arrowed).

Treatment for acute renal failure secondary to urethral obstruction involves analgesia and relieving the obstruction followed by fluid diuresis, correction of electrolyte imbalances, secondary gastrointestinal disturbances and urinary tract infection. The options available for relieving the obstruction include urethral catheterization, urethrotomy, or placement of a cystostomy catheter. Urethral catheterization of the male ferret is complicated by the J-shaped os penis, the narrow diameter of the penile urethra and the acute bend of the urethra at the pelvic canal (Figure 27.14). Initial catheterization may be aided by use of retrograde flushing through a blunt needle placed in the urethral orifice opening to dilate the urethra and allow for placement of a closed-ended urinary catheter (see also Chapter 18). A tube cystostomy has also been advocated as a means of providing urine outflow and relieving the immediate cause of acute renal failure (Nolte *et al.*, 2002).

Marsupialization of large periprostatic cysts or prostatic abscesses has been advocated as a method of immediate treatment while addressing underlying adrenal disease (Orcutt, 2001). See Chapter 23 for further details of surgical techniques. Marsupialization allows for immediate decompression of fluid-filled structures applying pressure on the urethra as well as drainage external to the abdominal cavity, thus avoiding peritonitis that has been associated with simple debulking of infected prostatic tissues. Regardless of which method the clinician uses to relieve urethral obstruction secondary to ferret prostatic disease, long-term management involves addressing the underlying adrenal disease.

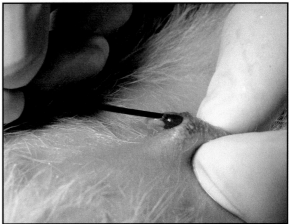

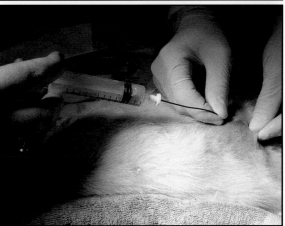

27.14 The author uses a 3 French, 11 cm open-ended silicone urinary catheter to catheterize and flush the urethra in cases of obstruction secondary to calculi, viscous pyuria or prostatomegaly.

Urinary tract neoplasia

Urinary tract neoplasia is generally considered rare in ferrets. An archive of 1525 ferret neoplasms compiled over a 10-year period (1990–2000) at the Armed Forces Institute of Pathology (Washington, DC) and a commercial pathology laboratory demonstrated seven cases of primary or secondary neoplasia involving the kidneys or bladder (Williams and Weiss, 2004).

Transitional cell carcinoma has been reported in the bladder (Bell and Moeller, 1990) and is the most commonly reported primary tumour of the ferret kidney, usually arising in the renal pelvis. Renal cell carcinomas and adenomas have also been reported in the ferret (Li *et al.*, 1998). Papillary tubular cystadenomas are benign and have only been reported once as an incidental finding (Li and Fox, 1998). The ferret kidney may also be the site of metastatic disease. In a retrospective study on malignant lymphoma in the ferret (Li *et al.*, 1998), stage IV lymphoma had invaded the kidneys in eight out of 18 ferrets. In a study of 31 ferrets with confirmed lymphoma, 19% had abnormal renal values on blood chemistry analysis (Antinoff, 2007).

Clinical signs of urinary tract neoplasia include haematuria, dysuria, incontinence, abdominal effusion, anorexia, lethargy and weight loss. Abdominal palpation, radiography, urinalysis, ultrasonography and ultrasound-guided needle biopsy can be used to refine the diagnosis. Renal neoplasms generally present as cystic areas on ultrasound examination and may be mistaken for renal cysts, a more common and benign finding in many exotic mammals.

Primary renal tumours may be treated with nephrectomy and surgical excision. These tumours are often resistant to chemotherapy in human patients and little exists in the literature for chemotherapeutic use in domestic animals. Ferret transitional cell carcinomas may respond to surgical excision, radiation therapy and chemotherapy based upon the location of the mass.

References and further reading

Antinoff N (2007) Lymphoma in ferrets: review and preliminary findings. *Proceedings AEMV Scientific Program*, 99–100

Batchelder MA, Bell JA, Erdman SE *et al.* (1999) Pregnancy toxemia in the European ferret (*Mustela putorius furo*). *Laboratory Animal Science* **49**(40), 372–379

Bell JA (2004) Ferrets: periparturient and neonatal diseases. In: *Ferrets, Rabbits and Rodents: Clinical Medicine and Surgery, 2nd edn*, ed. KE Quesenberry and JW Carpenter, pp. 50–57. WB Saunders, Philadelphia

Bell JA (1999) Ferret nutrition. *Veterinary Clinics of North America: Exotic Animal Practice* **2**(1), 169–192

Bell RC and Moeller RB (1990) Transitional cell carcinoma of the renal pelvis in a ferret. *Laboratory Animal Science* **40**(5), 537–538

Besch-Williford CL (1987) Biology and medicine of the ferret. *Veterinary Clinics of North America: Small Animal Practice* **17**(5), 1155–1183

Bodri MS (2000) Theriogenology question of the month. *Journal of the American Veterinary Medical Association* **217**(10), 1465–1466

Brown SA (1997) Ferrets: neoplasia. In: *Ferrets, Rabbits and Rodents: Clinical Medicine and Surgery*, ed. EV Hillyer and KE Quesenberry, pp. 99–114. WB Saunders, Philadelphia

Coleman GD, Chavez MA and Williams BH (1998) Cystic prostatic disease associated with adrenocortical lesions in the ferret (*Mustela putorius furo*). *Veterinary Pathology* **35**, 547–549

Dillberger JE (1985) Polycystic kidneys in a ferret. *Journal of the American Veterinary Medical Association* **186**(1), 74–75

Dutton MA (1996) Treatment of cystine bladder urolith in a ferret (*Mustela putorius furo*). *Exotic Pet Practice* **1**(8), 7

Esteves ML, Marini RP, Ryder EB, Murphy JL and Fox JG (1994) Estimation of glomerular filtration rate and evaluation of renal function in ferrets (*Mustela putorius furo*). *American Journal of Veterinary Research* **55**(1), 166–172

Fisher PG (2006) Ferret behavior. In: *Exotic Pet Behavior, Birds, Reptiles and Small Mammals*, ed. T Bradley Bays *et al.*, pp. 163–205. Elsevier, Philadelphia

Fox JA, Parson RC and Bell JA (1998) Diseases of the genitourinary system. In: *Biology and Diseases of the Ferret*, ed. JG Fox, pp. 247–272. Williams and Wilkins, Baltimore

Fox JG and Bell JA (1998) Growth, reproduction, and breeding. In: *Biology and Diseases of the Ferret, 2nd edn*, ed. JG Fox, pp. 211–246. Williams and Wilkins, Baltimore

Garner MM, Raymond JT, O'Brien TD *et al.* (2007) Amyloidosis in the black-footed ferret (*Mustela nigripes*) (abstract). *Journal of Zoo and Wildlife Medicine* **38**(1), 32–41

Gentz EJ and Veatch JK (1995) Cystic ovarian remnant in a ferret. *Journal of Small Exotic Animal Medicine* **3**(2), 45–47

Henthorn PS, Liu J, Gidalevich T *et al.* (2000) Canine cystinuria: polymorphism in the SLC3A1 gene and identification of a nonsense mutation in cystinuric Newfoundland dogs. *Human Genetics* **107**(4), 295–303

Jekl V, Hauptman K, Jeklova E *et al.* (2006) Hydrometra in a ferret – case report. *Veterinary Clinics of North America: Exotic Animal Practice* **9**, 695–700

Kawasaki TA (1994) Normal parameters and laboratory interpretation of disease states in the domestic ferret. *Seminars in Avian and Exotic Pet Practice* **3**(1), 40–47

Kruger JM, Osborne CA, Lulich JP *et al.* (1996) Inherited and congenital diseases of the feline lower urinary tract. *Veterinary Clinics of North America: Small Animal Practice* **26**(2), 265–279

Lekcharoensuk C, Osborne CA, Lulich JP *et al.* (2001) Association between dietary factors and calcium oxalate and magnesium ammonium phosphate urolithiasis in cats. *Journal of the American Veterinary Medical Association* **219**(9), 1228–1237

Lewington JH (2007) *Ferret Husbandry, Medicine and Surgery, 2nd edn.* Saunders/Elsevier, Philadelphia

Li X and Fox JG (1998) Neoplastic diseases. In: *Biology and Diseases of the Ferret*, ed. JG Fox, pp. 405–447. Williams & Wilkins, Baltimore

Li X, Fox JG, Erdman SE, Lipman NS and Murphy JC (1996) Cystic urogenital anomalies in ferrets (*Mustela putorius furo*). *Veterinary Pathology* **33**, 150–158

Li X, Fox JG and Padrid PA (1998) Neoplastic diseases in ferrets: 574 cases (1968–1997). *Journal of the American Veterinary Medical Association* **212**(1), 1402–1406

McLain DE, Harper SM, Roe DA *et al.* (1985) Congenital malformations and variations in reproductive performance in the ferret: effects of maternal age, color and parity. *Laboratory Animal Science* **35**, 251–255

Miller BJ and Anderson SH (1989) Failure of fertilization following abbreviated copulation in the ferret (*Mustela putorius furo*). *Journal of Experimental Zoology* **249**, 85–89

Morrisey JK and Ramer JC (1999) Ferrets: clinical pathology and sample collection. *Veterinary Clinics of North America: Exotic Animal Practice* **2**(3), 553–564

Neal J, Murphy BD, Moger WH and Oliphant LW (1977) Reproduction in the male ferret: gonadal activity during the annual cycle; recrudescence and maturation. *Biology of Reproduction* **17**, 380–385

Nolte DM, Carberry CA, Gannon KM and Boren FC (2002) Temporary tube cystostomy as a treatment for urinary obstruction secondary to adrenal disease in four ferrets. *Journal of the American Animal Hospital Association* **38**(6), 527–532

Orcutt C (2001) Treatment of urogenital disease in ferrets. *Exotic DVM* **3**(3), 31–37

Orcutt CJ (2003) Ferret urogenital diseases. *Veterinary Clinics of North America: Exotic Animal Practice* **6**(1), 113–138

Osborne CA, Snaderson SL, Lulich JP *et al.* (1999) Canine cystine urolithiasis cause, detection treatment and prevention. *Veterinary Clinics of North America: Small Animal Practice* **29**(1), 193–211

Palmore WP and Bartos KD (1987) Food intake and struvite crystalluria in ferrets. *Veterinary Research Communications* **11**, 519–526

Patterson MM, Rogers AB, Schrenzel MD *et al.* (2003) Alopecia attributed to neoplastic ovarian tissue in two female ferrets. *Comparative Medicine* **53**(2), 213–217

Peter AT, Bell JA, Manning DD and Bosu WTK (1990) Real-time ultrasonographic determination of pregnancy and gestational age in ferrets. *Laboratory Animal Science* **40**(1), 91–92

Plotnick AN (1996) The role of omega-3 fatty acids in renal disorders. *Journal of the American Veterinary Medical Association* **209**(1), 906–910

Plotnick AN (2007) Feline chronic renal failure: long-term medical management. *Compendium on Continuing Education for the Practicing Veterinarian* **29**(6), 342–350

Pollock CG (2004) Ferret: urogenital diseases. In: *Ferrets, Rabbits and Rodents: Clinical Medicine and Surgery, 2nd edn*, ed. KE Quesenberry and JW Carpenter, pp. 41–49. WB Saunders, Philadelphia

Quesenberry KE and Orcutt C (2004) Basic approach to veterinary care. In: *Ferrets, Rabbits and Rodents: Clinical Medicine and Surgery, 2nd edn*, ed. KE Quesenberry and JW Carpenter, pp. 286–298. WB Saunders, Philadelphia

Richardson JA and Balabuszko RA (2000) Managing ferret toxicosis. *Exotic DVM* **2**(4), 23–26.

Rosenbaum MR, Affolter VK *et al.* (1996) Cutaneous epitheliotropic lymphoma in a ferret. *Journal of the American Veterinary Medical Association* **209**(8), 1441–1444

Williams BH (2004) Pathology of the domestic ferret (*Mustela putorius furo*). In: *2004 C.L. Davis ACVP Symposium Pathology of Non-Traditional Pets*, pp. 103–132

Williams BH and Weiss CA (2004) Ferrets: neoplasia. In: *Ferrets, Rabbits and Rodents, Clinical Medicine and Surgery, 2nd edn*, ed. KE Quesenberry and JW Carpenter, pp. 91–106. WB Saunders, Philadelphia

Williams ES, Thorne TE, Kwiatkowski DR, Lutx K and Anderson SL (1992) Comparative vaginal cytology of the estrous cycle of black-footed ferrets (*Mustela nigripes*), Siberian polecats (*M. eversmanni*), and domestic ferrets (*M. putorius furo*). *Journal of Veterinary Diagnostic Investigation* **4**, 38–44

28

Ferrets: nervous and musculoskeletal disorders

William Lewis

Introduction

Diseases of the nervous and musculoskeletal systems in ferrets are rarely reported. A few cases have been reported in the USA, but this does not necessarily reflect what is seen in private practice as many unusual and interesting conditions undoubtedly go unreported. All cases should be approached in a logical and systematic manner. The adage that 'you will miss more by not looking than by not knowing' holds true. Although a list of differential diagnoses exists for ferrets, it may be wise to broaden one's thoughts and include conditions seen in other species to ensure that the diagnosis is not missed.

Neurological examination

There are very few published data on neurological examinations in ferrets. Performing a valid neurological examination may prove difficult or impossible in ferrets that are very aggressive, playful or uncooperative. An attempt should be made to perform as much of an examination as possible and extrapolate from what is known about canine and feline neurology.

Assessment of cranial nerves

Cranial nerve assessment may prove difficult, but certain procedures or tests may be carried out to attempt to localize lesions. In the absence of any published data on the validity of cranial nerve assessment in the ferret, results should be interpreted with care. Figure 28.1 indicates tests for assessing cranial nerve function based on those used in canine and feline patients.

Postural reflex assessments may be attempted but it may prove difficult to perform a full examination. A continuous head tilt indicates a problem in the vestibular system. In the author's experience, hopping, wheelbarrowing, hemi-standing, hemi-walking and extensor postural thrust tests are difficult or impractical. Reflexes such as the patella and biceps reflexes may also prove difficult to perform, although the anal reflex may be assessed readily.

Assessment of lower and upper motor neurons

Lower motor neurons (LMNs) are efferent neurons connecting the central nervous system (CNS) to an effector muscle or gland. Signs of LMN lesions include

Cranial nerve	Method of assessment
CN I	Place a swab soaked in alcohol under the nose
CN II and III	Pupillary light reflex
CN II and VII	The menace reflex can be used but is often suppressed in ferrets
CN III, IV and VI	Note symmetry of eyes and pupils
CN V ophthalmic branch	Response to touching medial canthus of the eye
CN V maxillary branch	Response to touching lateral canthus of the eye
CN III, IV, VI and VII	Move head from side to side and observe vestibular eye movements
CN V	With bilateral paralysis there will be a dropped jaw. With unilateral paralysis there will be decreased jaw tone
CN VI	The retractor bulbi muscle is tested with the palpebral and corneal reflex
CN V and VII	Touch and pinch the nose and lower jaw
CN VII	Check the symmetry of the face
CN VIII	The cochlear part is evaluated by testing the response to a loud noise. Lesions affecting the vestibular portion are usually unilateral and produce ataxia, nystagmus and a head tilt to the side of the lesion
CN IX and X	Evaluated by stimulating the back of the pharynx to induce a gag reflex
CN XI	Palpate the trapezius muscle and parts of the sternocephalicus and brachycephalicus for symmetry
CN XII	Palpate the trapezius and brachycephalic muscles for symmetry
CN XII	Wet the nose and evaluate the ability of the tongue to extend forward

28.1 Cranial nerve examination.

paralysis, loss of muscle tone and reflexes and muscle atrophy if present for longer than a week.

Upper motor neurons (UMNs) form the motor system in the brain that controls the LMNs. They are responsible for the initiation and maintenance of normal movements and the maintenance of tone in extensor muscles to support the body against gravity. UMN lesions produce signs caudal to the lesion. The main sign is paresis with increased extensor tone and normal or exaggerated reflexes. In dogs, UMN signs are more common than LMN signs in clinical patients, and this also seems to be the case in ferrets.

Other diagnostic tests

Most cases will require further diagnostic tests such as a cerebrospinal fluid (CSF) tap, myelography, computed tomography (CT) or a magnetic resonance imaging (MRI) scan to achieve a definitive diagnosis. It may be more prudent to refer such cases to a specialist neurologist. In many cases a firm diagnosis may only be achieved post mortem and with histopathological examination.

Various tests and procedures that may be considered in the evaluation of a patient exhibiting nervous or musculoskeletal clinical signs include haematology, biochemistry, serology, radiography, ultrasonography, fine-needle aspiration and cytology, and histopathology.

Haematology, biochemistry and standard radiographical views should be considered the basic minimum. Other tests would then be performed as necessary. (See also Chapters 18 and 19.)

CSF taps are performed using a 20 or 22 gauge spinal needle. The procedure is identical to that for dogs and cats and may be performed under general anaesthesia in either the atlanto-occipital area or the lumbar region (Figures 28.2a,b). It is a specialized procedure and requires skill and experience to perform. Ultrasonography may be used to help guide the needle (Figure 28.2c). Iohexol can be used at 0.25–0.5 ml/kg for myelography (see Chapter 18 for further details). For peripheral nerve and muscular defects, the patient may need to be referred for electromyelography (EMG) or nerve conduction velocity (NCV) tests.

Differential diagnoses

Insulinomas (see Chapter 30) and bacterial meningitis/encephalitis are the most common causes of neurological disease in ferrets (Williams, 2003). If the diagnosis is not immediately obvious, it would be prudent to try to rule out these two conditions before pursuing further diagnostics.

Differential diagnoses for ferrets presented with apparent neurological or musculoskeletal clinical signs are listed in Figure 28.3.

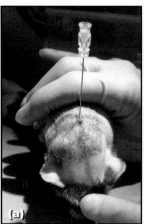
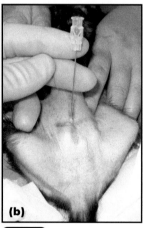
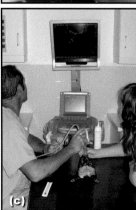

28.2

(a) Positioning of spinal needle for cervical CSF tap.
(b) Positioning of spinal needle for lumbar CSF tap.
(c) Ultrasound guidance may be used for CSF tap.

Signs that are *not* due to primary nervous system or musculoskeletal disease

Hypoglycaemia caused by: insulinoma, food deprivation; anorexia; vomiting; sepsis; other metabolic disorders
Hypocalcaemia (especially lactating jills)
Pregnancy toxaemia
Thromboembolism
Hepatic failure
Renal failure
Hypoxia
Anaemia
Cardiac disease
Proliferative bowel disease
Splenomegaly
Caudal abdominal masses
Cystic calculi
Peritonitis
Prostatomegaly
Urinary obstruction

Nervous and musculoskeletal diseases reported in the ferret

Extensor rigidity/hyperreflexia
Neoplasia:
- Central nervous system: astrocytoma; primitive neuroepithelial tumour; granular cell tumour; meningioma; metastatic disease
- Peripheral nervous system: malignant peripheral nerve sheath tumour; schwannoma
- Other neoplasia: chordoma; plasma cell myeloma; lymphoma; chondroma/chondrosarcoma; osteoma/osteosarcoma; squamous cell carcinoma; leiomyosarcoma; rhabdomyosarcoma; other sarcoma

Otitis media/interna
Infectious diseases: distemper; rabies; Aleutian disease; leptospirosis; listeriosis; toxoplasmosis; cryptococcosis; other bacterial meningitis/encephalitis
Systemic granulomatous inflammatory syndrome (SGIS)
Neuronal ceroid lipofuscinosis
Spinal trauma
Spinal abscess
Intervertebral disc prolapse
Megaoesophagus
Botulism
Other toxins: liquid potpourri; lead; chocolate; nicotine; bromethalin
Fractures
Osteomyelitis

28.3 Differential diagnoses for ferrets presented with apparent neurological or musculoskeletal clinical signs. (continues) ▶

Differential diagnoses for paresis, paraparesis and paralysis in the ferret
Spinal trauma/abscess
Other musculoskeletal trauma
Intervertebral disc prolapse
Aleutian disease
Hypocalcaemia
Insulinoma
Myelitis
Thromboembolism
Neoplasia (primary or secondary)
Disseminated idiopathic myositis (DIM)
Systemic granulomatous inflammatory syndrome (SGIS)
Toxicity, including botulism

28.3 (continued) Differential diagnoses for ferrets presented with apparent neurological or musculoskeletal clinical signs.

Specific conditions

Extensor rigidity/hyperreflexia

This is a progressive ascending dysfunction of the spinal nerves that begins as a paresis or paralysis. It most commonly affects the rear limbs and may be progressive or may regress completely. The aetiology is unknown. Some ferrets have clinical signs consistent with epizootic catarrhal enteritis, which may include a profuse green mucoid diarrhoea that may progress to a loose grainy stool. Diagnosis is presumed based on clinical signs. There are no spinal cord or brain lesions visible on histopathology and the pathophysiology of the condition is unknown.

Disseminated idiopathic myositis (DIM)/myofasciitis

This devastating disease was first reported in the USA in 2003 (Garner *et al.*, 2007). It is characterized by fever and an extremely high neutrophil count. The onset of illness is acute; it typically affects ferrets 3–21 months of age, but does not appear to be contagious. Clinical signs include lethargy, anorexia and a reluctance to move. Affected animals may exhibit signs of pain when being handled. Ataxia and paresis may occur. There is marked pain over the lumbar area and the ferret may find it easier to eat soft food. Tachycardia and heart murmurs may be present. Enlargement of individual lymph nodes may be seen without a generalized lymphadenopathy. Seizures may occur. The disease lasts from days to months and all patients eventually die.

Neutrophil counts may be elevated and are in the region of 40,000–60,000/μl (in some cases as high as 100,000/μl). Haematology reveals a mild to moderate anaemia, which becomes regenerative. Biochemistry is normal and there is no elevation of CK. The most significant finding is a suppurative myositis of all muscles in the body, including cardiac muscle. All tests for viruses have proved negative and to date no aetiological agent has been identified. In the report by Garner *et al.* (2007), the only commonality was that all of the ferrets in the study had received one dose of a commercial canine distemper vaccine (Fervac-D,

United Vaccines Inc.) but there is no current evidence to suggest that this condition is related to vaccine reaction (Peter Fisher, personal communication). However, Schoemaker *et al.* (2005) managed to induce an identical disease to this in an entire group of ferrets administered an experimental castration vaccine that contained an aluminium adjuvant.

Treatment with antibiotics, antifungals, steroids, NSAIDs, vitamins and antihistamines has not resulted in any improvement.

Confirmation is by biopsy of rear leg or lumbar muscles and histopathology, which reveals a widely disseminated suppurative to pyogranulomatous polymyositis involving most muscles, including the periocular and cardiac muscles. The oesophagus is the organ that is most severely affected. The lumbar and rear limb muscles are also severely affected. Myeloid hyperplasia of the spleen and/or bone marrow is a prominent feature.

Neoplasia of the central nervous system

Brain neoplasms are rarely reported in ferrets, astrocytomas being the most common. Other reported tumours include primitive neuroepithelial tumours, granular cell tumours and meningiomas (Xiantang and Fox, 1998).

Lewington (2007) reported an adenocarcinoma of the paranasal sinuses metastasizing to the brain. Initial clinical signs were exophthalmos and sneezing. The eye was ulcerated and the optic disc was red and swollen. Ultrasonography revealed a retrobulbar mass. A CT scan revealed tumours in the brain and paranasal sinuses. Post-mortem examination and histopathology confirmed this to be an adenocarcinoma originating in the paranasal sinuses.

Neoplasia of the peripheral nervous system

Benign and malignant peripheral nerve sheath tumours have been reported (Williams, 2003). Malignant peripheral nerve sheath tumours may occur anywhere on the body. They are clinically obvious and signs depend on which part of the body is affected. The head seems to be the area most commonly affected and the eyelids appear to be the most common site of origin. Treatment is by surgical excision with repeat surgeries often being required for a cure.

Neoplasia of the musculoskeletal system

Tumours reported to affect the musculoskeletal system include squamous cell carcinomas of the mandible, leiomyosarcomas, osteosarcomas, rhabdomyosarcomas and sarcomas affecting muscles and the humerus (Chesterman and Pomerance, 1965; Li *et al.*, 1998; Lewington, 2007).

Chordoma

Chordomas commonly occur near the tip of the tail (Figure 28.4) but may also affect the thoracic or cervical spine. Metastases are extremely rare. Those on the tail tip should be removed by amputating two intervertebral spaces cranial to the mass. Thoracic or cervical chordomas require an MRI scan for diagnosis. Clinical signs include motor dysfunction and loss

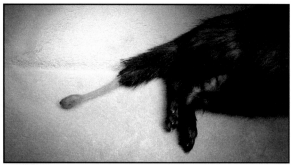

28.4 Chordoma on tail tip. (Courtesy of Peter Fisher.)

of conscious proprioception and perception of pain in the hind limbs. Segmental reflexes are not affected. Treatment involves decompressive surgery, which may not be successful. Immunohistochemical staining of biopsy samples should be used to differentiate this condition from chondrosarcoma. (See also Chapter 24.)

Plasma cell myeloma
A case of plasma cell myeloma of the lumbar vertebra has been reported (Methiyapun *et al.*, 1985). The patient was presented with an 8-month history of slowly progressive paraparesis, rear limb paralysis, absent patellar reflex and no central recognition of pain terminally. The diagnosis was confirmed on postmortem examination: a 3 x 3 x 4 cm lobulated firm light-tan mass occupied the body of the sixth lumbar vertebra (L6) and invaded the bone marrow, adjacent bone, muscles and vertebral canal.

Lymphoma
Lymphoma is a common condition in ferrets and may metastasize to the vertebrae and cause osteolytic lesions and hind limb paresis (see Chapter 30 for further details).

Osteoma
Osteomas of the skull of ferrets present as firm hard bony masses arising from the zygomatic arch, parietal or occipital bone (Figure 28.5). Most cases are non-symptomatic. They are benign neoplasms and any clinical signs that occur are related to physical compression or displacement of normal structures. They are readily visible on radiographs. Biopsy may be attempted with Jamshidi needles. In clinical cases, surgical excision would be expected to be curative.

Osteosarcoma and rhabdomyosarcoma
Osteosarcomas of flat bones are locally destructive and may be difficult to treat. Those involving a limb (Figure 28.6) should be treated by amputation. Osteosarcomas have also been reported on the ribs, thoracic vertebrae and maxilla. Two ferrets with infiltrative osteosarcomas of the rib and maxilla were euthanased due to the aggressiveness of their tumours; no evidence of metastasis was seen (Wilber and Williams, 1997) . There has been a report of a humerus sarcoma and an osteosarcoma of the thoracic vertebrae in a 4-year-old ferret with acute-onset lameness (Lewington, 2007).

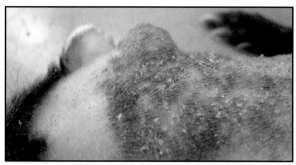

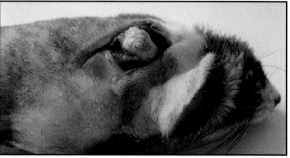

28.5 Osteoma of the skull.

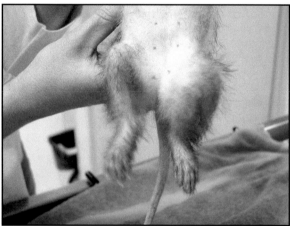

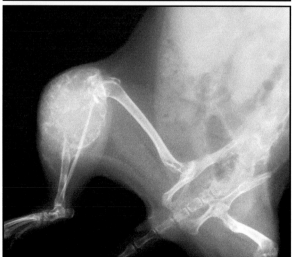

28.6 Osteosarcoma of the tibia. (Courtesy of Peter Fisher.)

Rhabdomyosarcomas are malignant tumours of skeletal muscle and should be treated by radical excision wherever possible.

Otitis interna

Otitis interna is an uncommon condition in ferrets. Clinical signs include head tilt, circling and nystagmus, which may be horizontal or rotatory. Infection usually spreads from an otitis media and may also occur secondary to infection with ear mites. Radiography or MRI may be used to confirm the diagnosis. Bacterial cultures should be performed and treatment should mimic that of canine and feline patients.

Distemper

Clinical cases in unvaccinated ferrets result in 100% mortality (see Chapter 17 for details on vaccination). Signs include hyperexcitability, excessive salivation, muscle tremors, convulsions and death. Histopathology shows a non-suppurative encephalomyelitis. (See Chapter 31 for further details.)

Rabies

Rabies is extremely rare in ferrets. Experimentally infected ferrets showed a mean incubation period of 33 days and morbidity period of 4–5 days (Niezgoda et al., 1997). Paralysis, ataxia, cachexia, bladder atony, fever, hyperactivity, tremors and parasthaesia were seen. Viral antigen was detected in the brain tissue of all clinically rabid ferrets. Not all ferrets appear to seroconvert. In this study group of 55 ferrets only one had virus present in the salivary glands. (See also Chapter 31.)

Aleutian disease

Aleutian disease is caused by a parvovirus and is not commonly seen in ferrets, though up to 30% of ferrets in the USA may test positive. It is of most concern in mink that are homozygous for the Aleutian (blue) gene. Wild mink in the UK may act as a reservoir of infection, which occurs by inhalation or ingestion of virus shed in saliva, faeces or urine. It is an immune complex-mediated disorder causing signs such as mild incoordination, posterior ataxia, ascending paresis, tremors and paraplegia. Ferrets may remain infected but asymptomatic or the disease may be self-limiting. Treatment involves supportive care.

Diagnosis is based on typical clinical signs, a positive countercurrent immunoelectrophoresis (CIEP) test and raised gammaglobulin levels, which may be greater than 20% of the total serum protein concentration. Histopathology reveals perivascular cuffing with lymphocytes and possibly plasma cells, non-suppurative meningitis, astrocytosis, mononuclear cell infiltration and focal malacia of the spinal cord and brain. See Chapter 31 for further details.

Listeriosis

Listeria monocytogenes is rarely reported in ferrets and its prevalence is unknown. The organism is transmitted by the ingestion of contaminated food or by inhalation via aerosols. Clinical signs and pathology have not been described in the ferret, but they can be assumed to be similar to those in other species. Diagnosis is by the culture of CSF. Treatment is with penicillin or ampicillin. Experimentally the organism has been recovered from the lungs, spleen and pleural fluid of ferrets.

Toxoplasmosis

Toxoplasmosis has been recorded after exposure to cat faeces or raw meat containing cysts of *Toxoplasma gondii*. Ferrets may become infected or may act as intermediate hosts. Early work showed that *Toxoplasma* isolated from ferrets was morphologically, biologically and serologically indistinguishable from that found in rabbits in England (Lainson, 1957). There is a case report of 30% of 750 neonatal ferrets dying without clinical signs on a fur farm in New Zealand, where multifocal necrosis associated with *Toxoplasma*-like organisms was observed in lung, heart and liver (Thornton and Cook, 1986). As in other species, clinical signs depend on the organs involved and may include anorexia, lethargy, corneal oedema, retinitis, iritis, blindness, ataxia, fever, anaemia, hepatitis, CNS signs, respiratory disease and diarrhoea. The diagnosis involves ELISA tests for IgG and IgM as well as *T. gondii*-specific antigens in the serum (Lewington, 2007). Treatment is usually with sulphonamides and should be continued for at least 2 weeks and for a short time after cessation of clinical signs (Bell, 1994). (See Chapter 21 for dosages; note that sulfaquinoxaline is toxic to ferrets.) An example of treatment would be pyrimethamine (0.5–1 mg/kg per day) plus sulfadiazine (60 mg/100 ml drinking water or 60 mg per 100 g of food).

Cryptococcosis

Cryptococcosis is a rare disease of ferrets caused by *Cryptococcus neoformans*, with single-case reports from the UK, Australia and the USA. It starts as a serous or purulent unilateral or bilateral nasal discharge, which may contain traces of blood. The organism then spreads to the lungs, brain and abdomen. Clinical signs may include stiffness around the neck, incoordination, ataxia and death. Diagnosis requires the analysis of CSF and antigen tests. Encapsulated budding spores of *Cryptococcus* can be visualized microscopically if the CSF is mixed with Indian ink. The diagnosis may be confirmed by isolating the organism, by culturing the CSF or by histopathology. The prognosis is poor, but treatment of confirmed cases may be attempted with antifungal drugs such as amphotericin B, itraconazole, ketoconazole or fluconazole. For dose rates, see Chapter 21.

Systemic granulomatous inflammatory syndrome (SGIS)

SGIS is an emerging disease which was first seen in Spain in 2005 (Martinez et al., 2006). Nine ferrets were affected with ages ranging from 5 to 38 weeks (median of 18 weeks). All nine cases were seen by the same clinician. Brown or yellow–green diarrhoea was usually the first clinical sign seen. In some cases this progressed to a haemorrhagic diarrhoea. Other clinical signs included lethargy, anorexia, weight loss, hindlimb weakness, tremors, convulsions and death. In some cases splenomegaly and non-regenerative anaemia were seen. Mesenteric lymphadenopathy was detected in all cases by abdominal palpation and was confirmed by exploratory laparotomy, radiography or post-mortem examination. Haematology was variable but non-specific, but hyperglobulinaemia with a polyclonal gammopathy was detected in all cases. The globulin levels were greater than 42 g/l and the gammaglobulins were greater than 18 g/l in all cases. The rest of the biochemical parameters that were measured were within the normal range. Various treatments were tried, including glucocorticoids, anabolic steroids, antibiotics, antiprotozoals, cytotoxic drugs, NSAIDs and nutritional support. All nine ferrets eventually died or were euthanased.

In the work done by Martinez *et al.* (2006) a specific immunohistological reaction using the monoclonal antibodies directed towards feline coronavirus could be seen in macrophages. This is similar to the well known reaction that is found in granulomas in cases of feline infectious peritonitis (FIP). The histopathological and immunohistochemical findings suggested that the aetiology of this condition is a coronavirus. This requires further investigation, as Koch's postulates have not been fulfilled.

This condition is now being diagnosed with more frequency (D Perpinan, personal communication, 2007). It has subsequently been diagnosed in the USA, The Netherlands, France and Spain (D Perpinan, personal communication, 2008).

Neuronal ceroid lipofuscinosis

This is a rare condition causing hindlimb paresis which progresses to incontinence, behavioural changes and blindness. It is an inherited disease with an enzyme deficiency causing accumulation of macromolecules within neurons. The diagnosis is confirmed at post-mortem examination on histopathology, which reveals typical intracytoplasmic granules in the neurons of the brain, spinal cord and peripheral ganglia. There is no treatment and affected animals should be euthanased.

Spinal trauma

Spinal injury is usually a result of trauma. Diagnosis involves clinical history of trauma, radiography and/or MRI. Treatment is on an individual basis, depending on the severity and location of the lesion. Prognosis varies from good to hopeless, depending on the extent of the lesion.

Spinal abscesses

Spinal abscesses have been found in six out of seven ferrets undergoing post-mortem examination for hindquarter paralysis (J Chitty, personal communication).

Intervertebral disc prolapse

Prolapse of an intervertebral disc may result in paraplegia. The diagnosis may be confirmed on MRI scan or myelography. A hemilaminectomy may be performed to remove the extruded disc material. Decompressive surgery has been successful in one case (Lu *et al.*, 2004) and the treated animal made a good recovery. This ferret had exhibited paraplegia with increased muscle tone in the pelvic limbs. The withdrawal reflexes were intact but deep pain perception was reduced bilaterally. There was a normal panniculus reflex.

Megaoesophagus

Megaoesophagus is a rare acquired disease in ferrets that should be considered in any patient exhibiting regurgitation or difficulty in swallowing. Regurgitation should be differentiated from vomiting. It may be associated with gastritis, gastric acid reflux and oesophagitis. Patients may show distress while eating and may choke, cough, regurgitate or extend the neck postprandially.

The aetiology is poorly understood in most cases but it appears to be an acquired rather than a congenital condition (Harms and Andrews, 1993; Blanco *et al.*, 1994). Some cases have been histopathologically linked to underlying gastritis with associated gastric acid reflux and oesophagitis (M Burgess and M Garner, unpublished clinical and histopathological data from clinical cases, 1995–2005).

The diagnosis may be confirmed on radiography. A barium oesophagram will reveal a dilated cervical and thoracic oesophagus, which may measure up to 2 cm in diameter (Figure 28.7). Barium sulphate can be administered at 10 ml/kg body weight or mixed with food.

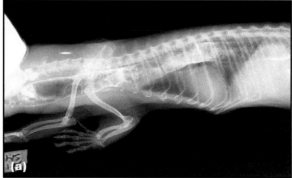

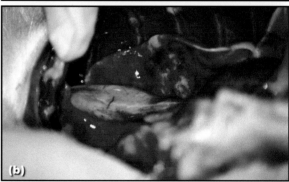

28.7 **(a)** Barium study showing megaoesophagus in a ferret that had ear mites and a head tilt. **(b)** Dilated oesophagus at post-mortem examination.

Cases that occur as a result of reflux oesophagitis carry a better prognosis and some success has been achieved in treating them with H2 receptor blockers such as ranitidine or famotidine. Treatment may be required for several weeks or longer. Sucralfate may aid the healing of gastric and oesophageal ulcers. (see Chapter 21). Affected ferrets should be fed a gruel such as Hills a/d from a height (Burgess, 2007). See also Chapter 25.

In many cases debilitation eventually occurs due to dehydration, malnutrition and secondary aspiration pneumonia. Antibiotics should be administered and the use of a gastrotomy tube may prove helpful. The author has seen a single case of megaoesophagus that began with an otitis externa caused by ear mites (Figure 28.8). This progressed to a purulent otitis externa and media with a head tilt. After a few days in hospital the ferret started regurgitating food and developed respiratory disease. A barium study revealed megaoesophagus and the patient succumbed to aspiration pneumonia.

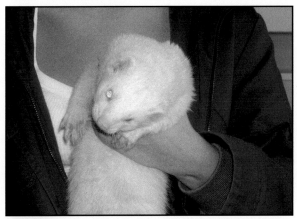

28.8 Ferret with ear mites and head tilt that went on to develop megaoesophagus.

Botulism

Clostridium botulinum Type C toxin is fatal to ferrets. Experimentally, ferrets are susceptible to infection by *C. botulinum* Types A and B, highly susceptible to Type C and refractory to Type E (Moll and Brandly, 1951; Harrison and Borland, 1973). Hungry working ferrets may eat dead rats, rabbits or birds which may be a source of the toxin. It is advisable to ensure that ferrets are well fed prior to working. Feeding ferrets in the evening and early morning will prevent hoarding and decay of food during the day, when ferrets usually sleep. Food should also be limited to what is required. Paralysis starts with the hind limbs and moves forwards, but sensation does remain. The temperature is normal but respiration is affected by partial paralysis of the intercostal muscles and diaphragm. The prognosis is poor, though patients treated very early with penicillin, force feeding and vitamins may be cured (Lewington, 2007).

Other toxins

A number of toxic substances have been shown to cause neurological signs in ferrets, including:

- Liquid potpourri
- Chocolate (contains caffeine and theobromine): toxicity results in CNS stimulation, tremors, seizures and death
- Nicotine: may result in respiratory paralysis and death
- Bromethalin: causes hyperexcitability, muscle tremors, seizures, forelimb extensor rigidity, ataxia, CNS depression, loss of vocalization, paresis, paralysis and death
- Organophosphates: ferrets are susceptible to organophosphate-induced neurotoxicity. Signs

include increasing trunk and hindlimb ataxia culminating in fore- and hindlimb paralysis. Histopathology reveals widespread axonal degeneration extending from the brainstem and cerebellum into midbrain and forebrain areas
- Cannabis: coma has been reported after ingestion (Richardson and Balabuszko, 2000)
- Ibuprofen: causes ataxia, depression, coma and tremors
- Copper: toxicosis has been reported (Fox *et al.*, 1994) and was suspected to be congenital.

Seizures

Seizures are a common reason for middle-aged and older ferrets being presented for veterinary attention. An insulinoma would be the first condition to rule out. Seizures may also be caused by CNS infection, trauma, inflammation, neoplasia, liver or kidney failure and toxins (see above). Although primary (idiopathic) epilepsy has not been reported (Antinoff, 2003), it could occur and management would mimic that of canine or feline patients.

A full clinical examination should be performed, including a neurological examination. A complete blood profile including haematology and biochemistry should be obtained, radiographs should be taken and a thorough cardiac workup should be performed. If possible an MRI or CT scan should be performed and a sample of CSF obtained. If the cause of the seizure is hypoglycaemia, intravenous fluids containing 2.5–10% dextrose should be administered and a diagnosis of insulinoma pursued (see Chapter 30). If an insulinoma is not the cause of the seizures, they should be controlled initially with diazepam using boluses of 0.5–1 mg/kg given intravenously; if this does not control the seizures it may be necessary to use phenobarbitone and/or potassium bromide. Long-term treatment may prove necessary and there should be regular monitoring of serum drug levels. A diagnosis should be pursued wherever possible.

In cases of suspected organosphosphate or carbamate toxicity, atropine sulphate can be used at 0.2–0.5 mg/kg to effect, i.e. mydriasis and reduced salivation. This dose may need to be repeated at 3–6-hour intervals for 1–2 days (Lewington, 2007).

Pregnancy toxaemia

This may occur in young primiparous jills in late gestation. Neurological signs occur when hepatic lipidosis is severe enough to cause hepatic encephalopathy (see Chapter 27).

Nutritional hyperparathyroidism

Nutritional hyperparathyroidism has been reported but is now extremely rare, due to the availability of commercial ferret diets. It may result from a lack of calcium, phosphorus or vitamin D. Clinical signs in kits include weight loss, reluctance to move and an inability to support their body weight. The bones are soft and may be fractured easily. The parathyroid glands are grossly hyperplastic and microscopically the bones are osteoporotic with typical lesions of osteodystrophia fibrosa.

Acknowledgement

The author is grateful for personal communications with Peter Fisher, David Perpinan, John Chitty and John Lewington. Special thanks to Richard Doyle and the nursing staff at The Wylie Veterinary Centre for help with clinical cases.

References and further reading

Antinoff A (2003) Musculoskeletal and neurologic diseases. In: *Ferrets, Rabbits and Rodents: Clinical Medicine and Surgery, 2nd edn*, ed. KE Quesenberry and JW Carpenter. WB Saunders, Philadelphia

Bell JA (1994) Parasites of domesticated pet ferrets. *Compendium on Continuing Education for the Practicing Veterinarian* **16**, 617–620

Blanco MC, Fox JG, Rosenthal K *et al.* (1994) Megaoesophagus in nine ferrets. *Journal of the American Veterinary Medical Association* **205**, 444–447

Burgess ME (2007) Ferret gastrointestinal and hepatic diseases. In: *Ferret Husbandry, Medicine and Surgery 2nd edn*, ed. JH Lewington, pp. 203–223. Saunders Elsevier, Oxford

Chesterman FC and Pomerance A (1965) Spontaneous neoplasms in ferrets and polecats. *Journal of Pathology and Bacteriology* **89**, 529–534

Fox JG (1998) Mycotic diseases. In: *Biology and Diseases of the Ferret, 2nd edn*, ed. JG Fox, pp. 397–398. Lippincott Williams and Wilkins, Baltimore

Fox JG and McLain D E (1998) Nutrition. In: *Biology and Diseases of the Ferret, 2nd edn,* ed. J G Fox, pp. 167–168. Lippincott Williams and Wilkins, Baltimore

Fox JG, Zeman DH and Mortimer JD (1994) Copper toxicosis in sibling ferrets. *Journal of the American Veterinary Medical Association* **205**, 1154–1156

Garner MM, Ramsell K, Schoemaker NJ *et al.* (2007) Myofasciitis in the domestic ferret. *Veterinary Pathology* **44**, 25–38

Greenlee PG and Stephens E (1984) Meningeal cryptococcosis and congestive cardiomyopathy in a ferret. *Journal of the American Veterinary Medical Association* **184**, 840

Harms C and Andrews GA (1993) Megaoesophagus in a domestic ferret. *Laboratory Animal Science* **43**, 5

Harrison SG and Borland ED (1973) Deaths in ferrets (*Mustela putorius*) due to *Clostridium botulinum* type C. *Veterinary Record* **93**, 576

Lainson R (1957) Symposium on Toxoplasmosis. III. The demonstration of Toxoplasma in animals, with particular reference to members of the Mustelidae. *Transactions of the Royal Society for Medical Hygiene* **51**, 111

Lewington JH (1982) Isolation of *Cryptococcus neoformans* from a ferret. *Australian Veterinary Journal* **58**, 124

Lewington JH (2007) *Ferret Husbandry, Medicine and Surgery, 2nd edn.* Saunders Elsevier, Oxford

Li X, Fox J and Padrid PA (1998) Neoplastic diseases in ferrets: 574 cases (1968–1997). *Journal of the American Veterinary Medical Association* **212**, 1402–1406

Lu D, Lamb CR , Patterson-Kane JC and Cappello R (2004) Treatment of a prolapsed lumbar intervertebral disc in a ferret. *Journal of Small Animal Practice* **45**(10): 501–503

Malik R, Alderton B, Finlaison D *et al.* (2002) Cryptococcosis in ferrets; a diverse spectrum of clinical cases. *Australian Veterinary Journal* **80**, 749–755

Martinez J, Ramis AJ, Reinacher M and Perpinan D (2006) Detection of feline peritonitis virus-like antigen in ferrets. *Veterinary Record* **158**, 523

Methiyapun S, Myers RK and Pohlenz JFL (1985) Spontaneous plasma cell myeloma in a ferret. *Veterinary Pathology* **22**, 517–519

Moll T and Brandly CA (1951) Botulism in mouse, mink and ferret with special reference to susceptibility and pathological alterations. *American Journal of Veterinary Research* **12**, 355

Niezgoda M, Briggs DJ, Shadduck J *et al.* (1997) Pathogenesis of experimentally-induced rabies in domestic ferrets. *American Journal of Veterinary Research* **58**, 1327–1331

Perpinan D and Lopez C (2008) Clinical aspects of systemic granulomatous inflammatory syndrome in ferrets (*Mustela putorius furo*). *Veterinary Record* **162**(6), 180–183

Richardson J and Balabuszko R (2000) Managing ferret toxicoses. *Exotic DVM* **2**(4), 23–26

Schoemaker NJ, Lumeij JT and Rijnberk A (2005) Current and future alternatives to surgical neutering in ferrets to prevent hyperadrenocorticism. *Veterinary Medicine* **100**, 484–496

Skulski G and Symmers WSC (1954) Actinomycosis and torulosis in the ferret. *Journal of Comparative Pathology* **64**, 306

Thornton RN and Cook TG (1986) A congenital Toxoplasma-like disease in ferrets (*Mustela putorius furo*). *New Zealand Veterinary Journal* **34**, 31

Wilber J and Williams B (1997) Osteosarcoma in two domestic ferrets (*Mustela putorius furo*). *Veterinary Pathology* **34**, 487

Williams BH (2003) Neoplasia. In: *Ferrets, Rabbits and Rodents: Clinical Medicine and Surgery, 2nd edn*, ed. KE Quesenberry and JW Carpenter, pp. 91–106. WB Saunders, St Louis

Xiantang L and Fox JG (1998) Neoplastic diseases. In: *Biology and Diseases of the Ferret, 2nd edn*, ed. JG Fox, pp. 405–447. Williams and Wilkins, Baltimore

29

Ferrets: ophthalmology

Fabiano Montiani-Ferreira

Anatomy

The anatomy of the ferret eye is largely similar to that of other carnivores. However, the size of the ferret eye is proportionally and absolutely small, having an axial length of about 7 mm.

Developmentally, there is one important difference between ferrets and other carnivores. Ferret kits, just like puppies, are born with their eyelids closed, but ferret eyelids open at 4 weeks of age instead of about 2 weeks as in most breeds of dogs.

The conjunctiva lines the posterior face of the eyelids, the entire semilunar fold of the conjunctiva (third eyelid) and the exposed sclera before terminating at the corneal limbus (corneoscleral junction). Ferrets have a well developed third eyelid covered by tightly adherent conjunctiva on its bulbar and palpebral surfaces and it is usually either non-pigmented (whitish) or pigmented at the margin. The third eyelid is reinforced by a T-shaped piece of cartilage that has a gland (superficial gland of the semilunar fold of the conjunctiva) at its base that is responsible for secreting part of the aqueous layer of the tear film. There is no deep gland of the third eyelid.

The corneal surface of the ferret is large, as it is in other species adapted for night vision. Adult ferret corneas have the same layers as other carnivores (Figure 29.1) but are about half the thickness of adult dog corneas. The uveal tract is composed of the iris, the ciliary body and the choroid. A striking anatomical peculiarity is the ferret pupil, which is ovoid and horizontally oriented, somewhat similar in shape to an American football or a rugby ball (Figure 29.2). The irides are thin (as observed using light microscopy) and usually brownish in colour, or red/pink in albinos.

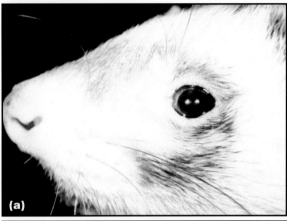

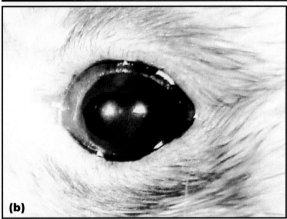

29.2 **(a)** Detail of a typical small ferret eye with its brown iris. **(b)** Detail of the ferret's pupil, clearly demonstrating that it is ovoid in shape and horizontally oriented.

Ferrets have a well developed reflective tapetum lucidum cellulosum, which is rich in zinc and cysteine. It is present in both the pigmented and the albinotic eye. Ferrets have holangiotic retinas (where the inner retina is nourished by the retinal circulation and the outer retina receives nourishment and oxygen from the adjacent choriocapillaris) similar to those in dogs. The optic disc is small and poorly myelinated.

29.1 Photomicrograph of a 5 μm thick histological paraffin-embedded section of a ferret's cornea. Note the presence of an epithelium (Ep), a stroma (St), a posterior limiting membrane (also called Descemet's membrane, Dmt) and an endothelium (arrowed). The ferret's corneal epithelium is about 4–5 cells thick. Gomori's Trichromic stains collagen tissue blue; thus it is possible to see how rich in collagen the corneal stroma is. (Bar size: 350 μm; stain: Gomori's Trichromic; original magnification: ×400).

The bony orbit is conical and relatively deep and its caudolateral margin is incomplete (open) (Figure 29.3). This incomplete portion is closed by an orbital ligament, which is a fibrous tissue band that extends from the zygomatic process of the frontal bone to the frontal process of the zygomatic bone.

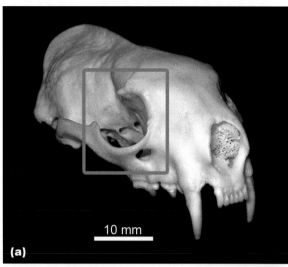

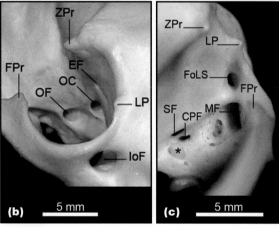

29.3 Adult male ferret skull and bony orbit elements.
(a) Right rostrodorsolateral view of the skull without the jaw. **(b)** Close-up of the right rostrodorsolateral view of the orbit (rectangular area of (a)).
(c) Caudodorsolateral view of the orbit. CPF = caudal palatine foramen; EF = ethmoidal foramen; FoLS = fossa of the lacrimal sac; FPr = frontal process of the zygomatic bone; IoF = infraorbital foramen; LP = lacrimal process; MF = maxillary foramen; OC = optic canal; OF = orbitorotundum foramen; SF = sphenopalatine foramen; ZPr = zygomatic process of the frontal bone. Note the exposure of the apical end of the palatine root (asterisk) of the superior first (and unique) molar tooth through the pterygopalatine surface of the maxillary bone, on the floor of the pterygopalatine fossa. (Courtesy of Marcello Machado.)

Ferrets have a retrobulbar venous plexus that is similar to that of rodents. This has been suggested as a site for blood collection (Fox *et al.*, 1984), but the author has no experience in using this site. There is a risk of damaging the eye bulb and the procedure is potentially painful and would require anaesthesia for restraint. Therefore it is generally not recommended in veterinary practice, but is used primarily in laboratory animals.

Restraint and ophthalmic examination

A protocol for ophthalmic examination is shown in Figure 29.4. Physical restraint is often necessary to perform a proper ophthalmic examination in the ferret, due to the restless nature of the species. In the author's experience, one of the best ways to immobilize the head for an eye examination is to have an assistant gently hold the ferret by its scruff and then suspend the animal with its legs off the table while

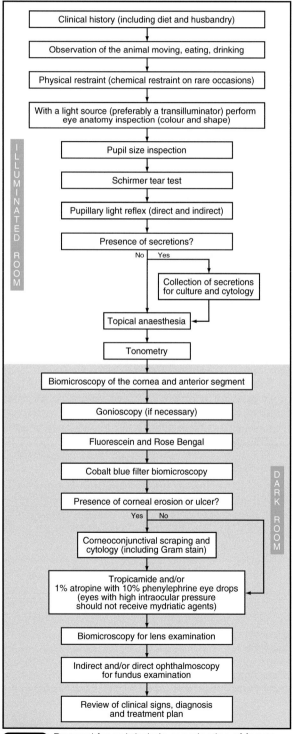

29.4 Protocol for ophthalmic examination of ferrets. (Modified from Montiani-Ferreira, 2001.)

supporting most of its dorsum with the forearm. However, in order to prevent iatrogenic intraocular pressure (IOP) alterations it is essential to avoid applying too much pressure in the neck region (and thus the jugular veins). Therefore, the assistant's other hand should support some of the animal's weight, thus not leaving all the weight to be supported by the scruff. A conscious effort should be made to minimize patient stress during examination and for this reason frequent breaks are helpful. (See also Chapter 18 for restraint techniques.)

The ferret eye is rather small, which means that a source of magnification is indispensable for its examination. A portable handheld slit lamp biomicroscope is the best option for this purpose. Careful and thorough examination of the eye is the key to ophthalmological diagnosis. The transparent nature of many of the ocular structures permits direct visualization of disease processes, allowing diagnosis and close monitoring of progression or resolution of lesions. The eye offers direct visualization of blood vessels and contains the only part of the central nervous system (the retina) that can be directly examined.

Most diagnostic procedures used in dogs and cats can be used to examine the ferret eye. Unfortunately, the palpebral fissure in the young ferret is not wide enough to accommodate commercially available Schirmer tear tests, thus preventing accurate measurement of tear production in young patients. The test can be performed in most adult ferrets (Figure 29.5a). The corneal surface of the adult ferret is also large enough and suitable for intraocular pressure evaluation using a Tono-Pen XL (Figure 29.5b). Figure 29.6

Test	Mean value	Standard deviation	Confidence interval
Schirmer tear test (mm/min)	5.31	± 1.32	4.2–6.4
Intraocular pressure (mmHg)	14.50	± 3.27	12.8–16.2
Corneal thickness (mm)	0.337	± 0.020	0.327–0.347

29.6 Mean reference values of Schirmer tear test, intraocular pressure and central corneal thickness of non-sedated, unstressed ferrets. Note the 95% confidence interval for each test. (Data from Montiani-Ferreira *et al.*, 2006.)

gives mean reference values of Schirmer tear test, intraocular pressure and central corneal thickness of non-sedated, unstressed ferrets.

Ophthalmic diseases

Congenital and neonatal disorders
Even though congenital conditions are not commonly seen by the ophthalmologist, some eye disorders of this nature have already been reported in the ferret and include microphthalmia, cataracts, corneal dermoids and persistent fetal intraocular vasculature (PFIV).

Persistent fetal intraocular vasculature
PFIV is an eye anomaly attributed to the persistence of embryonal vascular vestiges within the eye that did not undergo normal involution during the prenatal or early postnatal period of ocular development. It has been detected in a colony of genetically related ferrets (Lipsitz *et al.*, 2001).

Ophthalmia neonatorum
Some neonatal ophthalmic disorders have also been reported, the most common of them probably being ophthalmia neonatorum. This condition occurs when microorganisms proliferate at the corneoconjunctival surface before the eyelids open, causing an accumulation of ocular discharge in the conjunctival sac. The eyelids appear distended, with or without exterior drainage. Often more than one individual in a litter is affected.

In general, this disease is diagnosed in kits aged a few days to 3 weeks old. In most cases the condition is not noticed until the accumulation of infectious exudate causes the eyelid to bulge. Several microorganisms may cause this condition but bacterial infection is probably the most common. Although details of the route for infection have not yet been confirmed, *Escherichia coli* mastitis in the jill appears to contribute to the formation of ophthalmia neonatorum in kits.

Regardless of the causative organism or route of infection, ophthalmia neonatorum should be treated by manually or surgically opening the adhered eyelids in order to drain the infectious exudate, which is usually mucopurulent. At this point, a sample of the exudate should be collected with a sterile swab and submitted for culture and antimicrobial sensitivity

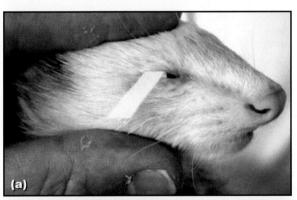
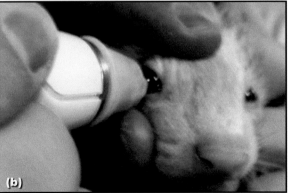

29.5 Demonstration of selected ophthalmic procedures. **(a)** Use of a commercial Schirmer tear test strip. **(b)** Use of Tono-Pen XL (Mentor, Santa Barbara, California).

tests. Then the corneoconjunctival surface should be flushed with sterile saline solution. Finally, treatment with an antibiotic ointment should be initiated 4 times a day until accumulation of secretion inside and outside the conjunctival sac has stopped. The choice of the antibiotic should be guided by the sensitivity results or, alternatively, an empirical choice of a broad-spectrum antibiotic such as tobramycin or ciprofloxacin can be made.

Possible sequelae to the disease are symblepharon (conjunctival adhesion to adjacent tissues), corneal perforation, fibrosis and blindness.

Conjunctivitis

Conjunctivitis in ferrets is commonly caused by a viral or bacterial infection and it often represents an ocular manifestation of a systemic disease such as distemper virus infection, human influenza virus infection, salmonellosis or mycobacteriosis.

Bacterial conjunctivitis

Bacteria can frequently be cultured at low numbers from the normal conjunctival sac (most isolates are Gram-positive, e.g. *Staphylococcus* spp., *Coryne-bacterium* spp.), which should be remembered when evaluating bacterial culture results from the conjunctiva. Primary bacterial conjunctivitis in ferrets is not very common but it is a possible aetiology. Bacterial conjunctivitis is more commonly the result of a predisposing factor that allows an overgrowth of the normal conjunctival bacterial flora or alters the environment, allowing growth of potential pathogens not normally part of the flora.

Clinical signs in the ferret are usually similar to those of other species, with blepharospasm, mucopurulent ocular discharge and conjunctival hyperaemia being the most common. Conjunctival scrapings can aid the diagnosis, as neutrophils, bacteria, and neutrophils with intracellular bacteria are often seen. Additionally, virus isolation or serological titres can be helpful for diagnosing influenza-related conjunctivitis.

Topical therapy with a broad-spectrum antibiotic 4–6 times a day is usually curative. If several animals are affected, or if the initial therapy fails, culture and sensitivity tests are indicated. It is important to arrive as close as possible to an accurate diagnosis, because the prognosis differs depending on the cause of the conjunctivitis: for instance, canine distemper virus is usually fatal whereas ferrets infected with human influenza virus usually recover (Miller, 1997).

Conjunctivitis and systemic disease

Viral disease: Ocular signs of canine distemper virus infection in ferrets, especially conjunctivitis, might be the first signs of this systemic disease. The ocular signs include mucopurulent oculonasal discharge, blepharitis, ankyloblepharon, photophobia, keratoconjunctivitis sicca (dry eye) and corneal ulcers. Conjunctivitis with a mucopurulent ocular and nasal discharge typically develops in 7–10 days post infection. In the case of distemper virus, conjunctivitis is usually associated with a secondary bacterial infection in concert with decreased tear production

(lacrimal adenitis), creating a mucopurulent discharge. Other systemic signs include an erythematous skin rash involving the chin, inguinal region and foot pads. Although the clinical signs are suggestive, definitive diagnosis can be facilitated by serum antibody titres or immunofluorescent antibody testing of conjunctival or blood smears. Canine distemper virus in ferrets is almost invariably fatal; most animals die within 12–35 days post exposure (depending on the specific strain involved), with or without symptomatic therapy (see Chapter 31).

Human influenza virus can cause mild pneumonia and nasal and ocular discharge in ferrets. The disease tends to be self-limiting and runs its course in about 5 days. Treatment is not usually required.

Salmonellosis: *Salmonella* spp. have been reported as causing conjunctivitis in ferrets but usually cause systemic signs such as haemorrhagic diarrhoea and fever.

Mycobacteriosis: Conjunctival swelling and proliferation of the nictitans caused by infection with *Mycobacterium genavense* has been reported in ferrets, which also presented with generalized lymphadenopathy. Response to treatment is variable and reports are rare. Drugs with potential to treat this condition include chloramphenicol ophthalmic ointment, twice a day for 60–90 days, combined with one or more systemic drugs such as rifampicin, clofazimine or clarithromycin.

Lucas *et al.* (2000) reported that two ferrets were treated with a regimen of rifampicin (30 mg), clofazimine (12.5 mg) and clarithromycin (31.25 mg) all given orally, once a day, suspended in a highly palatable gel (Energel, Veterinary Companies of Australia, Artarmon). One of the ferrets was doing well 18 days after starting therapy; compliance with dosing was facilitated by delivering the antimicrobial agents in Energel, which the ferret ingested readily despite the suspended medication. There were no discernible adverse side-effects of the antimicrobial agents at that time and the ferret was reportedly doing well several weeks later. The owners reported that they continued the medication for 2–3 months, until the ferret became inappetent. At that time, the ferret was thought to be clinically cured. Ten months after the initiation of treatment, the ferret lost weight and developed polydipsia. The animal's condition deteriorated rapidly and renal failure was diagnosed on the basis of azotaemia, hyperphosphataemia and isosthenuria. End-stage renal disease was observed grossly at necropsy, following euthanasia. It is important to remember that this conjunctival disease was reported in these two ferrets only as part of disseminated mycobacteriosis, thus special attention to the systemic disease should be given.

Ferrets are susceptible to a number of mycobacterial infections, including *M. avium*, *M. bovis*, *M. genavense*, *M. microti* and *M. celatum*. *M. bovis* is probably the most important cause of mycobacteriosis in ferrets, and ferrets appear to be less susceptible to *M. avium* than to *M. bovis*. Ferrets are an important wildlife reservoir of *M. bovis* in New Zealand, and prevalence rates for tuberculosis in feral ferrets are as high as 32%. Ferrets with tuberculosis have been implicated in the transmission of *M. bovis* to both humans and domestic livestock (Saunders and Thomsen, 2006).

Foreign bodies: Other causes of conjunctivitis and ocular surface disease include foreign bodies, husbandry issues such as the use of dusty and dirty bedding, use of red cedar shavings as bedding and nutritional deficiencies such as of biotin or vitamin A.

Because ferrets are curious about their environment and like to search around and hide in corners and holes, accidents with foreign bodies are a common occurrence. Foreign bodies may become trapped in the conjunctival sac, causing conjunctivitis and corneal irritation or ulcers. Treatment involves gently removing the foreign body with fine forceps and treating with topical broad-spectrum antibiotics. Some foreign bodies may penetrate through the conjunctiva, leaving a sinus that discharges into the conjunctival sac. Treatment involves surgical curettage and removal of the foreign body as well as treating with systemic topical broad-spectrum antibiotics.

Corneal disease

Corneal ulcers

Corneal ulcers are probably the most common of all corneal diseases in the ferret. Traumatic lesions are a particularly common cause of corneal ulcers. However, as for other species, the aetiology of corneal ulceration is often multifactorial.

If corneal lesions are suspected, the use of fluorescein dye will show whether the epithelium has been breached and will help in determining the nature of the defect (Figure 29.7). For instance, in chronic non-healing ulcers (also called indolent ulcers or recurrent erosions) fluorescein dye will underrun the surrounding non-adherent epithelium around the defect. Fluorescein dye is also useful in assessing tear drainage to the nares.

The usual recommended treatment for superficial corneal ulcerations is similar to that for other species, including eye drops of a broad-spectrum antibiotic at least 6 times a day; and an ophthalmic ointment formulation of the same antibiotic should be used at night. Both antibiotic formulations should be used for at least 10 days. If iridocyclospasm is present, a topical parasympathetic blocking agent such as a 1% atropine solution, once a day for about 3–5 days, should be added to the protocol. Time intervals between eye drops should be of about 5 minutes to allow for complete corneal absorption.

Treatment can be adapted for each patient using culture and sensitivity tests, which can then be used to direct the antibiotic choice. Besides the standard topical treatment, chronic non-healing ulcers (recurrent erosions) may require debridement with a cotton swab to promote healing. The procedure is best performed under topical anaesthesia. With the aid of a dry sterile cotton swab, the clinician should remove all loose epithelium by rubbing outwards

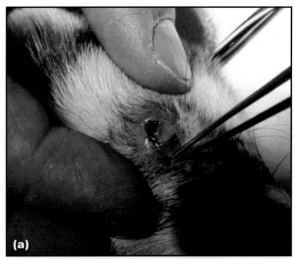

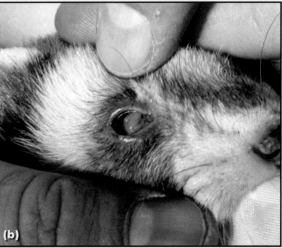

29.7 Large chronic non-healing corneal ulceration of the right eye of a ferret. Note **(a)** the corneal oedema and **(b)** the presence of non-adherent epithelium surrounding the main central defect. Fluorescein dye clearly under-ran the surrounding loose epithelium in this case. (Courtesy of Giuseppe Visigalli.)

from the edge of the defect. Deep or melting ulcers should preferably be treated with surgery, typically a conjunctival pedicle graft technique combined with aggressive topical treatment.

Keratitis

Several other corneal diseases have been reported in the ferret and other mustelids, including exposure keratitis secondary to exophthalmos. Ferrets with diets deficient in riboflavin were reported to have developed corneal vascularization and opacification (Miller, 1997; Good, 2002). Degeneration of corneal endothelium leading to progressive corneal oedema has been reported in mink. Some cases seem to respond to a symptomatic treatment using 5% sodium chloride solution, 2–4 times a day (van der Woerdt, 2004).

A lymphoplasmacytic keratitis reported in a ferret was believed to be associated with multicentric lymphoma (Ringle *et al.*, 1993). The infiltrative lesion (lymphocytes and plasma cells) that was present in the cornea of this ferret resembled corneal lesions reported in mink with Aleutian disease. Ferrets with antibodies to the Aleutian disease virus (ADV), which is a parvovirus, are believed to be more susceptible to concurrent disease because of immunosuppression. The exact mechanism by which the ADV affects the immune system is still poorly characterized. Interference with the immune system could cause the ferret to be more susceptible to viral enteritis, canine distemper virus, lymphoma and other diseases. Thus, Aleutian disease should be considered in any ferret with lymphoplasmacytic infiltration of any organ, including the cornea (see Chapter 31).

Uveitis

- Anterior uveitis (iridocyclitis) is inflammation of the iris and ciliary body.
- Posterior uveitis (choroiditis) is inflammation of the choroid.
- Chorioretinitis is inflammation of the posterior uvea in addition to inflammation of the retina, which is a more frequent diagnosis than choroiditis alone.
- Panuveitis is inflammation of the entire uveal tissue.

Uveitis of any kind in ferrets is not as frequently diagnosed as it is in dogs and cats. The two most common aetiologies of uveitis in ferrets are traumatic and secondary to ulcerative keratitis by way of the reflex axonal pathway. Lens-induced uveitis in ferrets appears to be relatively mild in comparison with that seen in dogs.

Ferrets are susceptible to a number of infections that are well known causes of uveitis and retinochoroiditis in other species. These include toxoplasmosis, cryptococcosis, histoplasmosis, blastomycosis and coccidioidomycosis, but the resulting uveitis and/or other ophthalmic disease has not yet been properly characterized. Uveitis is the primary ocular lesion in mink with experimentally induced Aleutian disease, thus this disease might also be considered in ferrets with uveitis. Other causes of uveitis in ferrets include septicaemia and neoplasia, such as lymphosarcoma.

Because the presence of uveitis might indicate a systemic disease, additional diagnostic testing should always be performed when this condition is recognized. This testing should include conjunctival cytology, complete blood count, serum biochemistry panel, urinalysis, thoracic radiographs and abdominal ultrasonography as well as PCR and serology for infectious agents.

Treatment for uveitis in ferrets is similar to that in other small animals. Topical steroids are used in cases of uveitis in which corneal ulceration is not present. It is worth remembering that steroids can predispose an ulcerated cornea to secondary bacterial or fungal infections. The frequency of application varies directly with the severity of disease and can range from once daily to once hourly. Topical nonsteroidal ophthalmic solutions are also available. These too should be used with caution in cases of corneal ulceration as they have been implicated in retardation of corneal healing and secondary infections. Topical 1% atropine drops to relieve ciliary spasm caused by the release of prostaglandins during

uveitis may also be a useful adjunct therapy. This is used to relieve pain and also to minimize the potential for posterior synechia formation in the miotic eye. Caution should be used in cases where secondary glaucoma is a concern.

Systemic steroids at anti-inflammatory doses are still the cornerstone of the treatment of uveitis, but it is necessary to recognize that steroid use could aggravate the underlying cause of the uveitis. Systemic non-steroidal anti-inflammatory drugs can be used when appropriate for the patient, mainly when systemic steroids are contraindicated.

It is always best to diagnose the inciting cause of uveitis or at least rule out causes for which steroid use is contraindicated. Thus, when possible, the underlying cause must be identified and treated first. One should keep in mind that topical treatment only treats the anterior uvea. If there are concurrent posterior uveal signs, such as retinal oedema, retinal detachment, active retinitis or chorioretinitis, optic neuritis or retinal haemorrhages, then systemic treatment (usually steroids) is the only effective means to treat the condition. Prognosis is fair for acute uncomplicated cases but it is worse in cases where the condition is severe and chronic and, especially, in the presence of synechia and secondary glaucoma.

Cataracts

The opacification of the lens, lens capsule or both (cataracts) is fairly common in ferrets (Figure 29.8). Progressive cataract formation has been reported in two genetically unrelated populations of ferrets: Miller *et al.* (1993) evaluated three groups of ferrets for the presence of cataracts by use of slit-lamp biomicroscopy. The authors demonstrated that in certain ferret populations slowly progressive cataracts can form spontaneously with high frequency, citing a 47% incidence of cataracts in young ferrets. The mechanism of cataractogenesis in ferrets is unknown and may be multifactorial; causes for cataracts in ferrets may have genetic or nutritional components.

The general aetiology of cataracts is the same as for most animals and includes congenital causes and nutritional imbalances. Because congenital cataracts are suspected to be inherited, affected ferrets should be excluded from breeding programmes. Dietary factors may play an important role in the development of some cataracts and dietary disorders seem to be a more commonly reported cause of cataracts in ferrets than in other small animals. Reports indicate that a diet high in fat or deficient in vitamin E, vitamin A or protein may promote cataract formation in ferrets (Miller, 1997; Good, 2002).

Treatment for cataracts is strictly surgical and is considered as feasible in the ferret. Even though their small eyes and shallow anterior chambers make lens extraction difficult, reports indicate successful surgical treatment of cataracts in ferrets by means of an extracapsular or phacoemulsification technique (van der Woerdt, 2004). If surgical treatment is not chosen to correct the disease, there should be monitoring for the onset of secondary complications such as lens-induced uveitis (Figure 29.8b), subluxation, luxation and glaucoma.

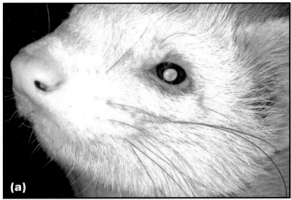

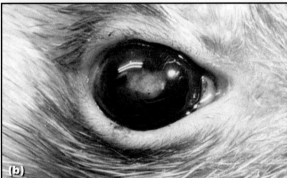

29.8 Cataracts in ferrets. **(a)** Mature cataracts. **(b)** Hypermature cataracts and lens-induced uveitis. Note the small size of the lens due to reabsorption of the lens cortex. The lens cortical material is reabsorbed faster than the nucleus. Note the presence of a blood clot and pigment in the anterior surface of the lens. Lens-induced uveitis typically affects ferrets with mature or hypermature ('resorptive') cataracts. (a, courtesy of Paolo Selleri; b, courtesy of Yasutsugu Miwa.)

Lens luxations and subluxations have been described in the ferret and they can occur as a primary condition to the non-cataractous lens or secondary to chronic cataracts. Lens-induced uveitis can usually be controlled with topical application of 1% prednisolone acetate twice a day (van der Woerdt, 2004). Lens luxation should be corrected by intracapsular lens extraction to prevent the development of glaucoma.

Glaucoma

Glaucoma is caused by a group of conditions rather than a single disease entity. All of these conditions (i.e. malformations, uveitis, neoplasia) lead to an impairment of the aqueous humour outflow system. This, in turn, leads to an elevation of pressure within the eye that is damaging to axoplasmic flow in the optic nerve head, resulting in retinal degeneration and loss of vision. A rise in intraocular pressure (IOP) also causes pain, which in turn can cause the ocular tissues to become hyperaemic. This means that glaucoma must be considered as a differential diagnosis for a red or watery eye.

Glaucoma is infrequently reported in ferrets. Nevertheless, primary glaucoma and glaucoma secondary to lens-induced uveitis are believed to occur. Neoplastic disease is also a possibility. Intraocular neoplasia can cause glaucoma by infiltrating the drainage angle or by causing inflammation and adhesions (Figure 29.9).

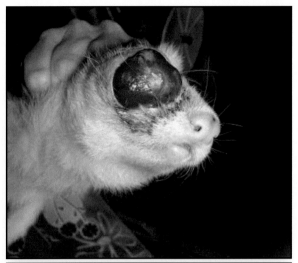

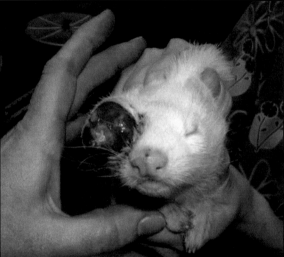

29.9 Chronic glaucoma has led to a massive buphthalmia and forward displacement of the globe of the right eye. Due to the magnitude of the globe enlargement, it was believed to be possibly secondary to an intraocular neoplastic disease. Further diagnostic tests were not possible at the time because the owners declined the recommendation of enucleation and/or histopathological analysis. Thus, the actual cause of this massive globe enlargement was unknown. The case was lost to follow-up care. (Courtesy of Angela Duke.)

A tonometer, an instrument that measures the IOP of an eye, is essential for the diagnosis and treatment of glaucoma. The most popular among veterinary ophthalmologists for small and exotic animals is an applanation tonometer called Tono-Pen XL (see Figure 29.5b).

The normal range of IOP in the ferret is 12–17 mmHg (Montiani-Ferreira et al., 2006) and represents a delicate balance between production of aqueous humour and its subsequent drainage from the anterior chamber. In normal ferrets there is usually no more than 5 mmHg difference in IOP between the left and right eyes of an individual.

In chronic cases of glaucoma, an absolute globe enlargement can take place. The condition occurs more quickly in young animals. If this condition has already developed by the time of presentation, the eye will probably be blind. If, despite intensive treatment, an eye becomes irreversibly blind with an elevated IOP, enucleation or evisceration should be discussed with the owners (see also Chapter 23).

An eye with uncomplicated severe iridocyclitis will typically have a low IOP. If the IOP is elevated or even towards the top of the normal range, the clinician should monitor for increases as the inflammation is suppressed. If there are no signs of active inflammation and the IOP surpasses the top of the normal range, the clinician should add anti-glaucoma medication to the treatment regime.

Although there are anecdotal reports about the use of topical beta-blockers (0.5% timolol maleate), carbonic anhydrase inhibitors (2.0% dorzolamide), parasympathomimetic agents (1.0% pilocarpine) and prostaglandin analogues (0.005% latanoprost) to treat glaucoma in ferrets, there are no scientific data supporting the efficacy of these agents in this species. The author suggests using the fixed combination of dorzolamide–timolol with one drop in the affected eye two or three times a day (q8–12h).

In one case of bilateral glaucoma in a 7-year-old neutered male ferret (Good, 2002), a diode laser was used to perform unilateral trans-scleral cyclophoto-coagulation to control the pressure in one of the two affected eyes that had been unresponsive to medical therapy. After 3 months of follow-up, the pressure was controlled with alternate-day application of a topical steroid.

Since the majority of glaucomas will not be controlled permanently with medication, clients should be advised that a surgical procedure might be indicated. If a clinician does not have the required expertise or equipment to monitor and treat cases of glaucoma, early referral should be considered before irreversible loss of vision occurs. There should be no waiting until globe enlargement (buphthalmia) is seen. Referral is no longer an emergency once buphthalmia has occurred, because vision has already been permanently lost for most of these buphthalmic cases.

Retinal atrophy

Progressive retinal atrophy (PRA) is reportedly fairly commonly in ferrets. It is a collective term used to describe several hereditary retinal diseases that appear clinically similar. Clinical signs are progressive loss of vision that may not be noticed until the disease is advanced, decreased pupillary light reflexes and mydriasis. Cataracts may or may not be present. Fundus examination reveals marked hyper-reflectivity and vascular attenuation, indicating retinal thinning. Suspected causes are still under investigation but include genetic factors and nutritional (e.g. taurine and vitamin A) deficiencies. Atrophy associated with taurine deficiency was well noted in reviews but not reported in the primary literature. As with cataracts, affected animals should not be bred.

Exophthalmos

Exophthalmos is the proper nomenclature for a pathological protrusion or prominence of the eye. In this condition a normal-sized globe is displaced rostrally within the orbit. This is not the same condition as buphthalmos, in which the globe itself is enlarged. Exophthalmos should also be differentiated from proptosis, which is a sudden (often traumatic) forward displacement of the globe that traps the eyelid margins behind the equator of the globe. The clinician should always look for eyelid margins. If the eyelid margins are visible, the condition can be defined as exophthalmos. If the eyelid margins are not visible, it is a case of proptosis (Figure 29.10).

Retrobulbar diseases, which are a common cause of exophthalmos in most species, are occasionally seen in ferrets. Possible clinical signs of retrobulbar disease are progressive exophthalmos, protrusion of the third eyelid and inability to retropulse the globe.

Neoplastic disease should always be considered during the preparation of a list of differential diagnoses for exophthalmos. There are several reported causes of exophthalmos secondary to orbital neoplastic disease in ferrets (Figure 29.11), such as lymphosarcoma. The diagnosis of retrobulbar lymphosarcoma can be confirmed by cytological examination of a sample collected from the retrobulbar area obtained by fine-needle aspiration. Ultrasonography is useful to aid needle guidance and sample collection.

Exophthalmos	Buphthalmos	Proptosis
Normal sized globe protrudes from the orbit	Ocular radii (corneal and scleral) increased, making the whole globe enlarged	Globe protrudes from the orbit
Examined from above: globe is positioned rostrally	Examined from above: enlarged globe is not displaced at the equatorial region	Examined from above: globe is positioned rostrally
Resists retropulsion	Retropulses normally	Resists retropulsion but degree of resistance depends on the retrobulbar tissue oedema and/or damage and the integrity of the bony orbit
Normal globe and corneal diameter	Increased globe and corneal diameter	Usually normal globe and corneal diameter
Often visual	Usually blind	May be visual or blind
Eyelid margins visible	Eyelid margins visible	Eyelid margins not visible
Common aetiology: retrobulbar disease	Common aetiology: glaucoma (primary or secondary)	Common aetiology: trauma

29.10 Clinical signs and medical manoeuvres that may help to differentiate between exophthalmos, buphthalmos and proptosis in ferrets.

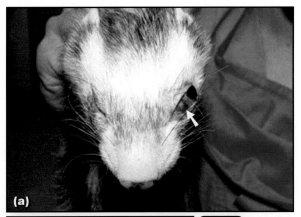

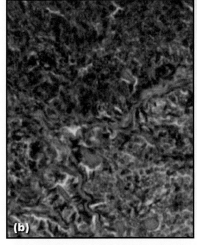

29.11

Exophthalmos in the left eye of a ferret due to an orbital tumour. **(a)** Note the soft tissue proliferation near the medial canthus region (arrowed). **(b)** The neoplastic tissue was diagnosed as adenocarcinoma originating from paranasal sinus epithelium. (Courtesy of Yasutsugu Miwa.)

Zygomatic salivary gland mucocele is another reported condition causing exophthalmos in ferrets. A retrobulbar abscess, even though not yet reported in ferrets, should be considered as a possible cause of exophthalmos, because it is a common cause of the condition in other species.

If available, a computed tomography scan is especially helpful in diagnosing retrobulbar disease.

Acknowledgements

The author wishes to thank Dr Gillian Shaw (The Johns Hopkins University, Baltimore, Maryland) for her help in the preparation of this chapter, the colleagues who have contributed with experience or photographs and Linda Harrison (*Exotic DVM*). Dr Marcello Machado contributed as co-author to the section on basic anatomical features of the ferret eye and supplied related figures.

References and further reading

Aboelela SW and Robinson DW (2004) Physiological response properties of displaced amacrine cells of the adult ferret retina. *Visual Neuroscience* **21**, 135–144

Bell JA (1997) Periparturient and neonatal diseases. In: *Ferrets, Rabbits, and Rodents*, ed. EV Hillyer and KE Quesenberry, pp. 53, 55, 62. WB Saunders, Philadelphia

Besch-Williford CL (1987) Biology and medicine of the ferret. *Veterinary Clinics of North America: Small Animal Practice* **17**, 1155–1183

Braekevelt CR (1981) Fine structure of the tapetum lucidum in the domestic ferret. *Anatomy and Embryology* **163**, 201–214

Chen B, Boukamel K and Kao JP (2005) Spatial distribution of inhibitory synaptic connections during development of ferret primary visual cortex. *Experimental Brain Research* **160**, 496–509

Davidson MGD (1985) Ophthalmology of exotic pets. *Compendium on Continuing Education for the Practicing Veterinarian* **7**, 724–737

Duval-Hudelson KA (1990) Coccidiodomycosis in three European ferrets. *Journal of Zoo and Wildlife Medicine* **21**, 353–357

Fox JG, Hewes K and Niemi SM (1984) Retro-orbital technique for blood collection from the ferret (*Mustela putorius furo*). *Laboratory Animal Science* **34**, 198–199

Gaarder JE and Kern TJ (2001) Ocular disease in rabbits, rodents, reptiles and other small exotic animals. In: *Fundamentals of Veterinary Ophthalmology, 3rd edn*, ed. D Slatter, pp. 593–599. WB Saunders, Philadelphia

Good KL (2002) Ocular disorders of pet ferrets. *Veterinary Clinics of North America: Exotic Animal Practice* **5**, 325–339

Gorham JR (1949) Salmonella infections in mink and ferret. *American Journal of Veterinary Research* **10**, 183–192

Hadlow WJ (1987) Chronic corneal oedema in aged ranch mink. *Veterinary Pathology* **24**, 323–329

Hernández-Guerra AM, Rodilla V and López-Murcia MM (2007) Ocular biometry in the adult anesthetized ferret, *Mustela putorius furo*. *Veterinary Ophthalmology* **10**, 50–52

Hoar RM (1984) Use of ferrets in toxicity testing. *Journal of the American College of Toxicologists* **3**, 325–330

Hoffmann KP, Garipis N and Distler C (2004) Optokinetic deficits in albino ferrets (*Mustela putorius furo*): a behavioral and electrophysiological study. *Journal of Neuroscience* **24**, 4061–4069

Kern TJ (1989) Ocular disorders of rabbits, rodents and ferrets. In: *Current Veterinary Therapy X*, ed. RW Kirk and JD Bonagura, pp. 681–685. WB Saunders, Philadelphia

Lenhard A (1985) Blastomycosis in a ferret. *Journal of the American Veterinary Medical Association* **186**, 70–72

Lewington JH (2000) *Ferret Husbandry, Medicine and Surgery*. Butterworth-Heinemann, Oxford

Liets LC, Olshausen BA, Wang GY *et al.* (2003) Spontaneous activity of morphologically identified ganglion cells in the developing ferret retina. *Journal of Neuroscience* **23**, 7343–7350

Lipsitz L, Ramsey DT, Render JA, Bursian SJ and Auelrich RJ (2001) Persistent fetal intraocular vasculature in the European ferret (*Mustela putorius*): clinical and histological aspects. *Veterinary Ophthalmology* **4**, 29–33

Lucas J, Lucas A, Furber H *et al.* (2000) Clinical *Mycobacterium genavense* infection in two aged ferrets with conjunctival lesions. *Australian Veterinary Journal* **78**, 685–689

Manger PR, Nakamura H and Valentiniene S (2004) Visual areas in the lateral temporal cortex of the ferret (*Mustela putorius*). *Cerebral Cortex* **14**, 676–689

Marini RP, Adkins JA and Fox JG (1989) Proven or potential zoonotic diseases of ferrets. *Journal of the American Veterinary Medical Association* **195**, 990–994

Miller PE (1997) Ferret ophthalmology. *Seminars in Avian and Exotic Pet Medicine* **6**, 146–151

Miller PE, Marlar AB and Dubielzig RR (1993) Cataracts in a laboratory colony of ferrets. *Laboratory Animal Science* **43**, 562–568

Miller PE and Pickett JP (1989) Zygomatic salivary gland mucocele in a ferret. *Journal of the American Veterinary Medical Association* **194**, 1437–1438

Montiani-Ferreira F, Mattos BC and Russ HH (2006) Reference values for selected ophthalmic diagnostic tests of the ferret (*Mustela putorius furo*). *Veterinary Ophthalmology* **9**, 209–213

Montiani-Ferreira F, Petersen-Jones S, Cassotis N *et al.* (2003) Early postnatal development of central corneal thickness in dogs. *Veterinary Ophthalmology* **6**, 19–22

Morris JA and Coburn DR (1948) The isolation of *Salmonella typhimurium* from ferrets. *Journal of Bacteriology* **55**, 419–420

Ringle MJ, Lindley DM and Krohne SG (1993) Lymphoplasmacytic keratitis in a ferret with lymphoma. *Journal of the American Veterinary Medical Association* **203**, 670–672

Ryland LM and Bernard SL (1983) A clinical guide to the pet ferret. *Compendium on Continuing Education for the Practicing Veterinarian* **5**, 25–32

Ryland LM and Gorham JR (1978) The ferret and its diseases. *Journal of the American Veterinary Medical Association* **173**, 1154–1158

Saunders GK and Thomsen BV (2006) Lymphoma and *Mycobacterium avium* infection in a ferret (*Mustela putorius furo*). *Journal of Veterinary Diagnostic Investigation* **18**(5), 513–515

Tjalve H and Frank A (1984) Tapetum lucidum in the pigmented and albino ferret. *Experimental Eye Research* **38**, 341–351

van der Woerdt A (2004) Ophthalmologic diseases in small pet mammals. In: *Ferrets, Rabbits and Rodents: Clinical Medicine and Surgery, 2nd edn*, ed. KE Quesenberry and JW Carpenter, pp. 421–428. WB Saunders, Philadelphia

Wen GY, Sturman JA and Shek JW (1985) A comparative study of the tapetum, retina and skull of the ferret, dog and cat. *Laboratory Animal Science* **35**, 200–210

30

Ferrets: endocrine and neoplastic diseases

Nico J. Schoemaker

Introduction

The two most common endocrine diseases in ferrets (insulinoma and hyperadrenocorticism) are also the most common neoplastic diseases. Endocrine and neoplastic diseases are therefore highly linked. The combination of an insulinoma and an adrenal tumour is frequently seen. It is even possible that these ferrets have additional concurrent lymphoma. The combination of other tumours is also possible (Figure 30.1).

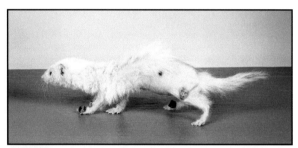

30.1 A 7½-year-old neutered female ferret with a history of progressive hair loss of more than 1 year and formation of skin masses over a period of 6 months. Ultrasonography confirmed a left adrenal enlargement, and histology confirmed the skin masses to be sebaceous epitheliomas. (© Nico J Schoemaker)

Endocrinology

Reproductive endocrinology

Gonadal activity in ferrets has a seasonal character in both genders. When day length exceeds 12 hours, reproductive activity is promoted. The pineal hormone melatonin plays a central role in the regulation of these changes. Plasma and pineal gland concentrations of melatonin are significantly higher during the dark phase of the day (scotophase) compared with the light phase (photophase). Hence, under natural light conditions the breeding season in the northern hemisphere is approximately from March until September. In ferrets that are kept indoors, the photophase is artificially lengthened by keeping the ferrets in a lightened room when it has become dark outside. It is therefore not uncommon to encounter jills that are already in heat in February. During the breeding season gonadotrophin-releasing hormone (GnRH) stimulates the production of the gonadotrophic hormones, luteinizing hormone (LH) and follicle-stimulating hormone (FSH), which stimulate the gonads to produce either oestradiol or testosterone. The latter two hormones exert a negative feedback on the hypothalamus and pituitary gland, thereby preventing an excessive secretion of GnRH, LH and FSH (Figure 30.2).

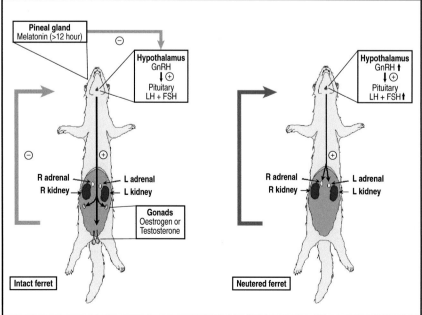

30.2 The regulation of reproductive endocrinology in intact ferrets, the consequences of neutering on this process, and the possible role it plays in the development of hyperadrenocorticism in this species. High melatonin concentrations for >12 h/day suppress the release of GnRH. When this suppression is lost, GnRH is released in a pulsatile fashion, resulting in the release of luteinizing hormone (LH) and follicle-stimulating hormone (FSH) which, in turn, stimulate the release of oestrogen and testosterone. This exerts a negative feedback on the hypothalamus and pituitary gland. When ferrets are neutered this negative feedback is lost, resulting in an increased release of the gonadotrophins, which may activate their respective receptors in ferret adrenal glands if they are present.

Persistent oestrus

Ferrets, like cats and rabbits, are induced ovulators. Jills need the most stimulation of all three species to ovulate. A firm stimulation, in the form of dragging by the scruff of the neck and mating, is necessary for ovulation. When ovulation does not occur, oestradiol levels will remain high until the end of the oestrous season. These continued high levels of oestradiol can lead to bone marrow suppression resulting in a pancytopenia, which is potentially lethal. Some ferrets will already show this pancytopenia within the first oestrous season.

Clinical signs

Pancytopenia may result in the occurrence of subcutaneous and mucosal petechiae or ecchymoses (Figure 30.3). In albino ferrets, the anaemia may be easily detected by observing the pale coloration of the eyes. Naturally, the nasal planum and mucous membranes will also be pale. In some ferrets, abdominal enlargement may be observed due to the formation of a mucometra (Figure 30.4).

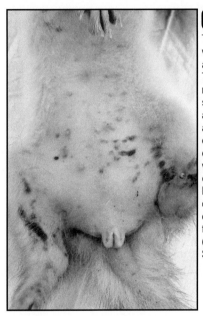

30.3 This female ferret was presented for an elbow luxation. The owner had not noticed the swollen vulva, abdominal alopecia and ecchymoses. The elbow luxation was most likely due to a haematoma that occurred as a consequence of thrombocytopenia. (© Nico J Schoemaker)

Diagnosis

Although blood is commonly collected from ferrets from the jugular vein or the cranial vena cava, it is advisable to collect blood from the cephalic or saphenous vein in ferrets suspected of having a pancytopenia. Due to the thrombocytopenia a large vein may continue to bleed, which may remain unnoticed. External pressure can also be applied more easily to the smaller veins of the extremities. Diagnosis of a mucometra is fairly easy by means of ultrasonography.

Treatment

The treatment of ferrets with pancytopenia due to persistent oestrus should address two aspects. One is to decrease the bone marrow suppression by oestradiol and the other is to provide supportive care and increase circulating blood cells.

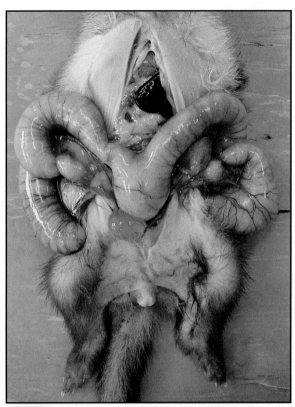

30.4 A female ferret at post-mortem examination showing a mucometra following persistent oestrus. Note the swollen pale vulva. (© Nico J Schoemaker)

Ovariohysterectomy would be ideal, as the source of oestradiol production would be removed. Due to the anaemia and thrombocytopenia, however, these patients are very poor surgical candidates. Ovariohysterectomy is also likely to increase the chance of the ferret developing hyperadrenocorticism later in life (see below). It would therefore be best to stimulate ovulation by giving 100 IU human chorionic gonadotrophin (hCG) intramuscularly, which may need to be repeated in 1–2 weeks.

A blood transfusion can easily be given to ferrets as these animals do not have any blood types. A blood transfusion should be given to those that have a PCV below 15%. Unfortunately, a thrombocytopenia cannot be addressed by providing fresh blood, as the platelets are destroyed during blood collection. Further supportive care may consist of hand-feeding, supplementing the diet with vitamins and minerals and giving broad-spectrum antibiotics to prevent secondary infections that may develop due to concurrent leucopenia. Prognosis is usually guarded to poor.

Prevention

Until recently, ovariohysterectomy was advised within the first year of life before the oestrous season had begun (usually in the first two months of the year). Independent observations, however, have provided support for the hypothesis that hyperadrenocorticism in ferrets (see later) is mediated by increased secretion of gonadotrophic hormones after neutering (Schoemaker *et al.*, 2000, 2002b). Potential alternatives are the use of progestogens, slow-release GnRH implants, GnRH antagonists or immunization against GnRH. Mating jills with a vasectomized hob has also been common practice in the UK for many years. Of the progestogens, proligestone (14α, 17α propylidene-dioxy progesterone) has been used for many years in the UK. The presumptive mode of action of proligestone is the suppression of the secretion of gonadotrophic hormones, thereby preventing ovarian cyclicity. Usually a single dose (50 mg/kg i.m.) at the beginning of the oestrous season is reported to be sufficient to suppress oestrus throughout the entire season. Only in a minority of cases is a repeat injection necessary after 2 months. In a trial (unpublished data) in the Netherlands, however, many ferret owners (14 out of 28) were unhappy with this type of oestrus prevention. The biggest problem was that some ferrets became pseudopregnant several days before the efficacy of the drug wore out. During this period the jills became very territorial and started to bite their cage mates and in some cases even their owners. Once the ferrets came into oestrus again, their normal behaviour would return.

Pseudopregnancy is also likely to occur after mating with a vasectomized hob. This technique is therefore not preferred for ferrets kept indoors as pets. Further studies are needed to find suitable alternatives for surgical neutering in ferrets. Research on the use of depot GnRH implants is ongoing in the Netherlands and seems to show promising results.

Endocrine diseases

Of the endocrine diseases known in dogs and cats, the following have never been documented in ferrets: growth hormone deficiency or growth hormone excess, diabetes insipidus, hypo- and hyperthyroidism, hypo- and hyperparathyroidism and spontaneous hypoadrenocorticism (Addison's disease). Although these diseases should not be high on the differential diagnosis list, they may not be ruled out.

Hyperadrenocorticism

Hyperadrenocorticism, also referred to as adrenocortical disease, or adrenal gland disease, is considered to be one of the most common diseases in ferrets. Since the first description of this disease (Fox et al., 1987), much information has become available. Hyperadrenocorticism in ferrets is different from Cushing's disease in dogs and cats. In the latter species, elevated plasma cortisol concentrations are characteristic for hyperadrenocorticism, while in ferrets, plasma androstenedione, 17α-hydroxyprogesterone and oestradiol concentrations are increased. The term hyperandrogenism might therefore be a more suitable description of this disease in ferrets.

In approximately 85% of ferrets with hyperadrenocorticism, one adrenal gland is enlarged without atrophy of the contralateral adrenal gland, while in the remaining 15% of cases there is bilateral enlargement (Weiss and Scott, 1997). After unilateral adrenalectomy in the case of unilateral enlargement, the disease may recur due to enlargement of the contralateral adrenal gland. Histological changes of the adrenals range from (nodular) hyperplasia to adenoma and adenocarcinoma. The histological diagnosis, however, does not provide any prognostic information. No functional pituitary tumours have been found in ferrets with hyperadrenocorticism.

Aetiology

In the USA, where ferrets are commonly neutered at the age of 6 weeks, it has been postulated that adrenal tumours may develop in ferrets due to this early neutering practice. The prevalence of hyperadrenocorticism in Dutch ferrets, however, has been reported to be 0.55% (95% confidence interval: 0.2–1.1%), and it can therefore also be considered very common. Since ferrets are neutered at a much older age (>6 months) in the Netherlands, it is unlikely that neutering at an early age is the most important factor in the development of these tumours. In the same report a linear correlation was found between age at neutering and age at time of diagnosis of hyperadrenocorticism (Schoemaker et al., 2000). Based on these findings it was hypothesized that increased concentrations of gonadotrophins, which occur after neutering due to the loss of negative feedback, persistently stimulate the adrenal cortex, resulting in adrenocortical hyperplasia and tumour formation. Strong support for this hypothesis may be found in the fact that the depot GnRH agonists, leuprolide acetate and deslorelin, can be used successfully to treat ferrets with hyperadrenocorticism, and that luteinizing hormone receptors (LH-R) have been detected in the adrenal glands of ferrets with hyperadrenocorticism. These receptors are considered to be functional, because plasma concentrations of adrenal androgens increase after intravenous injection of a GnRH agonist (Schoemaker et al., 2002b).

It has been proposed that ferrets kept indoors have a higher chance of developing hyperadrenocorticism compared with ferrets housed outdoors (Wagner et al., 2001, 2005). Since indoor ferrets will be more under the influence of light, and thus gonadotrophins, compared with ferrets that are housed outdoors, this aetiological factor has the same endocrine background as described above. The fact that adrenal gland disease is less common in the UK may therefore be explained by the fact that many ferrets are still being kept outdoors without being neutered.

A genetic background can play a role in the aetiology of this disease as well. Ferret owners have especially blamed a specific breeding facility in the USA, which provides an estimated 80% of all American ferrets, for the high occurrence of hyperadrenocorticism in American ferrets. If this claim were to be accurate, then why is the prevalence of hyperadrenocorticism so high in the Netherlands, where ferrets do not have the same genetic background as ferrets from this facility?

In humans a hereditary syndrome occurs in which multiple endocrine neoplasias are seen. Three different syndromes are recognized (MEN1, MEN2a and MEN2b). In ferrets, insulinomas and adrenal gland tumours are frequently seen simultaneously, suggesting that a condition similar to MEN in humans exists in the ferret. Research is in progress to determine whether this is indeed the case.

Clinical signs

The most prominent signs of hyperadrenocorticism in ferrets are symmetrical alopecia (Figure 30.5), vulvar swelling in neutered jills, recurrence of sexual behaviour after neutering in hobs, and pruritus. The skin itself is usually not affected, though some excoriations may be seen. The alopecia usually begins in spring, which coincides with the start of the breeding season, and may disappear without treatment. The next year the alopecia usually returns, but may not resolve spontaneously at the end of the breeding season. Other concurrent signs include urinary obstruction in males, due to peri-prostatic or peri-urethral cysts, and prostatic enlargement. Occasionally mammary gland enlargement in jills is also seen. Most cases of hyperadrenocorticism in the Netherlands are seen in ferrets >3 years; >80% are over 5 years of age. In the USA, more and more ferrets are already diagnosed with hyperadrenocorticism at 2 years. Although polyuria and polydipsia are reported in ferrets with hyperadrenocorticism, it is not clear whether adrenal hormone production is responsible for these signs, or if these (possibly elderly) ferrets have concurrent kidney disease. Initially it was reported that the majority of ferrets with adrenocortical disease were females. Noticing the enlarged vulva may contribute to this (false) sex predilection. A study performed in the Netherlands could not detect a sex predilection (Schoemaker *et al.*, 2000).

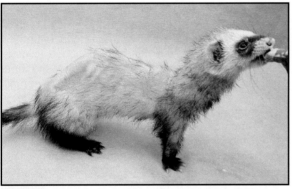

30.5 A female ferret with typical alopecia on the dorsum and flanks as seen in ferrets with hyperadrenocorticism. (© Nico J Schoemaker)

Diagnosis

The clinical signs are the most important tool in diagnosing hyperadrenocorticism in ferrets. During abdominal palpation enlarged adrenal glands may be palpated. The right adrenal gland is more difficult to palpate due to the overlying right caudal liver lobe. Different diagnostic tests are available for further confirmation of the diagnosis. The results of ACTH stimulation tests and dexamethasone suppression tests are not considered diagnostic in ferrets. In the USA a serum adrenal panel is performed at the University of Tennessee. This panel consists of androstenedione, oestradiol and 17α-hydroxyprogesterone (dehydroepiandrosterone sulfate is currently no longer incorporated). Elevation of one or more of these hormones is considered diagnostic for hyperadrenocorticism. In the author's opinion, androstenedione is the most sensitive indicator of all these hormones. Since hormone concentrations in intact female ferrets are identical to those in hyperadrenocorticoid ferrets (Quesenberry and Rosenthal, 2003), it is likely that this hormone panel does not aid in differentiating between a ferret with hyperadrenocorticism and one with an active ovarian remnant. In another study it was shown that plasma concentrations of ACTH and α-MSH in hyperadrenocorticoid ferrets (0.2–58.3 pmol/l (median 9.9 pmol/l) and 6–88.8 pmol/l (median 27.6 pmol/l), respectively) did not significantly differ from those of healthy neutered ferrets (2.9–22 pmol/l and 4.8–108 pmol/l, respectively) (Schoemaker *et al.*, 2002a). Based on these findings it is concluded that plasma hormone analysis is not an important tool for diagnosing hyperadrenocorticism in ferrets.

The urinary corticoid–creatinine ratio (UCCR), in combination with a high-dose dexamethasone suppression test (HDDST), is one of the most powerful tools for diagnosing Cushing's disease in dogs. In ferrets with adrenocortical disease the UCCR is also higher than the reference value of 2.1×10^{-6} (Schoemaker *et al.*, 2004). With an HDDST it is possible to show that hyperadrenocorticism is of non-pituitary origin. The UCCR, however, is also increased in intact ferrets during the breeding season, as well as in jills with an active ovarian remnant. The UCCR is therefore not considered to be of use in diagnosing hyperadrenocorticism in ferrets.

An abdominal ultrasound examination is one of the most useful tools for diagnosis. It is possible to determine whether one or both adrenal glands are affected, or whether an ovarian remnant is present. In addition, other abdominal organs can be evaluated during the same procedure. All of these results are of great value prior to surgery, so that the owner can be informed about the potential surgical risks that may be encountered.

To be able to distinguish an adrenal gland from an abdominal lymph node, specific landmarks need to be used. The left adrenal gland is located ventrolateral to the aorta, at the level of and/or immediately caudal to the origin of the cranial mesenteric artery. The right adrenal gland is more cranial and is attached to the dorsolateral surface of the caudal vena cava, at the level of, and/or immediately cranial to, the origin of the cranial mesenteric artery, and lies adjacent to the caudomedial aspect of the caudate process of the caudate liver lobe. Locating these structures during an ultrasound examination enables visualization of the adrenal glands in nearly 100% of cases. The adrenal glands of ferrets with hyperadrenocorticism have a significantly increased thickness (>3.9 mm), a rounded appearance, a heterogenous structure and an increased echogenicity, and sometimes contain signs of mineralization (Kuijten *et al.*, 2007).

The most important differential diagnoses include a non-ovariectomized female or the presence of active remnant ovaries. The author has also seen a ferret with severe alopecia and pruritus due to a food allergy. Hormone analysis in blood and urine, as well as abdominal ultrasonography, could not confirm the presence of a hyperfunctioning adrenal gland. Changing the diet in this ferret resolved the alopecia.

Treatment

The treatment of choice used to be surgery (see also Chapter 23). The left adrenal gland can be removed fairly easily, and only the phrenicoabdominal vein needs to be ligated. Resection of the right adrenal gland is more difficult, due to its dorsolateral attachment to the caudal vena cava and close proximity to the liver. During resection, either a part of the adrenal needs to be left attached to the vena cava, or part of the wall of the vein has to be removed. Some veterinary surgeons have ligated the caudal vena cava, but there is a great risk of hypertension distal to ligation which may lead to acute kidney failure. In cases of bilateral adrenocortical tumours, different surgical protocols have been proposed. Some advise the removal of the largest adrenal gland and part of the other affected gland. Others advise removal of both adrenal glands. When removing both glands there is a chance of inducing an Addisonian crisis. No accurate documentation of these cases, including an ACTH stimulation test to confirm the diagnosis, has been published. Short-term treatment with cortisone and fludrocortisone seems to be sufficient in most cases.

Different medical treatments have been proposed for hyperadrenocorticism in ferrets. Ketoconazole, which inhibits the steroid biosynthetic pathway in different species, was found to be ineffective. Mitotane (o,p'-DDD) has for long been the treatment of choice in dogs with pituitary-dependent hyperadrenocorticism. The mode of action of this drug is to destroy the adrenocortical layer, whereby the greatest affinity is for the cells of the zona fasciculata. This drug was found to be effective in a few ferrets at an initial dose of 50 mg once daily for a week, followed by 50 mg every second or third day. Due to the potential side effects, however, this drug is seldom used.

The most effective drugs to date are the depot GnRH-agonists of which leuprolide acetate is the most well known. Deslorelin implants (Suprelorin, Virbac) are now commercially available and are likely to become the drug of choice. The Lupron 30-day depot formulation is given at a monthly dose of 100 μg i.m. for ferrets weighing <1 kg and 200 μg i.m. for ferrets >1 kg. This drug will suppress adrenocortical hormone release for at least 1 month in ferrets and may last up to 3 months.

For many owners (and veterinary surgeons) it is difficult to understand why a depot GnRH-agonist would work in the treatment of hyperadrenocorticism since the increased release of GnRH and gonadotrophins, which occurs after neutering, is responsible for the disease in the first place. To explain this, it is important to realize that hormones produced by the hypothalamus and pituitary gland are released in a pulsatile fashion. For the release of gonadotrophins, a pulsatile release of GnRH is necessary. By giving a depot injection or implant with a GnRH-agonist, this pulsatile release is blocked, resulting in a single release of gonadotrophins followed by baseline concentrations. As a result, there is a cessation of hormone secretion by the adrenal glands and disappearance of clinical signs. In the author's experience, however, the tumour does not decrease in size. It has even been suggested that with the use of a deslorelin implant the tumour may continue to grow (Wagner et al., 2005). Further research is necessary to confirm the latter statement. In the author's experience, most ferrets respond very well to the treatment with a GnRH-agonist and will eventually die from a disease unrelated to hyperadrenocorticism.

Melatonin has also been proposed as a therapeutic option for hyperadrenocorticoid ferrets. The suggested mechanism behind this drug is that melatonin suppresses the release of GnRH (see Figure 30.2). Carter et al. (1982), however, demonstrated that ferrets kept under 8 hours light to 16 hours darkness (8L:16D) come into oestrus only 7 weeks later than ferrets exposed to long photoperiods (14L:10D). When ferrets kept under long photoperiods (14L:10D) received melatonin (1 mg/day) 8 hours after the onset of light, they came into oestrus only 7 weeks later than ferrets kept under similar conditions that received oil injections. It can therefore be questioned whether melatonin is capable of sufficiently suppressing the release of gonadotrophins. In studies using either daily administration of 0.5 mg melatonin orally or a subcutaneously placed implant containing 5.4 mg melatonin, there was alleviation of clinical signs in the ferrets with hyperadrenocorticism (Murray, 2005; Ramer et al., 2006). However, in the study in which melatonin was given orally, hormone concentrations in general rose and the tumours continued to grow. This treatment may therefore pose a risk to the ferret as their condition deteriorates, which may remain undetected by the owner. Another point to consider is that melatonin can be purchased in drugstores in the USA. Home medication with melatonin may therefore delay the initial presentation of ferrets with hyperadrenocorticism to veterinary surgeons.

In recent years trilostane, a 3β-hydroxysteroid dehydrogenase (3β-HSD) blocker, has become an important drug for treating pituitary-dependent hyperadrenocorticism in dogs. When looking at the biosynthetic pathways of adrenocortical steroids (Figure 30.6) it is tempting to speculate that this drug would be very effective in treating ferrets with hyperadrenocorticism as well (3β-HSD is necessary for the synthesis of androstenedione and 17α-hydroxyprogesterone). In an unpublished case, 5 mg trilostane was given orally once daily to a jill with hyperadrenocorticism. Within a month the owner complained that the alopecia and vulval swelling in the ferret increased. Plasma hormone analysis showed a decreased 17α-hydroxyprogesterone concentration, but increased concentrations of androstenedione, oestradiol and dehydroepiandrosterone sulphate. These results can be explained by the fact that a decrease of 3β-HSD may lead to an activation of 17,20-lyase, and thus the androgen pathway. Therefore, more research is necessary before this drug can be safely used in practice in ferrets.

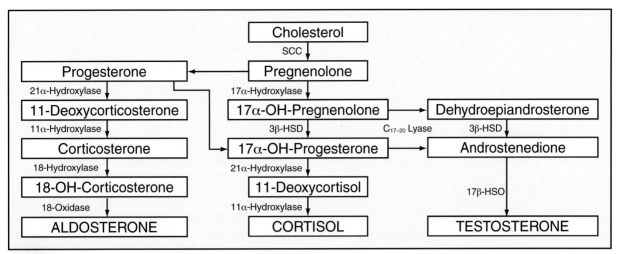

30.6 Major biosynthetic pathways of adrenocortical steroid synthesis. SCC = side chain cleavage; 3β-HSD = 3β-hydroxysteroid dehydrogenase; 17β-HSO = 17β-hydroxysteroid oxidase.

Insulinoma

Insulinomas are small tumours of the pancreatic beta cells. These microadenomas, sometimes referred to as islet cell tumours, produce an excess of insulin, resulting in hypoglycaemia. There is an equal distribution of insulinomas among the sexes and the median age at which ferrets are affected is 5 years (range 2–8 years).

Clinical signs

Clinical signs vary from slight incoordination and weakness in the hind limbs to complete collapse and coma. In humans, adrenaline is released in the early stages of hypoglycaemia. This may explain the nausea, which can also be seen in ferrets with insulinoma, in the form of salivation and pawing at the mouth. Besides these signs of nausea, owners may notice a glazed look in the eyes of their ferrets. Signs are most often seen when the ferret has not eaten for some time. Usually these signs resolve spontaneously, especially when the ferret is provided with some food or a calorie-rich beverage.

Diagnosis

Blood glucose concentrations <3.4 mmol/l (60 mg/dl), after withholding food for 4 hours, are considered diagnostic when ferrets display the above-mentioned signs. In ferrets with blood glucose concentrations between 3.4 and 4.2 mmol/l (60–75 mg/dl), the author advises prolonging the fast by another 2 hours. In most cases the blood glucose will then drop to below 3.4 mmol/l. Digital point-of-care (POC) glucometers, manufactured for use by human diabetic patients, seem very practical for obtaining quick results, but they are plasma calibrated. This calibration process has been found to be inaccurate for dogs and cats, which explains why different glucose values are measured from venous plasma, venous blood or capillary blood. The glucose concentration measured from venous plasma by an official laboratory should be considered the gold standard. Glucose concentrations measured with the POC meters in venous and capillary blood are, respectively, 75% and 70% of those from venous plasma. If one wants to use these

POC glucometers for measuring glucose concentrations in ferrets, new reference ranges have to be established for these specific meters. Plasma insulin concentrations can also be measured and are usually increased, but concentrations within the reference range may also be seen.

As insulinomas are usually very small (1–2 mm), it is not possible to visualize the primary tumour by use of diagnostic imaging techniques. In dogs, insulinomas are always malignant and quickly metastasize to the liver. These metastases can be seen on ultrasonography. Adenocarcinoma of the pancreas has been reported in ferrets. The great majority of insulinomas, however, are benign and do not metastasize (Weiss *et al.*, 1998). Diagnostic imaging in the form of radiography or ultrasound examination is therefore not routinely advised.

Treatment

Surgery is seemingly the best therapeutic option, as in this way excess production of insulin is prevented. Multiple tumours may be present, of which some can be so small that they remain undetected during surgery. In addition, it may be possible that some insulinomas cannot be removed due to their location near the pancreatic ducts in the body of the pancreas. Instead of a pancreatic nodulectomy, partial pancreatectomy is advised in order to remove as many undetectable islet tumours as possible and thus increase the survival time post surgery (see also Chapter 23). A mean disease-free state after surgery of about 1 year and a survival time of 22 months can be achieved in this manner (Weiss *et al.*, 1998). There is a chance of inducing diabetes mellitus if too large a portion of the pancreas is removed and it should be stressed that this has to be prevented, since the medical management of insulinoma is far easier than that of diabetes mellitus.

Medical management of insulinomas may be preferred by owners because of the age of the ferret or financial restrictions. Prednisolone and diazoxide are the drugs described for treating insulinomas. Prednisolone, of which the most important action is gluconeogenesis, is advised in most textbooks as the drug of first choice. Although the treatment protocol seems to be very effective in practice, side effects should be taken into consideration. The author, for instance, has seen a case of iatrogenic Cushing's disease in a ferret with long-term treatment with prednisolone. In addition, gluconeogenesis results in an increase of glucose. Increasing glucose by gluconeogenesis has the potential contraindicated risk of stimulating the secretion of insulin. Diazoxide, which is registered for treating human insulinoma patients, inhibits insulin release. The author therefore prefers this drug over prednisolone. Expense is often given as reason why prednisolone is chosen over diazoxide. Although the drug is certainly more expensive than prednisolone, the low dose needed by a ferret makes this a very affordable option. Compounding with methylcellulose also eases administration.

Treatment with diazoxide is started at a dose of 5 mg/kg orally q12h. The effect of treatment may be evaluated based on resolution of clinical signs as well as plasma glucose concentrations. Blood should be collected 4 hours after giving the diazoxide. During this period food should be withheld. The dose of diazoxide may be gradually increased. Prednisolone can be added to the treatment protocol at 0.2–1 mg/kg orally q24h in case of insufficient response to treatment. The author usually starts to add prednisolone to the treatment protocol when diazoxide at 15 mg/kg q12h is not able to control the hypoglycaemia. There are no real upper limits for the dosages of diazoxide and prednisolone. The only limiting factor may be the development of side effects such as vomiting and anorexia. Medical management, as described above, is usually sufficient to control hypoglycaemia for a period of 6–18 months, though the author has seen ferrets survive up to 2 years on medical treatment.

Prognosis
Prognosis is considered better in ferrets than in dogs, in which metastases are very common. Although metastases are rare in ferrets, multiple tumours and recurrent signs are common. Recurrent signs are probably due to the development of new tumours rather than metastasis of the earlier tumour.

Prevention
Based on the natural carnivorous diet of mustelids, it has been suggested that diets high in carbohydrates contribute to the development of insulinoma in ferrets (Finkler, 2004). Some veterinary surgeons therefore advise feeding a diet high in protein (42–55%), high in fat (18–30%), low in carbohydrates (8–15%) and low in fibre (1–3%) (all percentages on a dry matter basis). In the Netherlands it has also become popular to feed commercial balanced diets based on entire prey animals. Although the theory behind this advice sounds very plausible, there is no scientific evidence to back up any claims that these diets would indeed prevent the occurrence of insulinoma in ferrets.

Diabetes mellitus
Diabetes mellitus has been documented in ferrets, but is considered rare. It is most often seen after debulking of the pancreas for beta cell tumour removal. Clinical signs are identical to those seen in dogs and cats, with polyuria and polydipsia as the most prominent. Plasma glucose concentrations >22 mmol/l are considered suspicious for diabetes mellitus. Regulation has been attempted, starting with 0.1 IU of protamine Hagedorn insulin twice daily. Regulation of blood glucose concentrations in ferrets is difficult (Quesenberry and Rosenthal, 2003).

Neoplastic conditions

The most common neoplastic conditions in ferrets are adrenocortical tumours, insulinoma and lymphoma, but any type of tumour may be diagnosed. Only after an accurate diagnosis has been made can appropriate treatment be started. It is therefore necessary to follow a protocol to establish the type of neoplasm.

Diagnosis
Clinical examination
As with any patient, a thorough clinical examination is performed first. External masses can either be seen or palpated. It is important to record aspect, location, size and involvement of connecting tissues. For instance: is the skin tumour located within the skin or is there involvement of underlying structures? Indications of internal masses can be obtained during an abdominal palpation, or during auscultation of the thorax. Laboured breathing and coughing may also be seen (see Chapter 18).

Diagnostic imaging
The most common diagnostic imaging techniques for private practice are radiography and ultrasonograpy. Thoracic radiographs may reveal mediastinal masses as well as lung metastases. Ultrasonography is especially helpful in locating abdominal masses and may be very useful in determining the extent of mediastinal masses (see also Chapter 19).

Computed tomography and magnetic resonance imaging are more advanced imaging techniques. The resolution and limited availability of the equipment may be limiting factors. This may also be true for scintigraphy, whereby the distribution of radiopharmaceutical agents in specific tissues can be visualized using a gamma camera. The close proximity of both thyroid glands in ferrets may be an additional limiting factor when attempting to visualize possible thyroid tumours. This technique has been used to diagnose metastasis of bone tumours in ferrets (Antinoff and Hahn, 2004).

Cytology
Cytological evaluation of fine-needle aspiration samples is extremely useful in determining the origin of the tumour. An experienced cytologist can distinguish normal tissue from neoplastic tissue, with further classification into benign or malignant. The cell type can then be classified into epithelial or mesenchymal. This information, combined with the location of sample collection, will often result in a presumptive diagnosis. Histological evaluation of the tissue is necessary for confirmation of the diagnosis.

The procedure for fine-needle aspiration biopsy is the same as in other animals, though with a smaller needle than in dogs and cats. To obtain slides of good quality, the sample needs to be taken with a needle of at least 22 gauge.

Histology

Histological evaluation of tissue provides a more accurate diagnosis. The preferred surgical technique is an excisional biopsy in which enough margin is taken to prevent leaving part of the tumour behind. When cytology is indicative of a malignant tumour, a wider margin around the tumour is advised. If the entire tumour cannot be removed, an incisional biopsy can assist in deciding what therapeutic options are best suitable for that type of tumour (see also Chapter 23). Other types of biopsy are those performed during an endoscopic examination and so-called Tru-Cut biopsies. With the latter type of biopsy needle, fine pieces of tissue can be obtained. As the needle is thick, blood clotting times should be checked prior to performing this type of biopsy.

Besides routine staining, immunohistochemistry can be used to further specify the exact origin of cells. This technique is especially helpful for determining the type of lymphoma.

Lymphoma

Lymphomas are the third most common tumours found in ferrets and can be found in juvenile as well as adult ferrets. The disease in juvenile ferrets has been reported to be much more aggressive than in adult ferrets, though in one report this was stated not to be the case in the authors' practice (Antinoff and Hahn, 2004). A transmission study has been performed in which cells and cell-free inocula from a ferret with lymphoma were given to healthy ferrets. All inoculated ferrets developed lymphoma, suggesting that at least certain types of lymphoma are transmittable (Erdman et al., 1995). Feline leukaemia virus and Aleutian disease virus were both ruled out as possible causes.

Clinical signs

Clinical presentation of ferrets with lymphomas is often non-specific and may include loss of appetite, weight loss and peripheral lymph node enlargement. Although it has been reported that these signs may wax and wane for years, one may question whether an accurate diagnosis was made in most of those cases. More severe signs, as seen in juvenile ferrets, may include dyspnoea and coughing caused by pleural effusion and mediastinal masses.

Diagnosis

There is considerable controversy over diagnosing lymphoma in ferrets. Some authors state that cytological samples have to be submitted to pathologists with knowledge of ferrets to avoid missing the diagnosis. This may be due to the definition used for lymphoma in ferrets. Every pathologist will agree that finding atypical lymphocytes in any organ or lymph node leads to the diagnosis of (malignant) lymphoma. Finding large numbers of lymphocytes (normal or abnormal) in organs in which they are not commonly found is open for debate.

Radiographs can be useful in detecting masses in the anterior mediastinum and pleural effusion. With ultrasound examination, a more precise diagnosis can be made in the thoracic as well as the abdominal cavity. In addition, ultrasonography is very useful as a guiding tool for performing FNA, which is essential for confirming the diagnosis, though false-negative diagnoses (reactive lymph nodes) do occur. A full-thickness biopsy or surgical removal of an enlarged external lymph node is therefore recommended.

Histologically, lymphomas of juvenile and young adult ferrets are often immunoblastic with a high mitotic index, while lymphomas of adult ferrets are mixed cell lymphomas with a much lower mitotic index. Immunohistochemical staining can help to distinguish a reactive lymph node from a mixed cell lymphoma. There are two commonly used markers: CD3 is a T-cell marker, while CD79a is a B-cell marker. A reactive lymph node will contain both types of cell, while in lymphoma only one cell type will be found. These stains can be performed on cytological samples as well as histological samples.

Staging lymphomas in ferrets helps in determining which treatment protocol should be advised. The staging scheme used in ferrets is similar to the one used for dogs:

- Stage 1: One single site involved
- Stage 2: Two or more non-contiguous sites on the same side of the diaphragm
- Stage 3: Multiple lymphatic sites on both sides of the diaphragm (spleen, lymph nodes)
- Stage 4: Multiple sites on both sides of the diaphragm, including non-lymphatic tissue or bone marrow involvement.

Stage 1 has the best prognosis, while stage 4 has the poorest prognosis.

Treatment

Just as in the other companion animals, it is not possible to provide a clear-cut treatment protocol for lymphoma in ferrets. Surgery (splenectomy, lymph nodectomy) is the preferred treatment protocol in stage 1 cases. In stage 2 cases, surgery may also be of supplemental use. Stage 3 cases are predominantly managed through chemotherapy protocols, but supplemental surgery may be of use. Ferrets with stage 4 lymphoma seem to respond poorly to chemotherapy.

Different chemotherapy protocols have been developed for ferrets with lymphoma (see Chapter 21). It needs to be understood that administration of glucocorticoids to ferrets may result in resistance of lymphoid cells. Ferrets receiving glucocorticoids for treating insulinoma or immune-mediated diseases may therefore be refractory to chemotherapy. Temporary remission is seen with most chemotherapy protocols, but curing the disease is not likely. Radiation therapy has also been used as a complementary treatment option.

In cases where the owner declines these advanced treatment modalities, glucocorticosteroids may be used as an alternative to chemotherapy. Ferrets often respond well to these steroids initially but the duration of effect is limited. The author will start treatment with a dose of dexamethasone at 1 mg/kg s.c., followed by prednisolone at 1 mg/kg orally q12h.

Splenomegaly

Splenomegaly is a very common finding in ferrets but is seldom of clinical importance. It can be found in healthy ferrets as well as in animals with seemingly unrelated diseases. During abdominal palpation the spleen can easily be detected and in severe cases extends all the way to the pelvic inlet. The total blood count and differential white cell count of ferrets with splenomegaly does not show any abnormalities. The most common histological diagnosis of these enlarged spleens is extramedullary haemopoiesis.

Tumours of the spleen, however, do occur. Therefore, when a ferret is presented with non-specific signs and a large spleen is palpable on physical examination, abdominal ultrasonography is recommended. In the case of lymphoma, the spleen usually has an irregular aspect and hypoechoic areas. An ultrasound-guided biopsy is mandatory to confirm the diagnosis prior to surgery.

The only indication for splenectomy is when the spleen contains a tumour (e.g. lymphoma) or if the spleen is so large that it causes discomfort; otherwise the spleen should be left in place.

Integumentary tumours

Sebaceous epitheliomas and mast cell tumours are the most common integumentary tumours seen in ferrets. In a recent survey on the distribution of different neoplasms (n = 1525) submitted for histological evaluation, a total of 275 integumentary tumours were submitted (18% of all submitted neoplasias) (Williams and Weiss, 2003). Almost 40% of these tumours were sebaceous epitheliomas, while another 30% were mast cell tumours.

Sebaceous epitheliomas are of basal cell origin. Although multiple epitheliomas are frequently present, and the neoplasias have an irregular appearance, the tumour is considered benign. The tumours only involve the skin and not the subcutis, making them fairly easy to remove surgically.

It is important to realize that mast cell tumours in ferrets are benign. This is in sharp contrast to mastocytoma in dogs and cats. The tumours in ferrets do not infiltrate the dermis and can therefore easily be excised. Premedication with antihistamines and wide surgical margins are not considered necessary. After surgery, mast cell tumours may, over time, reappear at a different site. This is no indication of a poor prognosis, and these tumours may be removed as well.

Chordoma

The next most common tumour found in ferrets is the chordoma (3.6% of 1525 submitted neoplasms) (Williams and Weiss, 2003). A chordoma is a skeletal neoplasm originating from mesoderm-derived notochord. Chordomas are locally aggressive, destroying the vertebrae, but seldom metastasize. The great majority of these tumours (91%) are found at the tip of the tail (Figure 30.7), making them fairly easy to

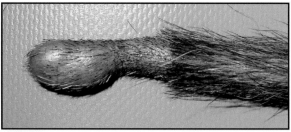

30.7 Typical presentation of a chordoma in a ferret. These tumours can easily be removed when they are present at the tip of the tail. (© Nico J Schoemaker)

remove. If the tumour is located further up the spinal column, no therapy is possible. During progression of the disease pathological fractures occur, making euthanasia inevitable.

The above-described tumours comprise more than 80% of tumour types found in ferrets. The remaining 20% represent tumours from other tissues which are also found in the other species. As described above, cytological and/or histological examination is necessary to determine the origin of the mass.

Treatment of neoplastic conditions

A good overview of available treatment options for oncological cases in exotic animal medicine has been published (Graham *et al.*, 2004). When surgery is technically possible, it is one of the most definitive treatment options. A common phrase used by an oncological surgeon is: 'When in doubt, cut it out.' Debulking of tumours is also commonly used as palliative treatment option. Besides the conventional surgical techniques, cryosurgery and laser surgery should be considered.

Chemotherapy is the next treatment modality. This can be performed systemically as well as intralesionally. Radiation therapy can be combined with chemotherapy or used as a single treatment option. More recent treatment options include photodynamic therapy, immunotherapy and the use of certain non-steroidal anti-inflammatory drugs.

Besides addressing the actual tumour during the treatment regimen, the veterinary surgeon should provide optimal support for the animal. Proper nutrition, especially in cachexic patients, is essential. Oesophageal feeding tubes are well accepted by ferrets and facilitate feeding high quality liquid diets such as feline convalescence support.

In conclusion, neoplasms are commonly found in ferrets. The diagnosis should be based on cytological and histological results. Some tumours are easily treated by practitioners. For more complicated cases it is advisable to refer these patients to a specialized centre where advanced oncological knowledge and treatment options are present.

References and further reading

Antinoff A and Hahn K (2004) Ferret oncology: diseases, diagnostics, and therapeutics. *Veterinary Clinics of North America: Exotic Animal Practice* **7**, 579–625
Carter DS, Herbert J and Stacey PM (1982) Modulation of gonadal activity

by timed injections of melatonin in pinealectomized or intact ferrets kept under two photoperiods. *Journal of Endocrinology* **93**, 211–222

Erdman SE, Reimann KA, Moore FM *et al.* (1995) Transmission of a chronic lymphoproliferative syndrome in ferrets. *Laboratory Investigation* **72**, 539–546

Finkler MR (2004) A nutritional approach to the prevention of insulinomas in the pet ferret. *Exotic Mammal Medicine and Surgery* **2**(2), 1–5

Fisher PG and Lennox A (2003) Therapeutic options for ferret lymphoma: a review. *Exotic Mammal Medicine and Surgery* **1**(2), 1–5

Fox JG, Pequet-Goad ME, Garibaldi BA *et al.* (1987) Hyperadrenocorticism in a ferret. *Journal of the American Veterinary Medical Association* **191**, 343–344

Graham JE, Kent MS and Théon A (2004) Current therapies in exotic animal oncology. *Veterinary Clinics of North America: Exotic Animal Practice* **7**, 757–781

Kuijten AM, Schoemaker NJ and Voorhout G (2007) Ultrasonographic visualization of the adrenal glands of healthy and hyperadrenocorticoid ferrets. *Journal of the American Animal Hospital Association* **43**, 78–84

Murray J (2005) Melatonin implants: an option for use in the treatment of adrenal disease in ferrets. *Exotic Mammal Medicine and Surgery* **3**(1), 1–6

Quesenberry KE and Rosenthal KL (2003) Endocrine diseases. In: *Ferrets, Rabbits and Rodents: Clinical Medicine and Surgery, 2nd edn*, ed. KE Quesenberry and JW Carpenter, pp. 79–90. WB Saunders, Philadelphia

Ramer JC, Benson KG, Morrisey JK *et al.* (2006) Effects of melatonin administration on the clinical course of adrenocortical disease in domestic ferrets. *Journal of the American Veterinary Medical Association* **229**, 1743–1748

Schoemaker NJ (2003) Hyperadrenocorticism in ferrets. PhD thesis, online at http://igitur-archive.library.uu.nl/dissertations/2003-1128-094343/inhoud.htm

Schoemaker NJ, Mol JA, Lumeij JT *et al.* (2002a) Plasma concentrations of adrenocorticotrophic hormone and alpha-melanocyte-stimulating hormone in ferrets (*Mustela putorius furo*) with hyperadrenocorticism. *American Journal of Veterinary Research* **63**, 1395–1399

Schoemaker NJ, Schuurmans M, Moorman H *et al.* (2000) Correlation between age at neutering and age at onset of hyperadrenocorticism in ferrets. *Journal of the American Veterinary Medical Association* **216**, 195–197

Schoemaker NJ, Teerds KJ, Mol JA, *et al.* (2002b) The role of luteinizing hormone in the pathogenesis of hyperadrenocorticism in neutered ferrets. *Molecular and Cellular Endocrinology* **197**, 117–125

Schoemaker NJ, Wolfswinkel J, Mol JA *et al.* (2004) Urinary excretion of glucocorticoids in the diagnosis of hyperadrenocorticism in ferrets. *Domestic Animal Endocrinology* **27**, 13–24

Wagner RA, Bailey EM, Schneider JF *et al.* (2001) Leuprolide acetate treatment of adrenocortical disease in ferrets. *Journal of the American Veterinary Medical Association* **218**, 1272–1274

Wagner RA, Piché CA, Jöchle W *et al.* (2005) Clinical and endocrine responses to treatment with deslorelin acetate implants in ferrets with adrenocortical disease. *American Journal of Veterinary Research* **66**, 910–914

Weiss CA and Scott MV (1997) Clinical aspects and surgical treatment of hyperadrenocorticism in the domestic ferret: 94 cases (1994–1996). *Journal of the American Animal Hospital Association* **33**, 487–493

Weiss CA, Williams BH and Scott MV (1998) Insulinoma in the ferret: clinical findings and treatment comparison of 66 cases. *Journal of the American Animal Hospital Association* **34**, 471–475

Williams BH and Weiss CA (2003) Neoplasia. In: *Ferrets, Rabbits and Rodents: Clinical Medicine and Surgery, 2nd edn*, ed. KE Quesenberry and JW Carpenter, pp. 91–106. WB Saunders, Philadelphia

31

Ferrets: systemic viral diseases

Anna Meredith

Introduction

Ferrets are subject to a number of important viral diseases. This chapter deals with the three important systemic viral diseases of ferrets; distemper, parvovirus (Aleutian disease) and rabies. Other viral diseases encountered in ferrets are mentioned elsewhere in the book: influenza virus (Chapter 26), coronavirus and rotavirus (Chapter 25). Vaccination protocols for ferrets are also discussed in Chapter 17.

Distemper

Canine distemper virus (CDV) is an RNA virus of the genus *Morbillivirus* (family Paramyxoviridae), closely related to human measles virus. There is only one serotype, but several strains that cause different clinical presentations. CDV occurs worldwide and mortality in ferrets approaches 100% in unvaccinated animals. Infection with CDV is relatively uncommon in pet ferrets, because of both ferret and dog vaccination, but unvaccinated dogs and wild canids, mustelids and procyonids can act as reservoirs of the disease. CDV was responsible for an epizootic in the highly endangered black-footed ferret (*Mustela nigripes*) in the USA in 1985. In Europe epidemics have been reported in polecats, stone martens, weasels and badgers. CDV does not infect humans, and measles virus does not infect ferrets.

Transmission

CDV is transmitted by aerosol and direct contact with infected animals, body fluids or via contaminated fomites. Virus is shed in ocular and nasal secretions, saliva, urine and faeces. An infected animal sheds virus from approximately 7 days post infection, just prior to or coincident with the development of clinical signs.

Pathogenesis

Virus replication after infection occurs primarily in the respiratory epithelium and lymphoid tissue of the nasopharynx. The virus is then carried in the peripheral white blood cells to the liver, kidneys, gastrointestinal tract, bladder and brain. Spread of virus is associated with pyrexia and leucopenia due to viral-associated loss of T and B lymphocytes.

Clinical signs

Clinical signs (Figure 31.1) appear after an incubation period of 7–10 days. Ferrets typically exhibit a catarrhal phase followed by a fatal neurotropic phase. Initial signs are anorexia, pyrexia, conjunctivitis and a serous nasal discharge. A characteristic erythematous and pruritic rash occurs on the chin and spreads to the inguinal area. Hyperkeratosis of the footpads is not a consistent feature of the disease in ferrets, but may be seen in some animals. Melaena may also be seen. Some ferrets die at this stage due to secondary

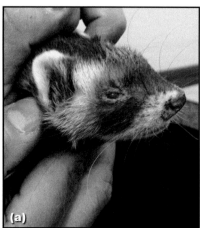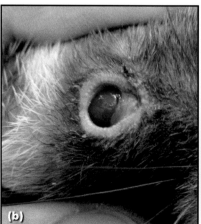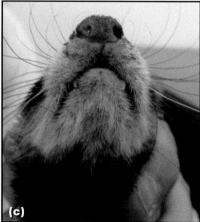

31.1 A case of ferret distemper. **(a,b)** Ocular and nasal discharge leading to crusting around the eyes and nose. **(c)** Nasal discharge and characteristic chin rash. (Courtesy of O Contreras and B Portillo Lopez.) (continues) ▶

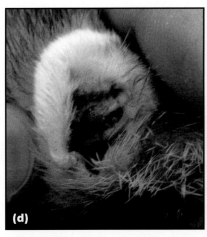 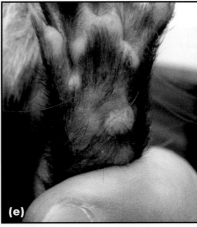

31.1 (continued) A case of ferret distemper. **(d)** This ferret also had aural discharge and crusting. **(e)** Swelling and crusting of the footpads. (Courtesy of O Contreras and B Portillo Lopez.)

bacterial infections, typically pneumonia. The neurotropic phase is characterized by hyperexcitability, muscle tremors, hypersalivation, seizures and coma. Death usually occurs in 12–16 days with a ferret-adapted strain of CDV, but can take a longer course of 21–35 days if infection is with a wild canine strain (Fox *et al.*, 1988). Hypothermia may be seen in moribund animals.

Diagnosis
A history of possible exposure, clinical signs and severe leucopenia are suggestive of CDV in an unvaccinated ferret. Diagnosis in the live ferret is generally obtained by immunofluorescence testing of blood smears, buffy coat or conjunctival scrapings. Inclusion bodies may also be seen on smears of conjunctival scrapes or buffy coat. However, these cytological tests are not very sensitive, especially early in the course of the disease, or in animals with a prolonged clinical course. Molecular techniques have been developed, such as reverse transcriptase polymerase chain reaction (RT-PCR) and nested PCR (N-PCR) on peripheral blood mononuclear cells, but these are not commercially available. Serum antibody tests can be used, such as serum neutralization and enzyme-linked immunosorbent assay (ELISA), but animals that die of CDV often do not have antibodies, and in dogs antibody titres vary inversely with the severity of the disease.

Post-mortem diagnosis includes suggestive gross lesions of thymic atrophy and pneumonia, and demonstration of round eosinophilic intracytoplasmic and occasionally intranuclear inclusion bodies in epithelial cells of the respiratory tract and other organs. The virus can be demonstrated by negative stain transmission electron microscopy, or via immunofluorescence or immunohistochemistry.

Treatment
There is no effective treatment for distemper and the disease is invariably fatal in ferrets. Supportive care may be attempted – fluid therapy, antibiosis, nutritional support – but there are no published reports of successful treatment of naturally occurring distemper in the ferret. Blair *et al.* (1998) reported treating a young ferret in the catarrhal phase, but only achieved prolonged and improved quality of life until the

neurotropic phase developed and the animal was euthanased. Rodeheffer *et al.* (2007) showed that, in experimental infection, ferrets given high doses (30 mg) of vitamin A prior to infection did not develop typical signs of distemper compared with control vitamin A-depleted animals. The ferrets given vitamin A only exhibited a mild rash and recovered uneventfully. This is similar to results seen with vitamin A therapy in humans with measles, and suggests that vitamin A has antiviral actions. The effects of vitamin A in treating established cases of distemper have not been reported, but this does provide an interesting therapeutic possibility.

Barrier nursing and strict disinfection practices should be employed in suspected cases, as infected animals will be a source of virus for other ferrets and for dogs. CDV is easily killed by heat, light and all commonly used disinfectants.

Prevention
The mainstay of prevention is vaccination. Both monovalent and multivalent vaccines may be used. Availability of vaccines varies between countries; for example, in the USA only one monovalent modified live vaccine is currently marketed and licensed specifically for ferrets. Purevax Ferret Distemper vaccine® (Merial) is a recombinant canary pox vector vaccine that has no adjuvant or entire virus and the manufacturers report an adverse reaction incidence of 0.3%. Moore *et al.* (2005) reported an overall incidence of 1% of adverse reactions to distemper vaccines in the USA. Another canine modified live CDV vaccine (primate cell line attenuated) has been assessed in ferrets in the USA (Galaxy-D®, Schering Plough Animal Health) and although it is effective in preventing distemper in ferrets challenged with CDV, the duration of immunity and incidence of reactions are not known and it is not FDA approved. The vaccination schedule is generally one dose at 8 weeks of age and then every 3 weeks for a total of three vaccinations, followed by annual boosters (Langlois, 2005).

In the UK and many other countries, no monovalent vaccines are available and multivalent modified live canine vaccines have to be used (containing distemper, canine parvovirus, canine adenovirus 2 and canine parainfluenza, e.g. Nobivac DHPPi®,

Intervet Ltd), which are not licensed for use in ferrets, but appear to be safe and effective. There is some debate about the dose and volume given, varying between one-sixth and one-half that of the canine recommendations (Lewington, 2000), and will depend on the viral isolate used, so individual manufacturers' advice should always be sought. The schedule for multivalent vaccines generally follows that of dogs, i.e. one dose at 6–8 weeks, one at 12–14 weeks, followed by annual boosters.

Postvaccinal distemper infections have occurred in black-footed ferrets given modified live CDV vaccine of chicken-embryo tissue culture origin (Carpenter *et al.*, 1976) and also in domestic ferrets vaccinated with CDV of canine kidney cell origin (Kauffman *et al.*, 1982).

Due to the risk of adverse reactions, it is recommended that all ferrets are observed for 25 minutes following vaccination, as this is the time period within which reported reactions have occurred (Greenacre, 2003), at least for adjuvant-based vaccines. Clinical signs reported are hyperaemia, hypersalivation and vomiting with or without diarrhoea. Moore *et al.* (2005) found that the risk of adverse reactions was associated with an increase in the number of distemper vaccines an animal had received. If adverse reactions are encountered, adrenaline, antihistamines, fluids and oxygen should be administered as required.

Vaccination site-associated sarcomas have been reported in ferrets (see Chapter 24), but the convention is still to administer vaccines subcutaneously in the interscapular region. Although the number of reports of sarcomas is very small, it may be more prudent to give vaccines subcutaneously in the rear limb, or at least to note on the animal's records where the vaccine was given. If a mass is still apparent at the inoculation site more than 2 months after vaccination, a recommendation in cats is that it should be removed with wide margins and submitted for histopathology (Danielle Gunn-Moore, personal communication), and this could also be applicable to ferrets.

Aleutian disease

Aleutian disease virus (ADV) is a parvovirus that affects both mink and ferrets. It is so called because when first discovered in the 1940s in the USA it affected the Aleutian genotype (blue coat colour) of mink most severely. There are several strains of ADV and at least three strains have been identified in ferrets that are distinct from the mink strains (Porter *et al.*, 1982). These ferret strains are believed to be mutant strains of the mink virus. Ferrets can also be infected with the mink strain.

Aleutian disease has been reported in ferrets in the USA, UK, New Zealand, Sweden, Canada and Japan. In the UK one survey of 445 ferrets found an incidence of 8.5% of seropositive ferrets (Welchman *et al.*, 1993) and in the USA approximately 10% of 500 ferrets in a shelter were seropositive (Hillyer, 1997). However, clinical disease is relatively rare.

Transmission

Transmission of ADV can occur via aerosol, by direct contact with infected saliva, urine, blood or faeces, or via fomites. Vertical transmission can occur in mink; this has not been reported in ferrets but is suspected to occur.

Pathogenesis

Aleutian disease is an immune complex-mediated condition, but the exact mechanism of interaction of the virus with the host immune system is poorly understood. Outcome of infection depends on the strain of ADV and the immune status and genotype of the host. In the classic form of the disease in mink, immune complexes are deposited in major organs (kidneys, liver, spinal cord, gastrointestinal tract, bladder) and cause a plasmacytic/lymphocytic infiltration of these organs, glomerulonephritis and vasculitis. Infection is associated with the presence of non-neutralizing antibodies, and many ferrets can be seropositive without going on to develop clinical disease.

Clinical signs

Severe disease and death are seen in Aleutian mink, but infection in non-Aleutian mink and ferrets is generally either asymptomatic or much milder. The clinical signs seen in ferrets are typically hindlimb ascending paresis or paralysis (which may or may not progress cranially) (Figure 31.2), chronic wasting, lethargy, melaena, hepatomegaly, splenomegaly and twitching or seizures. Some ferrets can develop a severe form of the disease and die. Onset of clinical signs is extremely variable, but most ferrets that exhibit clinical signs are between 2 and 4 years old (Langlois, 2005). Immunocompetent adult animals can be persistently infected and persistently shed virus without disease, or can develop clinical signs later in life. Immunosuppression probably plays a role in the development of disease. Affected animals are immunosuppressed, making them more susceptible to other infectious diseases.

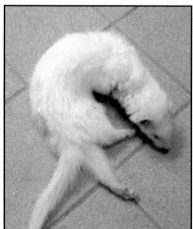

31.2
Severe hindlimb paresis in a suspected case of Aleutian disease.

Diagnosis

Hypergammaglobulinaemia is a feature of Aleutian disease and is considered pathognomonic in mink, but is more variable in ferrets and may or may not be present. Definitive diagnosis in the live animal is difficult and a presumptive diagnosis can be based on clinical signs, the presence of serum antibodies to ADV, hypergammaglobulinaemia and the presence of lymphoplasmacytic inflammation in tissue biopsy samples. Where hypergammaglobulinaemia is present, gamma globulins typically make up more than 20% of the total serum protein. Serum antibodies are detected using counter-current immunoelectrophoresis (CIEP), or the immunofluorescent antibody (IFA) or enzyme-linked immunosorbent assay (ELISA) tests. The commercial availability of these tests may vary according to country. A positive result indicates exposure but does not give definitive confirmation that the clinical signs seen are due to ADV. PCR techniques are also described for blood and tissue.

At post-mortem examination, gross lesions are either absent or non-specific, with hepatomegaly, splenomegaly and mesenteric lymphadenopathy reported.

Histological findings include lymphoplasmacytic infiltration in multiple organs, including the liver, periportal fibrosis, bile duct hyperplasia and membranous glomerulonephrosis. In animals with neurological signs a lymphoplasmacytic meningitis and perivascular lymphocytic cuffing are seen.

Treatment

There is no specific treatment for Aleutian disease, and therapy is symptomatic and supportive. Anti-inflammatory and immunosuppressive drugs may be useful; cyclophosphamide has been used to suppress lesions in mink for up to 16 weeks, but virus titres did not decrease. Syringe feeding, fluid therapy and covering antibiosis may be given, and mildly affected ferrets can make a full recovery, though those with severe clinical signs rarely improve.

Prevention and control

There is no vaccine for Aleutian disease and, given the immune-mediated nature of the disease, vaccination is probably contraindicated. In mink, experimental vaccination exacerbated the severity of the disease. Infected ferrets are a source of virus for other in-contact ferrets and strict hygiene practices should be employed when dealing with suspected cases. Formalin, sodium hydroxide and phenolic disinfectants are effective at killing ADV (Shen *et al.*, 1981) and products active against other parvoviruses are likely to be effective. In breeding and colony situations, serological testing and isolation or culling of seropositive animals may be indicated, along with cessation of breeding and disinfection. In the pet situation, this is generally not practical and culling of clinically normal seropositive animals is not acceptable, though it should be remembered that they are a potential source of virus to other animals. As the incidence of clinical disease is low, even in seropositive ferrets, the most practical approach is generally good hygiene and prevention of other conditions that may cause immunosuppression.

Rabies

Rabies is an acute fatal encephalomyelitis caused by viruses of the genus *Lyssavirus* (family Rhabdoviridae). Classic rabies is caused by *Lyssavirus* serotype/genotype 1 (rabies virus). Ferrets are susceptible to rabies but in the USA fewer than 30 cases have been reported since 1958 to the US Centers for Disease Control, so the incidence is low. There are no reports of human rabies due to a ferret bite. Ferrets have been shown to be susceptible to experimentally induced rabies with European bat lyssaviruses (EBLV) (Vos *et al.*, 2004), but virus transmission to other hosts seems unlikely.

Pathogenesis

Rabies virus must contact nerve endings and enter nerve fibres to cause infection and this occurs primarily by contact with infected saliva after a bite from a rabid animal. More rarely, infection can occur after contact with the conjunctiva or olfactory mucosa.

Clinical signs

Rabies in ferrets has been studied experimentally (Niezgoda *et al.*, 1997) and the incubation period is approximately 1 month, after which clinical signs of ascending paralysis, ataxia, tremors, paraesthaesia, hyperactivity, anorexia, cachexia, bladder atony, constipation, fever and hypothermia are reported. Aggression is not a consistent feature. Severity of the disease and whether or not virus is excreted in saliva vary depending on the type and dose of the rabies variant given (Langlois, 2005).

Diagnosis

In countries where rabies is present (not the UK), rabies should be considered as a differential diagnosis in any unvaccinated ferret that has access to the outdoors that develops neurological signs or alterations in personality. *In vivo* diagnosis is not possible, but if suspected the animal should be euthanased and the head or whole carcass submitted to the appropriate laboratory, where diagnosis is based on direct immunofluorescent antibody testing of brain tissue.

Prevention

Effective seroconversion and protective response to inactivated (killed) rabies vaccine has been demonstrated in ferrets (Hoover *et al.*, 1989; Rupprecht *et al.*, 1990). Killed vaccines are approved in some countries for use in ferrets (e.g. ImRab3® (Mérial) in the US). In many countries vaccines are not specifically licensed for ferrets but there are some data on their use (e.g. Nobivac Rabies, Intervet; Rabisin, Mérial). The protocol is for one vaccination at 3 months of age or older, followed by annual boosters. In the UK rabies vaccination is a requirement for ferrets travelling within the EU under the Pet Travel Scheme. One report exists of an adverse reaction to rabies vaccination (Greenacre, 2003).

References and further reading

Blair EM, Chambers MA and King HA (1998) Treating distemper in a young ferret. *Veterinary Medicine* **93**(7), 655–658

Carpenter JW, Appel MJ, Erickson RC and Novilla MN (1976) Fatal vaccine-induced canine distemper virus infection in black-footed ferrets. *Journal of the American Veterinary Medical Association* **169**(9), 961–964

Davidson M (1986) Canine distemper virus infection in the domestic ferret. *Compendium on Continuing Education for the Practicing Veterinarian* **8**, 448–453

Fox JG, Pearson RC and Gorham JR (1988) Viral and chlamydial diseases. In: *Biology and Diseases of the Ferret, 2nd edn*, ed. JG Fox, pp. 217–234. Williams and Wilkins, Baltimore

Greenacre CB (2003) Incidence of adverse events in ferrets vaccinated with distemper or rabies vaccine: 143 cases (1995–2001). *Journal of the American Veterinary Medical Association* **223**(5), 663–665

Greene CE and Appel MJ (1998) Canine distemper. In: *Infectious Diseases of the Dog and Cat, 2nd edn*, ed. CE Greene, pp. 9–22. WB Saunders, Philadelphia

Hillyer EV (1997) Aleutian disease. In: *Ferrets, Rabbits and Rodents: Clinical Medicine and Surgery*, ed. EV Hillyer and KE Quesenberry, pp. 71–76. WB Saunders, Philadelphia

Hoover JP, Baldwin CA and Rupprecht CE (1989) Serologic response of domestic ferrets (Mustela putorius furo) to canine distemper and rabies virus vaccines. *Journal of the American Veterinary Medical Association* **194**(2), 234–238

Kauffman CA, Bergman AG and O'Connor RP (1982) Distemper virus infection in ferrets: an animal model of measles-induced immunosuppression. *Clinical and Experimental Immunology* **47**(3), 617–625

Langlois I (2005) Viral diseases of ferrets. *Veterinary Clinics of North America: Exotic Animal Practice* **8**(1), 139–160

Lewington JH (2000) *Ferret Husbandry, Medicine and Surgery*. Butterworth Heinemann, Oxford

Moore GE, Glickman NW, Ward MP et al. (2005) Incidence of and risk factors for adverse events associated with distemper and rabies vaccine administration in ferrets. *Journal of the American Veterinary Medical Association* **226**(6), 909–912

Niezgod M et al. (1997) Pathogenesis of experimentally induced rabies in domestic ferrets. *American Journal of Veterinary Research* **58**(11), 1327–1331

Oshima K, Shen DT, Henson JB and Gorham JR (1978) Comparison of the lesions of Aleutian disease in mink and hypergammaglobulinaemia in ferrets. *American Journal of Veterinary Research* **39**, 653–657

Porter HG, Porter DD and Larsen AE (1982) Aleutian disease in ferrets. *Infection and Immunity* **36**(1), 379–386

Rodeheffer C, von Messling V, Milot S et al. (2007) Disease manifestations of canine distemper virus infection in ferrets are modulated by vitamin A status. *Journal of Nutrition* **137**(8), 1916–1922

Rupprecht CE, Gilbert J, Pitts R, et al. (1990) Evaluation of an inactivated rabies virus vaccine in domestic ferrets. *Journal of the American Veterinary Medical Association* **196**(10), 1614–1616

Shen DT, Leendertsen LW and Gorham JR (1981) Evaluation of chemical disinfectants for Aleutian disease virus of mink. *American Journal of Veterinary Research* **42**(5), 838–840

Stephensen CB et al. (1997) Canine distemper virus (CDV) infection of ferrets as a model for testing Morbillivirus vaccine strategies. *Journal of Virology* **71**(2), 1506–1513

Une Y, Wakimoto Y, Nakano Y, Konishi M and Nomura Y (2000) Spontaneous Aleutian disease in a ferret. *Journal of Veterinary Medical Science* **62**(5), 553–555

Vos A, Müller T, Cox J, et al. (2004) Susceptibility of ferrets (*Mustela putorius furo*) to experimentally induced rabies with European Bat Lyssaviruses (EBLV). *Journal of Veterinary Medicine Bulletin of Infectious Diseases and Veterinary Public Health* **51**(2), 55–60

Welchman D deB, Oxenham M and Done SH (1993) Aleutian disease in domestic ferrets: diagnostic findings and survey results. *Veterinary Record* **132**(19), 479–484

Williams ES (2001) Canine distemper. In: *Infectious Diseases of Wildlife, 3rd edn.*, ed. ES Williams and IK Barker, pp. 50–59. Manson Publishing/The Veterinary Press, London

Williams ES et al. (1988) Canine distemper in black-footed ferrets (*Mustela nigripes*) from Wyoming. *Journal of Wildlife Diseases* **24**(3), 385–398

Wimsatt J, Jay MT, Innes KE, Jessen M and Collins JK (2001) Serologic evaluation, efficacy, and safety of a commerical modified-live canine distemper vaccine in domestic ferrets. *American Journal of Veterinary Research* **62**(5), 736–740

Differential diagnoses based on clinical signs

Myomorph rodents: mice [M], rats [R], hamsters [H] and gerbils [G]

Clinical sign	Differential diagnoses	Further investigations
Abdominal distension	Ileus Gastric tympany ('bloat') [G] Ascites, e.g. associated with a hepatopathy (see below) Neoplasia Intussusception Colorectal impaction Tyzzer's disease or other clostridial enteropathy Cryptosporidiosis Proliferative ileitis [H] Bacterial enteritis (e.g. salmonellosis) Antibiotic-associated enterocolitis [H,G] Abdominal mass (see below) Pregnancy Obesity Organomegaly	CBC and blood biochemistry; radiography, contrast studies; ultrasonography; peritoneal tap; exploratory surgery
Abdominal mass	Foreign body Impaction Neoplasia Hepatomegaly Uterine hyperplasia/neoplasia Pyometra Metritis Cystic ovarian disease Polycystic disease Abdominal fat Fetus(es) Abscess	CBC and blood biochemistry; radiography, contrast studies; ultrasonography; ultrasound-guided FNA; exploratory surgery/biopsy
Alopecia	Barbering Dermatophytosis Fur mites (*Myobia musculi, Myocoptes musculinus* and *Radfordia affinis* [M]; *Radfordia ensifera* [R]; *Acarus farris* [G]) *Demodex* mite [H,G] Hormonal (hyperadrenocorticism [H,G], cystic ovarian disease [H,G]) Nutritional disease Epitheliotropic lymphoma [H]	Impression smears – cytology; skin scrape – deep and superficial; microscopic examination of hair; fungal culture; skin biopsy
Anaemia	Renal disease Any chronic disease Lead toxicity [G]	CBC and blood biochemistry; serum lead levels (sample volume may be a problem in an anaemic animal); radiography; ultrasonography
Anorexia	Dental disease Any systemic disease, especially gastrointestinal, amyloidosis, renal failure [R] Pain Any stressor	CBC and blood biochemistry; dental examination; radiography – skull and body; ultrasonography
Ascites	Abdominal neoplasia Liver disease Cardiac disease Renal disease Enteric disease Amyloidosis [H,G]	CBC and blood biochemistry; peritoneal tap and cytology; radiography; ultrasonography; liver FNA/biopsy ▶

Clinical sign	Differential diagnoses	Further investigations
Dermatitis	Ectoparasites – fur mites, *Notoedres muris* [R], *Notoedres notoedres* [H], *Polyplax serrata* [M,R], pinworms [M,R] Bacterial dermatitis (usually secondary *Staphylococcus aureus*, *Streptococcus* spp., *Corynebacterium* spp.) Dermatophytosis Self-trauma – fight wounds, bites Viral infection (mousepox [M], sialodacryoadenitis virus [M,R]) Immune complex vasculitis [R] Injection site reaction (enrofloxacin)	Impression smears – cytology; skin scrape – deep and superficial; microscopic examination of hair; bacterial culture; fungal culture; skin biopsy; histology; serology
Diarrhoea	Nutritional/dietary factors Environmental stressors Antibiotic-induced enterotoxaemia Bacterial enteritis – Tyzzer's disease (*Clostridium piliforme*), salmonellosis, *Lawsonia intracellularis* [H]) Viral enteritis – mouse hepatitis virus [M], rotavirus [M,R] Candidiasis Cestodiasis Helminthiasis Protozoal enteritis Liver disease Gastric stasis/ileus	Dietary history; faecal analysis – culture, parasitology; radiography/contrast studies; post-mortem examination; histology; serology
Dyspnoea / collapse	Any respiratory disease (see below) Cardiac disease [H,G] Severe pain Gastric tympany [G] Megaoesophagus [R]	Radiography; echocardiography; ECG; CBC and blood biochemistry
Facial swelling	Facial/dental abscess Cellulitis Coronaviruses: sialodacryoadenitis virus (SDAV); Parker's rat coronavirus [R] Neoplasia, e.g. Zymbal's gland tumour [R] Cheek pouch disease [H]	Skull radiography; dental examination; fine-needle aspiration; histopathology; serology
Haematuria	Cystitis Urolithiasis Bladder neoplasia Uterine hyperplasia/neoplasia Pyometra Renal infarcts Ovarian cystic disease [G] Disseminated intravascular coagulation	Urinalysis – dipstick, culture, cytology; CBC and biochemistry; radiography/contrast studies; ultrasonography
Lower respiratory signs	Bacterial pneumonia (*Mycoplasma pulmonis*, esp. [R], *Pasteurella pneumotropica*, *Streptococcus penumoniae*, CAR *Bacillus*, *Corynebacterium* spp.) Viral pneumonia (Sendai virus – young animals) Parasitic pneumonia (*Pneumocystis carinii* – immunodeficient [M,R]) Pulmonary abscess Pulmonary neoplasia – primary or secondary Cardiac disease [H,G]	Radiography; pleural fluid analysis and culture; bronchoalveolar lavage; ultrasound-guided biopsy; echocardiography; serology
Neurological signs	Otitis media and interna – *Pseudomonas aeruginosa/Mycoplasma pulmonis*, *Pasteurella pneumotropica*, *Streptococcus pneumoniae* [R] Heat stroke Trauma CNS neoplasia (pituitary adenoma [R]) Aural cholesteatomas [G] Epilepsy [G] Lead toxicity [G]	Neurological examination; radiography (skull, spine); CBC and blood biochemistry; serology; MRI/CT scan
Paresis/paralysis	Lymphocytic choriomeningitis virus (LCMV) Mouse poliovirus infection (Theiler's meningoencephalitis virus) Murine encephalomyelitis virus Spontaneous degeneration of the spinal cord and peripheral nerves (radiculoneuropathy) [R] Streptomycin toxicity [G] Spinal trauma (fracture/luxation)	Neurological examination; radiography; serology; MRI/CT scan
Rectal prolapse	Usually occurs secondary to diarrhoea or straining, e.g. proliferative ileitis or other cause of severe enteritis; helminthiasis	Faecal analysis – culture, parasitology; post-mortem examination ▶

Clinical sign	Differential diagnoses	Further investigations
Subcutaneous mass	Abscess Seroma Haematoma Mammary neoplasia Lymphoma [H] Other neoplasia Galactocele Injection reaction	Ultrasonography; fine-needle aspiration; biopsy
Testicular swelling	Orchitis Epididymitis Testicular neoplasia NB: Open inguinal canal, testicles can appear swollen but may be normal in these species	Ultrasonography; fine-needle aspiration; bacterial culture; histology
Torticollis	Otitis media/interna *Clostridium piliforme* (Tyzzer's disease), Neoplastic disease of the nervous system (glioblastoma, astrocytoma, pituitary adenoma) Aural cholesteatomas [G] Aural papilloma/polyp [G] Meningitis Cerebral abscess Trauma	Aural examination/endoscopy; skull radiography; bacterial culture; CBC and blood biochemistry; MRI/CT scan
Urinary incontinence/ urine scald	Cystitis Urolithiasis Posterior paralysis/paresis (see above) Renal failure Diabetes mellitus	Urinalysis; radiography; ultrasonography; CBC and blood biochemistry
Upper respiratory signs	*Mycoplasma pulmonis* Other bacterial URT disease, e.g. *Pasteurella pneumotropica* Coronaviruses [R] Fungal URT disease High environmental ammonia levels Allergic/irritant rhinitis Foreign body Neoplasia Dental disease	Radiography; endoscopy; bacterial culture; fungal culture; serology
Vaginal discharge	Pyometra, e.g *Mycoplasma pulmonis* Mucometra [M] Metritis Uterine hyperplasia/neoplasia Dystocia Normal oestrous cycle [H]	Culture and cytology of discharge; radiography; ultrasonography; exploratory surgery
Weight loss	Dental disease Any infectious or metabolic disease Neoplasia Bullying	Dental examination; radiography; ultrasonography; CBC and biochemistry; urinalysis; appropriate serology; faecal sample; MRI/CT scan

Hystricomorph rodents: guinea pigs [GP], chinchillas [C] and degus [D]

Clinical sign	Differential diagnoses	Further investigations
Abdominal distension	Cystic ovarian disease [GP] Gastric bloat Ileus Ascites Organomegaly Pregnancy Abdominal mass (see below)	CBC and blood biochemistry; radiography, contrast studies; ultrasonography; peritoneal tap; exploratory surgery ▶

Appendix 1 Differential diagnoses based on clinical signs

Clinical sign	Differential diagnoses	Further investigations
Abdominal mass	Neoplasia Abscess Lymphadenopathy – e.g yersiniosis, lymphoma/lymphosarcoma [GP] GI foreign body Gastric trichobezoar Impaction Uterine hyperplasia/neoplasia Pyometra/metritis Cystic ovarian disease Abdominal fat Pregnancy	CBC and blood biochemistry; radiography, contrast studies; ultrasonography; ultrasound-guided FNA; exploratory surgery/biopsy
Alopecia	Barbering/fur chewing Stress Ectoparasites (*Trixacarus, Gliricola porcelli, Gyropus ovalis, Demodex caviae, Chirodiscoides caviae* [GP]) Dermatophytosis Fur slip [C] Cystic ovarian disease (bilateral symmetric) [GP] Pregnancy- and lactation-associated [GP] Hyperadrenocorticism (bilateral symmetric) [GP]	Examination of plucked hair; cellophane tape test; skin scrapes; Wood's lamp; radiography; ultrasonography; serum/saliva cortisol levels; ACTH stimulation test
Anaemia	Renal disease Any chronic disease Lead toxicity Hypovitaminosis C [GP]	CBC and blood biochemistry; serum lead levels; bone marrow biopsy
Anorexia	Any systemic disease – infectious/metabolic Oral disease Dental disease Hypovitaminosis C [GP] Change in diet Pregnancy toxaemia Pyometra	CBC and blood biochemistry; radiography; ultrasonography
Ascites	Abdominal neoplasia Liver disease Cardiac disease Renal disease Enteric disease	CBC and blood biochemistry; peritoneal tap and cytology; radiography; ultrasonography; liver FNA/biopsy
Dermatitis	Ectoparasites (*Trixacarus, Gliricola porcelli, Gyropus ovalis, Demodex caviae, Chirodiscoides caviae* [GP]) Bacterial dermatitis Dermatophytosis Allergic dermatitis Pododermatitis Hypovitaminosis C [GP] Dental disease (moist dermatitis)	Cellophane tape test; impression smears – cytology; skin scrape – deep and superficial; microscopic examination of hair; bacterial culture; fungal culture/Wood's lamp; skin biopsy; histology; radiography (pododermatitis); dental examination
Diarrhoea	Nutritional/dietary factors Environmental stressors Antibiotic-induced enterotoxaemia (*Clostridium difficile*) Bacterial enteritis – Tyzzer's disease (*Clostridium piliforme*), *C. perfringens, Salmonella* spp., *Escherichia coli, Yersinia pseudotuberculosis, Pseudomonas aeruginosa, Listeria monocytogenes* Candidiasis Protozoal enteritis Liver disease Gastric stasis/ileus	Dietary history; faecal analysis – culture, parasitology; radiography/contrast studies; post-mortem examination; histology; serology
Dyspnoea / collapse	Cardiovascular disease Respiratory disease (e.g. *Bordetella bronchispeptica. Streptococcus pneumoniae*, pulmonary neoplasia; see URT signs below) Pregnancy toxaemia Heat stroke Choke [C] Hypovitaminosis C [GP] Any severe metabolic disease	Radiography; bronchoalveolar lavage and cytology/culture; echocardiography; endoscopy (choke)

▶

338

Clinical sign	Differential diagnoses	Further investigations
Facial swelling	Dental disease Dental abscess Cervical lymphadenitis [GP] Abscess Neoplasia	Skull radiography; dental examination; FNA and cytology; histopathology; CT/MRI scan
Haematuria	Cystitis Urolithiasis Bladder neoplasia Uterine hyperplasia/neoplasia Pyometra Renal infarcts Ovarian cystic disease [GP] Disseminated intravascular coagulation	Urinalysis – dipstick, culture, cytology; CBC and biochemistry; radiography/contrast studies; ultrasonography
Lower respiratory signs	Bacterial pneumonia Parasitic pneumonia (*Pneumocystis carinii* – immunodeficient [GP]) Pulmonary abscess Pulmonary neoplasia – primary or secondary Cardiac disease Mediastinal disease – e.g. lymphoma/lymphosarcoma [GP]	Radiography; pleural fluid analysis and culture; bronchoalveolar lavage; ultrasound-guided biopsy; echocardiography; serology
Neurological signs	Heat stress Pregnancy toxaemia Trauma Hypocalcaemia Systemic bacterial infections *Clostridium piliforme* (Tyzzer's disease) Toxoplasmosis Lymphocytic choriomeningitis virus (LCMV) Vitamin E deficiency Hypervitaminosis D Osteoarthritis Vitamin C deficiency Lead toxicosis [C] *Frenkelia* [C] Herpesvirus 1 infections (human herpesvirus) [C] Otitis media/interna Epilepsy [C,D]	Neurological examination; radiography (skull, spine); CBC and blood biochemistry; serology; MRI/CT scan; (*Toxoplasma*, LCMV); serum lead levels
Paresis/paralysis	Spinal trauma (fracture/luxation) Spondylosis/spondylitis Spinal abscess Osteoarthritis (infectious and spontaneous) Histoplasmosis [GP] Iatrogenic (intramuscular drug administration) Vitamin D deficiency	Neurological examination; radiography; CBC and blood biochemistry; MRI/CT scan; serology
Subcutaneous mass	Abscess Seroma Haematoma Lymphoma [GP] Benign trichoepithelioma [GP] Other neoplasia Injection reaction	Ultrasonography; fine-needle aspiration; biopsy
Testicular swelling	Orchitis Epididymitis Testicular neoplasia Do not confuse with rectal faecal impactions in older male [GP]	Ultrasonography; fine-needle aspiration; bacterial culture; histology
Torticollis	Otitis media and interna Meningitis *Baylisascaris* Severe reactions to *Trixicarus caviae* infections [GP] Streptococcal lymphadenitis – [GP] Ototoxicity Gentamicin toxicity [GP] Listeriosis [C] Thiamine deficiency [C] Aflatoxicosis [C] Cerebral abscess	Aural examination/endoscopy; skull radiography; bacterial culture; CBC and blood biochemistry; MRI/CT scan ▶

Appendix 1   Differential diagnoses based on clinical signs

Clinical sign	Differential diagnoses	Further investigations
Urinary incontinence/ urine scald	Cystitis Urolithiasis Posterior paralysis/paresis (see above) Obesity Renal failure, e.g. chronic interstitial nephritis [GP] Diabetes mellitus	Urinalysis; radiography; ultrasonography; CBC and blood biochemistry
Upper respiratory signs	*Bordetella bronchiseptica* [GP] *Chlamydophila caviae* [GP] *Streptococcus zooepidemicus* [GP] Other bacterial URT disease, e.g. *Streptococcus pneumoniae* [GP] High environmental ammonia levels Allergic/irritant rhinitis Adenovirus [GP] Fungal URT disease Foreign body Neoplasia / polyps Dental disease Choke [C]	Radiography; endoscopy; bacterial culture; fungal culture; serology; conjunctival scraping (*Chlamydophila*)
Vaginal discharge	Pyometra, e.g. *Bordetella bronchiseptica*, haemolytic *Streptococcus* Vaginitis Metritis Uterine hyperplasia/neoplasia Dystocia Mucometra [GP] Ovarian cystic disease [GP]	Culture and cytology of discharge; radiography; ultrasonography; exploratory surgery
Weight loss	Dental disease Any infectious or metabolic disease Neoplasia Bullying, e.g. housed with rabbits [GP]	Dental examination; radiography; ultrasonography; CBC and biochemistry; urinalysis; appropriate serology; faecal sample; MRI/CT scan

Ferrets

Clinical sign	Differential diagnoses	Further investigations
Abdominal distension	Splenomegaly Polycystic kidneys/renal cyst GI foreign body Neoplasia Ascites (see below)	CBC and blood biochemistry; radiography, contrast studies; ultrasonography; peritoneal tap; exploratory surgery; pregnancy and abdominal mass (see below)
Abdominal mass	Neoplasia Abscess/granuloma Lymphadenopathy Splenomegaly GI foreign body Pyometra/mucometra (incl. stump) Urinary tract obstruction Hydronephrosis Polycystic kidneys/renal cyst	CBC and blood biochemistry; radiography, contrast studies; ultrasonography; ultrasound-guided fine-needle aspiration; exploratory surgery
Alopecia	Hyperadrenocorticism Hyperoestrogenism Seasonal Telogen defluxion (stress) Mast cell tumour *Sarcoptes scabiei*	Examination of plucked hair; examination for fleas; radiography; ultrasonography; CBC; serum adrenal hormone panel
Anaemia	Ticks, fleas Lead toxicity Renal disease Gastrointestinal bleeding (ulceration) Neoplasia Aleutian disease Hyperoestrogenism Any chronic disease	CBC and blood biochemistry; ectoparasite examination; faecal occult blood; serum lead levels; endoscopy; CIEP/ELISA (Aleutian disease); bone marrow biopsy

▶

Clinical sign	Differential diagnoses	Further investigations
Anorexia	Ginigivitis/periodontal disease Tooth root abscess Pain Any systemic disease	CBC and blood biochemistry; oral/dental examination; radiography; ultrasonography
Ascites	Right-sided congestive heart failure Neoplasia Haemoabdomen (trauma, neoplasia) Hypoalbuminaemia (GI disease, liver disease) Polycystic disease (liver, renal)	Radiography; echocardiography; abdominal ultrasonography; peritoneal tap; liver fine-needle aspiration/biopsy
Dermatitis	Ectoparasites (*Sarcoptes scabiei, Otodectes cyanotis*, fleas) Dermatophytosis Bacterial pyoderma Canine distemper virus Atopy Food hypersensitivity	Cellophane tape test; impression smears – cytology; skin scrape – deep and superficial; microscopic examination of hair; bacterial culture; fungal culture/Wood's lamp; skin biopsy; histology; immunofluorescence testing of blood smears, buffy coat or conjunctival scrapings, PCR (CDV); intradermal allergen testing; food elimination tests
Diarrhoea	Dietary indiscretion Bacterial, primary or secondary: *Helicobacter mustelae, Lawsonia intracellularis/Desulfovibrio, Campylobacter jejuni* Mycobacteriosis Viral: ferret enteric coronavirus (FEVC), rotavirus, canine distemper virus Parasitic: coccidiosis, giardiasis, cryptosporidiosis Inflammatory bowel disease Gastrointestinal neoplasia	Dietary history; faecal analysis – culture, parasitology, coronavirus isolation; PCR; radiography/contrast studies; exploratory surgery; histology; post-mortem examination
Dyspnoea/ collapse	Pneumonia (viral, bacterial, fungal, aspiration) Primary or metastatic neoplasia Congestive heart failure (CHF) Arrhythmia/syncope Pleural effusion (neoplasia, CHF, heartworm disease) Pneumothorax – usually secondary to trauma Diaphragmatic hernia Hypoglycaemia Metabolic acidosis/pregnancy toxaemia Anaemia Compressive lesions (abscesses, neoplastic masses) Insulinoma Hypocalcaemia (especially lactating jills) Thromboembolism Hepatic failure Renal failure Hypoxia	CBC and biochemistry; blood glucose; blood gas/electrolytes; radiography; echocardiography, electrocardiography, thoracic ultrasonography
Facial swelling	Abscess Neoplasia Salivary mucocele Allergic reaction (e.g. vaccination)	Skull radiography; dental examination; fine-needle aspiration and cytology; histopathology; CT/MRI
Haematuria	Urolithiasis Cystitis Bladder neoplasia Prostatic disease	Urinalysis – dipstick, culture, cytology; CBC and biochemistry; radiography/contrast studies; ultrasonography
Hypersalivation	Oral/tongue or GI foreign body Dental disease Hypoglycaemia/insulinoma Gastroenteritis	Oral/dental examination; blood glucose; faecal analysis – culture, parasitology, coronavirus isolation; PCR; radiography/contrast studies; histology

▶

Appendix 1 Differential diagnoses based on clinical signs

Clinical sign	Differential diagnoses	Further investigations
Lower respiratory signs	Pleural effusion – cardiac disease, lymphoma, other neoplasia, infection, heartworm Pulmonary oedema – cardiac disease, heartworm, electrocution Pneumonia: bacterial, viral, fungal Mediastinal mass Pneumothorax Aspiration pneumonia (megaoesophagus)	Radiography; pleural fluid analysis and culture; bronchoalveolar lavage; ultrasound-guided biopsy; echocardiography; serology
Neurological signs	Hypoglycaemia Canine distemper Aleutian disease Rabies Leptospirosis Toxoplasmosis Cryptococcosis Other bacterial meningitis/encephalitis Extensor rigidity/hyperreflexia CNS neoplasia Otitis interna Systemic granulomatous inflammatory syndrome Neuronal ceroid lipofuscinosis Spinal trauma Spinal abscess Intervertebral disc prolapse Botulism Other toxicity	Neurological examination; radiography/ myelography; CBC and blood biochemistry; CSF analysis – cytology, culture; CIEP/ELISA (Aleutian disease); serology; MRI/CT scan; serology (*Toxoplasma*); serum lead levels; post-mortem examination; histology
Paresis/paralysis	Spinal trauma/abscess Other musculoskeletal trauma Intervertebral disc prolapse Insulinoma (hypoglycaemia) Aleutian disease Hypocalcaemia Myelitis Thromoboembolism Neoplasia (primary or secondary) Disseminated idiopathic myositis Systemic granulomatous inflammatory syndrome Toxicity, including botulism	Neurological examination; blood glucose; CBC and biochemistry; CIEP/ELISA (Aleutian disease); radiography/myelography; MRI/CT scan; muscle biopsy/histology (DIM)
Subcutaneous mass	Abscess *Actinomyces* spp. (lumpy jaw) Salivary mucocele Seroma Haematoma Neoplasia Injection reaction	Fine-needle aspiration; ultrasonography; biopsy
Swollen vulva	Normal oestrus Hyperoestrogenism Adrenal gland disease/hyperadrenocorticism Ovarian remnant (spayed jill) Vaginitis	Ultrasonography; CBC; serum adrenal hormone panel
Testicular swelling	Abscess Neoplasia Orchitis	Ultrasonography; fine needle aspiration; biopsy
Torticollis	Ear mite (*Otodectes cyanotis*) Otitis interna Vestibular disease	Aural examination/endoscopy; skull radiography; bacterial culture; MRI/CT scan
Upper respiratory signs	Primary upper respiratory disease (viral, bacterial, fungal, neoplasia, foreign body, hypersensitivity) Space-occupying masses compressing respiratory tract (e.g. abscess, lymphadenopathy, neoplasia) Congestive heart failure	CBC; radiography; echocardiography, electrocardiography; tracheal wash – cytology, bacterial and fungal culture/sensitivity; CT scan

Clinical sign	Differential diagnoses	Further investigations
Vomiting/ regurgitation	Gastroenteritis Oesophageal obstruction GI obstruction Megaoesophagus Insulinoma Any metabolic disturbance	Radiography, including contrast studies; endoscopy; ultrasonography; blood glucose; blood gas/electrolytes; histopathology; exploratory surgery; CBC and biochemistry
Weight loss	Cardiovascular disease Aleutian disease Megaoesophagus Dental disease Chronic GI foreign body (non-obstructive) Endoparasites Proliferative/inflammatory bowel disease Gastroenteritis Neoplasia Systemic disease	Radiography, including contrast studies; endoscopy; ultrasonography; blood glucose; CIEP/ELISA (Aleutian disease); histopathology; faecal analysis; exploratory surgery; CBC and biochemistry

Appendix 2

Conversion tables

Biochemistry

	SI unit	Conversion	Non-SI unit
Alanine aminotransferase	IU / l	x 1	IU / l
Albumin	g / l	x 0.1	g / dl
Alkaline phosphatase	IU / l	x 1	IU / l
Aspartate aminotransferase	IU / l	x 1	IU / l
Bilirubin	µmol / l	x 0.0584	mg / dl
Calcium	mmol / l	x 4	mg / dl
Carbon dioxide (total)	mmol / l	x 1	mEq / l
Cholesterol	mmol / l	x 38.61	mg / dl
Chloride	mmol / l	x 1	mEq / l
Cortisol	nmol / l	x 0.362	ng / ml
Creatine kinase	IU / l	x 1	IU / l
Creatinine	µmol / l	x 0.0113	mg / dl
Glucose	mmol / l	x 18.02	mg / dl
Insulin	pmol / l	x 0.1394	µIU / ml
Iron	µmol / l	x 5.587	µg / dl
Magnesium	mmol / l	x 2	mEq / l
Phosphorus	mmol / l	x 3.1	mg / dl
Potassium	mmol / l	x 1	mEq / l
Sodium	mmol / l	x 1	mEq / l
Total protein	g / l	x 0.1	g / dl
Thyroxine (T4) (free)	pmol / l	x 0.0775	ng / dl
Thyroxine (T4) (total)	nmol / l	x 0.0775	µg / dl
Tri-iodothyronine (T3)	nmol / l	x 65.1	ng / dl
Triglycerides	mmol / l	x 88.5	mg / dl
Urea	mmol / l	x 2.8	mg of urea nitrogen / dl

Temperature

	SI unit	Conversion	Conventional unit
	°C	(x 9/5) + 32	°F

Haematology

	SI unit	Conversion	Non-SI unit
Red blood cell count	10^{12} / l	x 1	10^6 / µl
Haemoglobin	g / l	x 0.1	g / dl
MCH	pg / cell	x 1	pg / cell
MCHC	g / l	x 0.1	g / dl
MCV	fl	x 1	µm^3
Platelet count	10^9 / l	x 1	10^3 / µl
White blood cell count	10^9 / l	x 1	10^3 / µl

Hypodermic needles

	Metric	Non-metric
External diameter	0.8 mm	21 G
	0.6 mm	23 G
	0.5 mm	25 G
	0.4 mm	27 G
Needle length	12 mm	1/2 inch
	16 mm	5/8 inch
	25 mm	1 inch
	30 mm	1 1/4 inch
	40 mm	1 1/2 inch

Suture material sizes

Metric	USP
0.1	11/0
0.2	10/0
0.3	9/0
0.4	8/0
0.5	7/0
0.7	6/0
1	5/0
1.5	4/0
2	3/0
3	2/0
3.5	0
4	1
5	2
6	3

Index

Page numbers in *italic* type indicate figures.

Index

Index

Index

Index

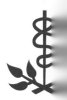

BSAVA Manuals

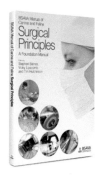
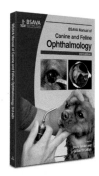
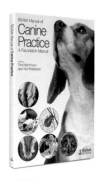
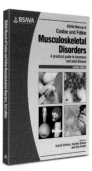
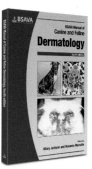
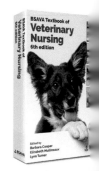

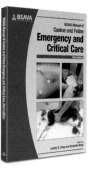
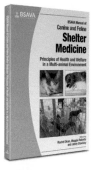
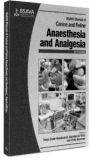
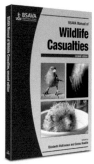
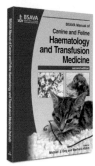
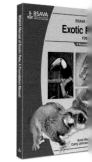

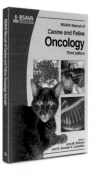
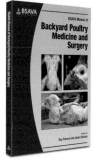
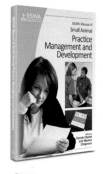
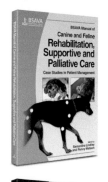
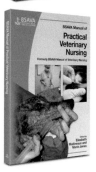
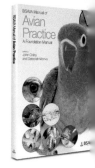

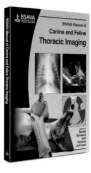
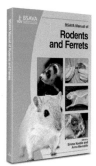
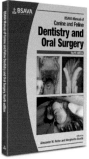
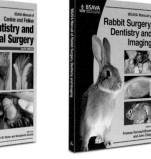
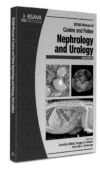
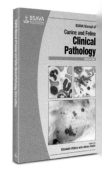

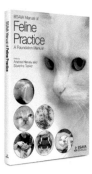
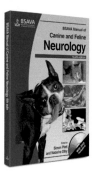
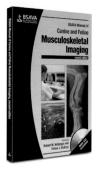
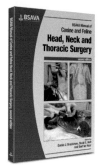
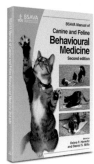
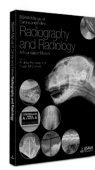

Tel: 01452 726700   Fax: 01452 726701
Email: administration@bsava.com   Web: www.bsava.com